Drug Handbook for Massage Therapists

Drug Handbook for Massage Therapists

Jean M. Wible
RN, BSN, NCTMB, CHTP

Wolters Kluwer | Lippincott Williams & Wilkins
Health

Philadelphia • Baltimore • New York • London
Buenos Aires • Hong Kong • Sydney • Tokyo

Acquisitions Editor: John Goucher
Managing Editor: Linda G. Francis
Marketing Manager: Nancy Bradshaw
Production Editor: Gina Aiello
Creative Director: Doug Smock
Compositor: International Typesetting & Composition

351 West Camden Street
Baltimore, MD 21201

530 Walnut Street
Philadelphia, PA 19106

Printed in the United States of America

9 8 7 6 5 4 3 2 1

Library of Congress Cataloging-in-Publication Data

Wible, Jean M.
Drug handbook for massage therapists / Jean M. Wible.
p. ; cm.
Includes bibliographical references and index.
ISBN-13: 978-0-7817-6309-7 (alk. paper)
ISBN-10: 0-7817-6309-6 (alk. paper)
1. Drugs—Handbooks, manuals, etc. 2. Massage therapy—Handbooks, manuals, etc. I. Title.
[DNLM: 1. Drug Therapy—Handbooks. 2. Pharmaceutical Preparations—administration & dosage—Handbooks. 3. Massage—Handbooks. QV 735 W632d 2009]
RM301.12.W52 2008
615.8'22—dc22

2007043323

DISCLAIMER

Care has been taken to confirm the accuracy of the information present and to describe generally accepted practices. However, the author, editors, and publisher are not responsible for errors or omissions or for any consequences from application of the information in this book and make no warranty, expressed or implied, with respect to the currency, completeness, or accuracy of the contents of the publication. Application of this information in a particular situation remains the professional responsibility of the practitioner; the clinical treatments described and recommended may not be considered absolute and universal recommendations.

The author, editors, and publisher have exerted every effort to ensure that drug selection and dosage set forth in this text are in accordance with the current recommendations and practice at the time of publication. However, in view of ongoing research, changes in government regulations, and the constant flow of information relating to drug therapy and drug reactions, the reader is urged to check the package insert for each drug for any change in indications and dosage and for added warnings and precautions. This is particularly important when the recommended agent is a new or infrequently employed drug.

Some drugs and medical devices presented in this publication have Food and Drug Administration (FDA) clearance for limited use in restricted research settings. It is the responsibility of the health care provider to ascertain the FDA status of each drug or device planned for use in their clinical practice.

To purchase additional copies of this book, call our customer service department at **(800) 638-3030** or fax orders to **(301) 223-2320.** International customers should call **(301) 223-2300.**

Visit Lippincott Williams & Wilkins on the Internet: http://www.lww.com. Lippincott Williams & Wilkins customer service representatives are available from 8:30 am to 6:00 pm, EST.

Preface

Drug Handbook for Massage Therapists is the first-of-its-kind drug reference book for the profession. It offers clear, consistent, and practical information on drugs as it specifically relates to massage therapy.

The book is set up so that it can be used quickly and easily and in any setting, from a spa to a wellness center to a medical setting. It addresses contraindications, whether and how the drug may affect the application of massage, and how to individualize massage sessions.

The introductory chapter, "Drug Assessment for Massage Therapy," offers a series of questions to be answered based on deductive reasoning that is adaptable for clients taking one drug or many drugs. These questions will help the therapist design a massage session that will accommodate the medication being used as well as the condition and needs of the client. Although the final determination of the safety of massage or any massage technique for the client always is the responsibility of the individual massage therapist, this book gives practical information and guidelines to inform practitioners as they design their massage sessions.

The main body of the book, of course, is the Alphabetical Listing of Drugs.

Drug entries appear alphabetically by generic name for quick reference. The generic name is followed by a pronunciation guide and a list of the brand or trade names for that drug (i.e., the drug listed alphabetically as "furosemide" followed by the pronunciation (fyoo-ROH-seh-mighd) and then the brand names "Apo-Furosemide, Furoside, Lasix, Lasix Special, Myrosemide, Novo-Semide, Uritol"). If you know either the brand name or the generic name, you can find it quickly using the index toward the back of the book. (Note that the mention of a brand name in no way implies endorsement of that product or guarantees its legality.)

Each entry also identifies the drug class, based on drug action in the body.

The "Drug Actions" section of each entry explains the drug's effect on the body. It is important for the massage therapist to determine whether and how the drug's action will change how the massage affects the body. A discussion of how to assess the action of a drug and its implications on massage may be found in the introductory chapter, "Drug Assessment for Massage Therapy."

Each entry also contains, under "Use," a listing of the diseases, disorders, or symptoms the drug would be used to treat. Although short descriptions of the diseases or disorders are provided in the text or in the glossary at the back of the book, this book is not intended to give details on diseases or disorders. Please check more complete reference books if you require complete information on a client's condition (for example, Ruth Werner's *A Massage Therapist's Guide to Pathology*, 4th Ed., 2008).

Side effects—unwanted and undesirable effects of a drug caused by the action of the drug or its breakdown—are listed. Not all side effects will be experienced by all clients; some will experience only a few, and some will experience no side effects. Some side effects may be serious and even life-threatening and require immediate intervention by a physician. In these cases, massage is contraindicated. Other side effects are simply annoying but can be tolerated and may even disappear after the drug has been taken for some time.

This book does not differentiate between the different kinds of side effects. It is up to the massage therapist to ask the client about any side effects as part of intake and assessment.

For each drug, a table is provided with the following information:

- Onset: amount of time for drug action to begin in the body
- Peak: amount of time for the strongest action of the drug on the body
- Duration: amount of time for the action of the drug on the body to be finished

These items are provided for each possible route of the drug's entrance into the body, e.g., oral or intravenous (I.V.—direct injection of a drug into a vein).

The "Massage Considerations" section in each entry (signaled by the small hand next to the heading) addresses in a quick list what, if any, cautions, contraindications, and changes in the application of massage may exist for a client taking this drug. It addresses what a massage therapist can do to individualize a session for the best possible outcomes for the client.

Some medications have serious implications for massage therapy, others require just a few small changes in the application of massage, and some have few or no implications for massage therapy. This section lets the massage therapist review a list of the drugs a client is taking and know what it means for the client's massage.

The following implications are addressed as needed:

- Any contraindications or cautions to massage or specific massage techniques
- Whether a physician consultation is needed
- The effect of massage on the absorption of the drug and the best time to give massage
- The action of the drug in the body and whether this affects how the body reacts to massage
- Side effects that would affect how the massage should be given
- When appropriate, the types of massage strokes that would be most effective for this client

The Appendix contains definitions for all abbreviations used in this book, as well as abbreviations commonly used in the medical profession. A glossary and an alphabetical index—containing both generic and brand names of drugs—complete the book.

A Note About Herbal Medicines: This book is designed to cover medications regulated by the Food and Drug Administration as prescription or over-the-counter drugs. Herbal medications are regulated differently, as supplements.

With so many herbal products on the market, it would be impossible to cover them in this text, and picking and choosing a few to discuss seemed insufficient. The reader is directed to use a complete, up-to-date reference on the subject for information on herbal medications.

As a teacher of massage therapists and massage therapy students, I have often been asked what medications mean with regard to massage. I hope that this book will to some extent answer that question in a format that is quick and easy to use as well as be an aid to improving and expanding the practice of massage in all settings.

—Jean Wible

Reviewers

Dr. Nicole Benge
Rising Spirit Institute
Dallas, Georgia

Lucy Keefer, CMT
Baltimore, Maryland

Robert Peterson-Wakeman, MSc
Saskatoon, Saskatchewan, Canada

Wendy Stone, MS, LMT
Muscular Therapy Institute
Cambridge, Massachusetts

Contents

Drug Assessment for Massage Therapy

As with any discipline, massage therapy utilizes basic tools to achieve its effects. These include effleurage, pétrissage, vibration, friction, tapotement, traction, stretching, and rocking. Variations in how these are applied give us deep tissue massage, sports massage, myofascial massage, and other techniques. Speed, depth, direction, and intention all affect how the massage will physiologically change the body.

The general effects of massage are relaxation, increased blood circulation, warmth to the areas worked and softening of tissues. More specific effects occur from the mechanical working of the soft tissues and movement of body fluids. Massage also has systemic effects mediated through the central nervous system (CNS). The release of neurochemicals into the body brings about changes that affect the entire body through the autonomic nervous system (ANS) and its branches, the parasympathetic nervous system (PNS) and sympathetic nervous system (SNS). Other effects of massage occur on the local level and are also mediated through the CNS as reflex arcs. Each of the different strokes have all these effects; some, however, have stronger systemic effects on the CNS or stronger mechanical effects. Others have stronger local effects on the CNS.

Knowing which strokes have which effect will help to determine whether or not the action of an individual drug will interfere with or increase the actions of these techniques or not. The following table describes the strongest effects of each of the massage strokes.

Massage Actions/ Effects	Strongest Strokes for This Effect	How Effect Works Physiologically
Mechanical, local	• Effleurage • Pétrissage • Friction	• Warms local area • Softens tissue • Brings blood/lymph circulation to the area
Mechanical, systemic	• Effleurage (circulatory) • Tapotement (nervous system)	• Physically increases systemic blood and lymph flow • Physically stimulates the peripheral and central nervous systems
Local (somatic), reflex	• Touch/compression • Friction • Vibration/Shaking • Stretching/Traction	• Stimulates local sensory receptors in muscles, tendons and ligaments • CNS reflex response to the above stimulation causes muscle tonus (contraction and relaxation) to change
Systemic (autonomic), reflex	• Effleurage • Friction • Rocking • Tapotement	• Stimulates the ANS to change levels of neuroendocrine substances • These chemical changes affect the whole body through the PNS and SNS actions.

When looking at the effect a particular drug may have on the application of massage, there are several aspects to be explored:

- Does the action of the drug suggest caution (use with care until client response is determined) for any specific type of massage stroke or technique?
- Does the action of the drug contraindicate (do not use) any specific type of massage stroke or technique?
- Does the action of the drug contraindicate massage completely (do not give any kind of massage)?

Once these are determined, the action of the drug on the effect of massage in the body can be looked at as well.

- Does the action of the drug increase the actions/effects or decrease the actions/effects of certain massage strokes?
- Does the action of the drug have no effect on the actions of massage on the body?
- If there are effects from the drug, which strokes should be used or not used?
- How can the strokes be applied differently so as to achieve the desired effects?

- Is the absorption of the drug affected by massage? How can this be avoided?
- Does the client have any side effects from the drug?
- If yes, do these side effects caution or contraindicate any massage strokes or techniques?
- Or can massage application be changed to balance or aid with these side effects?

An additional question is what effect the drug administration route (for example, oral, or intramuscular) may have on the massage; in many cases while there is no massage caution or contraindication for the drug, massage of an injection site may be contraindicated.

Once these questions are answered, an individualized session can be given to the client using the most effective and safest strokes and techniques. The Massage Considerations sections in this book quickly answer these questions for the massage therapist.

The massage therapist will be able to look up the drugs that the client is taking, see what massage strokes should or should not be used, how to change application of massage when necessary and when to consult with the physician.

This book deals with the effects of drugs on massage and is not intended to discuss the implications of various diseases or conditions. It is noted when the client condition may or will have implications; in those cases, you should refer to an appropriate pathology text.

Massage can be given in a safer and more effective manner when knowledge, assessment skills, and the art of massage come together. This book is intended to help with that on-going process.

A

abacavir sulfate (uh-BACK-ah-veer SUL-fayt)

Ziagen

Drug Class: Antiviral, specifically antiretroviral

Drug Actions

Reduces the symptoms of HIV-1/AIDS infection

Use

- HIV-1 infection
- Acquired Immune Deficiency Syndrome (AIDS)

Side Effects

Gastrointestinal: loss of appetite, nausea, vomiting, diarrhea.
Nervous System: insomnia, sleep disorders, headache, fever.
Skin: rash.
Other: liver toxicity, metabolic acidosis, fatal hypersensitivity reaction.

Onset, Peak, and Duration

Route	Onset	Peak	Duration
Oral	Unknown	Unknown	Unknown

Massage Considerations

- There are no contraindications to massage for a client taking this drug. There may be cautions and contraindications to massage related to the client condition.
- This drug acts directly on the virus in the cells and prevents growth of the virus. It does not affect how the body will react to massage.
- Side effects of nausea may contraindicate massage if the massage increases this side effect.
- All massage techniques are appropriate for this client depending on the individual's condition. Because the client may be on this drug for a long time, support for the immune system and stress reduction using systemic reflex and systemic mechanical strokes of effleurage, friction, and rocking (if the client is experiencing nausea, do not use rocking, as this may increase this side effect).

---

abciximab (ab-SIKS-ih-mahb)

ReoPro

Drug Class: Platelet-aggregation inhibitor to prevent blood clotting

Drug Action

Inhibits platelets from forming blood clots

Use

- To prevent blood clots during and after cardiac catheterization
- Unstable angina

Side Effects

Cardiovascular: hypotension, bradycardia, peripheral edema, easy bruising, chest pain.
Gastrointestinal: nausea, vomiting, abdominal pain.
Nervous System: hypesthesia, headache, confusion, pain.
Other: back pain, anemia, abnormal vision, bleeding, blood disorders, pleural effusion, pleurisy, pneumonia.

Onset, Peak and Duration

Route	Onset	Peak	Duration
I.V.	Almost immediate	Almost immediate	24 hr

Massage Considerations

- Physician approval should be obtained prior to any massage being given.
- Massage is contraindicated if any blood clots are present. If the drug is given for prevention of blood clots, deep tissue massage is contraindicated.
- The drug acts directly on platelets and clotting factors and will not affect how the body receives massage.
- Side effects of concern for the massage therapist are bruising, hypotension, hypesthesia and nausea. Massage should be gentle in order to prevent bruising. Massage can increase the side effect of hypotension. Stimulate the client with light, rapid effleurage; also, care is required in getting the client off the table at the end of the session. Hypesthesia means the client may not be able to give good feedback about depth and pressure.

Firm but light strokes should be utilized. If nausea is present, rocking and shaking strokes are contraindicated and if severe, massage should not be given.
- The client will benefit from local mechanical and local reflex strokes. These include gentle pétrissage, gentle friction, light compression, and some firm but gentle effleurage.

acarbose (ay-KAR-bohs)

Precose

Drug Class: Antidiabetic

Drug Action

Delays carbohydrate digestion and glucose absorption. Lowers blood sugar especially after a meal.

Use

- Type 2 (non-insulin dependent) diabetes mellitus not controlled by diet, insulin, or other drugs

Side Effects

Gastrointestinal: flatulence, abdominal pain, diarrhea.

Onset, Peak, and Duration

Route	Onset	Peak	Duration
Oral	Unknown	1 hr	2–4 hr

 Massage Considerations

- There are no contraindications or cautions for a client taking this drug. There may be cautions or contraindications to massage related to the client condition.
- The drug works to delay breakdown of carbohydrates in digestion and subsequent movement of glucose into the blood stream. Massage may increase digestion due to its parasympathetic system stimulation. Massage should not be given for at least 2 hours following a meal when this drug is being taken.
- The side effect of flatulence may be helped by gentle effleurage of the stomach and abdomen.

acebutolol (as-ih-BYOO-tuh-lol)

Sectral

Drug Class: Beta blocker antihypertensive, antiarrhythmic

Drug Action

Lowers blood pressure and heart rate and restores normal sinus rhythm

Use

- Hypertension
- Suppression of premature ventricular contractions in heart arrhythmias
- Stable angina

Side Effects

Cardiovascular: hypotension, chest pain, edema, bradycardia, heart failure.
Gastrointestinal: upset stomach, flatulence, constipation, nausea, diarrhea, vomiting, abdominal blood clot.
Nervous System: fatigue, dizziness, headache, insomnia, fever.

Skin: rash.
Other: arthralgia, myalgia, cough, impotence, type 2 diabetes mellitus, shortness of breath, bronchospasm.

Onset, Peak, and Duration

Route	Onset	Peak	Duration
Oral	1–1 1/2 hr	2 1/2 hr	Up to 24 hr

Massage Considerations

- There are no cautions or contraindications for massage in clients taking this drug. There may be cautions or contraindications to massage related to the client's individual condition.
- This drug, although selective to beta receptors, does stimulate the sympathetic nervous system. When the goal of massage is relaxation, the affect of massage may be lessened and/or take longer to achieve. The use of systemic reflex strokes such as slow, rhythmic effleurage and rocking can help counteract this effect of the drug.
- The side effects of concern are hypotension, dizziness, constipation, flatulence, and nausea. Stimulation at the end of the session with rapid effleurage and tapotement can prevent dizziness and care should be taken when changing position. Effleurage of the abdomen can help with constipation and flatulence. Rocking or shaking strokes should be avoided if nausea is present and if severe, massage should not be given.

---

acetaminophen (APAP, paracetamol) (as-ee-tuh-MIH-nuh-fin)

Abenol; Aceta Elixir; Acetaminophen Uniserts; Aceta Tablets; Actamin; Actimol; Aminofen; Anacin-3; Anacin-3 Children's Elixir; Anacin-3 Children's Tablets; Anacin-3 Extra Strength; Anacin-3, Infants'; Apacet Capsules; Apacet Elixir; Apacet Extra Strength Caplets; Apacet, Infants'; Apo-Acetaminophen; Arthritis Pain Formula Aspirin Free; Atasol Caplets; Atasol Drops®; Atasol Elixir; Atasol Tablets; Banesin; Dapa; Dapa X-S; Datril Extra-Strength; Dorcol Children's Fever and Pain Reducer; Dymadon; Exdol; Feverall Junior Strength; Feverall Children's Sprinkle Caps; Genapap Children's Elixir; Genapap Children's Tablets; Genapap Extra Strength Caplets; Genapap, Infants'; Genapap Regular Strength Tablets; Genebs Extra Strength Caplets; Genebs Regular Strength Tablets; Genebs X-Tra; Halenol Elixir; Liquiprin Infants' Drops; Meda Cap; Neopap; Oraphen-PD; Panadol; Panadol, Children's; Panadol Extra Strength; Panadol, Infants'; Panadol Maximum Strength Caplets; Redutemp; Ridenol Caplets; Robigesic; Rounox; Snaplets-FR; St. Joseph Aspirin-Free Fever Reducer for Children; Suppap-120; Suppap-325; Suppap-650; Tapanol Extra Strength Caplets; Tapanol Extra Strength Tablets; Tempra†; Tempra D.S.; Tempra, Infants'; Tempra Syrup; Tylenol Arthritis Strength; Tylenol Children's Elixir; Tylenol Children's Chewable Tablets; Tylenol Extended Relief; Tylenol Extra Strength Caplets; Tylenol Infants' Drops; Tylenol Junior Strength Caplets; Valorin; Valorin Extra

Drug Class: Nonopioid pain reliever, fever reducer

Drug Action

May produce analgesic effect by blocking pain impulses, probably by inhibiting prostaglandin or other substances that sensitize pain receptors. May relieve fever by action in hypothalamic heat-regulating center.

Use

- Mild pain or fever
- Osteoarthritis

Side Effects

Cardiovascular: serious blood disorders.
Gastrointestinal: liver damage, jaundice.
Skin: rash, hives.
Other: hypoglycemia.

Onset, Peak, and Duration

Route	Onset	Peak	Duration
Oral and Rectal	Unknown	1–3 hr	1–3 hr

 Massage Considerations

- There are no cautions or contraindications to massage for the client taking this drug except in the case of fever and active, acute infection. No massage should be given until the client has recovered from the acute phases of illness.
- The drug acts to decrease pain sensation. Caution should be used with deep tissue massage. The client may not be able to give accurate feedback of depth and pressure.

---

acetazolamide (ah-see-tuh-ZOH-luh-mighd)

Acetazolam, Apo-Acetazolamide, Diamox, Diamox Sequels

Drug Class: Adjunct therapy for open-angle glaucoma, anticonvulsant, agent for management of edema, and for prevention and treatment of acute mountain sickness

Drug Action

Lowers intraocular pressure, controls seizure activity, and may improve respiratory function

Use

- Glaucoma
- Edema in heart failure
- Prevention or amelioration of acute mountain sickness
- Adjunct treatment of seizures
- Drug-induced edema

Side Effects

Cardiovascular: none.
Gastrointestinal: nausea, altered taste, vomiting, anorexia.
Nervous System: drowsiness, paresthesia, confusion.
Skin: rash.
Urinary: crystalluria, kidney stones, hematuria.
Other: blood disorders, acidosis, hypokalemia, hyperuricemia, abscesses at injection site, transient myopia, pain at injection site.

Onset, Peak, and Duration

Route	Onset	Peak	Duration
Oral:			
Tablets	1–1 1/2 hr	2–4 hr	8–12 hr
Capsules	2 hr	8–12 hr	18–24 hr
I.V.	2 min	15 min	4–5 hr

Massage Considerations

- There are no cautions or contraindications related to this drug. There may be cautions or contraindications to massage related to the client condition.
- The action of the drug does not affect how the body will receive massage.
- The side effects of concern to the massage therapist are drowsiness and paresthesia. The client may relax very deeply and quickly and may need some stimulating effleurage or tapotement at the end of the massage.
- Paresthesia could prevent the client from giving good feedback on depth and pressure. Deep tissue massage should be given with great caution.

---

acetylcysteine (as-ee-til-SIS-teen)

Mucomyst, Mucomyst-10, Mucosil-10, Mucosil-20, Parvolex

Drug Class: Mucolytic, antidote for acetaminophen overdose

Drug Action

Increases production of respiratory tract fluids to help liquefy and reduce viscosity of tenacious secretions. Also, restores glutathione in liver to treat acetaminophen toxicity.

Use

- pneumonia
- bronchitis
- tuberculosis
- cystic fibrosis
- emphysema
- atelectasis (adjunct)
- complications of thoracic and cardiovascular surgery
- acetaminophen toxicity
- prevention of acute renal failure related to radiographic contrast media

Side Effects

Gastrointestinal: nausea, vomiting, stomatitis.
Skin: rash.
Other: hemoptysis, bronchospasm, runny nose.

Onset, Peak, and Duration

Route	Onset	Peak	Duration
Oral, I.V., inhalation	Unknown	Unknown	Unknown

 Massage Considerations

- There are no contraindications to massage for the client taking this drug.
- The action of the drug does not affect how the body responds to massage. Because the drug loosens and thins respiratory secretions, tapotement over the back and chest could bring on coughing and expectoration of mucous secretions. Tapotement should only be done if the setting is appropriate for this outcome.
- There are no side effects of concern to the massage therapist for clients taking this drug.

---

acyclovir sodium (ay-SIGH-kloh-veer SOH-dee-um)

Acyclovir, Acihexal, Avirax, Zovirax

Drug Class: Antiviral

Drug Action

Kills susceptible viruses

Use

- initial and recurrent episodes of herpes simplex virus (HSV-1 and HSV-2) infections
- initial genital herpes
- intermittent therapy for recurrent genital herpes
- long-term suppressive therapy for recurrent genital herpes
- chickenpox
- acute herpes zoster (shingles)
- herpes simplex encephalitis
- recurrent herpes labialis (cold sores)

Side Effects

Cardiovascular: hypotension.
Gastrointestinal: nausea, vomiting, diarrhea.
Nervous System: headache, encephalopathic changes (including lethargy, obtundation, tremor, confusion, hallucinations, agitation, seizures, coma, headache [with I.V. dosage]).
Skin: itching, rash, vesicular eruptions.
Urinary: hematuria.
Other: inflammation, phlebitis at injection site.

Onset, Peak, and Duration

Route	Onset	Peak	Duration
Oral	Unknown	Unknown	Unknown
I.V.	Immediate	Immediate	Unknown

 Massage Considerations

- Massage is contraindicated for the client taking this drug if open lesions of active infection are present. If the drug is taken to prevent outbreaks and there is no current rash or open lesions, then massage may be given.
- The side effects of hypotension and itching are of concern to the massage therapist. Stimulating strokes such as rapid effleurage and tapotement may be needed at the end of the massage and care should be taken when the client is changing position. If itching is present, determine if massage helps it or worsens it. Stop massage if the itching is increased.

adalimumab (ay-da-LIM-yoo-mab)

Humira

Drug Class: Antirheumatic

Drug Actions

A recombinant human monoclonal antibody that blocks human inflammatory and immune responses. Reduces signs and symptoms of rheumatoid arthritis.

Use

- Moderately to severely active rheumatoid arthritis

Side Effects

Cardiovascular: hypertension.
Gastrointestinal: nausea, abdominal pain.
Nervous System: headache.
Skin: rash.
Urinary: urinary tract infection, hematuria.
Other: hypercholesterolemia, hyperlipidemia, upper respiratory tract infection, bronchitis, malignancy, flu syndrome, accidental injury, allergic reactions, injection site reactions (erythema, itching, hemorrhage, pain, swelling), sinusitis, back pain.

Onset, Peak, and Duration

Route	Onset	Peak	Duration
Subcutaneous Injection	Variable	Variable	Unknown

 Massage Considerations

- There are no contraindications to massage for the client taking this medication. There are some cautions to consider.
- These clients have some decreased immune system function; therefore, it will be essential that they do not become exposed to infections either from the massage therapist or from clients in the office before them. Schedule the client as the first appointment of the day; reschedule the appointment if you have a cold or other infection on that day.
- Physician approval should be obtained before massage therapy for this client.
- The absorption of this drug may be increased by massage since it is given as a subcutaneous injection. The site of injection should not be massaged for 48 hours.
- There are no side effects of concern to the massage therapist.

adefovir dipivoxil (uh-DEF-uh-veer dih-pih-VOCKS-ul)

Hepsera

Drug Class: Antiviral

Drug Action

Inhibits hepatitis B virus growth

Use

- Chronic hepatitis B infection

Side Effects

Gastrointestinal: upset stomach, flatulence, nausea, abdominal pain, diarrhea, vomiting.
Nervous System: headache, asthenia (muscle weakness), fever.
Skin: itching, rash.
Urinary: renal failure, renal insufficiency, hematuria, glycosuria.
Other: liver enlargement, liver failure, lactic acidosis, sinusitis, pharyngitis, cough.

Onset, Peak, and Duration

Route	Onset	Peak	Duration
Oral	Unknown	1–4 hr	Unknown

Massage Considerations

- There are no cautions or contraindications to massage for the client taking this drug.
- The side effects of concern to the massage therapist are nausea, flatulence and itching.
- If nausea and/or itching are severe, massage may be contraindicated.
- If itching is mild, use of systemic reflex techniques such as rocking and shaking may be used along with compression strokes.
- Avoid effleurage and pétrissage if they worsen the symptom.
- If nausea is present, rocking and shaking strokes should be avoided.

---

adenosine (uh-DEN-oh-seen)

Adenocard

Drug Class: Antiarrhythmic (treats irregular heart rhythms)

Drug Action

Restores normal heart rhythm

Use

- conversion of paroxysmal supraventricular tachycardia (PSVT) to a normal heart rhythm

Side Effects

Cardiovascular: facial flushing, headache, hypotension, chest pressure or pain, palpitations.
Gastrointestinal: nausea.
Nervous System: apprehension, dizziness, heaviness in arms, burning sensation, numbness, tingling in arms.
Skin: sweating.
Other: groin pressure, back and neck pain, metallic taste, blurred vision, tightness in throat, shortness of breath, hyperventilation.

Onset, Peak, and Duration

Route	Onset	Peak	Duration
I.V.	Immediate	Immediate	Extremely short

Massage Considerations

- This drug is given when the client is having life-threatening heart arrhythmias. Massage is completely contraindicated at this time and until client is recovered and the physician has given a release for massage to be done.

albuterol sulfate (salbutamol sulfate) (al-BYOO-ter-ohl SUHL-fayt)

AccuNeb, Airomir, Asmol CFC-free, Proventil, Proventil HFA, Proventil Repetabs, Ventolin, Ventolin CFC-free, Ventolin HFA, Ventolin Obstetric injection, Ventolin Rotacaps, Volmax

Drug Class: Adrenergic (mimics sympathetic nervous system effects) bronchodilator

Drug Action

Relaxes bronchial and uterine smooth muscle by acting on $beta_2$-adrenergic receptors. Improves respiration by opening the airway passages.

Use

- Prevention of exercise-induced bronchospasm
- To prevent or treat bronchospasm in patients with reversible obstructive airway disease

Side Effects

Cardiovascular: palpitations, rapid heart rate, tachycardia, hypertension.
Gastrointestinal: heartburn, nausea, vomiting.
Nervous System: tremor, nervousness, dizziness, insomnia, headache.
Other: drying of nose and throat, hypokalemia, weight loss, muscle cramps, bronchospasm.

Onset, Peak, and Duration

Route	Onset	Peak	Duration
Oral	15–30 min	2–3 hr	6–12 hr
Inhalation	5–15 min	1–1 $^1/_2$ hr	3–6 hr

 Massage Considerations

- There are no contraindications to massage for the client taking this medication. Cautions depend on the client's condition.
- The drug acts on the sympathetic nervous system (SNS) receptors and stimulates them. Although the drug targets the receptors in the lungs, there are some system-wide effects and stimulation of the SNS.
- Massage techniques aimed at relaxation may not be as effective and/or may take longer to have their effect.
- The systemic reflex strokes such as effleurage, rocking, and shaking will be the most affected by the drug. They may need to be applied for longer periods for relaxation to occur.
- Tapotement and rapid effleurage aimed at stimulation will have a more rapid and intense effect and should be used sparingly to avoid overstimulation.
- Side effects of concern to the massage therapist are nervousness, dizziness and insomnia. These come mostly from the systemic effects of the drug described above and may be approached in the same manner as previously explained. Care should be taken when the client changes positions and is getting off the table if dizziness is a problem.
- If relaxation and stress reduction are the goal of the massage session, then utilizing systemic reflex strokes for a good part of the session and longer than usual will be helpful. These include long, slow, firm effleurage, rocking, and gentle shaking. Mechanical strokes also will help with local muscle relaxation. These are pétrissage and compression.

alefacept (ALE-fuh-sept)

Amevive

Drug Class: Immunosuppressive

Drug Action

Reduces symptoms of psoriasis

Use

- Moderate to severe chronic plaque psoriasis in candidates for systemic therapy or phototherapy

Side Effects

Cardiovascular: coronary artery disorder, heart attack.
Gastrointestinal: nausea.
Nervous System: dizziness.
Skin: itching.
Other: pharyngitis, muscle pain, cough, lymphopenia, infection, chills, malignancy, hypersensitivity reaction, antibody formation, injection site pain, inflammation, bleeding, edema, or mass.

Onset, Peak, and Duration

Route	Onset	Peak	Duration
I.V., I.M.	Unknown	Unknown	Unknown

 Massage Considerations

- Massage may be contraindicated during the course of treatment with this drug. A physician release is required to do any massage.
- Take extra care not to expose this client to any possible infections as the immune system function will be decreased in clients taking this drug. Schedule the client in his or her own home or as the first client of the day. Cancel the session if you have a cold or other infection. The individual client's condition may require further cautions.
- Massage may increase the rate of absorption of this drug when given by IM injection. Site of injection should be avoided for as long as the physician requires, at least 24 hours. If the drug is given by I.V. injection, absorption rates will not be affected, but the site of I.V. injection should not be massaged.
- Side effects of concern to the massage therapist are dizziness, itching, and muscle pain. Care should be taken when the client is changing positions. Itching and muscle pain may contraindicate massage if they are severe. If not, gentle compression, pétrissage, rocking, and shaking may help relax the client without increasing the side effects.

alemtuzumab (ah-lem-TOO-zeh-mab)

Campath

Drug Class: Monoclonal antibody antineoplastic

Drug Action

Destroys leukemic cells and stops progression of leukemia

Use

- B-cell chronic lymphocytic leukemia in patients treated with alkylating drugs, and for whom fludarabine therapy has failed.

Side Effects

Cardiovascular: hypotension, edema, hypertension, tachycardia, supraventricular tachycardia.
Gastrointestinal: anorexia, nausea, stomatitis, constipation, upset stomach, vomiting, diarrhea, ulcerative stomatitis, mucositis, abdominal pain.
Nervous System: insomnia, sleepiness, headache, dizziness, fatigue, tremor, fever, depression, muscle weakness.
Skin: itching, increased sweating, hives, rash.
Other: runny nose, pharyngitis, muscle pain, back pain, cough, nose bleeds, blood disorders, purpura, bronchitis, pneumonitis, bronchospasm, sepsis, herpes simplex, rigors, chills, candidiasis.

Onset, Peak, and Duration

Route	Onset	Peak	Duration
I.V.	Unknown	Unknown	Unknown

 Massage Considerations

- Massage is contraindicated for the client taking this drug without the approval of the physician.
- This client has a serious cancer and if massage is given the massage therapist needs to protect the client against exposure to infection. Timing of the massage should be planned with the physician. If possible, the massage should be given prior to receiving the drug. Client condition may require further adjustments to massage protocols.
- Massage does not affect the rate of absorption of this I.V.-administered drug. The site of injection should be avoided if the client has a permanent I.V.-access device such as a hep-lock or central line. If the client has a port-a-cath (access device implanted under the skin), gentle effleurage may be done over the site when not in use.
- The drug acts to kill the cancerous cells but also has systemic toxic effects. Massage needs to be gentle and supportive. Deep tissue massage is generally contraindicated.
- Side effects may be severe and may contraindicate massage if the massage worsens symptoms. Clients may need shortened sessions or only local massage on tension spots such as the neck and shoulders rather than a full body massage.
- The most effective strokes for this client will be mechanical and local reflex strokes such as gentle pétrissage, compression, gentle friction, and vibration. Rocking may be effective if the client is not experiencing nausea or dizziness. The protocol will ultimately be determined by the client condition.

alendronate sodium (ah-LEN-droh-nayt SOH-dee-um)

Fosamax

Drug Class: Treats osteoporosis

Drug Action

Increases bone mass

Use

- Osteoporosis in postmenopausal women; to increase bone mass in men with osteoporosis. Prevention of osteoporosis in postmenopausal women

- Corticosteroid-induced osteoporosis, given with calcium and vitamin D supplements. Postmenopausal women not receiving estrogen replacement therapy
- Paget's disease of bone

Side Effects

Gastrointestinal: nausea, constipation, gas, acid reflux, altered taste, abdominal pain, diarrhea, esophageal ulcer, vomiting, dysphagia, abdominal distention, gastritis.
Nervous System: headache.
Other: muscle pain.

Onset, Peak, and Duration

Route	Onset	Peak	Duration
Oral	1 mo	3–6 mo	3 wk after therapy

 Massage Considerations

- There is no contraindication to massage for the client taking this drug.
- There is a caution for deep tissue massage depending on the severity of the osteoporosis. If severe, massage may be contraindicated. Deep tissue massage should be done with great caution in mild to moderate osteoporosis and not at all for severe.
- The side effects of concern to the massage therapist are nausea, constipation, gas, and acid reflux. If nausea is severe and worsened by massage, then no massage should be given. If mild, avoid rocking and shaking techniques. Gas and constipation may be helped by gentle abdominal massage. If acid reflux is severe, client may not be able to lie flat. The massage therapist should position with pillows or tilted table.

alfentanil hydrochloride (al-FEN-tah-nil high-droh-KLOR-ighd)

Alfenta

Drug Class: Opioid narcotic analgesic (pain reliever), adjunct to anesthetic, primary anesthetic

Drug Action

Binds with opiate receptors in nervous system, altering perception of and emotional response to pain through unknown mechanism. Enhances anesthesia and relieves pain.

Use

- Adjunct to general anesthetic
- Monitored analgesic care (pain control)
- Primary anesthetic

Side Effect

Cardiovascular: hypotension, hypotension with position changes, hypertension, bradycardia, tachycardia.
Gastrointestinal: nausea, vomiting.
Nervous System: blurred vision, headache, anxiety, agitation, confusion.
Skin: itching.
Other: intraoperative muscle movement, chest wall rigidity, bronchospasm, respiratory depression, hypercapnia.

Onset, Peak, and Duration

Route	Onset	Peak	Duration
I.V.	1 min	$1\frac{1}{2}$–2 min	5–10 min

Massage Considerations

- Massage is contraindicated when this drug is used as an anesthetic or an adjunct to anesthesia. When used for pain control, deep tissue massage should be used with great caution or not at all, as client's perception of pain is altered and feedback about depth and pressure may not be accurate.
- This drug acts on pain perception in the nervous system. It has a sedative effect as well. This will increase the relaxing effects of massage significantly. Using stimulating strokes and increasing speed of strokes throughout the massage will allow for relaxation without increasing sedation. These strokes include rapid effleurage, pétrissage, and tapotement.
- The side effects of concern to the massage therapist are itching and hypotension. Itching should be reported to the physician as the drug may need to be stopped and massage may need to be withheld. Hypotension may be avoided with the earlier-mentioned change in application of massage. Care should be taken when client is getting on and off the table or out of a bed.

alfuzosin hydrochloride (al-FYOO-zoe-sin)

UroXatral

Drug Class: Selective postsynaptic alpha$_1$-adrenergic antagonist

Drug Action

Drug exhibits selectivity for alpha$_1$-adrenergic receptors in the lower urinary tract. Blockade of these adrenoreceptors can cause smooth muscle in the bladder, neck, and prostate to relax. Improves urine flow and reduces symptoms of benign prostatic hypertrophy.

Use

- Benign prostate hypertrophy

Side Effects

Cardiovascular: orthostatic hypertension, angina.
Gastrointestinal: constipation, nausea, abdominal pain.
Nervous System: dizziness, headache, fatigue, pain.
Urinary: impotence.
Other: sinusitis, pharyngitis, upper respiratory tract infection, bronchitis.

Onset, Peak, and Duration

Route	Onset	Peak	Duration
Oral	Unknown	8 hr	Unknown

Massage Considerations

- There are no cautions or contraindications to massage for clients taking this drug.
- The drug acts to block specific receptors in the sympathetic nervous system. Although specific for the urinary tract, there may be some systemic effects. Massage may have increased relaxing effects. Simply using stimulating strokes such as rapid effleurage and

tapotement throughout or at the end of the massage may counteract this effect and help the client relax without feeling too tired and drowsy.

- Side effects of concern to the massage therapist are orthostatic hypotension, dizziness, fatigue, nausea and constipation.
- Low blood pressure, dizziness, and fatigue may be helped by the changes noted above.
- Nausea, if severe, may contraindicate massage. If mild, avoid rocking and shaking techniques.
- Constipation may be aided by gentle abdominal massage.

---

allopurinol (al-oh-PYOOR-ih-nol)

Allorin, Apo-Allopurinol, Capurate, Zyloprim

allopurinol sodium

Aloprim

Drug Class: Antigout drug

Drug Action

Reduces uric acid production by inhibiting the necessary biochemical reactions

Use

- Gout, primary or secondary to hyperuricemia
- Hyperuricemia secondary to malignancies
- Prevention of acute gouty attacks
- Prevention of uric acid nephropathy during cancer chemotherapy
- Recurrent calcium oxalate kidney stones

Side Effects

Gastrointestinal: nausea, vomiting, diarrhea, abdominal pain.
Nervous System: drowsiness, headache.
Skin: severe rash with raised, red and draining lesions, sometimes with necrosis.
Urinary: renal failure, uremia.
Other: cataracts, retinopathy, severe furunculosis of nose, agranulocytosis, anemia, aplastic anemia, thrombocytopenia, hepatitis.

Onset, Peak, and Duration

Route	Onset	Peak	Duration
Oral	2–3 days	$^1/_2$–2 hr	1–2 wk
I.V.	Unknown	$^1/_2$ hr	Unknown

Massage Considerations

- There are no contraindications to massage for the client taking this drug.
- Caution should be used at the site of any acutely inflamed joint with no traction to the joint(s) involved and no deep tissue massage or friction to the affected area(s).
- Side effects of concern to the massage therapist are drowsiness and nausea. Stimulating strokes at the end of the massage will help the client to feel less drowsy and more alert. Nausea may contraindicate massage if it is severe. If mild, avoid rocking and shaking techniques.

almotriptan malate (AL-moh-trip-tan MAH-layt)

Axert

Drug Class: Antimigraine drug

Drug Action

Binds selectively to various serotonin receptors, primarily serotonin$_{1B/1D}$ receptors, resulting in cranial vessel constriction, which inhibits migraine headache
Blocks neuropeptide release to the pain pathways to prevent migraine headaches

Use

- Acute migraine with or without aura

Side Effects

Cardiovascular: coronary artery vasospasm, transient myocardial ischemia, heart attack, ventricular tachycardia, ventricular fibrillation.
Gastrointestinal: nausea, dry mouth.
Nervous System: paresthesia, headache, dizziness, sleepiness.

Onset, Peak, and Duration

Route	Onset	Peak	Duration
Oral	1–3 hr	1–3 hr	3–4 hr

 Massage Considerations

- There are no contraindications to massage for clients taking this drug.
- Caution should be used with deep tissue massage as the client may not be able to give accurate feedback about depth, pressure and pain with massage. The client's condition (severe headache, nausea) may require that massage not be given until the migraine has stopped.
- Side effects of concern to the massage therapist are dizziness, sleepiness, paresthesia and nausea. Slightly more rapid strokes and stimulating strokes throughout the massage and at the end of massage will help counteract dizziness and sleepiness.
- Paresthesia, or altered sensation, will prevent the client from giving accurate feedback to the massage therapist. When present, caution should be taken with depth and pressure of all strokes. Nausea, if severe, may contraindicate massage. If mild, avoid rocking, shaking, and vibratory techniques.

alosetron hydrochloride (a-LOE-se-tron high-droh-KLOR-ighd)

Lotronex

Drug Class: Gastrointestinal drug for irritable bowel syndrome

Drug Action

Relieves pain and decreases frequency of loose stools caused by irritable bowel syndrome (IBS)

Use

- IBS in women with severe diarrhea

Side Effects

Cardiovascular: arrhythmias, hypertension.
Gastrointestinal: constipation, nausea, gas, hemorrhoids, abdominal discomfort and pain, abdominal distention, viral gastrointestinal infections, proctitis, ileus, perforation, ischemic colitis, small bowel mesenteric ischemia.
Nervous System: headache, sedation, abnormal dreams, anxiety, sleep and depressive disorders.
Skin: acne, rash, folliculitis.
Urinary: frequency, urinary tract infection, excessive urination.
Other: photophobia, sore throat, runny nose, bacterial ear, nose, and throat infections, cough.

Onset, Peak, and Duration

Route	Onset	Peak	Duration
Oral	Unknown	1 hr	Variable

 Massage Considerations

- There are no contraindications to massage for the client taking this drug.
- Massage of the abdomen should be done only lightly and with caution if diarrhea or pain is present.
- A release from the physician should be obtained, as this is a drug with serious adverse effects used only in clients who have not responded to other treatments.
- The side effects of concern to the massage therapist are constipation, gas, nausea, anxiety and sedation. Constipation and gas may be helped by gentle abdominal massage. If the client is anxious, systemic reflex strokes such as rocking and slow, rhythmic effleurage may help. If sedation is a problem, stimulate the client at the end of the massage with tapotement and rapid effleurage. Nausea will contraindicate massage if it is severe. If mild, avoid rocking, shaking and vibratory techniques.
- The most effective strokes for this client will be the systemic reflex strokes described above with stimulation at the second half of the massage. This will help with stress reduction but not increase gastric motility (which is increased when the parasympathetic nervous system is activated by massage) and bring the body back into a good balance between the parasympathetic and the sympathetic nervous system.

---

alprazolam (al-PRAH-zoh-lam)

Apo-Alpraz, Novo-Alprazol, Nu-Alpraz, Xanax, Xanax XR

Drug Class: Benzodiazepine antianxiety agent

Drug Action

Probably potentiates effects of Gamma-aminobutyric acid (GABA), an inhibitory neurotransmitter, and depresses central nervous system at limbic and subcortical levels of brain. Decreases anxiety.

Use

- Anxiety
- Panic disorders
- Social phobias

Side Effects

Cardiovascular: hypotension, palpitations, chest pain.
Gastrointestinal: dry mouth, constipation, nausea, decreased or increased appetite, diarrhea, vomiting, abdominal pain.

Nervous System: drowsiness, light-headedness, sedation, sleepiness, memory impairment, fatigue, anxiety, headache, dizziness, tremor, restlessness, irritability, difficulty speaking, impaired coordination, depression, mental impairment, ataxia, paresthesia, dyskinesia, emergence of anxiety between doses, hypesthesia, lethargy, confusion, agitation, nightmare, fainting, akathisia, mania, suicidal thoughts.
Skin: increased sweating, itching, dermatitis.
Urinary: difficulty urinating.
Other: sore throat, nasal congestion, runny nose, painful menstruation, premenstrual syndrome, painful joints, muscle pain, increased or decreased weight, hot flushes, sexual dysfunction, blurred vision, limb and back pain, muscle rigidity, cramps, or twitch, upper respiratory tract infection, dyspnea, hyperventilation, influenza, injury, dependence.

Onset, Peak, and Duration

Route	Onset	Peak	Duration
Oral	Unknown	1–2 hr	Unknown
Oral extended	Unknown	Unknown	Unknown

 Massage Considerations

- There are no contraindications or cautions to massage for the client taking this drug.
- The drug has a sedating effect and may increase the relaxing effects of massage significantly. It also may decrease the accuracy of feedback to pressure and depth of the massage. Using slightly more rapid and stimulating stokes such as applying effleurage and pétrissage with more speed than usual and the use of tapotement throughout the massage is suggested to counteract these effects.
- Side effects of concern to the massage therapist are hypotension, dizziness, sedation, sleepiness and fatigue. These may be addressed as discussed earlier.
- Itching and nausea, if severe, may contraindicate massage. If mild, avoid rocking and shaking techniques for nausea and avoid effleurage for itching.
- Although all massage strokes and techniques are safe and appropriate for the client taking this drug, the systemic reflex stokes applied in a more stimulating manner are the best to use with a client taking this drug.
- If anxiety or restlessness are present, use rocking and slow effleurage but stimulate at the end of the massage.

---

alprostadil (al-PROS-tuh-dil)

Prostin VR Pediatric

Drug Class: Prostaglandin

Drug Action

Relaxes smooth muscle of ductus arteriosus. Improves cardiac circulation

Use

- Temporary maintenance of patent ductus arteriosus until surgery can be performed

Side Effects

Cardiovascular: flushing, hypotension, bradycardia, cardiac arrest, tachycardia.
Gastrointestinal: diarrhea.
Nervous System: fever, seizures.
Other: Diseminated Intravascular Coagulation (DIC), apnea, sepsis.

Onset, Peak, and Duration

Route	Onset	Peak	Duration
I.V.	5–10 min	20 min	1–3 hr

Massage Considerations

- Massage may be completely contraindicated for an infant taking this drug due to the seriousness of the cardiac condition present. No massage should be done without the consent and release from a physician.
- Effleurage, which moves blood and lymph mechanically, should only be used with great caution or not at all.
- The side effect of concern is hypotension; however, stimulating strokes are not appropriate. Because an infant would not be able to tell the massage therapist if they are dizzy or weak, observe the infant closely for restlessness and color.
- Massage strokes most appropriate for this client include gentle touch/compression, rocking techniques and pétrissage, mostly mechanical strokes.

aluminum hydroxide (uh-LOO-mih-num high-DROKS-ighd)

AlternaGEL, Alu-Cap, Alu-Tab, Amphojel, Dialume

Drug Class: Antacid

Drug Action

Reduces total acid load in GI tract, elevates gastric pH to reduce pepsin activity, strengthens gastric mucosal barrier, and increases esophageal sphincter tone.

Use

- Antacid; relief from peptic ulcer or gastric symptoms
- Hyperphosphatemia

Side Effects

Gastrointestinal: constipation, anorexia, intestinal obstruction.
Other: hypophosphatemia.

Onset, Peak, and Duration

Route	Onset	Peak	Duration
Oral	Varies: liquids more rapid than tablets or capsules	Unknown	20–60 min if fasting; 3 hr if taken 1 hr after meal

Massage Considerations

- There are no cautions or contraindications to massage for the client taking this drug.
- The side effect of concern for the massage therapist is constipation. If the client is experiencing this side effect, gentle massage of the abdomen may help.
- All massage strokes are appropriate for the client taking this drug.

amantadine hydrochloride (uh-MAN-tah-deen high-droh-KLOR-ighd)

Symadine, Symmetrel

Drug Class: Antiviral, antiparkinsonian

Drug Action

May interfere with influenza A virus penetration into susceptible cells. In parkinsonism, action is unknown. Protects against and reduces symptoms of influenza A viral infection and extrapyramidal symptoms.

Use

- Prophylactic or symptomatic treatment of influenza type A virus; respiratory tract illnesses in geriatric or debilitated patients
- Drug-induced extrapyramidal reactions
- Idiopathic parkinsonism, parkinsonian syndrome

Side Effects

Cardiovascular: orthostatic hypotension, peripheral edema, heart failure.
Gastrointestinal: nausea, constipation, dry mouth, anorexia, vomiting.
Nervous System: fatigue, dizziness, anxiety, irritability, insomnia, weakness, headache, difficulty concentrating, depression, confusion, psychosis, hallucinations, ataxia.
Skin: livedo reticularis.
Urinary: urine retention.
Other: none.

Onset, Peak, and Duration

Route	Onset	Peak	Duration
Oral			
Antiparkinsonian	48 hr	2–4 hr	Unknown
Antiviral	Unknown	Unknown	Unknown

 Massage Considerations

- Massage is contraindicated in the presence of active influenza infection. If the drug is given for Parkinson's syndrome or extrapyramidal symptoms, massage may be given with caution. No deep tissue massage should be used.
- Side effects of concern to the massage therapist are hypotension, nausea, constipation, fatigue, and dizziness. The use of mechanical strokes to stimulate the client such as rapid effleurage and tapotement at the end of the massage will help with hypotension, fatigue, and dizziness. If pronounced, apply massage in a more rapid and stimulating manner throughout the massage.
- Constipation may respond well to effleurage of the abdomen. If nausea is present and not worsened my massage, avoid rocking, shaking, and vibratory techniques.

amifostine (am-eh-FOS-teen)

Ethyol

Drug Class: Antimetabolite

Drug Action

Reduces toxic effects of cisplatin on renal tissue

Use

- To reduce cumulative renal toxicity from repeated administration of cisplatin in patients with advanced ovarian cancer or non–small cell lung cancer.
- To reduce moderate to severe dry mouth in patients undergoing postoperative radiation treatment for head or neck cancer.

Side Effects

Cardiovascular: hypotension, flushing or feeling of warmth, chills or feeling of coldness.
Gastrointestinal: nausea, vomiting.
Nervous System: dizziness, sleepiness.
Skin: rash.
Other: sneezing, hiccups, hypocalcemia, allergic reactions ranging from rash to rigors.

Onset, Peak, and Duration

Route	Onset	Peak	Duration
I.V.	5–8 min	Unknown	Unknown

 Massage Considerations

- Massage is contraindicated without the consent of the physician. The client taking this drug is often undergoing treatment for cancer and massage should be given with caution depending on the individual client's condition.
- Side effects of concern to the massage therapist are hypotension, nausea, dizziness and sleepiness. Nausea may contraindicate massage if severe or if massage worsens the symptom. If mild, avoid rocking, shaking, and vibratory strokes. Care should be taken when the client changes position and gets up from the table, bed, or chair.
- Slightly more rapid strokes and mechanical stimulating strokes such as effleurage and tapotement may be used with caution.
- Changes in massage application will be guided by the client's condition and not the drug itself, and massage protocols should be discussed with the physician.

---

amikacin sulfate (am-eh-KAY-sin SUL-fayt)

Amikin

Drug Class: Antibiotic

Drug Action

Kills susceptible bacteria and many aerobic gram-negative organisms (including most strains of Pseudomonas aeruginosa) and some aerobic gram-positive organisms. Ineffective against anaerobes

Use

- Serious infections caused by sensitive strains of pseudomonas aeruginosa, escherichia coli, proteus, klebsiella, serratia, enterobacter, acinetobacter, providencia, citrobacter, staphylococcus, meningitis
- Uncomplicated urinary tract infection
- Mycobacterium avium complex, with other drugs

Side Effects

Nervous System: headache, lethargy, neuromuscular blockade.
Urinary: nephrotoxicity.
Other: ototoxicity, hepatic necrosis, hypersensitivity reactions, anaphylaxis.

Onset, Peak, and Duration

Route	Onset	Peak	Duration
I.V.	Immediate	Immediate	8–12 hr
I.M.	Unknown	1 hr	8–12 hr

 Massage Considerations

- Massage is contraindicated in the presence of acute infection. If client is improving, massage may be given with caution depending on the client's condition.
- Massage may speed the rate of absorption of this drug when it is given by intramuscular injection (I.M.). The site of injection should not be massaged for at least 1 hour (peak time for blood levels of the drug).
- The side effect of concern to the massage therapist is lethargy. This severe form of fatigue may require a shortened session. A slightly more stimulating massage may be given if the client condition allows it.

---

amiloride hydrochloride (uh-MIL-uh-righd high-droh-KLOR-ighd)

Kaluril, Midamor

Drug Class: Diuretic, antihypertensive

Drug Action

Reduces blood pressure; promotes sodium and water excretion while blocking potassium excretion

Use

- Hypertension
- Edema caused by heart failure, usually in patients also taking thiazide or other potassium-wasting diuretics
- Lithium-induced polyuria

Side Effects

Cardiovascular: orthostatic hypotension, anorexia, diarrhea, vomiting, abdominal pain.
Gastrointestinal: nausea, constipation.
Nervous System: headache, weakness, dizziness.
Other: impotence, aplastic anemia, hyperkalemia.

Onset, Peak, and Duration

Route	Onset	Peak	Duration
Oral	2 hr	6–10 hr	24 hr

 Massage Considerations

- There is no contraindication to massage for the client taking this drug. The client's condition may require cautions and changes in massage protocols. Physician release may be obtained if there are questions.
- The action of the drug in the renal system is to increase production and excretion of urine. Because massage, especially systemic mechanical strokes that move fluid such as effleurage may increase urination, this stroke should be used sparingly.

- The side effects of concern to the massage therapist are hypotension, weakness, dizziness, and constipation. The use of tapotement and friction toward the end of the massage as mechanical stimulation may help if weakness, dizziness, and hypotension are experienced. Abdominal massage may help constipation.

---

amino acid infusions, crystalline (uh-MEEN-oh AS-id in-FYOO-zhuns)

Aminosyn, Aminosyn II, Aminosyn-PF, FreAmine III, Novamine, Travasol, Trophamine

amino acid infusions in dextrose

Aminosyn II with Dextrose

amino acid infusions with electrolytes

Aminosyn with Electrolytes, Aminosyn II with Electrolytes, FreAmine III with Electrolytes, ProcalAmine with Electrolytes, Travasol with Electrolytes

amino acid infusions with electrolytes in dextrose

Aminosyn II with Electrolytes in Dextrose

amino acid infusions for hepatic failure

HepatAmine

amino acid infusions for high metabolic stress

Aminosyn-HBC, BranchAmin, FreAmine HBC

amino acid infusions for renal failure

Aminess, Aminosyn-RF, NephrAmine, RenAmin

Drug Class: Parenteral nutritional therapy and caloric

Drug Action

Provides body with needed calories and protein

Use

- Total parenteral nutrition in patients who can't or won't eat
- Nutritional support in patients with cirrhosis, hepatitis, or hepatic encephalopathy
- Nutritional support in patients with high metabolic stress

Side Effects

Cardiovascular: flushing, hypervolemia, heart failure, worsening hypertension, thrombophlebitis, thrombosis.
Gastrointestinal: nausea, vomiting.
Nervous System: headache, dizziness, feeling of warmth.
Urinary: glycosuria, osmotic diuresis.
Other: fatty liver, rebound hypoglycemia, hyperglycemia, metabolic acidosis, alkalosis, hypophosphatemia, hyperosmolar hyperglycemic nonketotic syndrome, hyperammonemia, electrolyte imbalances, dehydration (if hyperosmolar solutions are used), pulmonary edema, chills, hypersensitivity reactions, tissue sloughing at infusion site caused by extravasation, catheter sepsis.

Onset, Peak, and Duration

Route	Onset	Peak	Duration
I.V.	Immediate	Immediate	Unknown

 Massage Considerations

- Massage is contraindicated without the consent of the physician. The client condition also may contraindicate massage. When massage is given, the client receiving this form of nutrition should not receive any deep tissue massage.
- Side effects of concern to the massage therapist are dizziness and nausea. The client receiving this drug is very ill and may be more prone to these symptoms.
- Minimize the systemic reflex strokes, such as effleurage, that can lower blood pressure. Both nausea and dizziness may be worsened by rocking and vibratory strokes. Avoid these if nausea and dizziness are present.
- The best strokes for this client are the mechanical strokes of pétrissage, gentle friction, and gentle touch/compression.

---

aminophylline (theophylline and ethylenediamine)

(uh-mih-NOF-il-in)

Aminophyllin, Phyllocontin, Phyllocontin-350, Somophyllin, Somophyllin-DF, Truphylline

Drug Class: Bronchodilator

Drug Action

Inhibits phosphodiesterase, the enzyme that degrades cAMP, thereby relaxing smooth muscle of bronchial airways and pulmonary blood vessels. Eases breathing.

Use

- Symptomatic relief of bronchospasm
- Chronic bronchial asthma
- Periodic apnea related to Cheyne-Stokes respirations
- Paroxysmal nocturnal dyspnea
- To reduce severe bronchospasm in infants with cystic fibrosis

Side Effects

Cardiovascular: flushing, hypotension, palpitations, tachycardia, extrasystole, arrhythmias.
Gastrointestinal: nausea, heavy feeling in stomach, bitter aftertaste, vomiting, anorexia, diarrhea.
Nervous System: nervousness, restlessness, dizziness, headache, insomnia.
Skin: hive, local irritation with rectal suppositories.
Other: increased respiratory rate, respiratory arrest.

Onset, Peak, and Duration

Route	Onset	Peak	Duration
Oral			
Tablets	15–60 min	2 hr	Varies
Extended-release solution	Unknown	4–7 hr	Varies
	15–60 min	1 hr	Varies
I.V.	15 min	Immediate	Varies
Rectal	Varies	Varies	Varies

 Massage Considerations

- There are no contraindications to massage for the client taking this drug.
- Cautions in applying massage will depend on client condition and a physician release should be obtained. Avoid stimulating strokes if the client is sensitive as it may trigger an asthma attack. Strong scents in oils, lotions, and candles also may trigger the client's breathing problems. Use with caution or not at all.
- Side effects of concern to the massage therapist are many and do affect how the body responds to massage. The drug has side effects of restlessness, nervousness, insomnia, dizziness, hypotension, and nausea.
- The client may have a hard time relaxing, and systemic reflex strokes may be less effective or take longer to have an effect. Rocking techniques and slow, rhythmic effleurage at the beginning of the massage may help with this problem. If nausea is a problem, rocking techniques may need to be avoided. Take extra care and stay with the client when they are getting off the table to be sure dizziness and hypotension are not present. Mild stimulation may be used with caution at the end of the session.
- The best approach to massage for this client is to use the systemic reflex strokes of effleurage, rocking, and friction for longer periods of time during the massage to relax the client and mechanical strokes such as pétrissage and compression to stimulate slightly. This will balance the parasympathetic and sympathetic nervous systems and allow the client to be relaxed but alert.
- Myofascial techniques for the neck, shoulders, chest and rib areas as well as diaphragm work may be helpful, but apply with caution until the client's response is verified.

---

amiodarone hydrochloride (am-ee-OH-dah-rohn high-droh-KLOR-ighd)

Cordarone, Cordarone X, Pacerone

Drug Class: Ventricular antiarrhythmic

Drug Action

Abolishes cardiac ventricular arrhythmia

Use

- recurrent ventricular fibrillation
- unstable ventricular tachycardia
- atrial fibrillation, angina
- hypertrophic cardiomyopathy
- supraventricular arrhythmias

Side Effects

Cardiovascular: hypotension, bradycardia, arrhythmias, heart failure, heart block, cardiac arrest.
Gastrointestinal: nausea, constipation, vomiting.
Nervous System: headache, fatigue, peripheral neuropathy, extrapyramidal symptoms.
Skin: sensitivity to light, blue-gray skin.
Urinary: none.
Other: corneal microdeposits, vision disturbances, hepatic dysfunction, hypothyroidism, hyperthyroidism, muscle weakness, severe pulmonary toxicity (pneumonitis, alveolitis), gynecomastia.

Onset, Peak, and Duration

Route	Onset	Peak	Duration
Oral	2–21 days	3–7 hr	Varies
I.V.	Unknown	Unknown	Unknown

 Massage Considerations

- Massage is contraindicated in the presence of serious, acute ventricular arrhythmias. When the drug is given to treat and prevent arrhythmias massage may be given with caution and with the release of the physician.
- Cautions will depend on the client condition.
- The side effects of concern to the massage therapist are hypotension, nausea, constipation, fatigue, and peripheral neuropathies. The presence of peripheral neuropathies will contraindicate deep tissue massage. The client will not be able to give accurate feedback and often will not even be aware of the lack of or change in sensation.
- Abdominal massage may help with constipation.
- Avoid rocking, shaking, and vibratory strokes and techniques if nausea is present. Care should be taken when the client is changing positions.

---

amitriptyline hydrochloride (am-ih-TRIP-tuh-leen high-droh-KLOR-ighd)

Apo-Amitriptyline, Endep, Tryptanol

Drug Class: Tricyclic antidepressant

Drug Action

Tricyclic antidepressant increases norepinephrine, serotonin, or both in central nervous system by blocking their reuptake by presynaptic neurons. Relieves depression.

Use

- depression
- anorexia or bulimia related to depression
- adjunctive therapy for neurogenic pain

Side Effects

Cardiovascular: orthostatic hypotension, tachycardia, ECG changes, hypertension, heart attack, arrhythmias.
Gastrointestinal: dry mouth, constipation, nausea, vomiting, anorexia, paralytic ileus.
Nervous System: drowsiness, dizziness, tremors, headache, excitation, weakness, confusion, CVA, nervousness, EEG alterations, seizures, extrapyrimidal reactions.
Skin: sweating, rash, hives, sensitivity to sunlight.
Urinary: urine retention.
Other: blurred vision, mydriasis, agranulocytosis, thrombocytopenia, hypersensitivity reactions, ringing in the ears.

Onset, Peak, and Duration

Route	Onset	Peak	Duration
Oral., I.M.	Unknown	2–12 hr	Unknown

 Massage Considerations

- There are no contraindications to massage for the client taking this drug. In general, there are no cautions for clients taking this drug. This will depend on the client's condition and the reason for taking the drug.
- Massage will affect the absorption rate of this drug when given by intramuscular injection. The injection site should not be massaged for up to 12 hours after the injection (time for the drug to reach peak effect).
- The action of the drug is to increase certain neurotransmitters in the brain. Massage has been shown to increase both norepinephrine and serotonin and may therefore enhance the action of the drug. This is a desirable outcome and does not change how massage may be applied. In cases of severe depression, a physician release will be required.
- The side effects of concern to the massage therapist are hypotension, nausea, constipation, dizziness, and drowsiness. Constipation may be helped by abdominal massage. If nausea is present, avoid rocking, shaking, and vibratory techniques. Using slightly stimulating techniques such as rapid effleurage and tapotement may help with hypotension, dizziness, and drowsiness.
- The massage strokes that will work best for this client are the systemic reflex strokes of effleurage, friction, and rocking. These will help increase the neurotransmittors and contribute to the easing of depression. Paired with slightly more stimulating mechanical strokes of pétrissage and compression, this protocol can assist the client to relaxed and alert state. If the client has depression with anxiety or nervousness, then do not use the stimulating strokes or limit their use.

---

amlodipine besylate (am-LOH-dih-peen BES-eh-layt)

Norvasc

Drug Class: Antianginal, antihypertensive

Drug Action

Reduces blood pressure and prevents angina

Use

- chronic stable angina
- vasospastic angina (Prinzmetal's [variant] angina)
- hypertension

Side Effects

Cardiovascular: dizziness, flushing, edema, palpitations.
Gastrointestinal: nausea, abdominal pain, dyspepsia.
Nervous System: headache, fatigue, sleepiness.

Onset, Peak, and Duration

Route	Onset	Peak	Duration
Oral	Unknown	6–9 hr	24 hr

 Massage Considerations

- There are no contraindications or cautions for massage for the client taking this drug. Cautions and contraindications may be present related to the client's condition. Consult a physician for any concerns.

- The side effects of concern to the massage therapist are nausea, dizziness, fatigue, and sleepiness. If these are present then mechanical stimulating strokes such as pétrissage, effleurage, and tapotement at the end of the session may help.
- If nausea is present, avoid rocking, shaking, and vibratory techniques.

---

amoxicillin and clavulanate potassium (uh-moks-uh-SIL-in and KLAV-yoo-lan-ayt poh-TAH-see-um)

Augmentin, Augmentin ES-600, Augmentin XR, Clavulin

Drug Class: Antibiotic

Drug Action

Kills susceptible bacteria

Use

- lower respiratory tract infections
- otitis media
- sinusitis
- skin and skin-structure infections
- urinary tract infection caused by susceptible strains of gram-positive and gram-negative organisms
- recurrent or persistent acute otitis media caused by *streptococcus pneumoniae, haemophilus influenzae,* or *moraxella catarrhalis*
- community-acquired pneumonia or acute bacterial sinusitis caused by confirmed, or suspected beta-lactamase producing pathogens (*H. influenzae, M. catarrhalis, H. parainfluenzae, K. pneumoniae,* or methicillin-susceptible *S. aureus*) and *S. pneumoniae* with reduced susceptibility to penicillin

Side Effects

Gastrointestinal: nausea, indigestion, vomiting, diarrhea, gastritis, stomatitis, glossitis, mucocutaneous candidiasis, abdominal pain, black "hairy" tongue, enterocolitis, pseudomembranous colitis.
Nervous System: anxiety, insomnia, dizziness, agitation, confusion, behavioral changes.
Other: vaginitis, vaginal candidiasis, anemia, thrombocytopenia, thrombocytopenic purpura, eosinophilia, leukopenia, agranulocytosis, hypersensitivity reactions (rash, urticaria, pruritus, angioedema, anaphylaxis), overgrowth of nonsusceptible organisms, serum sickness-like reactions (urticaria or skin rash accompanied by arthritis, arthralgia, myalgia and frequently fever).

Onset, Peak, and Duration

Route	Onset	Peak	Duration
Oral	Unknown	1–2 1/2 hr	6–8 hr
Oral			
Augmentin	Unknown	1–4 hr	Unknown
ES-600			
Augmentin XR	Unknown	1–6 hr	Unknown

 Massage Considerations

- Massage is contraindicated in the presence of acute, active infection. If the client is recovering, massage may be given with caution depending on the individual condition.

- The side effects of concern to the massage therapist are insomnia, dizziness, fatigue, and nausea. Stimulate the client gently with some rapid effleurage at the end of the session to combat fatigue and dizziness. Insomnia may be helped by the relaxing effects of massage in general. If nausea is present, avoid strokes that may worsen the symptom.
- The best strokes to be used with this client are the systemic reflex strokes such as effleurage and rocking, paired with gentle mechanical strokes. Avoid deep tissue massage and too much stimulation until client is completely recovered from the infection.

---

amoxicillin trihydrate (amoxycillin trihydrate)

(uh-moks-uh-SIL-in trigh-HIGH-drayt)

Alphamox, Amoxil, Apo-Amoxi, Cilamox, DisperMox, Moxacin, Novamoxin, Nu-Amoxi, Trimox

Drug Class: Antibiotic

Drug Action

Kills susceptible bacteria

Use

- systemic infections
- acute and chronic urinary tract infections caused by susceptible strains of gram-positive and gram-negative organisms
- uncomplicated gonorrhea
- endocarditis prophylaxis for dental procedures
- *helicobacter pylori* eradication to reduce the risk of duodenal ulcer with clarithromycin or lansoprazole
- postexposure prophylaxis to penicillin-susceptible anthrax
- Lyme disease
- acute complicated urinary tract infection in nonpregnant women

Side Effects

Gastrointestinal: nausea, vomiting, diarrhea.
Nervous System: seizures.
Other: anemia, thrombocytopenia, thrombocytopenic purpura, eosinophilia, leukopenia, agranulocytosis, hypersensitivity reactions (erythematous maculopapular rash, urticaria, anaphylaxis), overgrowth of nonsusceptible organisms.

Onset, Peak, and Duration

Route	Onset	Peak	Duration
Oral	Unknown	1–2 hr	6–8 hr

Massage Considerations

- Massage is contraindicated in acute, active infection. If the client is recovering, massage may be given with caution depending on the individual's condition.
- Nausea is the only side effect of concern to the massage therapist. Avoid strokes that may exacerbate this symptom.

amphotericin B (am-foh-TER-ah-sin bee)

Fungilin Oral, Fungizone Intravenous

Drug Class: Antifungal

Drug Action

Decreases activity of or kills susceptible fungi

Use

- Systemic fungal infections (histoplasmosis, coccidioidomycosis, blastomycosis, cryptococcosis, disseminated candidiasis, aspergillosis, mucormycosis)
- Fungal endocarditis
- Fungal septicemia
- Infections of gastrointestinal tract caused by *Candida albicans*
- Oral and perioral candidal infections
- Candidal cystitis
- Prophylaxis of fungal infection in bone marrow transplant recipients

Side Effects

Cardiovascular: hypotension, arrhythmias, asystole, phlebitis, thrombophlebitis.
Gastrointestinal: weight loss, nausea, anorexia, vomiting, diarrhea, stomach cramps, hemorrhagic gastroenteritis.
Nervous System: fatigue, headache, peripheral neuropathy, fever, seizures, peripheral nerve pain, paresthesia (with IV use).
Urinary: abnormal renal function with hypokalemia, azotemia, hyposthenuria, hypomagnesemia, renal tubular acidosis, nephrocalcinosis, permanent renal impairment, anuria, oliguria.
Other: normochromic normocytic anemia, thrombocytopenia, agranulocytosis, acute liver failure, hypokalemia, arthralgia, myalgia, burning, stinging, irritation, tissue damage with extravasation, pain at injection site, chills, generalized pain, anaphylactoid reactions.

Onset, Peak, and Duration

Route	Onset	Peak	Duration
Oral	Unknown	Unknown	Unknown
I.V.	Immediate	Immediate	Unknown

 Massage Considerations

- Massage is contraindicated in acute, active infection. If the client is recovering, massage may be given with caution depending on the client condition.
- Side effects of concern are hypotension, fatigue, nausea, and peripheral neuropathy. Use gentle stimulation with rapid effleurage or tapotement at the end of the session to combat hypotension and fatigue. Avoid strokes that increase nausea such as rocking, shaking, and vibration.
- If peripheral neuropathy is present, deep tissue massage is contraindicated or only used with great caution.

amphotericin B lipid complex (am-foe-TER-ah-sin bee LIP-id KOM-pleks)

Abelcet

Drug Class: Antifungal

Drug Action

Decreases activity of or kills susceptible fungi

Use

- Treatment of invasive fungal infections including *Aspergillus fumigatus, Candida albicans, C. guillermondii, C. stellatoideae, and C. tropicalis, Coccidioidomyces sp., Cryptococcus sp., Histoplasma sp., and Blastomyces sp.* in patients refractory to or intolerant of conventional amphotericin B therapy

Side Effects

Cardiovascular: hypotension, chest pain, cardiac arrest, hypertension.
Gastrointestinal: nausea, abdominal pain, diarrhea, vomiting, gastrointestinal hemorrhage.
Nervous System: headache, fever, pain.
Skin: rash.
Urinary: renal failure.
Other: anemia, leukopenia, thrombocytopenia, bilirubinemia, hypokalemia, dyspnea, respiratory disorder, respiratory failure, chills, infection, multiple organ failure, sepsis.

Onset, Peak, and Duration

Route	Onset	Peak	Duration
I.V.	Unknown	Unknown	Unknown

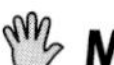 Massage Considerations

- Massage is contraindicated in acute, active infection. If the client is recovering, some massage may be given with caution depending on individual's condition.
- Side effects of concern are hypotension and nausea. Care when the client is changing positions and gentle stimulation at the end of the massage may help with hypotension. If nausea if present, avoid rocking, shaking, and vibratory strokes.

---

amphotericin B liposomal (am-foh-TER-ah-sin bee lye-po-SO-mal)

AmBisome

Drug Class: Antifungal

Drug Action

Decreases activity of or kills susceptible fungi. Treats visceral protozoal infections.

Use

- Empirical therapy for presumed fungal infection in febrile, neutropenic patients
- Systemic fungal infections caused by Aspergillus sp., Candida sp., or Cryptococcus sp. refractory to amphotericin B deoxycholate or in patients with renal impairment or unacceptable toxicity that precludes the use of amphotericin B deoxycholate
- Visceral leishmaniasis in immunocompetent patients and immunocompromized patients. Cryptococcal meningitis in HIV-infected patients

Side Effects

Cardiovascular: hypotension, chest pain, tachycardia, hypertension, edema, vasodilation.
Gastrointestinal: nausea, gastrointestinal hemorrhage, vomiting, abdominal pain, diarrhea.
Nervous System: anxiety, headache, insomnia, muscle weakness, confusion, fever, pain.
Skin: rash.
Urinary: blood in the urine.

Other: nosebleed, hepatomegaly, hyperglycemia, hypernatremia, hypocalcemia, hypokalemia, hypomagnesemia, back pain, dyspnea, hypoxia, pleural effusion, lung disorder, hyperventilation, chills, infection, anaphylaxis, sepsis, blood product infusion reaction, runny nose, itching, sweating, cough.

Onset, Peak, and Duration

Route	Onset	Peak	Duration
I.V.	Unknown	Unknown	Unknown

 Massage Considerations

- Massage is contraindicated in acute, active infections. If the client is recovering, massage may be given with caution depending on the client condition.
- Side effects of concern are hypotension, nausea, anxiety, insomnia, and itching. If itching or nausea is worsened by massage, no massage should be given. If mild, avoid effleurage strokes for itching and rocking and shaking techniques for nausea.
- Massage itself can help with anxiety and insomnia. Use systemic reflex strokes such as effleurage and rocking if appropriate to increase relaxation. If these strokes cannot be used, gentle friction at musculoskeletal junctions can also be used along with gentle compression.
- Care should be taken to support the client when changing positions if hypotension is a problem.

---

ampicillin (am-pih-SIL-in)

Apo-Ampi, Novo-Ampicillin, Nu-Ampi, Omnipen, Principen

ampicillin sodium

Ampicin, Ampicyn Injection, Omnipen-N, Penbritin, Polycillin-N, Totacillin-N

ampicillin trihydrate

Ampicyn Oral, D-Amp, Omnipen, Penbritin, Polycillin, Principen 250, Principen 500, Totacillin

Drug Class: Antibiotic

Drug Action

Kills susceptible bacteria, including non-penicillinase–producing gram-positive bacteria and many gram-negative organisms.

Use

- prophylaxis of neonatal group b streptococcus infections
- meningitis
- uncomplicated gonorrhea
- endocarditis prophylaxis for dental procedures
- enterococcal endocarditis.

Side Effects

Cardiovascular: vein irritation, thrombophlebitis.
Gastrointestinal: vomiting, diarrhea, glossitis, stomatitis, nausea.
Nervous System: seizures.
Skin: none.
Other: anemia, thrombocytopenia, thrombocytopenic purpura, eosinophilia, leukopenia, agranulocytosis, hypersensitivity reactions (maculopapular rash, urticaria, anaphylaxis), overgrowth of nonsusceptible organisms, pain at injection site.

Onset, Peak, and Duration

Route	Onset	Peak	Duration
Oral	Unknown	2 hr	6–8 hr
I.V.	Immediate	Immediate	Unknown
I.M.	Unknown	1 hr	Unknown

 Massage Considerations

- Massage is contraindicated in active, acute infection. If client is recovering, massage may be given with caution depending on the client's condition.
- Massage may affect the absorption rate of this drug when it is given by intramuscular injection (I.M.). Do not massage the site of injection for at least 1 hour (peak effect time).
- The only side effect of concern is nausea. If present, avoid strokes that may worsen the symptom such as rocking, shaking, or vibration.

---

ampicillin sodium and sulbactam sodium (am-pih-SIL-in SOH-dee-um and sul-BAC-tam SOH-dee-um)

Unasyn

Drug Class: Antibiotic

Drug Action

Kills susceptible bacteria.

Use

- Intra-abdominal, gynecologic, and skin and skin-structure infections caused by susceptible gram-positive, gram-negative, and beta-lactamase-producing strains
- Skin and skin-structure infections caused by susceptible organisms
- Pelvic inflammatory disease

Side Effects

Cardiovascular: vein irritation, thrombophlebitis.
Gastrointestinal: vomiting, diarrhea, glossitis, stomatitis, nausea.
Other: anemia, thrombocytopenia, thrombocytopenic purpura, eosinophilia, leukopenia, agranulocytosis, hypersensitivity reactions (erythematous maculopapular rash, urticaria, anaphylaxis), overgrowth of nonsusceptible organisms, pain at injection site.

Onset, Peak, and Duration

Route	Onset	Peak	Duration
I.V.	Immediate	Immediate	Unknown
I.M.	Unknown	Unknown	Unknown

 Massage Considerations

- Massage is contraindicated in acute, active infection. If the client is recovering, massage may be given with caution depending on the individual's condition.
- Massage may affect the absorption rate of this drug when it is given by intramuscular injection (I.M.). Because onset and peak action times are unknown, avoid massage to the injection site for at least 12 hours.
- The only side effect of concern is nausea. Avoid rocking, shaking, and vibratory techniques that may worsen the symptom.

amprenavir (am-PREH-nah-veer)

Agenerase

Drug Class: Antiviral

Drug Action

Reduces symptoms of HIV-1 infection

Use

- HIV-1 infection, with other antiretrovirals

Side Effects

Gastrointestinal: nausea, taste disorders, vomiting, diarrhea.
Nervous System: paresthesia, depressive or mood disorders.
Skin: rash, Stevens-Johnson syndrome.
Other: hypertriglyceridemia, hypercholesterolemia, hyperglycemia.

Onset, Peak, and Duration

Route	Onset	Peak	Duration
Oral	Unknown	1–2 hr	Unknown

Massage Considerations

- There are no absolute contraindications to massage for the client taking this drug. The client's condition may contraindicate massage if active infection, open rashes or Kaposi's sarcoma are present. Cautions and change to massage application will depend on the client condition.
- There is no caution or contraindication to massage for HIV infection with no symptoms.
- Side effects of concern are nausea and paresthesia. Avoid rocking, shaking, and vibratory strokes that may worsen nausea.
- If the client has paresthesia and cannot give accurate feedback regarding depth and pressure, deep tissue massage is contraindicated.

anakinra (ann-u-KIN-ruh)

Kineret

Drug Class: Immuno-regulatory drug; antirheumatic

Drug Action

Decreases inflammation and cartilage degradation and the progression of rheumatoid arthritis.

Use

- Moderate-to-severe active rheumatoid arthritis (RA) after one failure with disease-modifying antirheumatics

Side Effects

Gastrointestinal: nausea, abdominal pain, diarrhea.
Nervous System: headache.
Other: upper respiratory tract infection, sinusitis, neutropenia, infection (cellulitis, pneumonia, bone and joint), flulike symptoms, injection site reactions (erythema, ecchymosis, inflammation, pain).

Onset, Peak, and Duration

Route	Onset	Peak	Duration
Subcutaneous injection	Unknown	3–7 hr	Unknown

 Massage Considerations

- There is no contraindication to massage for the client taking this medication.
- Caution should be taken not to expose the client to infections as the immune system function is suppressed. Schedule as the first session of the day. Cancel session if you have any infection. Client condition will determine any other changes in massage protocols.
- Massage may affect the rate of absorption of this drug. No massage should be given to the site of injection and around it for at least 7 hours (peak time for drug absorption and action).
- The only side effect of concern is nausea. If present, avoid strokes that may exacerbate the symptom such as rocking, shaking, and vibratory techniques.

anastrozole (uh-NAS-truh-zohl)

Arimidex

Drug Class: Antineoplastic

Drug Action

Significantly lowers estradiol level hinders cancer cell growth

Use

- First-line treatment of postmenopausal women with hormone–receptor-positive or hormone–receptor-unknown locally advanced or metastatic breast cancer
- Advanced breast cancer in postmenopausal women with disease progression following tamoxifen therapy
- Adjuvant treatment of postmenopausal women with hormone–receptor-positive early breast cancer

Side Effects

Cardiovascular: chest pain, edema, thromboembolic disease.
Gastrointestinal: nausea, constipation, dry mouth, vomiting, diarrhea, abdominal pain, anorexia.
Nervous System: headache, dizziness, paresthesia, asthenia, depression.
Skin: sweating, rash.
Urinary: vaginal dryness.
Other: weight gain, increased appetite, increased cough, hot flushes, pharyngitis, pelvic pain, vaginal hemorrhage, back pain, bone pain, dyspnea, increased cough.

Onset, Peak, and Duration

Route	Onset	Peak	Duration
Oral	Unknown	Unknown	Unknown

Massage Considerations

- Massage is contraindicated without a release from a physician.
- Massage should be given with caution depending on the client condition. This drug can be toxic to the body and deep tissue massage should be used with caution or not at all.

- Side effects of concern are nausea, constipation, dizziness, and paresthesia. Avoid rocking, shaking, and vibratory techniques that may worsen nausea. Abdominal massage may help with constipation. Take care with change of position.
- If paresthesia is present use caution with depth and pressure, avoid deep tissue massage.

---

antihemophilic factor (AHF, Factor VIII) (an-tigh-hee-moh-FIL-ik FAK-tor)

Helixate FS, Hemofil M, Hyate:C, Koate-DVI, Kogenate, Kogenate FS, Monoclate-P, Recombinate, Refacto

Drug Class: Antihemophilic

Drug Action

Directly replaces deficient clotting factor that converts prothrombin to thrombin.
Allows blood clotting to occur.

Use

- Factor VIII deficiency
- Hemophilia A

Side Effects

Cardiovascular: flushing, hypotension, tachycardia, tightness in chest.
Gastrointestinal: nausea, vomiting.
Nervous System: headache, paresthesia, sleepiness, lethargy, fever, paresthesia, clouding or loss of consciousness.
Skin: rash, hives.
Urinary: none.
Other: visual disturbances, hemolysis (in patients with blood type A, B, or AB), hepatitis B, backache, wheezing, chills, hypersensitivity reactions, rigor, stinging at injection site, HIV.

Onset, Peak, and Duration

Route	Onset	Peak	Duration
I.V.	Immediate	1–2 hr	Unknown

 Massage Considerations

- Massage is contraindicated for the client taking this drug without physician release and involvement. If massage is given, deep tissue massage is contraindicated and circulatory strokes such as effleurage should not be used or used minimally. Tapotement is also contraindicated.
- Side effects of concern are hypotension, sleepiness, lethargy, nausea, and paresthesia. Have client change position slowly and with care. Apply massage a little more rapidly at the end of the session to stimulate the client.
- If nausea is present, avoid rocking, shaking, and vibratory strokes.
- Deep tissue massage is contraindicated with paresthesia.
- Massage strokes that would work well with this client are the systemic reflex strokes other than effleurage, such as rocking and gentle friction. Mechanical strokes will also work well such as pétrissage and compression/touch but should be applied gently.

anti-inhibitor coagulant complex (an-tigh-in-HIB-eh-tor koh-AG-yoo-lant KOM-pleks)

Autoplex T, Feiba VH Immuno

Drug Class: Antihemophilic

Drug Action

Allows blood clotting to occur

Use

- Prevention and control of hemorrhagic episodes in patients with hemophilia A for whom inhibitor antibodies to antihemophilic factor have developed
- Management of bleeding in patients with acquired hemophilia who have spontaneously acquired inhibitors to factor VIII

Side Effects

Cardiovascular: flushing, hypotension, transient chest discomfort, changes in pulse rate, heart attack, thromboembolism.
Gastrointestinal: nausea.
Nervous System: dizziness, headache, drowsiness, fever, lethargy.
Skin: rash, hives.
Other: Disseminated Intravascular Coagulation, risk of hepatitis B, dyspnea, chills, hypersensitivity reactions, risk of HIV, chills.

Onset, Peak, and Duration

Route	Onset	Peak	Duration
I.V.	10–30 min	Unknown	Unknown

 Massage Considerations

- Massage is completely contraindicated for the client taking this drug because it is given during hemorrhagic episodes (bleeding).

antithrombin III, human (ATIII, heparin cofactor I)

(an-tigh-THROM-bin three, HYOO-mun)

ATnativ, Thrombate III

Drug Class: Anticoagulant, antithrombotic

Drug Action

Prevents or decreases blood clotting

Use

- Thromboembolism from hereditary ATIII deficiency

Side Effects

Cardiovascular: vasodilation, lowered blood pressure.
Urinary: increased urination.

Onset, Peak, and Duration

Route	Onset	Peak	Duration
I.V.	Immediate	Unknown	4 days

 Massage Considerations

- Massage is completely contraindicated for clients taking this drug because of severe blood clotting disorder.

---

aprepitant (uh-pre-PI-tant)

Emend

Drug Class: Centrally-acting antiemetic

Drug Action

Inhibits nausea and vomiting caused by chemotherapy

Use

- Adjunct to corticosteroids and 5-HT_3–receptor antagonist for the prevention of both acute and delayed nausea and vomiting caused by chemotherapy, including cisplatin

Side Effects

Gastrointestinal: constipation, nausea, abdominal pain, anorexia, diarrhea, gastritis, vomiting.
Nervous System: dizziness, fatigue, headache, insomnia.
Skin: rash with hives, Stevens-Johnson syndrome.
Urinary: proteinuria.
Other: neutropenia, febrile neutropenia, angioedema, ringing in the ears, hiccups.

Onset, Peak, and Duration

Route	Onset	Peak	Duration
Oral	Unknown	4 hr	9–13 hr

 Massage Considerations

- There is no contraindication to massage for the client because they are taking this drug. The client's condition may contraindicate massage or require cautions such as shorter sessions and gentler work. A physician release and involvement is required.
- This drug acts on the central nervous system and lowers pain perception and nausea. Deep tissue massage is contraindicated.
- Side effects of concern are constipation, dizziness, fatigue, insomnia, and nausea.
- Constipation may be helped by gentle abdominal massage.
- To prevent increasing the side effects of dizziness and fatigue and yet relax the client to help with insomnia utilize gentle rocking, slow and rhythmic effleurage and gentle friction (systemic reflex strokes) along with more rapid mechanical strokes such as pétrissage and compression during the massage. This will relax yet increase alertness and well-being.
- The best strokes to use with this client are the systemic reflex strokes and mechanical strokes as noted earlier. As always, caution and changes in massage protocol will depend on the individual's condition.

aripiprazole (air-uh-PIP-rah-zol)

Abilify

Drug Class: Atypical antipsychotic

Drug Action

Decreases psychotic behaviors

Use

- Schizophrenia

Side Effects

Cardiovascular: orthostatic hypotension, peripheral edema, chest pain, hypertension, tachycardia, bradycardia.
Gastrointestinal: nausea, vomiting, anorexia, diarrhea, abdominal pain, esophageal dysmotility.
Nervous System: headache, anxiety, insomnia, dizziness, sleepiness, nervousness, akathisia, tremor, asthenia, depression, hostility, suicidal thoughts, manic behavior, confusion, abnormal gait, cogwheel rigidity, seizures, fever, tardive dyskinesia, cognitive and motor impairment, neuroleptic malignant syndrome.
Skin: dry skin, sweating, itching, rash, bruising, ulceration.
Urinary: incontinence.
Other: blurred vision, conjunctivitis, ear pain, anemia, weight gain, weight loss, hyperglycemia, neck pain, neck stiffness, muscle cramps, dyspnea, pneumonia, flulike syndrome, inability to regulate body temperature, runny nose, increased saliva.

Onset, Peak, and Duration

Route	Onset	Peak	Duration
Oral	Unknown	3–5 hr	Unknown

Massage Considerations

- Massage is contraindicated for the client taking this medication without the release and involvement of the physician. Active psychosis also contraindicates massage. Massage should be given with caution in clients who are on maintenance drug doses.
- Side effects of concern are hypotension, dizziness, nervousness, insomnia, sleepiness, and nausea, as well as itching. Approach hypotension and dizziness by taking care when the client changes position and gets off the table.
- Nervousness and insomnia can be addressed by using systemic reflex strokes such as rocking and effleurage for longer periods of time. If the client is sleepy, increase the speed of massage strokes slightly and use the mechanical strokes of effleurage, pétrissage, and friction. If itching is a problem, avoid effleurage.
- With nausea, avoid rocking and vibratory techniques.

arsenic trioxide (AR-sen-ik try-OX-ide)

Trisenox

Drug Class: Antineoplastic

Drug Action

Destroys promyelocytic leukemic cells

Use

- Acute promyelocytic leukemia (APL) in patients who have relapsed from or are refractory to retinoid and anthracycline chemotherapy

Side Effects

Cardiovascular: hypotension, flushing, hemorrhage, tachycardia, ECG changes, heart block, palpitations, edema, chest pain, facial edema, hypertension.
Gastrointestinal: nausea, constipation, dry mouth, vomiting, diarrhea, anorexia, abdominal pain, loose stools, oral blisters, fecal incontinence, gastrointestinal hemorrhage, abdominal tenderness or distention, bloody stools, oral candidiasis.
Nervous System: headache, insomnia, dizziness, tremor, sleepiness, anxiety, fatigue, weakness, fever, paresthesia, pain, seizures, coma, depression, agitation.
Skin: dry skin, itching, sweating, pallor, dermatitis, erythema.
Urinary: renal failure, renal impairment, oliguria, incontinence.
Other: nosebleeds, blurred vision, earache, facial and eyelid edema, sinusitis, nasopharyngitis, painful red eye, vaginal hemorrhage, bleeding between menstrual periods, leukocytosis, anemia, thrombocytopenia, neutropenia, lymphadenopathy, hypokalemia, hypomagnesemia, hyperglycemia, hypocalcemia, hypoglycemia, dry eyes, eye irritation, ringing in the ears, postnasal drip, acidosis, weight gain, weight loss, hyperkalemia, arthralgia, myalgia, bone pain, back pain, neck pain, limb pain, dyspnea, hypoxia, pleural effusion, wheezing, decreased breath sounds, crepitations, rales, hemoptysis, tachypnea, rhonchi, upper respiratory tract infection, drug hypersensitivity, erythema or edema at injection site, rigors, herpes simplex infection, bacterial infection, herpes zoster, sepsis.

Onset, Peak, and Duration

Route	Onset	Peak	Duration
I.V.	Unknown	Unknown	Unknown

 Massage Considerations

- Massage is contraindicated for the client taking this drug without the consent and involvement of the physician. If massage is to be given, caution should be used for all strokes depending on the client's condition. Deep tissue massage is contraindicated.
- Timing of the massage should be discussed with the physician and be prior to chemotherapy treatment if possible.
- This drug does not in essence change how the body responds to massage. However, it is toxic and massage should be given with caution.
- Side effects are many and are all of concern. The suggestions here will be helpful in approaching these effects.
- The best strokes for the client receiving this drug are systemic reflex strokes such as rocking and gentle friction. Effleurage should be limited or not used at all because of its circulatory effects, which could overwhelm the kidneys as they try to excrete the drug.
- Mechanical strokes such as compression and pétrissage should be applied gently.
- Client condition may indicate further changes in massage protocol such as shorter sessions.

---

asparaginase (L-asparaginase) (as-PAR-ah-jin-ays)

Elspar, Kidrolase

Drug Class: Antineoplastic

Drug Action

Kills leukemia cells

Use

- Acute lymphocytic leukemia (ALL) (with other drugs)

Side Effects

Gastrointestinal: nausea, weight loss, vomiting, anorexia, cramps, hemorrhagic pancreatitis.
Nervous System: drowsiness, nervousness, fever, chills, confusion, depression, hallucinations.
Skin: rash, hives.
Urinary: azotemia, renal impairment, uric acid nephropathy, glycosuria, polyuria, increased blood ammonia level.
Other: anemia, hypofibrinogenemia, thrombocytopenia, leucopenia, hepatotoxicity, hyperuricemia, hyperglycemia, anaphylaxis, fatal hyperthermia.

Onset, Peak, and Duration

Route	Onset	Peak	Duration
I.V.	Almost immediate	Almost immediate	23–33 days after stopping drug
I.M.	Almost immediate	4–24 hr after stopping drug	23–33 days

 Massage Considerations

- Massage is contraindicated without the consent and involvement of the physician. When massage is given, it should be with great caution and depend on the client condition. Deep tissue massage is contraindicated, and effleurage should be limited or not used at all.
- Massage may affect the absorption of this drug when it is given by intramuscular injection (I.M.). The site of the injection should not be massaged for 24 hours (peak effect time).
- This drug does not change how the body responds to massage, however, it's toxic and massage should be given with caution.
- Side effects are many and may be addressed by the massage suggestions here.
- The best strokes for this client will be systemic reflex and mechanical strokes. Rocking, gentle friction, pétrissage, and gentle touch/compression as well as some myofascial techniques may be used.

aspirin (acetylsalicylic acid) (AS-prin)

Ancasal, Arthrinol, Artria S.R., ASA, ASA Enseals, Aspergum, Aspro Preparations, Astrin, Bayer Aspirin, Bex Powders, Coryphen, Easprin, Ecotrin, Empirin, Entrophen, Halfprin, Measurin, Norwich Extra Strength, Novasen, Riphen-10, Sal-Adult, Sal-Infant, Sloprin, Supasa, Triaphen-10, Vincent's Powders, ZORprin

Drug Class: Salicylate nonopioid pain reliever, fever reducer, anti-inflammatory, antiplatelet drug

Drug Action

Produces analgesia by blocking prostaglandin synthesis (peripheral action). Exerts its anti-inflammatory effect by inhibiting prostaglandin synthesis; also may inhibit synthesis or action of other mediators of inflammatory response. Relieves fever by acting on hypothalamic heat-regulating center to cause peripheral vasodilation, which increases peripheral blood supply and promotes sweating, which leads to heat loss and to cooling by evaporation. In low doses, aspirin also appears to impede clotting by blocking prostaglandin synthesis, which prevents formation of platelet-aggregating substance thromboxane A_2.

Use

- Arthritis
- Mild pain or fever
- Prevention of thrombosis
- Reduction of risk of heart attack in patients with previous heart attack or unstable angina
- Kawasaki syndrome (mucocutaneous lymph node syndrome)
- Prophylaxis for transient ischemic attack (TIA)
- Transient Ischemic Attacks
- Prevention of reocclusion in coronary revascularization procedures
- Rheumatic fever
- Pericarditis after acute heart attack
- Cardiac stent implantation

Side Effects

Gastrointestinal: nausea, vomiting, gastrointestinal distress, occult bleeding, gastrointestinal bleeding.
Skin: easy bruising, rash, hives.
Urinary: transient renal insufficiency.
Other: hearing loss, prolonged bleeding time, thrombocytopenia, hepatitis, angioedema, hypersensitivity reactions, (anaphylaxis, asthma), Reye's syndrome, ringing in the ears.

Onset, Peak, and Duration

Route	Onset	Peak	Duration
Oral			
Buffered	5–30 min	1–2 hr	1–4 hr
Enteric-coated	5–30 min	4–8 hr	1-4 hr
Extended-release	5–30 min	1–2 hr	1–4 hr
Regular	5–30 min	25–40 min	1–4 hr
Solution	5–30 min	15–60 min	1–4 hr
Rectal suppositories	5–30 min	3–4 hr	1–4 hr

Massage Considerations

- There are no contraindications to massage for the client taking this drug. Deep tissue massage should be used with caution as the client may bruise easier and decreased pain perception may prevent accurate feedback.
- Massage does not affect the absorption of this drug unless applied topically. Avoid massage of this site for at least one hour.
- Side effects of concern are nausea and easy bruising. Avoid rocking, shaking, and vibratory techniques when nausea is present. Using caution with pressure and depth will prevent bruising.

atazanavir sulfate (att-uh-za-NUH-veer sul-FAYT)

Reyataz

Drug Class: Antiretroviral

Drug Action

Treats symptoms of HIV infection

Use

- HIV-1 infection

Side Effects

Gastrointestinal: nausea, abdominal pain, vomiting, diarrhea.
Nervous System: headache, fatigue, insomnia, dizziness, peripheral neuropathy, fever, pain, depression.
Skin: rash.
Urinary: none.
Other: hepatitis, jaundice or scleral icterus, lipidystrophy, lactic acidosis, lipohypertrophy, back pain, arthralgia, cough.

Onset, Peak, and Duration

Route	Onset	Peak	Duration
Oral	Unknown	2 $^1/_2$ hr	Unknown

Massage Considerations

- There is no contraindication to massage for the client taking this drug. Contraindications and cautions may exist related to the client condition.
- Side effects of concern are fatigue, insomnia, dizziness, peripheral neuropathies, and nausea. Fatigue, insomnia and dizziness may be addressed by giving a balancing massage of systemic reflex strokes and mechanical strokes in a slightly more rapid manner to stimulate while relaxing.
- Peripheral neuropathies contraindicate any deep tissue massage. Avoid strokes that would increase nausea such as rocking.

atenolol (uh-TEN-uh-lol)

Apo-Atenol, Noten, Nu-Atenol, Tenormin

Drug Class: Beta blocker antihypertensive, antianginal

Drug Action

Decreases blood pressure, relieves angina, and reduces cardiovascular mortality rate and risk of reinfarction after acute heart attack

Use

- Hypertension
- Angina pectoris
- To reduce CV mortality rate and risk of reinfarction in patients with acute heart attack
- To slow rapid ventricular response to atrial tachyarrhythmias after acute heart attack without left ventricular dysfunction and AV block

Side Effects

Cardiovascular: bradycardia, profound hypotension, intermittent claudication, second- or third-degree AV block.
Gastrointestinal: nausea, dry mouth, vomiting, diarrhea.
Nervous System: fatigue, fever, lethargy.
Skin: rash.
Urinary: none.
Other: increased risk of type 2 diabetes, dyspnea, bronchospasm.

Onset, Peak, and Duration

Route	Onset	Peak	Duration
Oral	1 hr	2–4 hr	24 hr
I.V.	5 min	5 min	12 hr

 Massage Considerations

- This drug blocks specific receptors of the sympathetic nervous system. Massage in general decreases the activity of the sympathetic nervous system so there may be some overlap of effects. This could make the client very drowsy and weak. Applying a more stimulating massage either throughout the session or just at the end will help bring the client back to alertness.
- The only side effect of concern is fatigue, which can be addressed as noted earlier.
- All strokes are appropriate for this client depending on the individual's condition. A physician consult may be required.

---

atomoxetine hydrochloride (ATT-oh-mocks-uh-teen high-droh-KLOR-ighd)

Strattera

Drug Class: Selective norepinephrine reuptake inhibitor

Drug Action

May relate to selective inhibition of the presynaptic norepinephrine transporter
Decreases symptoms of attention deficit hyperactivity disorder (ADHD)

Use

- Adjunct therapy for ADHD

Side Effects

Cardiovascular: orthostatic hypotension, tachycardia, hypertension, palpitations.
Gastrointestinal: constipation, nausea, decreased appetite, dry mouth, gas, abdominal pain, vomiting, gastroenteritis.
Nervous System: dizziness, headache, sleepiness, fatigue, insomnia, tremor, paresthesia crying, irritability, mood swings, pyrexia, sedation, depression, early morning awakening, paresthesia, abnormal dreams, sleep disorder.
Skin: increased sweating, itching, dermatitis.
Urinary: impotence, urinary retention, urinary hesitation, difficulty urinating, prostatitis.
Other: runny nose, sore throat, nasal congestion, sinus congestion, weight loss, cough, upper respiratory tract infections, decreased libido, hot flashes, ear infection, nasopharyngitis, mydriasis, sinusitis, arthralgia, myalgia, decreased libido, influenza, rigors, sexual dysfunction, menstrual dysfunction.

Onset, Peak, and Duration

Route	Onset	Peak	Duration
Oral	Rapid	1–2 hr	Unknown

Massage Considerations

- There are no cautions or contraindications to massage for the client taking this drug.
- Side effects of concern are constipation, nausea, dizziness, sleepiness, insomnia, paresthesia, and itching.
- Constipation may be helped by abdominal massage.
- Dizziness and sleepiness may be managed by stimulating the client gently at the end of the massage session.
- If paresthesia is present, deep tissue massage should not be done.
- Avoid effleurage if itching is present and avoid rocking and shaking strokes if nausea if present.

atorvastatin calcium (uh-TOR-vah-stah-tin KAL-see-um)

Lipitor

Drug Class: Anticholesterol

Drug Action

Lowers cholesterol and lipoprotein levels

Use

- Adjunct to diet to reduce elevated LDL, total cholesterol, apo B, and triglyceride levels and to increase HDL level in patients with primary hypercholesterolemia (heterozygous familial and nonfamilial) and mixed dyslipidemia
- Alone or as an adjunct to lipid-lowering treatments such as LDL apheresis to reduce total cholesterol and LDL cholesterol levels in patients with homozygous familial hypercholesterolemia
- Heterozygous familial hypercholesterolemia

Side Effects

Gastrointestinal: constipation, dyspepsia, flatulence, abdominal pain, diarrhea.
Nervous System: headache, asthenia, fever, malaise.
Skin: rash.
Urinary: none.
Other: sinusitis, pharyngitis, back pain, arthralgia, myalgia, infection, accidental injury, flu-like syndrome, hypersensitivity reaction.

Onset, Peak, and Duration

Route	Onset	Peak	Duration
Oral	Unknown	1–2 hr	Unknown

Massage Considerations

- There are no contraindications or cautions to massage for the client taking this drug. Any changes in massage application would be related to the client's condition.
- Side effects of concern are constipation and gas. Gentle abdominal massage may help to alleviate these symptoms.

atovaquone (uh-TOH-vuh-kwohn)

Mepron

Drug Class: Antiprotozoal

Drug Action

Kills *Pneumocystis carinii* protozoa

Use

- Prevention of *Pneumocystis carinii* pneumonia in patients who are intolerant to co-trimoxazole, including HIV-infected individuals
- Mild to moderate *P. carinii* pnuemonia in patients who can't tolerate cotrimoxazole
- Prevention of toxoplasmosis in HIV-infected patients

Side Effects

Gastrointestinal: nausea, abdominal pain, diarrhea, anorexia, gastritis, oral ulcers, vomiting.
Nervous System: dizziness, headache, insomnia, dreams, asthenia.
Skin: itching.
Other: cough, visual disturbances.

Onset, Peak, and Duration

Route	Onset	Peak	Duration
Oral	Unknown	1–8 hr (1st peak); 1–4 days (2nd peak)	Unknown

Massage Considerations

- Massage is contraindicated in acute, active infection. If client is recovering or taking the drug to prevent infection, then massage may be given with caution depending on the client's condition.
- Side effects of concern are nausea, itching, dizziness, and insomnia. Avoid strokes that could worsen nausea such as rocking. If itching is present, avoid effleurage. Assist client in changing positions if dizziness is a problem and stimulate at the end of the massage. Insomnia may be helped by the general relaxing effects of massage.
- Utilize systemic reflex strokes such as rocking and slow, rhythmic effleurage.
- Contact a physician with any questions.

atovaquone and proguanil hydrochloride (uh-TOH-vuh-kwohn and pro-GWAN-ill high-droh-KLOR-ighd)

Malarone, Malarone Pediatric

Drug Class: Antimalarial

Drug Action

Prevents and treats symptoms of malaria

Use

- Prevention of Plasmodium falciparum malaria in areas where chloroquine resistance has been reported
- Acute, uncomplicated P. falciparum malaria

Side Effects

Gastrointestinal: nausea, abdominal pain, diarrhea, anorexia, oral ulcers, gastritis, vomiting.
Nervous System: dizziness, headache, dreams, asthenia, hallucinations.
Skin: itching.
Other: cough, visual difficulties, anaphylaxis, flulike syndrome.

Onset, Peak, and Duration

Route	Onset	Peak	Duration
Oral	Unknown	Unknown	Unknown

Massage Considerations

- Massage is contraindicated in the presence of acute, active infection. If the client is taking the drug to prevent malaria, massage may be given.
- Side effects of concern are nausea, itching, and dizziness.
- If nausea is present, avoid rocking, shaking, and vibratory techniques that could worsen this symptom. If itching is a problem avoid effleurage.
- Assist the patient when changing position and getting off the massage table if dizziness is a problem.

atropine sulfate (AH-troh-peen SUL-fayt)

AtroPen Auto-Injector, Sal-Tropine

Drug Class: Anticholinergic, belladonna alkaloid antiarrhythmic, vagolytic

Drug Action

Increases heart rate, decreases secretions preoperatively, and slows GI motility. Antidote for anticholinesterase insecticide poisoning.

Use

- Symptomatic bradycardia, bradyarrhythmia (junctional or escape rhythm)
- Anticholinesterase insecticide poisoning
- Preoperatively for decreasing secretions and blocking cardiac vagal reflexes
- Adjunct in peptic ulcer disease; functional GI disorders such as irritable bowel syndrome

Side Effects

Cardiovascular: flushing, tachycardia, palpitations, angina, arrhythmias.
Gastrointestinal: dry mouth, thirst, constipation, nausea, vomiting.
Nervous System: headache, restlessness, ataxia, disorientation, hallucinations, delirium, coma, insomnia, dizziness, excitement, agitation, confusion.
Urinary: urine retention.
Other: blurred vision, leukocytosis, anaphylaxis, photophobia, dilated pupils.

Onset, Peak, and Duration

Route	Onset	Peak	Duration
Oral	$^1/_2$–1 hr	2 hr	4 hr
I.V.	Immediate	2–4 min	4 hr
I.M.	30 min	1–1 $^1/_2$ hr	4 hr
Subcutaneous Injection	Unknown	Unknown	4 hr

 Massage Considerations

- There are no contraindications to massage for the client taking this drug. The condition of the client may require contraindications or cautions.
- Massage may affect the absorption of this drug when it is given by intramuscular (I.M.) injection or subcutaneous (S.C.) injection. Do not massage the site of injection for at least $1\,^{1}/_{2}$ hours.
- This drug blocks the action of the parasympathetic nervous system. It may decrease the relaxing effects of massage and make the systemic reflex strokes less effective. The therapist may need to apply these strokes (effleurage, rocking, friction) for longer times than usual for the client to feel the effect.
- Side effects of concern are nausea, constipation, and restlessness. Avoid rocking and shaking and any strokes that may worsen nausea if this is a problem for the client. Constipation may be helped by abdominal massage. Restlessness may be addressed as described earlier.

---

auranofin (or-AN-uh-fin)

Ridaura

Drug Class: Antiarthritic

Drug Action

Relieves symptoms of rheumatoid arthritis

Use

- Psoriatic arthritis
- Active systemic lupus erythematosus
- Felty's syndrome
- Rheumatoid arthritis

Side Effects

Gastrointestinal: nausea, flatulence, diarrhea, abdominal pain, vomiting, stomatitis, enterocolitis, anorexia.
Nervous System: confusion, seizures.
Skin: rash, dermatitis, exfoliative dermatitis, itching.
Urinary: proteinuria, hematuria, glomerulonephritis, acute renal failure, nephrotic syndrome.
Other: thrombocytopenia, aplastic anemia, agranulocytosis, leukopenia, eosinophilia, jaundice, interstitial pneumonitis, metallic taste.

Onset, Peak, and Duration

Route	Onset	Peak	Duration
Oral	1–3 mo	2 hr	Unknown

 Massage Considerations

- There is no contraindication to massage for the client taking this drug. Contraindications and cautions may exist as a result of the client's condition.
- Side effects of concern to the massage therapist are nausea, flatulence, and itching.
- If nausea is present, avoid rocking, shaking, and vibratory techniques that may worsen the symptom.
- If flatulence is a concern, gentle abdominal massage may help.
- If itching is present, avoid effleurage.

aurothioglucose (or-oh-thigh-oh-GLOO-kohs)

Gold-50, Solganal

gold sodium thiomalate (gohld SOH-dee-um thee-oh-MAH-layt)

Myochrysine

Drug Class: Gold salt antiarthritic

Drug Action

Relieves signs and symptoms of rheumatoid arthritis

Use

- Rheumatoid arthritis
- Palindromic rheumatism
- Pemphigus

Side Effects

Cardiovascular: hypotension, bradycardia.
Gastrointestinal: nausea, metallic taste, stomatitis, difficulty swallowing, vomiting.
Nervous System: dizziness, System fainting, seizures.
Skin: increased sweating, photosensitivity reaction, rash, dermatitis.
Urinary: albuminuria, proteinuria, nephrotic syndrome, nephritis, acute tubular necrosis, acute renal failure.
Other: corneal gold deposition, corneal ulcers, thrombocytopenia, aplastic anemia, agranulocytosis, leukopenia, eosinophilia, hepatitis, jaundice, anaphylaxis, angioedema.

Onset, Peak, and Duration

Route	Onset	Peak	Duration
I.M.	Unknown	3–6 hr	Unknown

 Massage Considerations

- Massage may affect the absorption of this drug which is given by intramuscular (I.M.) injection. Do not massage the site of injection for at least 2 to 3 days, as drug may crystallize in the tissues and be absorbed slowly.
- Side effects of concern are hypotension, dizziness, and nausea. Stimulate the client with rapid effleurage and/or tapotement at the end of the session and assist in changing position if hypotension and dizziness are a problem.
- If nausea is present, avoid rocking and shaking, which may worsen the symptom.

azathioprine (ay-zuh-THIGH-oh-preen)

Azasan, Imuran, Thioprine

Drug Class: Immunosuppressant

Drug Action

Suppresses immune system activity

Use

- Immunosuppression in kidney transplantation
- Severe, refractory rheumatoid arthritis

Side Effects

Gastrointestinal: nausea, vomiting, esophagitis, anorexia, pancreatitis, steatorrhea, mouth ulceration.
Skin: itching, hair loss, rash.
Other: leucopenia, bone marrow suppression, anemia, pancytopenia, thrombocytopenia, hepatotoxicity, jaundice, arthralgia, muscle wasting, immunosuppression, infections, neoplasia.

Onset, Peak, and Duration

Route	Onset	Peak	Duration
Oral, I.V.	4–8 wk	1–2 hr	Unknown

 Massage Considerations

- Massage is contraindicated if the client is taking this drug for organ transplant until the physician has given a release.
- When massage is given, great caution must be taken to not expose the client to infection. Schedule the client as the first massage of the day and cancel the session if the massage therapist has any infection.
- Other contraindications and cautions may exist related to the client's condition. Always consult with a physician.
- Side effects of concern are nausea, itching, and hair loss. If the client is experiencing nausea avoid rocking, shaking, and vibratory techniques that could worsen the symptom. When itching is present, avoid effleurage. If the client is experiencing hair loss, do not massage the scalp.
- Client condition may require further changes in massage protocol.

---

azelastine hydrochloride (ah-zuh-LAST-een high-droh-KLOR-ighd)

Astelin, Optivar

Drug Class: Antihistamine

Drug Action

Relieves seasonal allergies

Use

- Seasonal allergic rhinitis, such as rhinorrhea, sneezing, and nasal itching
- Vasomotor rhinitis, such as rhinorrhea, nasal congestion, and postnasal drip

Side Effects

Gastrointestinal: bitter taste, dry mouth, nausea.
Nervous System: fatigue, headache, sleepiness, dizziness, dysesthesia.
Skin: itching.
Other: weight increase, transient eye burning, stinging, nasal burning, temporary eye blurring, conjunctivitis, eye pain, pharyngitis, rhinitis, paroxysmal sneezing, nosebleed, sinusitis, asthma, dyspnea, flulike symptoms.

Onset, Peak, and Duration

Route	Onset	Peak	Duration
Nasal	Unknown	2–3 hr	12 hr
Ophthalmic	3 min	Unknown	8 hr

Massage Considerations

- There are no contraindications or cautions to massage for the client taking this medication.
- Massage does not affect the absorption of this drug.
- This drug does not affect how the body responds to massage.
- Side effects of concern are nausea, itching, sleepiness, dizziness, and fatigue. If nausea is present avoid rocking and shaking techniques that could worsen the symptom. When itching is a problem, avoid effleurage.
- Sleepiness, dizziness, and fatigue may be helped by doing gently stimulating mechanical strokes such as rapid effleurage and tapotement at the end of the massage session.
- All strokes are appropriate for the client taking this drug.

---

azithromycin (uh-zith-roh-MIGH-sin)

Zithromax

Drug Class: Antibiotic

Drug Action

Hinders or kills susceptible bacteria, including many gram-positive and gram-negative aerobic and anaerobic bacteria.

Use

- Acute bacterial exacerbations of chronic obstructive pulmonary disease caused by *Haemophilus influenzae, Moraxella (Branhamella) catarrhalis,* or *Streptococcus pneumoniae;* uncomplicated skin and skin-structure infections caused by *Staphylococcus aureus, Streptococcus pyogenes, or Streptococcus agalactiae;* and second-line therapy for pharyngitis or tonsillitis caused by *S. pyogenes*
- Community-acquired pneumonia caused by *Chlamydia pneumoniae, H. influenzae, Mycoplasma pneumoniae, S. pneumoniae;* I.V. form is also used for *Legionella pneumophila, M. catarrhalis,* and *S. aureus*
- Nongonococcal urethritis or cervicitis caused by Chlamydia trachomatis
- Prevention of disseminated *Mycobacterium avium complex* (MAC) disease in patients with advanced HIV infection
- Disseminated MAC in patients with advanced HIV infection.
- Urethritis and cervicitis caused by *Neisseria gonorrhoeae*
- Pelvic inflammatory disease caused by *C. trachomatis, N. gonorrhoeae, or Mycoplasma hominis* in patients who require initial I.V. therapy
- Prophylaxis for sexual assault victims
- Genital ulcer disease caused by *Haemophilus ducreyi* (chancroid) in men
- Acute otitis media
- Pharyngitis, tonsillitis cause by *S. pyogenes*
- Chancroid
- Prophylaxis of bacterial endocarditis in penicillin-allergic patients at moderate-to-high risk
- Chlamydial ophthalmia neonatorum

Side Effects

Cardiovascular: palpitations, chest pain.
Gastrointestinal: nausea, flatulence, vomiting, diarrhea, abdominal pain, melena, cholestatic jaundice, pseudomembranous colitis.
Nervous System: dizziness, headache, fatigue, sleepiness.
Skin: photosensitivity, rash.
Urinary: nephritis.
Other: candidiasis, vaginitis, angioedema.

Onset, Peak, and Duration

Route	Onset	Peak	Duration
Oral	Unknown	2 $^1/_2$–4 $^1/_2$ hr	Unknown
I.V.	Unknown	Unknown	Unknown

 Massage Considerations

- Massage is contraindicated in acute, active infection. If the client is recovering or taking the drug to prevent infection, massage may be given with caution. Gentler, shorter sessions may be needed, depending on the client's condition.
- Side effects of concern to the massage therapist are nausea, flatulence, dizziness, fatigue, and sleepiness. When nausea is present, avoid strokes that could worsen symptoms such as rocking. Abdominal massage may help with flatulence.
- Dizziness, fatigue, and sleepiness may be helped by given stimulating mechanical strokes such as rapid effleurage and tapotement at the end of the session.

aztreonam (az-TREE-oh-nam)

Azactam

Drug Class: Antibiotic

Drug Action

Kills susceptible bacteria

Use

- Urinary tract infection
- Lower respiratory tract infections
- Septicemia
- Skin and skin-structure infections
- Intra-abdominal infections
- Surgical infections
- Gynecologic infections caused by various aerobic organisms
- Adjunct therapy to pelvic inflammatory disease or gonorrhea

Side Effects

Cardiovascular: hypotension.
Gastrointestinal: nausea, diarrhea, vomiting.
Nervous System: headache, insomnia, seizures, confusion.
Other: bad breath, altered taste, neutropenia, anemia, thrombocytopenia, pancytopenia, hypersensitivity reactions (rash, anaphylaxis); rash, thrombophlebitis at I.V. site; discomfort, swelling at I.M. injection site.

Onset, Peak, and Duration

Route	Onset	Peak	Duration
I.V.	Immediate	Immediate	Unknown
I.M.	Unknown	$^1/_2$–1 $^1/_4$ hr	Unknown

Massage Considerations

- Massage is contraindicated in acute, active infection. If the client is recovering, massage may be given with caution and gentle mechanical strokes would be the most appropriate.
- Massage may affect the absorption of the drug when it is given by intramuscular injection (I.M.). Do not massage the injection site for and least 1 $^1/_2$ hour.
- Side effects of concern to the massage therapist are hypotension and nausea. Care should be taken when the client is changing position or getting off the massage table if hypotension is a problem.
- Gentle stimulation with slightly more rapid effleurage at the end of the session may also help. If nausea is present, avoid strokes that could worsen the symptoms, such as rocking and shaking.

B

bacillus Calmette-Guérin (BCG), live intravesical

(bah-SIL-us kal-MET geh-RAN, in-trah-VES-ih-kal)

ImmuCyst, Pacis, TheraCys, TICE BCG

Drug Class: Vaccine antineoplastic, antituberculotic

Drug Action

Causes local inflammatory response. Decreases risk of superficial bladder tumors. Immunizes against tuberculosis.

Use

- In situ cancer of urinary bladder (primary and relapsed)
- Tuberculosis prevention

Side Effects

Cardiovascular: blood abnormalities, DIC (disemminated intravascular coagulation), anemia.
Gastrointestinal: nausea, vomiting, anorexia, diarrhea, mild abdominal pain, constipation.
Nervous System: fever, fatigue, headache, dizziness.
Skin: ulceration, rash, redness of injection site.
Urinary: hematuria, cystitis, tissue in urine, nephrotoxicity, painful urination, urinary frequency, urinary urgency, urinary incontinence, cramps, genital pain, urinary infection.
Other: chills, soreness of muscles and joints.

Onset, Peak, and Duration

Route	Onset	Peak	Duration
Directly into bladder, and intradermal (into first layer of the skin)	Unknown	Unknown	Unknown

 Massage Considerations

- The local area of injection of vaccine should not be massaged for 3–5 days. Massage does not affect absorption of the drug when instilled into the bladder.
- Once the vaccination area is healed, massage may be given with no further cautions.
- When used for bladder cancer treatment, a physician clearance should be received before doing any massage.
- No deep tissue or myofascial work should be done on the abdomen or low back when the drug is used for bladder cancer treatment.
- Gentle effleurage for these areas and Swedish work for the rest of the body are best. Some deep tissue in other areas may be done with caution depending on the client's general condition.
- Side effects of concern are soreness of muscles and joints, constipation, abdominal pain and cramping. The gentle Swedish work and abdominal effleurage described earlier will help these symptoms in many cases.
- Redness and rash are local contraindications to massage.
- Urinary symptoms such as frequency and urgency may require flexibility and allowing the client to go to the bathroom in the middle of a massage. No water fountains or music that could stimulate urination should be used. If work on the abdomen increases this side effect, avoid working on the area.
- All adverse reactions or severe side effects should be referred to the physician.
- Timing of the massage before or after instillation into the bladder should be discussed with the physician.

baclofen (BAH-kloh-fen)

Clofen, Kemstro, Lioresal, Lioresal Intrathecal

Drug Class: Skeletal muscle relaxant

Drug Action

Appears to reduce transmission of impulses from spinal cord to skeletal muscle. Relieves muscle spasms.

Use

- Spasticity in multiple sclerosis or spinal cord injury
- Spasticity in other neurological or musculoskeletal disorders

Side Effects

Cardiovascular: ankle edema, hypotension.
Gastrointestinal: vomiting, nausea, constipation.
Nervous System: confusion, convulsions, drowsiness, dizziness, headache, fatigue, hypotonis, numbness and tingling.
Skin: rash, itching, increased perspiration.
Urinary: frequency, incontinence.

Other: hyperglycemia, weight gain, nasal congestion, muscle rigidity or spasticity, rhabdomyolysis, dysarthria, dyspnea, sexual dysfunction, impotence, high fever, multiple organ-system failure.

Onset, Peak, and Duration

Route	Onset	Peak	Duration
Oral	1 hour	2–3 hr	Unknown
Into the spinal column	$^1/_2$–1 hr	4 hr	4–8 hr

Massage Considerations

- When drug is administered into the spinal column, massage is contraindicated until release from a physician is obtained.
- Because it is used with hypertonic or spastic muscle conditions, deep tissue massage is contraindicated. If other forms of massage worsened or brought on spasms, then massage could be contraindicated completely for this client.
- The best approach for a client taking this drug is to use gentle effleurage, rocking, and touch strokes either for systemic reflex relaxation or local mechanical effects. Pétrissage and touch/compression strokes should be gentle and used with caution. Myofascial work also would be helpful in some cases.
- Side effects of concern are hypotension, dizziness, and drowsiness. Care should be taken when positioning the client and getting on and off the table. Strokes that are too stimulating could increase spasticity so tapotement or rapid effleurage should not be used.
- Constipation may be helped by gentle effleurage of the abdomen.
- Numbness and tingling or paresthesia contraindicate deep tissue and itching may contraindicate massage completely if massage worsens this symptom.
- Urinary incontinence or frequency of urination may require the client to go to the bathroom in the middle of the massage; water fountains or music that could stimulate urination should not be used.

balsalazide disodium (bal-SAL-a-zide digh-SOH-dee-um)

Colazal

Drug Class: Anti-inflammatory

Drug Action

Decreases inflammation in the colon

Use

- Ulcerative colitis

Side Effects

Gastrointestinal: abdominal pain, anorexia, diarrhea, rectal bleeding, vomiting, constipation, cramps, heartburn, gas, frequent stools, dry mouth.
Nervous System: fever, dizziness, fatigue, headache, insomnia.
Other: liver toxicity, respiratory infection, flulike symptoms, hoarseness or loss of voice, runny nose, soreness of joints or muscles, cough.
Urinary: urinary infection.

Onset, Peak, and Duration

Route	Onset	Peak	Duration
Oral	Unknown	Unknown	Unknown

Massage Considerations

- Contraindications to massage are a result of the client condition and not the drug itself. If the client is having frequent, loose stools or abdominal pain, then abdominal massage may be contraindicated. Contact physician with any concerns.
- Deep tissue massage to the abdomen is contraindicated.
- The best strokes to use are systemic reflex and local mechanical strokes such as effleurage, rocking, and gentle compression.

basiliximab (ba-sil-IK-si-mab)

Simulect

Drug Class: Immunosuppressant

Drug Action

Prevents organ rejection

Use

- Prevention of acute organ rejection in renal transplant patients

Side Effects

Cardiovascular: hemorrhage, angina pectoris, arrhythmias, atrial fibrillation, heart failure, chest pain, abnormal heart sounds, aggravated hypertension, hypertension, leg or peripheral edema, general edema, hypotension, tachycardia, hypotension.
Gastrointestinal: abdominal pain, candidiasis, esophagitis, enlarged abdomen, gastroenteritis, GI disorder, GI hemorrhage, gum hyperplasia, melena, ulcerative stomatitis, vomiting, nausea, flatulence, constipation, upset stomach.
Nervous System: gastroenteritis, GI disorder, GI hemorrhage, gum hyperplasia, fever, agitation, depression, anxiety, dizziness, headache, hypesthesia, insomnia, neuropathy, paresthesia, tremor, fatigue.
Skin: cold sores, shingles, rash, ulcerations, acne, itching, cyst.
Urinary: abnormal renal function, albuminuria, bladder disorder, genital edema, hematuria, increased nonprotein nitrogen, oliguria, renal tubular necrosis, ureteral disorder, UTI, urine retention, impotence, dysuria, frequent urination.
Other: hematoma, polycythemia, purpura, thrombocytopenia, thrombosis.
acidosis, dehydration, diabetes mellitus, fluid overload, fluid and electrolyte abnormalities, weight gain, back pain, bone fracture, cramps, hernia, leg pain, abnormal chest sounds, bronchitis, bronchospasm, shortness of breath, pneumonia, pulmonary disorder, pulmonary edema, upper respiratory tract infection, accidental trauma, viral infection, infection, sepsis, surgical wound complications, rhinitis, sinusitis, anemia, muscle and joint aches, cramps, cough, colds.

Onset, Peak, and Duration

Route	Onset	Peak	Duration
Intravenous	Unknown	Immediate	Unknown

Massage Considerations

- Clients receiving this drug have just undergone renal transplant surgery. Massage is contraindicated soon after this surgery.
- A physician release is required before resuming massage.

---

becaplermin (be-KAP-ler-min)

Regranex

Drug Class: Tissue growth factor

Drug Action

Thought to promote proliferation of cells involved in wound repair and formation of new granulation tissue.

Use

- Diabetic neuropathic leg ulcers that extend into S.C. tissue or beyond and have adequate blood supply.

Side Effects

Skin: erythematous rash.
Other: cellulitis, infection, osteomyelitis.

Onset, Peak, and Duration

Route	Onset	Peak	Duration
Topical	Unknown	Unknown	Unknown

Massage Considerations

- Massage will be affected by the use of this drug.
- Massage is contraindicated at the site of the wound. The use of systemic reflex strokes and circulatory massage will help to promote healing.
- Effleurage and pétrissage above and below the wound site are especially beneficial.

---

beclomethasone dipropionate (bek-loh-METH-eh-sohn digh-proh-PIGH-uh-nayt)

Beclodisk, Becloforte Inhaler, QVAR, Vanceril, Vanceril Double Strength

Drug Class: Glucocorticoid anti-inflammatory, antiasthmatic

Drug Action

Decreases inflammation. Helps alleviate asthma symptoms

Use

- Asthma

Side Effects

Other: hoarseness, throat irritation, irritation of nasal passages and mucous, fungal infections of throat, fungal infections of mouth, bronchospasm, angioedema, adrenal insufficiency.

Onset, Peak, and Duration

Route	Onset	Peak	Duration
Inhalation	1–4 wk	Unknown	Unknown

Massage Considerations

- Any cautions or contraindications are a result of the client's condition and not because of the drug.
- Massage will not affect the absorption rate of this drug.
- All massage strokes and techniques may be used for a client taking this drug.

---

beclomethasone dipropionate monohydrate (bek-loh-METH-eh-sohn digh-proh-PIGH-uh-nayt mon-oh-HIGH-drayt)

Beconase AQ Nasal Spray, Vancenase AQ 84 mcg Double Strength, Vancenase Pockethaler

Drug Class: Glucocorticoid anti-inflammatory

Drug Action

Decreases nasal inflammation. Helps relieve nasal allergy symptoms.

Use

- Symptoms of seasonal or perennial allergies
- Prevention of recurrence of nasal polyps after surgical removal

Side Effects

Gastrointestinal: vomiting, nausea.
Nervous System: headache.
Other: nose bleeds, nasopharyngeal fungal infections, transient nasal burning, nasal congestion, sneezing, irritation of nasal mucosa.

Onset, Peak, and Duration

Route	Onset	Peak	Duration
Inhalation	5–7 days	≤3 wk	Unknown

Massage Considerations

- There is no caution or contraindication to massage for this client as a result of taking this drug. Any cautions are a result of the client's condition.
- Massage will not affect absorption of this drug.
- All strokes and techniques may be utilized.

benazepril hydrochloride (ben-AY-zuh-pril high-droh-KLOR-ighd)

Lotensin

Drug Class: Angiotensin converting enzyme (ACE) inhibitor antihypertensive

Drug Actions

Lowers blood pressure

Use

- Hypertension

Side Effects

Cardiovascular: symptomatic hypotension, angina, arrhythmias, palpitations, edema.
Gastrointestinal: nausea, vomiting, abdominal pain, constipation, upset stomach, gastritis, difficulty swallowing, increased salivation.
Nervous System: asthenia, headache, dizziness, light-headedness, anxiety, amnesia, depression, sleeplessness, nervousness, nerve pain, neuropathy, paresthesia, sleepiness, syncope.
Skin: rash, dermatitis, increased sweating, itching, sensitivity to light, purpura.
Urinary: impotence.
Other: hyperkalemia, weight gain, joint pain, arthritis, muscle pain, dry, persistent, tickling, nonproductive cough; shortness of breath, angioedema, hypersensitivity reactions.

Onset, Peak, and Duration

Route	Onset	Peak	Duration
Oral	≤1 hr	2–4 hr	24 hr

Massage Considerations

- There are no contraindications to massage for the client taking this drug. Any contraindications are a result of the client condition and not the drug itself.
- If you take the blood pressure before and/or after the session, any blood pressure readings outside of the normal range or the range given to you by the patient's physician would necessitate withholding massage and contacting the physician.
- Any side effects should be reported to the physician. Of the side effects noted, hypotension, dizziness, and lightheadedness require extra care in moving, positioning, and getting the client on and off the table. Stimulating strokes such as tapotement and rapid effleurage may be used at the end of the session to help prevent these or increased rate and speed of the massage throughout the session may be used if these side effects are severe.
- Constipation may be helped by doing abdominal massage.
- All strokes and types of massage may be utilized.

benztropine mesylate (BENZ-troh-peen MES-ih-layt)

Apo-Benztropine, Cogentin

Drug Class: Anticholinergic antiparkinsonian

Drug Actions

Thought to block central cholinergic receptors, helping to balance cholinergic activity in basal ganglia. Improves capability for voluntary movement and decreases involuntary, abnormal muscular activity

Use

- Drug-induced extrapyramidal disorders (except tardive dyskinesia)
- Acute dystonic reaction
- Parkinsonism

Side Effects

Cardiovascular: palpitations, tachycardia, paradoxical bradycardia, flushing.
Gastrointestinal: dry mouth, constipation, nausea, vomiting, epigastric distress.
Nervous System: disorientation, restlessness, irritability, incoherence, hallucinations, headache, sedation, depression, nervousness, confusion.
Urinary: urinary hesitancy, urine retention.
Other: dilated pupils, blurred vision, photophobia, difficulty swallowing, muscle weakness.

Onset, Peak, and Duration

Route	Onset	Peak	Duration
Oral	1–2 hr	Unknown	24 hr
I.V. or I.M. Injection	≤15 min	Unknown	24 hr

Massage Considerations

- There are no contraindications to massage related to this drug. The client's condition, however, may require cautions or contraindications.
- Because the drug blocks cholinergic activity, the sedating and relaxing effects of massage may be increased. Use of more rapid or stimulating strokes may be needed throughout the massage or at least at the end of the massage. Gentle tapotement, rapid effleurage, and pétrissage may be used. Care getting the client on and off the table and with positioning is essential.
- Any side effects should be reported to the physician.
- Constipation may be aided by abdominal massage.

---

17 beta-estradiol and norgestimate (17 bay-ta-eh-stray-DYE-ol nor-JES-ti-mate)

Ortho-Prefest

Drug Class: Combined synthetic estrogen and progestin

Drug Actions

Relieves menopausal hot flashes and vaginal dryness; reduces the severity of osteoporosis.

Use

- Moderate-to-severe vasomotor symptoms and vulvar and vaginal atrophy caused by menopause
- Prevention of osteoporosis in women with an intact uterus

Side Effects

Cardiovascular: edema.
Gastrointestinal: flatulence, nausea, abdominal pain, weight gain.
Nervous System: depression, dizziness, fatigue, pain, headache.
Urinary: dysmenorrhea, vaginal bleeding, vaginitis, decreased libido.
Other: arthralgia, myalgia, back pain, cough, upper respiratory tract infection, flulike symptoms, viral infection, breast pain, tooth disorder, pharyngitis, sinusitis.

Onset, Peak, and Duration

Route	Onset	Peak	Duration
Oral	Unknown	7 hr (estradiol),	Unknown
		2 hr (norgestimate)	

Massage Considerations

- There are no contraindications to massage for clients taking this medication.
- Caution should be used in applying deep tissue massage, especially to the lower extremities. There is a slight increase in the risk of blood clots for clients taking this medication. Any leg pain, swelling, redness, or heat should be immediately evaluated by a physician and massage withheld.
- Any side effects should be reported to the physician. Dizziness as a side effect requires care in positioning and in getting the client on and off the table.
- Flatulence may be relieved by abdominal massage.
- All types of massage strokes are useful with this client.

betamethasone (bay-tuh-METH-uh-sohn)

betamethasone acetate and betamethasone sodium phosphate

Celestone Chronodose, Celestone Soluspan

betamethasone sodium phosphate

Celestone Phosphate, Selestoject

Drug Class: Glucocorticoid anti-inflammatory

Drug Actions

Decreases inflammation, suppresses immune response; stimulates bone marrow; and influences protein, fat, and carbohydrate metabolism.

Use

- Conditions of severe inflammation
- For immunosuppression

Side Effects

Cardiovascular: heart failure, hypertension, edema, thromboembolism.
Gastrointestinal: peptic ulceration, GI irritation, increased appetite, pancreatitis.
Nervous System: euphoria, insomnia, psychotic behavior, pseudotumor cerebri, seizures.
Skin: hirsutism, delayed wound healing, acne, various skin eruptions.
Other: susceptibility to infections, acute adrenal insufficiency after stress (infection, surgery, or trauma) or abrupt withdrawal after long-term therapy, cataracts, glaucoma, low potassium, hyperglycemia, carbohydrate intolerance, muscle weakness, osteoporosis (long-term use), growth suppression in children.

Onset, Peak, and Duration

Route	Onset	Peak	Duration
Oral	Unknown	1–2 hr	3 $^{1}/_{4}$ days
I.V. I.M. or Into the Joint	Rapid	Unknown	7–14 days

Massage Considerations

- Although the absorption rates of this drug by of oral and I.V. routes are not affected by massage, I.M. or into-the-joint injections may increase or affect the absorption of this drug. The site of injection should not be massaged for at least 24 hours. It is best to check with the physician for the amount of time to avoid working the area, especially after injection into the joint.
- Clients who are on this medication less than 14 days have no contraindications or cautions related to the drug. If the client is taking this medication long-term for chronic conditions, there are multiple cautions for massage.
- Changes in metabolism and in the connective tissues of the body occur over time. Fatty deposits occur in various places on the body.
- Deep tissue massage should be applied only with great caution; myofascial techniques may be less effective and also should be applied with caution. Depth and pressure need to be lighter because of these tissue changes and to increased bone demineralization/osteoporosis that can occur as a side effect. These changes are more likely, the longer the client is on the drug.
- Side effects of susceptibility to infection are related to the immunosuppressant action of the drug. Be careful not to expose the client to infections; schedule the client first for the day, and cancel the session if you have a cold or other infection.
- Generally, systemic reflex strokes and circulatory massage strokes are the best to be used with these clients. Rocking, effleurage, gentle pétrissage, and gentle holding compression will have a good effect.

---

bethanechol chloride (beh-THAN-eh-kol KLOR-ighd)

Duvoid

Drug Class: Cholinergic agonist, urinary tract stimulant

Drug Actions

Directly stimulates cholinergic receptors, mimicking action of acetylcholine. Relieves urinary retention.

Use

- Acute urinary retention
- Chronic urinary retention
- To restore bladder function in patients with chronic neurogenic bladder
- Bladder dysfunction caused by phenothiazines
- To diagnose flaccid or atonic neurogenic bladder

Side Effects

Cardiovascular: bradycardia, hypotension, flushing, reflex tachycardia.
Gastrointestinal: abdominal cramps, diarrhea, excessive salivation, nausea, vomiting, belching, borborygmi, esophageal spasms.
Nervous System: headache, malaise.
Urinary: urinary urgency.
Skin: sweating.
Other: lacrimation, miosis, bronchoconstriction, increased bronchial secretions.

Onset, Peak, and Duration

Route	Onset	Peak	Duration
Oral	30–90 min	1 hr	1–6 hr
Subcutaneous Injection	5–15 min	5–30 min	2 hr

Massage Considerations

- Absorption of the drug is not affected by massage when the oral form is used. When the drug is given subcutaneously, the area of the injection should not be massaged for 2 hours so as not to increase the rate of absorption.
- There are no cautions or contraindications to massage for this drug.
- The side effect of hypotension requires care in positioning and getting the client on and off the table. Stimulating strokes at the end of the massage such as tapotement and rapid effleurage may help prevent problems with this.
- Urinary urgency may require that the client get up to go to the bathroom during the massage. Making the client feel comfortable about this and providing privacy and quick access are important. Also, avoid using flowing fountains or water music that may stimulate this response.
- All types of massage strokes are appropriate for this client.

bexarotene (bex-AHR-oh-teen)

Targretin

Drug Class: Tumor cell growth inhibitor

Drug Actions

Inhibits tumor growth in cutaneous T-cell lymphoma

Use

- Cutaneous effects of cutaneous T-cell lymphoma in patient's refractory to at least one previous systemic therapy

Side Effects

Cardiovascular: peripheral edema, chest pain, hemorrhage, hypertension, angina, heart failure, tachycardia.
Gastrointestinal: nausea, diarrhea, vomiting, anorexia, pancreatitis, abdominal pain, constipation, dry mouth, flatulence, colitis, dyspepsia, cheilitis, gastroenteritis, gingivitis, melena.
Nervous System: fever, headache, insomnia, asthenia, fatigue, syncope, depression, agitation, ataxia, CVA, confusion, dizziness, hyperesthesia, hypoesthesia, neuropathy.
Urinary: albuminuria, hematuria, incontinence, UTI, urinary urgency, dysuria, abnormal kidney function.
Skin: (P.O.) rash, dry skin, exfoliative dermatitis, hair loss, photosensitivity, itching, cellulitis, acne, skin ulcer, skin nodule; (Topical) contact dermatitis, pain, skin disorders.
Other: breast pain, infection, chills, flulike syndrome, sepsis, cataracts, pharyngitis, rhinitis, dry eyes, conjunctivitis, ear pain, blepharitis, corneal lesion, keratitis, otitis externa, visual field defect, abnormal blood profiles, bilirubinemia, liver failure, hyperlipemia, hypercholesteremia, hypothyroidism, hyperglycemia, hypoproteinemia, hypocalcemia, hyponatremia, weight change, arthralgia, myalgia, back pain, bone pain, myasthenia, joint degeneration.
Respiratory: pneumonia, dyspnea, hemoptysis, pleural effusion, bronchitis, cough, lung edema, hypoxia.

Onset, Peak, and Duration

Route	Onset	Peak	Duration
Oral, Topical	Unknown	Unknown	Unknown

Massage Considerations

- Clients taking this drug are being treated for cancer. A physician should be consulted before giving any massage. If skin involvement is extensive, massage may be totally contraindicated. If localized, the area of involvement should not receive massage. Cautions for massage depend very much on client condition rather than the use of the drug itself.
- The side effect of dizziness requires care in getting the client on and off the table.
- Constipation and flatulence may be relieved by gentle abdominal massage.
- As always, rash or any skin disorder is a local contraindication to massage. Joint degeneration contraindicates traction and caution in depth of massage with compression and friction at the site.
- The drug works on the tumor cells and therefore does not affect how the body receives massage. All strokes are appropriate depending on the client's condition.

---

bimatoprost (by-MAT-oh-prost)

Lumigan

Drug Class: Antiglaucoma drug, ocular antihypertensive

Drug Actions

Reduces intraocular pressure

Use

- To reduce elevated intraocular pressure (IOP) in patients with open-angle glaucoma ocular hypertension

Side Effects

Nervous System: headache, asthenia.
Skin: excessive and abnormal hair growth in women.
Other: infection, conjunctival hyperemia, growth of eyelashes, eye itching, ocular dryness, visual disturbance, ocular burning, foreign body sensation, eye pain, pigmentation of the periocular skin, ulceration of eyelids, cataract, superficial punctate keratitis, eyelid erythema, ocular irritation, eyelash darkening, eye discharge, tearing, photophobia, allergic conjunctivitis, asthenopia, increased iris pigmentation, conjunctival edema, gradual change in eye color, upper respiratory tract infection.

Onset, Peak, and Duration

Route	Onset	Peak	Duration
Into the Eye	4 hr	10 min	1 $\frac{1}{2}$ hr

Massage Considerations

- There are no cautions or contraindications to massage related to this drug.
- All types of massage are appropriate.

bisacodyl (bigh-suh-KOH-dil)

Bisac-Evac, Bisacodyl Uniserts, Bisacolax, Bisalax, Bisco-Lax, Carter's Little Pills, Correctol, Dacodyl, Deficol, Dulcolax, Durolax, Feen-a-Mint, Fleet Bisacodyl, Fleet Laxative, Fleet Prep Kit, Laxit, Modane, Theralax

Drug Class: Stimulant laxative

Drug Actions

Increases peristalsis, probably by acting directly on smooth muscle of intestine. Also promotes fluid accumulation in colon and small intestine. Relieves constipation.

Use

- Chronic constipation
- Preparation for childbirth, surgery, or rectal or bowel examination

Side Effects

Nervous System: tetany.
Gastrointestinal: nausea, vomiting, abdominal cramps, diarrhea (with high doses), burning sensation in rectum (with suppositories), protein-losing enteropathy (with excessive use), laxative dependence (with long-term or excessive use).
Other: alkalosis, hypokalemia, fluid and electrolyte imbalance, muscle weakness (with excessive use).

Onset, Peak, and Duration

Route	Onset	Peak	Duration
Oral	6–12 hr	Variable	Variable
Rectal	15–60 min	Variable	Variable

Massage Considerations

- There are no cautions or contraindications to massage for clients taking this drug.
- Clients should not take the rectal form of this drug prior to a massage because of the fairly rapid onset of action. It may make for abdominal cramps and urgency to evacuate bowel that could be uncomfortable during the massage.
- All types of massage strokes are appropriate.

bismuth subgallate (BIS-muth sub-GAL-ayt)

Devrom

bismuth subsalicylate

Children's Kaopectate, Extra Strength Kaopectate, Kaopectate (Regular), Maximum Strength Pepto-Bismol, Pepto-Bismol

Drug Class: Antidiarrheal

Drug Actions

Relieves diarrhea

Use

- To control fecal odors in colostomy, ileostomy, or incontinence
- Mild, nonspecific diarrhea

Side Effects

Gastrointestinal: temporary darkening of tongue and stools.
Other: toxicity (with high doses).

Onset, Peak, and Duration

Route	Onset	Peak	Duration
Oral	1 hr	Unknown	Unknown

 Massage Considerations

- There are no cautions or contraindications to massage for this drug.
- All massage strokes are appropriate.

---

bisoprolol fumarate (bis-OP-roh-lol FYOO-muh-rayt)

Zebeta

Drug Class: Beta blocker antihypertensive

Drug Actions

Decreases blood pressure

Use

- Hypertension
- Heart failure

Side Effects

Cardiovascular: bradycardia, peripheral edema, chest pain, heart failure.
EENT: pharyngitis, rhinitis, sinusitis.
Gastrointestinal: nausea, vomiting, diarrhea, dry mouth.
Nervous System: asthenia, fatigue, dizziness, headache, hypesthesia, vivid dreams, depression, insomnia.
Skin: sweating.
Other: pharyngitis, rhinitis, sinusitis, arthralgia, cough, shortness of breath.

Onset, Peak, and Duration

Route	Onset	Peak	Duration
Oral	Unknown	2–4 hr	24 hr

Massage Considerations

- As long as the client's blood pressure is under control, there are no cautions or contraindications to massage related to this drug.
- The side effect of dizziness requires care in getting the client on and off the table. Stimulating strokes such as tapotement or rapid effleurage at the end of the session may help prevent problems with this side effect.
- All strokes are appropriate for this client.

bleomycin sulfate (blee-oh-MIGH-sin SUL-fayt)

Blenoxane

Drug Class: Anticancer drug

Drug Actions

Kills selected types of cancer cells

Use

- Hodgkin's lymphoma
- Squamous cell carcinoma
- Non-Hodgkin's lymphoma
- Testicular cancer
- Malignant pleural effusion
- Prevention of recurrent pleural effusions
- To manage pneumothorax related to AIDS or Pneumocystis carinii pneumonia
- AIDS-related Kaposi's sarcoma

Side Effects

Gastrointestinal: stomatitis, prolonged anorexia, nausea, vomiting, diarrhea.
Nervous System: hyperesthesia of scalp and fingers, headache, fever.
Skin: reversible hair loss; erythema; vesiculation; hardening and discoloration of palmar and plantar skin; peeling of the skin of hands, feet, and pressure areas; hyperpigmentation; acne.
Other: hypersensitivity reactions (fever up to 106° F [41.1° C] with chills up to 5 hours after injection, anaphylaxis), leukocytosis, swelling of interphalangeal joints, pneumonitis, pulmonary fibrosis, fine crackles, shortness of breath, nonproductive cough.

Onset, Peak, and Duration

Route	Onset	Peak	Duration
I.V., I.M., Subcutaneous, Directly into the Lungs	Unknown	Unknown	Unknown

Massage Considerations

- The client taking this drug has cancer. The physician should always be consulted. There are no cautions or contraindications for massage related to the drug itself. Cautions and contraindications are related to the client's condition.
- Because absorption of the drug may be increased with massage in I.M and subcutaneous injections and the onset and peak of action are unknown, local contraindications to massage exist. The amount of time the area should be avoided will need to be discussed with the physician but should at least be 24 hours.
- The side effect of hyperesthesia (increased sensitivity to touch) if severe, may contraindicate massage in those areas affected. If mild to moderate, massage may need to be limited in that area with regard to depth, speed, and amount of time spent on the area.
- Hair loss requires sensitivity and contraindicates massage of the scalp if the client (or the massage therapist) are bothered by the hair coming out.
- Peeling of the skin may also be local contraindication or at least a local caution for massage. Minimize friction and strokes that rub the skin and may worsen the peeling.
- Use compression, traction, shaking, and light pétrissage.
- All strokes are appropriate depending on the client's condition.

bortezomib (bore-TEHZ-uh-mihb)

Velcade

Drug Class: Anticancer drug

Drug Actions

Destroys cancer cells

Use

- Multiple myeloma that's progressing after at least two therapies

Side Effects

Cardiovascular: edema, orthostatic, and postural hypotension.
Gastrointestinal: abdominal pain, constipation, decreased appetite, diarrhea, altered taste, dyspepsia, nausea, vomiting.
Nervous System: anxiety, asthenia, dizziness, dysesthesia, fever, headache, insomnia, paresthesia, peripheral neuropathy, rigors.
Urinary: dehydration.
Skin: rash, itching.
Other: herpes zoster, blurred vision, anemia, abnormal blood profiles, arthralgia, back pain, bone pain, limb pain, muscle cramps, myalgia, cough, shortness of blood, pneumonia, upper respiratory tract infection.

Onset, Peak, and Duration

Route	Onset	Peak	Duration
I.V.	Unknown	Unknown	Unknown

 Massage Considerations

- There are no cautions or contraindications related to the drug itself. However, a physician should be consulted, as the client's condition may require changes, cautions, and contraindications to massage.
- The side effects of dizziness and orthostatic and postural hypotension (drops in blood pressure with changes in position) require care with positioning and getting the client on and off the table. Use of stimulating strokes such as tapotement and rapid effleurage at the end of the session may help alleviate this side effect.
- Paresthesia and/or neuropathies that decrease the client's sensation and ability to give feedback require great caution up to and including contraindication for deep tissue massage
- Rash or itching may locally contraindicate massage.
- All strokes are appropriate depending on the client's condition.

bosentan (bow-SEN-tan)

Tracleer

Drug Class: Antihypertensive

Drug Actions

Increases exercise capacity and cardiac index. Decreases blood pressure, pulmonary arterial pressure, vascular resistance, and mean right arterial pressure.

Use

- Pulmonary arterial hypertension

Side Effects

Cardiovascular: hypotension, palpitations, flushing, edema, lower leg edema.
Gastrointestinal: dyspepsia.
Nervous System: headache, fatigue.
Skin: itching.
Other: nasopharyngitis, anemia, liver failure.

Onset, Peak, and Duration

Route	Onset	Peak	Duration
Oral	Unknown	3–5 hr	Unknown

Massage Considerations

- If blood pressure is controlled, there are no cautions or contraindications to massage for clients taking this drug. Because this drug is used for those with severe hypertension, it is appropriate to obtain physician approval for massage, and to obtain parameters for withholding massage if the blood pressure is elevated.
- The side effect of hypotension requires care in getting the client on and off the table. Stimulating strokes such as tapotement and rapid effleurage at the end the massage may help alleviate this side effect. Itching may be a local contraindication to massage if the side effect is aggravated by the massage. Using compression, shaking, traction, and minimizing use of strokes that rub such as friction and effleurage may help with this side effect.
- All strokes are appropriate for this client except as noted earlier.

bromocriptine mesylate (broh-moh-KRIP-teen MES-ih-layt)

Parlodel, Parlodel SnapTabs

Drug Class: Dopamine receptor agonist

Drug Actions

Inhibits secretion of prolactin and acts as dopamine-receptor agonist by activating postsynaptic dopamine receptors. Reverses amenorrhea and galactorrhea caused by hyperprolactinemia, increases fertility in women, improves voluntary movement in Parkinsonism, and inhibits prolactin and growth hormone release.

Use

- Parkinson's disease
- Acromegaly
- Amenorrhea and galactorrhea related to hyperprolactinemia
- Infertility or hypogonadism in women
- Premenstrual syndrome
- Cushing's syndrome
- Hepatic encephalopathy
- Neuroleptic malignant syndrome related to neuroleptic drug therapy

Side Effects

Cardiovascular: hypotension, orthostatic hypotension, hypertension, acute myocardial infarction (MI).
Gastrointestinal: nausea, vomiting, abdominal cramps, constipation, diarrhea.
Urinary: urine retention, urinary frequency.
Nervous System: confusion, hallucinations, uncontrolled body movements, dizziness, headache, fatigue, mania, delusions, nervousness, insomnia, depression, seizures, cerebrovascular accident (CVA), syncope.
Skin: coolness and pallor of fingers and toes.
Other: nasal congestion, tinnitus, blurred vision.

Onset, Peak, and Duration

Route	Onset	Peak	Duration
Oral	½–2 hr	1–3 hr	12–24 hr

 Massage Considerations

- This drug is used for multiple and very different reasons and disorders. The drug itself has no cautions or contraindications for massage; however, knowledge of the client's condition may require changes in application of massage.
- The action of the drug in stimulating dopaminergic activity may make the client less receptive to the relaxing effects of massage on the muscles and in general. This may require use of longer periods of work with slower rhythms with systemic reflex strokes that help to turn on the parasympathetic nervous system and allow the client to relax. Strokes such as slow, rhythmic effleurage, rocking, and gentle compression will be helpful.
- Side effects such as dizziness and hypotension require care in getting the client on and off the table. While using the slower strokes above during the massage, some more stimulating strokes may be needed at the end to avoid this problem. More rapid effleurage and tapotement may be useful.
- Constipation may respond well to abdominal massage.
- Urinary frequency may require that the client get up during the massage. Provide privacy and quick access to the bathroom. Avoid using water features or water music that might stimulate the need to urinate.
- The best strokes to use are those noted above that use the systemic reflex response to help the client reach relaxation and release muscle tension. These include rocking, shaking, compression (gentle), and effleurage.

brompheniramine maleate (brom-fen-IR-ah-meen MAL-ee-ayt)

Bromphen, Dimetane, Dimetapp Allergy, Nasahist B, ND-Stat

Drug Class: Antihistamine (H_1-receptor antagonist)

Drug Actions

Relieves allergy symptoms

Use

- Rhinitis, allergy symptoms

Side Effects

Cardiovascular: hypotension, palpitations.
Gastrointestinal: anorexia, nausea, vomiting, dry mouth and throat.

Nervous System: dizziness, tremors, irritability, insomnia, syncope, drowsiness, stimulation (especially in elderly patients).
Urinary: urine retention.
Skin: hives, rash, diaphoresis.
Other: local stinging, thrombocytopenia, agranulocytosis.

Onset, Peak, and Duration

Route	Onset	Peak	Duration
Oral., I.V., I.M., Subcutaneous Injection	15–60 min	2–5 hr (longer for P.O. extended-release)	4–8 hr

 Massage Considerations

- There are no cautions or contraindications for massage for the client taking this drug.
- When the drug is give by injection into the tissue, absorption rates could be increased by massage. The site of injection should not be massaged about 4–5 hours.
- The side effects of hypotension and dizziness require care in getting the client on and off the table, as does the sedation that the drug may cause. Using stimulation at the end of the massage with tapotement and rapid effleurage may help. The presence of rash or hives contraindicates massage in the local area. If severe, no massage should be given.
- All massage strokes are appropriate for this client.

---

budesonide (inhalation) (byoo-DES-oh-nighd)

Pulmicort Respules, Pulmicort Turbuhaler, Rhinocort Aqua

Drug Class: Glucocorticoid anti-inflammatory

Drug Actions

Decreases nasal and pulmonary congestion

Use

- Symptoms of seasonal or perennial allergic rhinitis and non-allergic perennial rhinitis
- Chronic asthma

Side Effects

Cardiovascular: facial edema.
Gastrointestinal: bad taste, dry mouth, dyspepsia, nausea, vomiting.
Nervous System: nervousness, headache.
Skin: rash, itching, contact dermatitis.
Other: hypersensitivity reactions, nasal irritation, nose bleed, pharyngitis, sinusitis, reduced sense of smell, nasal pain, hoarseness, weight gain, myalgia, cough, candidiasis, wheezing, shortness of breath.

Onset, Peak, and Duration

Route	Onset	Peak	Duration
Nasal Inhalation	10 hr	Unknown	Unknown
Oral Inhalation	24 hr	1–2 wk	Unknown

Massage Considerations

- There are no cautions or contraindications to massage for the client taking this drug.
- The side effects of rash, itching, or dermatitis may be a local contraindication. If severe, the massage should not be given and the physician contacted.
- All massage strokes are appropriate for this client.

---

budesonide (oral) (byoo-DES-oh-nighd)

Entocort EC

Drug Class: Corticosteroid anti-inflammatory

Drug Actions

Drug has significant glucocorticoid effects because of its high affinity for glucocorticoid receptors, which leads to improvement of Crohn's disease.

Use

- Mild to moderate active Crohn's disease

Side Effects

Cardiovascular: chest pain, dependent edema, facial edema, hypertension, palpitations, tachycardia, flushing.
Gastrointestinal: nausea, dyspepsia, abdominal pain, flatulence, vomiting, anus disorder, aggravated Crohn's disease, gastroenteritis, epigastric pain, fistula, glossitis, hemorrhoids, intestinal obstruction, tongue edema, dry mouth, tooth disorder, taste perversion, increased appetite, oral candidiasis.
Nervous System: headache, dizziness, asthenia, increased muscle movements paresthesia, syncope, tremor, vertigo, fatigue, malaise, agitation, confusion, insomnia, nervousness, sleepiness, migraine, fever, pain, sleep disorder.
Urinary: dysuria, frequency, nocturia, intermenstrual bleeding, menstrual disorder.
Skin: acne, alopecia, dermatitis, eczema, skin disorder, increased sweating, bruising.
Other: flulike syndrome, infection, pharyngitis, ear infection, eye abnormality, abnormal vision, sinusitis, voice alteration, neck pain, leukocytosis, anemia, hypercorticism, hypokalemia, weight gain, adrenal insufficiency, back pain, aggravated arthritis, cramps, myalgia, arthralgia, hypotonia, respiratory tract infection, bronchitis, shortness of breath, cough.

Onset, Peak, and Duration

Route	Onset	Peak	Duration
Oral	10 hr	$^1/_2$–10 hr	Unknown

Massage Considerations

- Long-term use of this drug (longer than 14 days) may cause changes in the connective tissue, fatty deposits in tissues, osteoporosis, and changes in metabolism. Deep tissue massage should be used with great caution. Myofascial techniques may not be as effective and the longer the client has been on the drug, the more caution should be used.
- Other side effects such as dizziness and sleepiness require care in getting the client on and off the table. Use of stimulating rapid effleurage may help. Tapotement may be used but only very lightly because of ease of bruising.
- Abdominal massage may be helpful with flatulence but should not be done if diarrhea is a problem.

- Loss of hair contraindicates massage of the scalp.
- The best massage strokes to use are gentle mechanical strokes and systemic reflex strokes such as rocking, effleurage, pétrissage, and gentle compression.

---

bumetanide (byoo-MEH-tuh-nighd)

Bumex, Burinex

Drug Class: Diuretic

Drug Actions

Promotes sodium and water excretion thus decreasing edema and lowering blood pressure

Use

- Postoperative edema
- Premenstrual syndrome edema
- Disseminated cancer edema
- Heart failure edema
- Edema in liver or kidney disease
- Hypertension
- Heart failure

Side Effects

Cardiovascular: volume depletion and dehydration, orthostatic hypotension, ECG changes.
Gastrointestinal: nausea.
Nervous System: dizziness, headache.
Urinary: renal failure, nocturia, polyuria, azotemia, frequent urination, oliguria.
Skin: rash.
Other: fluid and electrolyte imbalances, abnormal blood counts, hyperglycemia; impaired glucose tolerance, muscle pain and tenderness, transient deafness.

Onset, Peak, and Duration

Route	Onset	Peak	Duration
Oral	30–60 min	1–2 hr	4–6 hr
I.V.	3 min	15–30 min	3 $^1/_2$–4 hr
I.M.	40 min	Unknown	Unknown

Massage Considerations

- The site of I.M. injection of this drug should not be massaged at minimum 2 hours, because peak action is unknown, it is best to be cautious and massage could speed the rate of absorption.
- The drug itself does not affect how the body receives massage and does not bring with it any cautions or contraindications. The client's condition may require cautions and contraindications.
- Side effects of dizziness and orthostatic hypotension (drop in blood pressure with changes in position) require care in getting the client on and off the table. Stimulating strokes such as tapotement and rapid effleurage may be used at the end of the massage to help prevent any problems.
- Frequent urination may require that the client go to the bathroom in the middle of the massage. Privacy and easy access to the bathroom should be provided. Also, avoid use of fountains and water music that may stimulate the need to urinate.

- Rash is a local contraindication to massage.
- All massage strokes are appropriate for the client taking this drug depending on the client's condition.

---

buprenorphine hydrochloride (byoo-preh-NOR-feen high-droh-KLOR-ighd)

Buprenex, Subutex

buprenorphine hydrochloride and naloxone hydrochloride dihydrate

Suboxone

Drug Class: Opioid agonist-antagonist, opioid partial agonist, analgesic

Drug Actions

Binds with opiate receptors in CNS, altering perception of and emotional response to pain

Use

- Moderate to severe pain
- Opioid dependence
- Postoperative pain
- Pain
- Circumcision

Side Effects

Cardiovascular: hypotension, bradycardia, tachycardia, hypertension, Wenckebach block, cyanosis, flushing.
Gastrointestinal: nausea, vomiting, constipation, dry mouth.
Nervous System: dizziness, sedation, headache, confusion, nervousness, euphoria, vertigo, increased intracranial pressure, fatigue, weakness, depression, dreaming, psychosis, slurred speech, paresthesia.
Urinary: urine retention.
Skin: itching, sweating.
Other: injection site reactions, chills, withdrawal syndrome, blurred vision, double vision, visual abnormalities, ringing in the ears, conjunctivitis, respiratory depression, hypoventilation, shortness of breath.

Onset, Peak, and Duration

Route	Onset	Peak	Duration
I.V., I.M.	15 min	1 hr	6 hr
Under the Tongue	Unknown	Unknown	2–8 hr

Massage Considerations

- Massage may increase the rate of absorption of this drug when given I.M. The site should not be massaged for at least 1 hour after injection.
- Because this drug alters the perception of pain, it also will alter the perception of massage. Deep tissue massage should be used with great caution as the client will not be able to give accurate feedback on depth and pressure.

- Side effects of dizziness and hypotension require care in getting the client on and off the table. Sedation will increase the relaxing effects of the massage as well. Giving a slightly more stimulating massage throughout the session will help mitigate these effects. This can be done with increase in the rate and rhythm of strokes and use of rapid effleurage and tapotement toward the end of the session.
- Constipation may be helped by abdominal massage.
- Itching may contraindicate massage either locally or altogether if the massage aggravates this side effect. Locally, if mild, avoid effleurage and friction and use compression, shaking, and pétrissage that won't increase itching as much.
- Because of the alteration of perception caused by the drug, mechanical strokes will be the best to achieve results with this client. Pétrissage and effleurage will be most effective.

---

bupropion hydrochloride (byoo-PROH-pee-on high-droh-KLOR-ighd)

Wellbutrin, Wellbutrin SR, Wellbutrin XL, Zyban

Drug Class: Antidepressant, aid to smoking cessation

Drug Actions

Relieves depression; smoking deterrent.

Use

- Depression
- Aid to smoking cessation
- Attention deficit hyperactivity disorder

Side Effects

Cardiovascular: arrhythmias, hypertension, hypotension, palpitations, tachycardia.
Gastrointestinal: dry mouth, taste disturbance, increased appetite, constipation, dyspepsia, nausea, vomiting, anorexia.
Nervous System: fever, headache, movement disorders, seizures, agitation, anxiety, confusion, delusions, euphoria, hostility, impaired sleep quality, insomnia, sedation, sensory disturbance, syncope, tremor.
Urinary: impotence, menstrual complaints, urinary frequency.
Skin: itching, rash, cutaneous temperature disturbance, sweating.
Other: chills, decreased libido, auditory disturbance, blurred vision, hyperglycemia, weight gain or loss, arthritis.

Onset, Peak, and Duration

Route	Onset	Peak	Duration
Oral	1–3 wk	2 hr	Unknown
Wellbutrin SR	Unknown	3 hr	Unknown
Wellbutrin XL	Unknown	5 hr	Unknown

Massage Considerations

- There are no cautions or contraindications to massage for clients related to this drug.
- Side effects of sedation and hypotension require care in getting the client on and off the table. Using a slightly more stimulating massage throughout the session may help to prevent problems related to these side effects. Using more rapid effleurage, pétrissage, and tapotement are usually effective.

- Constipation may be helped by abdominal massage.
- Urinary frequency may require the client to go to the bathroom during the massage. Provide privacy and quick access to the bathroom and avoid using flowing fountains and water music that may stimulate the need to urinate.
- Itching may be a local contraindication to massage if the massage aggravates the effect. If severe, the physician should be contacted and massage withheld.
- Rash is also a local contraindication to massage and if severe, the physician should be contacted and massage withheld.

---

buspirone hydrochloride (byoo-SPEER-ohn high-droh-KLOR-ighd)

BuSpar

Drug Class: Anxiolytic

Drug Actions

May inhibit neuronal firing and reduce serotonin turnover in cortical, amygdaloid, and septo-hippocampal tissue. Relieves anxiety.

Use

- Anxiety disorders
- Short-term relief of anxiety

Side Effects

Gastrointestinal: dry mouth, nausea, diarrhea.
Nervous System: dizziness, drowsiness, nervousness, excitement, insomnia, headache, fatigue.

Onset, Peak, and Duration

Route	Onset	Peak	Duration
Oral	Unknown	40–90 min	Unknown

 Massage Considerations

- There are no cautions or contraindications to massage for the client taking this medication
- Side effects of dizziness and drowsiness may be increased by massage. Using stimulating strokes at the end of the massage such as rapid effleurage and tapotement may help. Care should be taken in getting the client on and off the table.
- All strokes are appropriate for this client.

---

busulfan (byoo-SUL-fan)

Busulfex, Myleran

Drug Class: Antineoplastic

Drug Actions

Kills selected type of cancer cell

Use

- Palliative treatment of chronic myelocytic (granulocytic) leukemia (CML)
- Before cell transplantation for chronic myelocytic leukemia
- Myelofibrosis

Side Effects

Cardiovascular: edema, chest pain, tachycardia, hypertension, hypotension, blood clot, vasodilation, heart rhythm abnormalities, cardiomegaly, ECG abnormalities, heart failure, pericardial effusion.
Gastrointestinal: cracking of skin around lips, nausea, ulcerations of mouth and tongue, vomiting, lack of appetite, diarrhea, abdominal pain and enlargement, painful digestion, constipation, dry mouth, rectal disorder, pancreatitis.
Nervous System: fever, headache, muscle weakness, pain, insomnia, anxiety, dizziness, depression, delirium, agitation, encephalopathy, confusion, hallucination, lethargy, sleepiness, seizures.
Urinary: painful urination, decreased urination, hematuria, hemorrhagic cystitis.
Skin: rash, itching, hair loss, exfoliative dermatitis, acne, skin discoloration, hyperpigmentation, absence of sweating.
Other: inflammation at injection site, Addison-like wasting syndrome, enlargement of breast tissue in men, (oral); chills, allergic reaction, graft versus host disease, infection, hiccup, rhinitis, nose bleed, pharyngitis, sinusitis, ear disorder, cataracts, blood disorders, anemia, jaundice, hepatic necrosis, hepatomegaly, hypomagnesemia, hyperglycemia, hypokalemia, hypocalcemia, hypervolemia, weight gain, hypophosphatemia, hyponatremia, back pain, myalgia, arthralgia, lung disorder, cough, shortness of breath, irreversible pulmonary fibrosis, alveolar hemorrhage, asthma, atelectasis, pleural effusion, hypoxia, hemoptysis.

Onset, Peak, and Duration

Route	Onset	Peak	Duration
Oral	1–2 wk	Unknown	Unknown
I.V.	Unknown	Unknown	Unknown

Massage Considerations

- This drug is used for clients with cancer and is toxic to cells. Consultation with a physician is important to coordinate care, and obtain contraindications related to the timing of massage and administration of the drug. Circulatory massage may tax the kidneys and liver as this drug is metabolized and excreted; this effect should be minimized by giving massage before administration of the drug and by minimizing use of strokes that move blood and lymph such as effleurage. Deep tissue massage should be used with great caution, again because of the toxicity to cells.
- Side effects of hypotension, dizziness, and lethargy/sleepiness require extra care in getting the client on and off the table. Because effleurage should be limited and tapotement may not be appropriate, simply stay with the client as he or she sits up until certain that they are steady.
- Constipation may be helped by abdominal massage.
- Hair loss may contraindicate scalp massage as this may increase rate of loss
- Rash and itching are local contraindications and, if severe, may contraindicate massage altogether.
- Massage strokes that are best for this client will be gentle rocking, gentle compression, pétrissage, and gentle friction. Myofascial techniques may be effective as well.

butorphanol tartrate (byoo-TOR-fah-nohl TAR-trayt)

Stadol, Stadol NS

Drug Class: Opioid agonist-antagonist; opioid partial agonist, adjunct to anesthesia

Drug Actions

Binds with opiate receptors in CNS, altering both perception of and emotional response to pain through unknown mechanism.

Uses

- Moderate to severe pain
- Labor for pregnant women at full term and in early labor
- Preoperative anesthesia or preanesthesia
- Adjunct to balanced anesthesia

Side Effects

Cardiovascular: palpitations, fluctuation in blood pressure.
Gastrointestinal: nausea, vomiting, constipation, dry mouth.
Nervous System: sedation, headache, vertigo, floating sensation, lethargy, confusion, nervousness, unusual dreams, agitation, euphoria, hallucinations, flushing, increased intracranial pressure.
Skin: rash, hives, clamminess, excessive sweating.
Other: double vision, blurred vision, nasal congestion (with nasal spray), respiratory depression.

Onset, Peak, and Duration

Route	Onset	Peak	Duration
I.V.	2–3 min	$^1/_2$–1 hr	2–4 hr
I.M.	10–30 min	$^1/_2$–1 hr	3–4 hr
Intranasal	≤15 min	1–2 hr	4–5 hr

 Massage Considerations

- Massage may increase the absorption rate of this drug when it is given I.M. The site of injection should not be massaged for at least an hour after administration.
- This drug alters the perception of pain and therefore the perception of massage. Deep tissue massage should be used with caution if at all.
- When this drug is used for anesthesia, massage is completely contraindicated.
- Side effects of sedation, lethargy, dizziness, and fluctuations in blood pressure require care in changing position and getting the client on and off the table. Use more rapid and stimulating strokes throughout the massage such as rapid effleurage and tapotement.
- Rash or hives are a contraindication to massage and should be reported to the physician.
- The best strokes to use with this client are generally as noted above. Slightly more rapid effleurage and pétrissage, shaking and vibration, gentle tapotement, and myofascial techniques will be useful.

C

calcitonin (salmon) (kal-sih-TOH-nin)

Miacalcin, Salmonine

Drug Class: Thyroid hormone, calcium and bone metabolism regulator

Drug Actions

Prohibits bone and kidney (tubular) resorption of calcium

Use

- Paget's disease of bone (osteitis deformans)
- Hypercalcemia
- Postmenopausal osteoporosis
- Osteogenesis imperfecta

Side Effects

Cardiovascular: facial flushing.
Gastrointestinal: transient nausea, unusual taste, diarrhea, anorexia, nausea with or without vomiting.
Nervous System: headache, weakness, dizziness, paresthesia.
Urinary: transient diuresis, urinary, frequency, nocturia.
Skin: rash.
Other: hand swelling, tingling, and tenderness; hypersensitivity reactions, inflammation at injection site, anaphylaxis, nasal symptoms (irritation, redness, sores) with intranasal use, rhinitis, nosebleed, hypocalcemia, hyperglycemia, hyperthyroidism, back pain, arthralgia.

Onset, Peak, and Duration

Route	Onset	Peak	Duration
I.V.	Immediate	Unknown	12 hr
I.M. S.C.	≤15 min	≤4 hr	8–24 hr
Intranasal	Rapid	30 min	1 hr

 Massage Considerations

- When this drug is given intramuscularly or subcutaneously, the injection site should not be massaged for about 4 hours because massage could speed the absorption of the drug.
- There are no cautions or contraindications related to the client taking this drug; however, client condition may require changes in how massage is done.
- The side effect of dizziness requires care in getting the client on and off the table.
- Stimulating strokes such as rapid effleurage and tapotement may be used at the end of the session.
- The side effect of urinary frequency may require the client to get up during the massage.
- Provide privacy and easy access to the bathroom. Avoid the use of water fountains or water music, which may stimulate the need to go to the bathroom.
- Rash and inflammation are local contraindications for massage; if severe, contact the physician and withhold massage.

- When paresthesia, or altered sensation, is present, deep tissue massage should be used with caution. If paresthesia is severe, no deep tissue massage should be given.
- All strokes and types of massage may be used for this client except as noted above.

---

calcitriol (1,25-dihydroxycholecalciferol) (kal-SIH-try-ohl)

Calcijex, Rocaltrol

Drug Class: Antihypocalcemic

Drug Actions

Raises calcium levels

Use

- Hypocalcemia in patients undergoing long-term dialysis
- Hypoparathyroidism and pseudohypoparathyroidism
- Hypoparathyroidism
- Management of secondary hyperparathyroidism and resulting metabolic bone disease in predialysis patients

Side Effects

Gastrointestinal: nausea, vomiting, constipation, metallic taste, dry mouth, anorexia.
Urinary: frequent urination.
Nervous System: headache, sleepiness.
Other: weakness, bone and muscle pain, conjunctivitis, photophobia, rhinorrhea.

Onset, Peak, and Duration

Route	Onset	Peak	Duration
Oral	2–6 hr	3–6 hr	3–5 days
I.V.	Immediate	Unknown	3–5 days

 Massage Considerations

- There are no cautions or contraindications for the client who is taking this drug; cautions or contraindications may exist, however, because of the client condition.
- Side effects of sleepiness require care in getting the client on and off the table.
- Stimulating strokes such as rapid effleurage and tapotement may be used at the end of the massage.
- Constipation may respond well to abdominal massage.
- Frequent urination, if a problem, may require the client to get up during the session.
- Provide privacy and quick access to the bathroom. Avoid water fountains and water music, which may stimulate the need to urinate.
- All strokes and types of massage may be used.

---

calcium acetate (KAL-see-um AS-ih-tayt)

Phos-Lo

calcium carbonate

Apo-Cal, Cal-Carb-HD, Calci-Chew, Calciday 667, Calci-Mix, Calcite 500, Calcium 600, Cal-Plus, Calsan, Caltrate, Caltrate 600, Chooz, Fem Cal, Florical, Gencalc 600,

Mallamint, Nephro-Calci, Nu-Cal, Os-Cal, Os-Cal 500, Os-Cal Chewable, Oysco, Oysco 500 Chewable, Oyst-Cal 500, Oystercal 500, Oyster Shell Calcium-500, Rolaids Calcium Rich, Super Calcium 1200, Titralac, Tums, Tums 500, Tums E-X

calcium chloride

Calciject

calcium citrate

Citrical, Citrical Liquitabs

calcium glubionate

Calcium-Sandoz, Neo-Calglucon

calcium gluconate

calcium lactate

calcium phosphate, dibasic

calcium phosphate, tribasic

Posture

Drug Class: Calcium supplement

Drug Actions

Replaces and maintains calcium levels

Use

- Hypocalcemic emergency
- Hypocalcemic tetany
- Adjunct in cardiac arrest
- Adjunct in magnesium intoxication
- During exchange transfusions
- Hyperphosphatemia in end-stage renal failure
- Dietary supplement

Side Effects

Cardiovascular: mild decrease in blood pressure; vasodilation, bradycardia, arrhythmias, and cardiac arrest with rapid intravenous injection.
Gastrointestinal: irritation, hemorrhage, constipation with oral use; chalky taste with intravenous use; hemorrhage, nausea, vomiting, thirst, abdominal pain with oral calcium chloride.
Nervous System: pain, tingling sensations, sense of oppression or heat waves with intravenous use; syncope with rapid intravenous injection.
Urinary: hypercalcemia, frequent urination, renal calculi.
Skin: local reactions including burning, necrosis, tissue sloughing, cellulitis, soft tissue calcification with intramuscular use.
Other: irritation (with subcutaneous injection); vein irritation with intravenous use.

Onset, Peak, and Duration

Route	Onset	Peak	Duration
Oral	Unknown	Unknown	Unknown
I.V.	Immediate	Immediate	$^1/_2$–2 hr

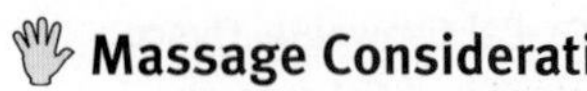

Massage Considerations

- When this drug is used in any of the serious conditions noted above, massage is absolutely contraindicated. When the drug is taken orally as a supplement, there are no cautions or contraindications for massage.
- Side effects of decrease in blood pressure require care in getting the client off the table, and using stimulation at the end of the massage may be helpful. Tapotement and rapid effleurage may be used for this.
- Constipation may be eased by regular abdominal massage.
- Any of the skin side effects are local contraindications and if severe may contraindicate massage completely.
- All types of massage and massage strokes may be used for the client taking this drug as a supplement.

---

calcium carbonate (KAL-see-um KAR-buh-nayt)

Alka-Mints, Amitone, Cal-Sup, Chooz, Equilet, Mallamint, Rolaids Calcium Rich, Titralac,Titralac Extra Strength, Titralac Plus, Tums, Tums E-X, Tums Extra Strength

Drug Class: Electrolyte, calcium supplement antacid

Drug Actions

Reduces total acid load in gastrointestinal tract, elevates gastric pH to reduce pepsin activity, strengthens gastric mucosal barrier, and increases esophageal sphincter tone.
Raises calcium level and relieves mild gastric discomfort.

Use

- Antacid
- Calcium supplement

Side Effects

Gastrointestinal: constipation, gastric distension, flatulence, rebound hyperacidity, nausea.

Onset, Peak, and Duration

Route	Onset	Peak	Duration
Oral:			
Fasting	≤20 min	Unknown	20–60 min
Nonfasting	≤20 min	Unknown	3 hr

Massage Considerations

- There are no cautions or contraindications to massage for the client taking this drug.
- The side effects of constipation, distention, and gas may be aided by regular abdominal massage.
- All massage types and strokes are appropriate for this client.

---

calcium polycarbophil (KAL-see-um pah-lee-KAR-boh-fil)

Equalactin, Fiberall, FiberCon, Fiber-Lax, FiberNorm, Mitrolan

Drug Class: Bulk laxative, antidiarrheal

Drug Actions

As a laxative, absorbs water and expands to increase bulk and moisture content of stool, which encourages peristalsis and bowel movement. As an antidiarrheal, absorbs free fecal water, thereby producing formed stools. Relieves constipation; relieves diarrhea caused by irritable bowel syndrome.

Use

- Constipation
- Diarrhea related to irritable bowel syndrome
- Acute nonspecific diarrhea

Side Effects

Gastrointestinal: abdominal fullness, increased gas, intestinal obstruction.
Other: laxative dependence with long-term or excessive use.

Onset, Peak, and Duration

Route	Onset	Peak	Duration
Oral	12–24 hr	≤3 days	Varies

Massage Considerations

- There are no cautions or contraindications to massage related to taking this drug.
- Side effects of fullness and gas may be aided by regular abdominal massage. No massage should be given with active diarrhea.
- All strokes and types of massage are appropriate.

---

calfactant (kal-FAK-tant)

Infasurf

Drug Class: Surfactant respiratory distress syndrome (RDS) agent

Drug Actions

Nonpyrogenic lung surfactant that modifies alveolar surface tension, thereby stabilizing the alveoli. Prevents RDS in premature infants or neonates with specific characteristics.

Use

- Confirmed RDS in neonates younger than 72 hours old
- Prevention of RDS in premature infants younger than 29 weeks' gestational age at high risk for RDS

Side Effects

Cardiovascular: bradycardia.
Other: airway obstruction, apnea, reflux of drug into endotracheal tube, dislodgment of endotracheal tube, hypoventilation, cyanosis.

Onset, Peak, and Duration

Route	Onset	Peak	Duration
Intratracheal	24–48 hr	Unknown	Unknown

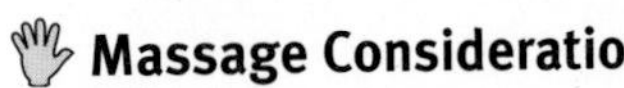

Massage Considerations

- Cautions and contraindications to massage do exist for the client taking this drug related to the client condition.
- Massage should only be done with great caution and by those trained in neonatal massage and with the direction of a physician.

---

candesartan cilexetil (kan-dih-SAR-ten se-LEKS-ih-til)

Atacand

Drug Class: Antihypertensive

Drug Actions

Dilates blood vessels and decreases blood pressure

Use

- Hypertension (alone or with other antihypertensives)

Side Effects

Cardiovascular: chest pain, peripheral edema.
Gastrointestinal: abdominal pain, diarrhea, nausea, vomiting.
Nervous System: dizziness, fatigue, headache.
Urinary: albuminuria.
Other: arthralgia, back pain, cough, bronchitis, upper respiratory tract infection, pharyngitis, rhinitis, sinusitis.

Onset, Peak, and Duration

Route	Onset	Peak	Duration
Oral	Unknown	3–4 hr	24 hr

Massage Considerations

- There are no cautions and contraindications to massage related to the client taking this drug; there may be cautions and contraindications related to the client condition.
- The action of the drug in lowering blood pressure, in conjunction with massage, may increase the incidence of the side effect of dizziness or low blood pressure or both. Care should be taken in getting the client on and off the table. Rapid effleurage and tapotement and even friction on the lower legs may help prevent this when given at the end of the massage.
- All strokes are appropriate for this client depending on his or her condition.

---

capecitabine (kape-SITE-a-been)

Xeloda

Drug Class: Antineoplastic

Drug Actions

Inhibits cell growth of selected cancer

Use

- Metastatic breast cancer
- First-line therapy for patients with metastatic colorectal cancer

Side Effects

Cardiovascular: edema.
Gastrointestinal: diarrhea, nausea, vomiting, stomatitis, abdominal pain, constipation, anorexia, intestinal obstruction, dyspepsia.
Nervous System: fever, dizziness, fatigue, headache, insomnia, paresthesia, peripheral neuropathy.
Skin: hand-and-foot syndrome, dermatitis, nail disorder, hair loss.
Other: dehydration, neutropenia, thrombocytopenia, leukopenia, anemia, lymphopenia. Hyperbilirubinemia, myalgia, limb pain, back pain, eye irritation.

Onset, Peak, and Duration

Route	Onset	Peak	Duration
Oral	Unknown	1 ½–2 hr	Unknown

 Massage Considerations

- This drug kills cells and therefore deep tissue massage is contraindicated for this client while taking this drug.
- Further cautions and contraindications may be present related to the client condition.
- Close communication with the physician is essential to coordinate care.
- Because this drug peaks in about 2 hours, massage should not be given for at least 2 hours after receiving this drug. However, because the duration of action is unknown, the timing of massage should be discussed with the physician and more than likely should be withheld for a longer period after the drug is given. The drug is often given daily for 2 weeks, with a week off. Massage may be given during the off week.
- Side effects of dizziness require care in getting the client on and off the table.
- Care should be taken with pressure in areas of neuropathy and altered sensation; if these conditions are severe, they may contraindicate massage completely.
- Gentle abdominal massage may help alleviate constipation.
- Hair loss may contraindicate scalp massage if the client is concerned or upset by hair coming out during massage or if the scalp is too sensitive.
- The type of massage strokes best used with this client are systemic reflex strokes for relaxation such as rocking, gentle shaking, gentle compression, and mechanical strokes such as gentle pétrissage. Effleurage and circulatory massage strokes should be limited because the body is already overtaxed in getting rid of this drug, and moving fluids faster into the liver and kidney is not appropriate.

---

captopril (KAP-toh-pril)

Capoten

Drug Class: ACE (angiotensin-converting enzyme) inhibitor antihypertensive, adjunct treatment of heart failure and diabetic nephropathy

Drug Actions

Reduces sodium and water retention, lowers blood pressure, and helps improve renal function adversely affected by diabetes.

Use

- Hypertension
- Heart failure
- Prevention of diabetic nephropathy
- Left ventricular dysfunction after heart attack

Side Effects

Cardiovascular: tachycardia, hypotension, angina pectoris, heart failure, pericarditis.
Gastrointestinal: anorexia, painful digestion.
Nervous System: fever, dizziness, fainting.
Urinary: proteinuria, nephrotic syndrome, membranous glomerulopathy, renal impairment (in patients with renal disease or those receiving high dosages), urinary frequency.
Skin: urticarial rash, maculopapular rash, itching.
Other: angioedema of face and limbs, leukopenia, agranulocytosis, pancytopenia, thrombocytopenia, hyperkalemia; dry, persistent, tickling, nonproductive cough.

Onset, Peak, and Duration

Route	Onset	Peak	Duration
Oral	15–60 min	30–90 min	6–12 hr

Massage Considerations

- There are no cautions or contraindications to massage for the client related to taking this drug. Cautions may exist related to the client condition.
- The action of this drug in lowering blood pressure may be increased with massage, and the side effects of hypotension and dizziness are more likely to occur. Use effleurage and tapotement at the end of the massage and take care in getting the client off the table. If this effect is severe, give a slightly more stimulating massage throughout by increasing the speed of the strokes.
- The side effect of urinary frequency may require the client to get up during the massage.
- Provide privacy and quick access to the bathroom. Avoid use of water fountains and water music, which may stimulate the need to urinate.
- The presence of rash or itching is a local contraindication to massage, if severe, massage may be completely contraindicated.

carbamazepine (kar-buh-MEH-zuh-peen)

Apo-Carbamazepine, Atretol, Carbatrol, Epitol, Novo-Carbamaz, Tegretol, Tegretol CR, Tegretol-XR, Teril

Drug Class: Anticonvulsant, analgesic

Drug Actions

May stabilize neuronal membranes and limit seizure activity by increasing efflux or decreasing influx of sodium ions across cell membranes in the motor cortex during generation of nerve impulses.

Use

- Generalized tonic-clonic and complex partial seizures, mixed seizure patterns
- Trigeminal neuralgia
- Bipolar affective disorder

- Intermittent explosive disorder
- Restless legs syndrome
- Chorea

Side Effects

Cardiovascular: heart failure, hypertension, hypotension, aggravation of coronary artery disease.
Gastrointestinal: nausea, vomiting, abdominal pain, diarrhea, anorexia, stomatitis, glossitis.
Nervous System: fever, dizziness, drowsiness, fatigue, ataxia, worsening of seizures (usually in patients with mixed seizure disorders, including atypical absence seizures).
Urinary: urinary frequency, urine retention, impotence, albuminuria, glycosuria.
Skin: excessive sweating, rash, hives, erythema multiforme, Stevens-Johnson syndrome.
Other: chills, water intoxication, aplastic anemia, agranulocytosis, eosinophilia, leukocytosis, thrombocytopenia, hepatitis, pulmonary hypersensitivity, conjunctivitis, dry mouth and pharynx, blurred vision, double vision, nystagmus.

Onset, Peak, and Duration

Route	Onset	Peak	Duration
Oral:			
Suspension	1 hr–days	1 ½ hr	Unknown
Tablets	1 hr–days	4–12 hr	Unknown

 Massage Considerations

- There are no cautions or contraindications to massage because a client is taking this medication. There may be cautions or contraindications related to the client condition. In rare instances, strokes that stimulate the nervous system such as tapotement or vibration may initiate seizure activity if the client is not well controlled. In these cases, massage would be contraindicated.
- The drug slows the reactivity of nerve impulses. This may cause a slowing of reflexes, and local reflex strokes such as stretching and compression may take longer to react and have the desired effect. Systemic reflex strokes such as effleurage and rocking may have increased effect, quickly leading to deep relaxation and increased chances of side effects such as dizziness and drowsiness.
- Side effects of dizziness, drowsiness, and hypotension require care in getting the client off the table. Stimulating strokes at the end of the session such as rapid effleurage may be used. If side effects are severe, using a more stimulating massage throughout the session may be needed, using slightly more rapid effleurage, friction, and pétrissage.
- Urinary frequency may require the client to go to the bathroom during the session.
- Provide privacy and quick access to the bathroom. Avoid the use of water fountains and water music, which may stimulate the need to urinate.
- Any rash or hives are a local contraindication to massage and should be reported to the physician. If severe, massage may need to be withheld.
- The best massage approach for this client would be using the mechanical strokes of effleurage, pétrissage, and friction and the systemic reflex strokes of effleurage applied in a more stimulating and rapid manner. Tapotement and vibration may be used if tolerated, but should be limited.

---

carbidopa and levodopa (kar-bih-DOH-puh and LEE-vuh-doh-puh)

Sinemet, Sinemet CR

Drug Class: Antiparkinsonian

Drug Actions

Unknown for levodopa. May be decarboxylated to dopamine, countering depletion of striatal dopamine in extrapyramidal centers. Carbidopa inhibits peripheral decarboxylation of levodopa without affecting levodopa's metabolism within the central nervous system. Therefore, more levodopa is available to be decarboxylated to dopamine in the brain. Improves voluntary movement.

Use

- Idiopathic Parkinson's disease
- Postencephalitic parkinsonism
- Symptomatic parkinsonism resulting from carbon monoxide or manganese intoxication

Side Effects

Cardiovascular: orthostatic hypotension, cardiac irregularities, flushing, hypertension.
Gastrointestinal: dry mouth, bitter taste, nausea, vomiting, anorexia, and weight loss at start of therapy; constipation; gas; diarrhea; epigastric pain.
Nervous System: abnormal and involuntary movements; involuntary grimacing, head movements, myoclonic body jerks, lack of muscle coordination, tremors, muscle twitching; bradykinetic episodes; psychiatric disturbances, memory loss, nervousness, anxiety, disturbing dreams, euphoria, malaise, fatigue, severe depression, suicidal tendencies, dementia, delirium, hallucinations.
Urinary: urinary frequency, urine retention, urinary incontinence, darkened urine, abnormal and painful erection of the penis.
Skin: dark perspiration, phlebitis.
Other: excessive and inappropriate sexual behavior, hemolytic anemia, spasms or twitching of the eyelid, blurred vision, double vision, pupil dilation or constriction, widening of eyelid fissures, activation of latent Horner syndrome, oculogyric crises (uncontrolled rapid eye movements), nasal discharge, excessive salivation, hepatotoxicity, hyperventilation, hiccups.

Onset, Peak, and Duration

Route	Onset	Peak	Duration
Oral:			
Regular-release	Unknown	40 min	Unknown
Extended-release	Unknown	2 ½ hr	Unknown

 Massage Considerations

- There are no cautions or contraindications related to the client taking this drug. The client condition may require changes and cautions in how massage is applied.
- Tapotement and vibration may exacerbate the nervous system effects of this drug and this disease and should be used with caution until the client's response to them has been established. Likewise, deep tissue massage should be used with caution because of the altered neuromuscular conditions.
- The drug increases dopamine or its effects, or both. Massage has been shown to slightly increase dopamine.
- Massage may help this drug to be more effective in improving voluntary movement and coordination.
- Coordinate with the physician; regular massage may allow for a decrease in the dose of medication.
- Side effects of orthostatic hypotension require care in moving the client.
- Stimulate the client gently at the end of the session with rapid effleurage and friction.
- Constipation and gas may be aided by regular abdominal massage.

- Urinary frequency may require the client to get up in the middle of the session. Provide privacy and quick access to the bathroom. Avoid water fountains and water music, which may stimulate the need to urinate.
- The best massage strokes and techniques to use are the mechanical strokes of effleurage, pétrissage, and friction. The reflex strokes, both local and systemic, may not be as effective. Myofascial techniques may be helpful for areas of tightness and gluteation.

---

carbidopa, levodopa, and entacapone (kar-bih-DOH-puh, LEE-vuh-doh-puh, and en-TAH-kah-pohn)

Stalevo

Drug Class: Antiparkinsonian

Drug Actions

Increases levodopa in the brain, which is converted to dopamine. Decreases symptoms of Parkinson's disease.

Use

- Idiopathic parkinsonism

Side Effects

Cardiovascular: hypotension, chest pain.
Gastrointestinal: nausea, diarrhea, abdominal pain, constipation, vomiting, dry mouth, painful digestion, gas, gastritis, gastrointestinal disorder, taste.
Nervous System: hallucinations, agitation, anxiety, asthenia, dizziness, abnormal movement, fatigue, hyperkinesia, hypokinesia, neuroleptic malignant syndrome, sleepiness, syncope.
Urinary: urine discoloration, nephrotoxicity.
Skin: sweating.
Other: bacterial infection, back pain, shortness of breath, anemia, blood abnormalities.

Onset, Peak, and Duration

Route	Onset	Peak	Duration
Oral	<1 hr	1–1 ½ hr	Unknown

Massage Considerations

- There are no contraindications to massage for the client taking this drug. There may be contraindications related to the client's condition. Tapotement and vibration may exacerbate the nervous system effects of both the drug and the disease and should be used with caution until the client's reaction to them is established. Deep tissue massage should be used with great caution because of the neuromuscular problems.
- The drug increases the amount and the effects of dopamine. Because massage has been shown to increase dopamine, it may increase the effectiveness of the drug. Coordinate with the physician to see if regular massage may decrease the dosage of medication needed.
- Side effects of dizziness, sleepiness, and hypotension require care in getting the client on and off the table. Use slightly more stimulating strokes such as rapid effleurage and friction at the end of the session. If side effects are severe, use a more stimulating and rapid application of strokes throughout the session.
- Constipation and gas may be helped by regular abdominal massage.
- The most effective strokes to use will be the mechanical strokes of effleurage, pétrissage, and friction. The reflex strokes, both local and systemic, may be less effective because of the problems with the neuromuscular connections related to this disease. Myofascial techniques may be helpful for areas of tightness and gluteation.

carboplatin (KAR-boh-plat-in)

Paraplatin, Paraplatin-AQ

Drug Class: Antineoplastic

Drug Actions

Impairs ovarian cancer cell replication

Use

- Palliative treatment of ovarian cancer
- Initial treatment of advanced ovarian cancer with cyclophosphamide

Side Effects

Cardiovascular: heart failure, embolism.
Gastrointestinal: constipation, diarrhea, nausea, vomiting.
Nervous System: dizziness, confusion, peripheral neuropathy, ototoxicity, central neurotoxicity, cerebrovascular accident.
Skin: hair loss.
Other: hypersensitivity reactions, abnormal blood profiles, anemia, bone marrow suppression, hepatotoxicity.

Onset, Peak, and Duration

Route	Onset	Peak	Duration
I.V.	Unknown	Unknown	Unknown

Massage Considerations

- This drug affects the cell replication in the body. Deep tissue massage should be used with great caution and in most cases would be contraindicated.
- Because the drug is toxic to cells, circulatory massage with effleurage that would move the fluids of the body more quickly through the already taxed liver and kidneys should be limited.
- Although onset, peak, and duration of action are unknown, about 70% of the drug is excreted within 24 hours. No massage should be given for at least 24 hours after the drug is administered. Timing of the massage should be coordinated with the physician.
- Because the drug is often given only once a month, massage would best be applied on the weeks that the drug is not being given.
- Side effects of dizziness require care in getting the client off the table. Use stimulating strokes of tapotement and friction at the end of the session to avoid this problem.
- Constipation may be helped by gentle abdominal massage but only if approved by the physician.
- Because the drug is used for ovarian cancer, abdominal surgery, or the presence of tumor may contraindicate abdominal massge.
- Hair loss would contraindicate scalp massage if the client is upset by the hair coming out during massage or if the scalp is tender.
- The best strokes for this client are the systemic reflex stroke of rocking and mechanical strokes of pétrissage and gentle friction. Local reflex strokes of stretching and gentle compression may also be effective. Myofascial techniques may be helpful for tightness and gluteation.

carisoprodol (kar-ih-soh-PROH-dol)

Soma

Drug Class: Skeletal muscle relaxant

Drug Actions

Appears to modify central perception of pain without modifying pain reflexes. Blocks interneuronal activity in descending reticular activating system and in spinal cord. Relieves musculoskeletal pain.

Use

- Adjunct in acute, painful musculoskeletal conditions

Side Effects

Cardiovascular: orthostatic hypotension, tachycardia, facial flushing.
Gastrointestinal: nausea, vomiting, increased bowel activity, epigastric distress.
Nervous System: fever, drowsiness, dizziness, abnormal movement, tremor, agitation, irritability, headache, depressive reactions, insomnia.
Skin: rash, itching.
Other: angioedema, anaphylaxis, eosinophilia, asthmatic episodes, hiccups.

Onset, Peak, and Duration

Route	Onset	Peak	Duration
Oral	≤30 min	≤4 hr	4–6 hr

 Massage Considerations

- Because this drug decreases the perception of pain, deep tissue massage should be used with great caution and may be contraindicated.
- This drug also affects the relay of nerve impulses to and from the spinal cord. Local reflex strokes such as stretching and compression may be ineffective.
- Because of the suppressive effect on the nervous system, systemic reflex strokes may have an increased effectiveness, and deep relaxation, dizziness, and drowsiness may be increased.
- Side effects of drowsiness, dizziness, and hypotension require care in moving the client.
- Stimulating strokes throughout the massage with more rapid effleurage and pétrissage and friction will help relax the client without having the side effects increased.
- Rash or itching is a local contraindication to massage and if severe may contraindicate massage completely.
- The best strokes to use are the mechanical strokes as noted above. Stimulating effleurage, pétrissage, and friction will relax muscles and the body while keeping the client alert.

carmustine (BCNU) (kar-MUHS-teen)

BiCNU, Gliadel

Drug Class: Antineoplastic

Drug Actions

Kills selected cancer cells

Use

- Hodgkin's disease
- Non-Hodgkin's lymphoma
- Multiple myeloma
- Recurrent glioblastoma and metastatic brain tumors
- Newly diagnosed high-grade malignant glioma
- Brain, breast, gastrointestinal tract, lung, and hepatic cancer
- Malignant melanomas

Side Effects

Cardiovascular: facial flushing.
Gastrointestinal: nausea beginning in 2 to 6 hours (can be severe), vomiting, anorexia, difficulty swallowing, esophagitis, diarrhea.
Nervous System: abnormal movement, drowsiness, brain edema, seizures.
Urinary: nephrotoxicity, renal impairment.
Skin: hyperpigmentation (if drug contacts skin).
Other: intense pain (at infusion site from venous spasm), cumulative bone marrow suppression (delayed 4 to 6 weeks, lasting 1 to 2 weeks), leukopenia, thrombocytopenia, acute leukemia or bone marrow dysplasia (may occur after long-term use), hepatotoxicity, possible hyperuricemia (in patients with lymphoma when rapid cell lysis occurs), pulmonary fibrosis, ocular toxicities.

Onset, Peak, and Duration

Route	Onset	Peak	Duration
I.V. wafer	Unknown	Unknown	Unknown

Massage Considerations

- This drug kills cells and is extremely potent. Deep tissue massage is contraindicated.
- Circulatory massage with effleurage that moves fluid more quickly through the body is also contraindicated because it may overwhelm the already taxed liver and kidney as they try to clear the drug from the body.
- Although the onset, peak, and duration of drug action is unknown, about 70% of the drug is excreted in urine in about 4 days. Although timing of the application of the massage should be discussed with the physician, no massage should be given for 4 to 5 days.
- Because the drug is given usually once every 6 weeks in most cases, massage may best be applied during the weeks that the drug is not given.
- Side effects of drowsiness require care in moving the client. Stimulate the client with shaking strokes and gentle tapotement.
- The best strokes to use with this client are the mechanical strokes of pétrissage and gentle friction and systemic reflex strokes of rocking. Local reflex strokes of stretching, gentle compression, and gentle friction may also be effective. Myofascial techniques may also be used.

---

carvedilol (kar-VAY-deh-lol)

Coreg

Drug Class: Alpha$_1$ and beta-blocker antihypertensive, adjunct treatment for heart failure

Drug Actions

Causes significant reductions in systemic blood pressure, pulmonary arterial pressure, pulmonary capillary wedge pressure, and heart rate.

Use

- Hypertension
- Mild to severe heart failure
- Left ventricular dysfunction following heart attack

Side Effects

Cardiovascular: hypotension, postural hypertension, edema, bradycardia, angina pectoris, peripheral edema, hypovolemia, fluid overload, atrioventricular block, hypertension, palpitation, peripheral vascular disorder, chest pain.
Gastrointestinal: diarrhea, vomiting, nausea, black, tarry feces, periodontitis, abdominal pain, painful digestion.
Nervous System: asthenia, fatigue, pain, dizziness, headache, malaise, fever, hypersthesia, paresthesia, syncope, sleepiness, cerebrovascular accident, depression, insomnia.
Urinary: impotence, abnormal renal function, albuminuria, hematuria, urinary tract infection.
Other: hypersensitivity reactions, infection, flulike syndrome, viral infection, injury, hyperglycemia, weight gain, weight loss, hypercholesterolemia, hyperuricemia, hypoglycemia, hyponatremia, glycosuria, hypervolemia, diabetes mellitus, hyperkalemia, gout, hypertriglyceridemia, arthralgia, back pain, muscle cramps, hypotonia, arthritis, purpura, anemia, thrombocytopenia, sinusitis, abnormal vision, blurred vision, pharyngitis, rhinitis, bronchitis, upper respiratory tract infection, cough, rales, shortness of breath, lung edema.

Onset, Peak, and Duration

Route	Onset	Peak	Duration
Oral	Unknown	1–2 hr	7–10 hr

 Massage Considerations

- There are no cautions or contraindications related to the client taking this medication; however, the client condition may require cautions and contraindications.
- This drug acts on specific receptors of the sympathetic nervous system but may have some blocking effects to the sympathetic nervous system in general. This may cause the relaxing effects of massage to be increased in some clients.
- The side effects of this may be dizziness, hypotension, and sleepiness. Giving stimulating strokes such as tapotement and rapid effleurage at the end of the session may help. If side effects are severe, use more rapid and stimulating strokes throughout the massage. Take care getting the client on and off the table.
- Hyperesthesia (increased sensitivity to any touch) may contraindicate massage if it is painful or uncomfortable for the client. Paresthesia will contraindicate deep tissue massage.
- All strokes and techniques may be used for the client taking this medication depending on the client overall condition.

---

caspofungin acetate (kas-poh-FUN-jin AS-ih-tayt)

Cancidas

Drug Class: Antifungal antibiotic

Drug Actions

Prevents fungi formation

Use

- Invasive aspergillosis

Side Effects

Cardiovascular: tachycardia, thrombophlebitis.
Gastrointestinal: nausea, vomiting, diarrhea, abdominal pain, anorexia.
Nervous System: headache, paresthesia, fever, chills.
Urinary: proteinuria, hematuria.
Skin: histamine-mediated symptoms (including rash, facial swelling, phlebitis, itching, sensation of warmth, erythema, and sweating).
Other: pain, myalgia, eosinophilia, anemia, tachypnea.

Onset, Peak, and Duration

Route	Onset	Peak	Duration
I.V.	Unknown	Unknown	Unknown

Massage Considerations

- Severe, active infection is a contraindication to massage. If massage is being given toward the end of treatment, cautions and contraindications will be dictated by the client condition.
- The side effect of paresthesia would be a caution for the use of deep tissue massage and if severe would contraindicate it.
- Any histamine-related side effect would contraindicate massage completely.

---

cefaclor (SEH-fuh-klor)

Ceclor, Ceclor CD

Drug Class: Antibiotic

Drug Actions

Hinders or kills susceptible bacteria

Use

- Respiratory, urinary tract, skin, and soft tissue infections
- Otitis media
- Acute uncomplicated urinary tract infection

Side Effects

Gastrointestinal: nausea, vomiting, diarrhea, anorexia, dyspepsia, abdominal cramps, pseudomembranous colitis, oral candidiasis.
Nervous System: dizziness, headache, sleepiness, malaise, fever.
Urinary: red and white cells in urine, vaginal candidiasis, vaginitis.
Skin: maculopapular rash, dermatitis.
Other: hypersensitivity reactions (serum sickness, anaphylaxis), transient leukopenia, lymphocytosis, anemia, eosinophilia, thrombocytopenia.

Onset, Peak, and Duration

Route	Onset	Peak	Duration
Oral	Unknown	30–60 min	Unknown

Massage Considerations

- There are no cautions or contraindications to massage for the client related to taking this drug. The client condition, with severe, active infection, may contraindicate massage.

- Rash or skin outbreaks are a local contraindication and should be reported immediately to the physician. If severe, massage may be contraindicated.
- Side effects of dizziness and sleepiness require care in moving the client.
- Stimulating effleurage or tapotement at the end of the massage should help.
- Except as noted above, all strokes and types of massage may be given depending on the client condition.

---

cefadroxil monohydrate (seh-fuh-DROKS-il MON-oh-HIGH-drayt)

Duricef

Drug Class: Antibiotic

Drug Actions

Hinders or kills susceptible bacteria

Use

- Urinary tract infections

Side Effects

Gastrointestinal: pseudomembranous colitis, nausea, anorexia, vomiting, diarrhea, glossitis, painful digestion, abdominal cramps, anal itching, spasms of anal sphincter, oral candidiasis.
Nervous System: dizziness, headache, malaise, paresthesia, seizures.
Urinary: genital itching, candidiasis.
Skin: rash.
Other: hypersensitivity reactions (serum sickness, anaphylaxis), abnormal blood profiles, shortness of breath.

Onset, Peak, and Duration

Route	Onset	Peak	Duration
Oral	Unknown	1–2 hr	Unknown

Massage Considerations

- There are no cautions or contraindications to massage for the client related to taking this medication.
- The side effect of dizziness may require care in getting the client on and off the table.
- Use stimulating strokes such as tapotement or rapid effleurage at the end of the session.
- The side effect of paresthesia requires caution when using deep tissue massage, and if deep tissue massage is severe its use locally may be contraindicated.
- Rash is a local contraindication to massage and should be reported to the physician immediately. If severe, massage should be withheld.
- All strokes and techniques may be used with this client except as noted above.

---

cefazolin sodium (sef-EH-zoh-lin SOH-dee-um)

Ancef, Zolicef

Drug Class: Antibiotic

Drug Actions

Hinders or kills susceptible bacteria

Use

- Serious infections of respiratory, biliary, and genitourinary tracts
- Skin, soft tissue, bone, and joint infections
- Septicemia
- Endocarditis
- Perioperative prophylaxis
- Perioperative prophylaxis in contaminated surgery

Side Effects

Gastrointestinal: pseudomembranous colitis, nausea, anorexia, vomiting, diarrhea, glossitis, painful digestions, abdominal cramps, anal itching, spasm of anal sphincter, oral candidiasis.
Nervous System: dizziness, headache, malaise, paresthesia.
Urinary: genital itching and candidiasis, vaginitis.
Skin: rash, hives, Stevens-Johnson syndrome.
Other: hypersensitivity reactions (serum sickness, anaphylaxis), abnormal blood profiles, shortness of breath.

Onset, Peak, and Duration

Route	Onset	Peak	Duration
I.V.	Immediate	Immediate	Unknown
I.M.	Unknown	1–2 hr	Unknown

Massage Considerations

- There are no cautions or contraindications to massage because a client is taking this medication. Severe infections and the client condition may require cautions and contraindications to massage.
- Side effects of dizziness require care in getting the client off the table, and stimulating strokes such as rapid effleurage and tapotement at the end of the session may help. Any paresthesias are a local caution for deep tissue massage and if severe may contraindicate deep tissue massage.
- Rash is a local contraindication to massage and should be reported to the physician immediately. If severe, massage should be withheld.
- All strokes and techniques for massage are appropriate for this client except as noted above.

cefdinir (SEF-dih-neer)

Omnicef

Drug Class: Antibiotic

Drug Actions

Kills susceptible bacteria

Use

- Mild to moderate infections for conditions of community-acquired pneumonia
- Uncomplicated skin and skin-structure infections
- Acute exacerbations of chronic bronchitis
- Acute bacterial otitis media
- Pharyngitis
- Tonsillitis
- Acute maxillary sinusitis

Side Effects

Gastrointestinal: abdominal pain, diarrhea, nausea, vomiting.
Nervous System: headache.
Urinary: vaginal candidiasis, vaginitis.
Skin: rash.

Onset, Peak, and Duration

Route	Onset	Peak	Duration
Oral	Unknown	2–4 hr	Unknown

 **Massage Considerations**

- There are no cautions or contraindications to massage because a client is taking this medication. However, severe infection and the client's condition may require cautions and contraindications.
- Side effects of rash are a local contraindication to massage and should be reported to the physician immediately. If severe, massage should be withheld.

---

cefditoren pivoxil (sef-da-TOR-en pa-VOX-ill)

Spectracef

Drug Class: Antibiotic

Drug Actions

Kills susceptible bacteria

Use

- Acute bacterial exacerbation of chronic bronchitis
- Pharyngitis
- Tonsillitis
- Uncomplicated skin and skin-structure infections

Side Effects

Gastrointestinal: abdominal pain, dyspepsia, diarrhea, nausea, vomiting, colitis, hepatic dysfunction (including cholestasis).
Nervous System: headache.
Urinary: vaginal candidiasis, hematuria, nephrotoxicity.
Skin: Stevens-Johnson syndrome, toxic epidermal necrolysis.
Other: hypersensitivity reactions (including serum sickness, rash, fever, anaphylaxis), anemia, hyperglycemia.

Onset, Peak, and Duration

Route	Onset	Peak	Duration
Oral	Unknown	1 $^1/_2$–3 hr	Unknown

 **Massage Considerations**

- There are no cautions or contraindications to massage because the client is taking this medication. There may be cautions or contraindications related to the client condition and the severity of the infection.
- Any side effects of skin or hypersensitivity are a contraindication to massage.

cefoperazone sodium (sef-oh-PER-ah-zohn SOH-dee-um)

Cefobid

Drug Class: Antibiotic

Drug Actions

Hinders or kills susceptible bacteria

Use

- Serious infections of respiratory tract
- Intra-abdominal, gynecologic, and skin infections
- Bacteremia
- Septicemia

Side Effects

Nervous System: headache, malaise, paresthesia, dizziness.
Gastrointestinal: pseudomembranous colitis, nausea, anorexia, vomiting, diarrhea, glossitis, painful digestion, abdominal cramps, tenesmus, anal itching, oral candidiasis.
Nervous System: headache, malaise, paresthesia, dizziness.
Urinary: genital itching and candidiasis.
Skin: rash, hives.
Other: hypersensitivity reactions (serum sickness, anaphylaxis); pain, induration, sterile abscesses, warmth, tissue sloughing at injection site; phlebitis, thrombophlebitis with intravenous injection, abnormal blood profiles, bleeding, shortness of breath.

Onset, Peak, and Duration

Route	Onset	Peak	Duration
I.V.	Immediate	Immediate	Unknown
I.M.	Unknown	1–2 hr	Unknown

Massage Considerations

- Although the drug itself does not caution or contraindicate massage, client condition, and severity of the infection may.
- Side effects of dizziness require care in getting the client on and off the table. Stimulating strokes such as rapid effleurage and tapotement at the end of the session may be helpful.
- Paresthesias are a local caution to deep tissue massage and if severe may contraindicate deep tissue massage completely.
- Any skin problems are a local contraindication to massage and should be reported to the physician immediately. If severe, massage should be withheld.

cefotaxime sodium (sef-oh-TAKS-eem SOH-dee-um)

Claforan

Drug Class: Antibiotic

Drug Actions

Hinders or kills susceptible bacteria

Use

- Perioperative prophylaxis in contaminated surgery
- Serious infections of lower respiratory and urinary tracts, central nervous system, skin, bone, and joints
- Gynecologic and intra-abdominal infections
- Bacteremia
- Septicemia
- Disseminated gonococcal infection
- Gonococcal ophthalmia
- Gonorrheal meningitis or arthritis

Side Effects

Gastrointestinal: pseudomembranous colitis, nausea, anorexia, vomiting, diarrhea, glossitis, painful digestion, abdominal cramps, tenesmus, anal itching, oral candidiasis.
Nervous System: headache, malaise, paresthesia, dizziness, elevated temperature.
Urinary: genital itching and candidiasis.
Skin: rash, hives.
Other: hypersensitivity reactions (serum sickness, anaphylaxis); pain, induration, sterile abscesses, warmth, tissue sloughing at injection site; phlebitis, thrombophlebitis with intravenous injection, abnormal blood profiles, shortness of breath.

Onset, Peak, and Duration

Route	Onset	Peak	Duration
I.V.	Immediate	Immediate	Unknown
I.M.	Unknown	30 min	Unknown

 Massage Considerations

- There are no cautions or contraindications to massage because the client in taking this drug. However, severity of the infection or the client condition may require cautions and contraindications.
- Side effects of paresthesia are a local caution to deep tissue and if severe may contraindicate its use completely.
- Dizziness requires care in getting the client on and off the table.
- Using stimulating strokes at the end of the massage, such as rapid effleurage and tapotement, may help.
- Skin reactions are a local contraindication to massage and should be reported to the physician immediately. If severe, massage should be withheld.

---

cefotetan disodium (SEF-oh-teh-tan die-SOH-dee-um)

Apatef, Cefotan

Drug Class: Antibiotic

Drug Actions

Hinders or kills susceptible bacteria

Use

- Serious urinary tract infections
- Lower respiratory tract infections
- Gynecologic, skin and skin-structure, intra-abdominal, and bone and joint infections
- Perioperative prophylaxis; used in contaminated surgery

Side Effects

Gastrointestinal: pseudomembranous colitis, nausea, anorexia, vomiting, diarrhea, glossitis, painful digestion, abdominal cramps, spasm of anal sphincter, anal itching.
Nervous System: headache, malaise, paresthesia, dizziness.
Urinary: genital itching and candidiasis, nephrotoxicity.
Skin: rash, hives.
Other: hypersensitivity reactions (serum sickness, anaphylaxis); elevated temperature; pain, induration, sterile abscesses, tissue sloughing at injection site; phlebitis, thrombophlebitis with intravenous injection, abnormal blood profiles, bleeding, shortness of breath.

Onset, Peak, and Duration

Route	Onset	Peak	Duration
I.V.	Immediate	Immediate	Unknown
I.M.	Unknown	1 1/2–2 hr	Unknown

 Massage Considerations

- Although there are no cautions or contraindication to massage because of the client taking this drug, the severity of the infection and the client condition may require altering how massage is applied and may even contraindicate it completely.
- Side effects of paresthesia are a local caution to deep tissue massage and if severe may contraindicate it completely.
- Dizziness requires care in getting the client on and off the table.
- Using stimulating strokes such as rapid effleurage and tapotement at the end of the session may help.
- Skin problems are a local contraindication to massage and should be reported to the physician immediately. If severe, massage should be withheld.

---

cefoxitin sodium (sef-OKS-ih-tin SOH-dee-um)

Mefoxin

Drug Class: Antibiotic

Drug Actions

Hinders or kills susceptible bacteria

Use

- Serious infections of respiratory and genitourinary tracts
- Skin, soft tissue, bone, and joint infections
- Bloodstream and intra-abdominal infections
- Prophylactic use in surgery

Side Effects

Cardiovascular: hypotension.
Gastrointestinal: pseudomembranous colitis, diarrhea.
Nervous System: fever.
Urinary: acute renal failure.
Skin: rash, hives.
Other: hypersensitivity reactions (serum sickness, anaphylaxis), phlebitis, thrombophlebitis with intravenous injection, abnormal blood profiles, shortness of breath.

Onset, Peak, and Duration

Route	Onset	Peak	Duration
I.V.	Immediate	Immediate	Unknown
I.M.	Rapid	20–30 min	<6 hr

 Massage Considerations

- Although there are no cautions or contraindications to massage related to the client taking this drug, client condition and severity of the infection may require cautions in the application of massage and may even contraindicate massage.
- Side effects of hypotension require care in getting the client off the table. Using stimulation at the end of the session with rapid effleurage and tapotement may help.
- Skin problems are a local contraindication to massage and should be reported to the physician immediately. If severe, massage should be withheld.

---

cefpodoxime proxetil (sef-poh-DOKS-eem PROKS-eh-til)

Vantin

Drug Class: Antibiotic

Drug Actions

Hinders or kills susceptible bacteria

Use

- Acute, community-acquired pneumonia
- Acute bacterial exacerbation of chronic bronchitis
- Uncomplicated gonorrhea in men and women
- Rectal gonococcal infections in women
- Uncomplicated skin and skin-structure infections
- Acute otitis media
- Pharyngitis or tonsillitis
- Uncomplicated urinary tract infections
- Mild to moderate acute maxillary sinusitis

Side Effects

Gastrointestinal: diarrhea, nausea, vomiting, abdominal pain.
Nervous System: headache.
Urinary: vaginal fungal infections.
Skin: rash.
Other: hypersensitivity reactions (anaphylaxis).

Onset, Peak, and Duration

Route	Onset	Peak	Duration
Oral	Unknown	2–3 hr	Unknown

 Massage Considerations

- There are no cautions or contraindications to massage because the client is taking this medication. There may be cautions or contraindications to massage related to client condition or the severity of infection.
- If rash is present, it is a local contraindication to massage and should be reported to the physician immediately. If severe, massage should be withheld.

cefprozil (SEF-pruh-zil)

Cefzil

Drug Class: Antibiotic

Drug Actions

Hinders or kills susceptible bacteria

Use

- Pharyngitis or tonsillitis
- Otitis media
- Secondary bacterial infections of acute bronchitis and acute bacterial exacerbation of chronic bronchitis
- Uncomplicated skin and skin-structure infections
- Acute sinusitis

Side Effects

Gastrointestinal: diarrhea, nausea, vomiting, abdominal pain.
Nervous System: dizziness, hyperactivity, headache, nervousness, insomnia.
Urinary: genital itching, vaginitis.
Skin: rash, hives.
Other: superinfection, hypersensitivity reactions (serum sickness, anaphylaxis), eosinophilia.

Onset, Peak, and Duration

Route	Onset	Peak	Duration
Oral	Unknown	Unknown	Unknown

 Massage Considerations

- There are no cautions or contraindications to massage because the client is taking this drug. Cautions and contraindications may exist, however, related to the client condition and severity of the infection.
- Side effects of dizziness require care in getting the client off the table. Using stimulation at the end of the massage with rapid effleurage and tapotement may help.
- Skin problems such as rash or hives are a local contraindication to massage and should be reported to the physician immediately. If severe, massage should be withheld.

ceftazidime (sef-TAZ-ih-deem)

Ceptaz, Fortaz, Tazicef, Tazidime

Drug Class: Antibiotic

Drug Actions

Hinders or kills susceptible bacteria

Use

- Serious infections of lower respiratory and urinary tracts
- Gynecologic, intra-abdominal, central nervous system, and skin infections
- Bacteremia
- Septicemia
- Uncomplicated urinary tract infection

- Complicated urinary tract infection
- Uncomplicated pneumonia or mild skin and skin-structure infection
- Bone and joint infection
- Empiric therapy in febrile patients with abnormally low neutrophils

Side Effects

Nervous System: headache, dizziness, seizures.
Gastrointestinal: pseudomembranous colitis, nausea, vomiting, diarrhea, painful digestion, abdominal cramps.
Nervous System: headache, dizziness, seizures.
Urinary: genital itching, candidiasis.
Skin: rash, hives.
Other: hypersensitivity reactions (serum sickness, anaphylaxis); elevated temperature; pain, induration, sterile abscesses, tissue sloughing at injection site; phlebitis, thrombophlebitis with intravenous injection, abnormal blood profiles, shortness of breath.

Onset, Peak, and Duration

Route	Onset	Peak	Duration
I.V.	Immediate	Immediate	Unknown
I.M.	Unknown	≤1 hr	Unknown

 Massage Considerations

- There are no cautions or contraindications to massage for the client taking this medication. However, severity of infection and the client condition may require changes in the application of massage and may even contraindicate massage completely.
- Side effects of dizziness require care in getting the client on and off the table. Using stimulating strokes such as rapid effleurage and tapotement at the end of the session may help.
- Rash and hives are local contraindications to massage and should be reported to the physician immediately. If severe, massage should be withheld.

---

ceftibuten (sef-tih-BYOO-tin)

Cedax

Drug Class: Antibiotic

Drug Actions

Hinders or kills susceptible bacteria

Use

- Acute bacterial exacerbation of chronic bronchitis
- Pharyngitis and tonsillitis

Side Effects

Gastrointestinal: nausea, vomiting, diarrhea, painful digestion, abdominal pain, loose stools, pseudomembranous colitis.
Urinary: toxic nephropathy, renal dysfunction.
Nervous System: headache, dizziness, aphasia, psychosis.
Hepatic: hepatic cholestasis.
Skin: Stevens-Johnson syndrome.
Other: allergic reaction, anaphylaxis, drug fever, hepatic cholestasis, abnormal blood profiles.

Onset, Peak, and Duration

Route	Onset	Peak	Duration
Oral	Unknown	2–4 hr	Unknown

Massage Considerations

- There are no cautions or contraindications to massage because the client is taking this drug. Client condition and severity of the infection may require cautions and even complete contraindication to massage.
- Side effects of dizziness require care in getting the client on and off the table. Use stimulating strokes such as rapid effleurage and tapotement at the end of the session to help prevent problems.

ceftizoxime sodium (sef-tih-ZOKS-eem SOH-dee-um)

Cefizox

Drug Class: Antibiotic

Drug Actions

Hinders or kills susceptible bacteria

Use

- Serious infections of lower respiratory and urinary tracts
- Gynecologic infections
- Bacteremia
- Septicemia
- Meningitis
- Intra-abdominal infections
- Bone and joint infections
- Skin infections
- Acute bacterial otitis media

Side Effects

Gastrointestinal: pseudomembranous colitis, nausea, anorexia, vomiting, diarrhea, glossitis, painful digestion, abdominal cramps, spasm of anal sphincter, anal itching.
Nervous System: fever; headache, malaise, paresthesia, dizziness.
Urinary: genital itching and candidiasis.
Skin: rash, hives.
Other: hypersensitivity reactions (serum sickness, anaphylaxis); induration, sterile abscesses, tissue sloughing at injection site; phlebitis, thrombophlebitis with intravenous injection, abnormal blood profiles, shortness of breath.

Onset, Peak, and Duration

Route	Onset	Peak	Duration
I.V.	Immediate	Immediate	Unknown
I.M.	Unknown	$^1/_2$–1 $^1/_2$ hr	Unknown

Massage Considerations

- Although no cautions or contraindications to massage exist simply because the client is taking this drug, cautions and contraindications may exist related to the client condition and severity of the infection involved.

- Side effects of paresthesia are a local caution for deep tissue massage and if severe may contraindicate deep tissue massage completely.
- Dizziness requires care in getting the client on and off the table. Using stimulating strokes such as rapid effleuage and tapotement may help. Rash or hives are local contraindications to massage and should be reported to the physician immediately. If severe, massage should be withheld.

---

ceftriaxzone sodium (sef-trigh-AKS-ohn SOH-dee-um)

Rocephin

Drug Class: Antibiotic

Drug Actions

Hinders or kills susceptible bacteria

Use

- Uncomplicated gonococcal vulvovaginitis
- Serious infections of lower respiratory and urinary tracts
- Gynecologic, bone, joint, intra-abdominal, and skin infections
- Bacteremia
- Septicemia
- Meningitis
- Preoperative prophylaxis
- Acute bacterial otitis media
- Persisting or relapsing otitis media in children
- Sexually transmitted epididymitis
- Pelvic inflammatory disease
- Anti-infectives for sexual assault victims
- Lyme disease

Side Effects

Nervous System: headache, dizziness, fever.
Gastrointestinal: pseudomembranous colitis, nausea, vomiting, diarrhea, painful digestion.
Urinary: genital itching and candidiasis.
Skin: phlebitis, rash.
Other: pain, induration, and tenderness at injection site; hypersensitivity reactions (serum sickness, anaphylaxis), abnormal blood profiles.

Onset, Peak, and Duration

Route	Onset	Peak	Duration
I.V.	Immediate	Immediate	Unknown
I.M.	Unknown	$1\,^1/_2$–4 hr	Unknown

Massage Considerations

- There are no cautions or contraindications to massage for the client related to taking this medication. There may be cautions or contraindications related to the client condition or the severity of the infection.
- Side effects of dizziness require care in getting the client on and off the table. Using stimulating strokes such as rapid effleurage and tapotement at the end of the session may help.

- Rash is a local contraindication to massage and should be reported to the physician immediately. If severe, massage should be withheld.

---

cefuroxime axetil (sef-yoor-OKS-eem AKS-eh-til)

Ceftin

cefuroxime sodium

Zinacef

Drug Class: Antibiotic

Drug Action

Hinders or kills susceptible bacteria, including many gram-positive organisms and enteric gram-negative bacilli.

Use

- Pharyngitis
- Tonsillitis
- Infections of urinary and lower respiratory tracts
- Skin and skin-structure infections
- Bone and joint infections
- Septicemia
- Meningitis
- Gonorrhea
- Perioperative prophylaxis
- Uncomplicated urinary tract infections
- Otitis media
- Acute bacterial maxillary sinusitis
- Secondary bacterial infection of acute bronchitis
- Early Lyme disease

Side Effects

Gastrointestinal: pseudomembranous colitis, nausea, anorexia, vomiting, diarrhea, glossitis, painful digestion, abdominal cramps, spasm of anal sphincter, anal itching.
Nervous System: headache, malaise, paresthesia, dizziness.
Urinary: genital itching and candidiasis.
Skin: rash, hives.
Other: hypersensitivity reactions (serum sickness, anaphylaxis); pain, induration, sterile abscesses, warmth, tissue sloughing at injection site; phlebitis, thrombophlebitis with intravenous injection, abnormal blood profiles, shortness of breath.

Onset, Peak, and Duration

Route	Onset	Peak	Duration
Oral	Unknown	2 hr	Unknown
I.V.	Unknown	Immediate	Unknown
I.M.	Unknown	15–60 min	Unknown

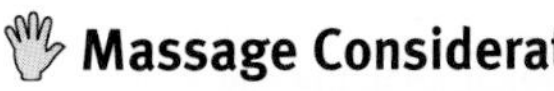

Massage Considerations

- There are no cautions or contraindications to massage related to a client taking this medication. However, the client condition or severity of the infections may require either cautions or even complete contraindications to massage.
- Side effects of paresthesia require local caution in applying deep tissue massage and if severe may contraindicate it completely. Dizziness requires care in getting the client on and off the table. Use stimulating strokes such as rapid effleurage and tapotement at the end of the session to conteract these effects.
- Rash and hives are a local contraindication to massage and should be reported to the physician immediately. If severe, massage should be withheld.

---

celecoxib (sel-eh-COKS-ib)

Celebrex

Drug Class: Anti-inflammatory

Drug Actions

Celecoxib is thought to selectively inhibit cyclooxygenase-2, resulting in decreased prostaglandin synthesis. Its anti-inflammatory effects along with its analgesic and antipyretic properties are thought to be related to a decrease in prostaglandin synthesis.

Use

- Relief of signs and symptoms of osteoarthritis
- Relief of signs and symptoms of rheumatoid arthritis
- Adjunct to familial adenomatous polyposis to reduce the number of adenomatous colorectal polyps
- Acute pain and primary dysmenorrhea

Side Effects

Cardiovascular: peripheral edema.
Gastrointestinal: abdominal pain, diarrhea, painful digestion, gas, nausea.
Respiratory: upper respiratory tract infection.
Nervous System: dizziness, headache, insomnia.
Skin: rash.
Other: accidental injury, hyperchloremia, hypophosphatemia, back pain, pharyngitis, rhinitis, sinusitis.

Onset, Peak, and Duration

Route	Onset	Peak	Duration
Oral	Unknown	3 hr	Unknown

Massage Considerations

- Because this drug reduces prostaglandins, it can decrease not only inflammation but the perception of pain. Deep tissue massage should be used with caution.
- A side effect of dizziness requires care in getting the client on and off the table. Using rapid effleurage and tapotement at the end of the session to stimulate the client may help.
- Peripheral edema, once determined by the physician to be related to the drug, may be helped by circulatory massage to the legs using long and slightly rapid effleurage moving toward the heart. Gentle lymphatic massage may also help.

- Gas may be aided by regular abdominal massage.
- Rash is a local contraindication to massage and should be reported to the physician immediately. If severe, massage should be withheld.
- All massage strokes and techniques may be used except as noted above.

cephalexin hydrochloride (sef-uh-LEK-sin high-droh-KLOR-ighd)

Keftab

cephalexin monohydrate

Apo-Cephalex, Biocef, Keflex, Novo-Lexin, Nu-Cephalex

Drug Class: Antibiotic

Drug Actions

Hinders or kills susceptible bacteria

Use

- Respiratory tract, gastrointestinal tract, skin, soft tissue, bone, and joint infections
- Otitis media

Side Effects

Gastrointestinal: pseudomembranous colitis, nausea, anorexia, vomiting, diarrhea, glossitis, painful digestion, abdominal cramps, anal itching, spasm of anal sphincter, oral candidiasis.
Nervous System: dizziness, headache, malaise, paresthesia.
Urinary: genital itching, candidiasis, vaginitis.
Skin: rash, hives.
Other: hypersensitivity reactions (serum sickness, anaphylaxis), abnormal blood profiles, shortness of breath.

Onset, Peak, and Duration

Route	Onset	Peak	Duration
Oral	Unknown	≤1 hr	Unknown

 Massage Considerations

- There are no cautions or contraindications to massage because the client is taking this medication. Cautions and contraindications may exist related to the client condition and severity of the infection.
- Side effects of dizziness require care in getting the client on and off the table. Using stimulating strokes such as rapid effleurage and tapotement at the end of the session may help.
- Paresthesia is a local caution for deep tissue massage and if severe may contraindicate it completely.
- Rash or hives are local contraindications to massage and should be reported to the physician immmediately. If severe, massage should be withheld.

cetrorelix acetate (set-RO-rel-icks AS-ih-tayt)

Cetrotide

Drug Class: Gonadotropin-releasing hormone (GnRH) analog infertility agent

Drug Actions

Drug competes with natural gonadatropin-releasing hormone for binding to membrane receptors on the gonadotrophic cells of the anterior pituitary and induces the production and release of luteinizing hormone and follicle-stimulating hormone (FSH). This results in the luteinizing hormone surge, which induces ovulation and increases fertility.

Use

- Infertility
- Inhibition of premature luteinizing hormone surges in women undergoing controlled ovarian stimulation

Side Effects

Gastrointestinal: nausea.
Nervous System: headache.
Urinary: ovarian hyperstimulation syndrome.
Other: anaphylaxis, local site reactions (including erythema, bruising, itching, and swelling).

Onset, Peak, and Duration

Route	Onset	Peak	Duration
S.C.	1–2 hr	1–2 hr	≥4 days

 Massage Considerations

- There are no cautions or contraindications to massage related to a client taking this drug.
- If there is tenderness or other reactions at the injection site, that local site should not be massaged.
- All strokes and techniques are appropriate for this client other than those related to the client condition.

---

chloral hydrate (KLOR-ŭl HIGH-drayt)

Aquachloral Supprettes, Noctec, Novo-Chlohydrate

Drug Class: General central nervous system depressant, sedative-hypnotic

Drug Actions

Promotes sleep and calmness

Use

- Sedation in adults
- Insomnia
- Preoperatively
- Premedication for electroencephalogram
- Alcohol withdrawal

Side Effects

Gastrointestinal: nausea, vomiting, diarrhea, gas.
Nervous System: hangover, drowsiness, nightmares, dizziness, abnormal movement, paradoxical excitement.
Other: hypersensitivity reactions, blood abnormalities.

Onset, Peak, and Duration

Route	Onset	Peak	Duration
Oral	≤30 min	Unknown	4–8 hr
Rectal	Unknown	Unknown	4–8 hr

Massage Considerations

- Massage is completely contraindicated for a client taking this drug in all cases except when it is taken for insomnia.
- The action of the drug is sedating, and this effect will increase the relaxing effects of massage.
- The drug duration of action is up to 8 hours. Schedule the client for the middle of the day to be sure the effects of the drug are out of the system.
- Some buildup and residual effects may still occur if the client uses the drug regularly. In this case, use deep tissue massage with caution because central nervous system depression interferes with perception of pain and pressure.
- Side effects of dizziness and drowsiness require care in getting the client on and off the table. Using stimulating strokes such as rapid effleurage and tapotement at the end of the session may help. If severe, use a more rapid and stimulating massage throughout the session.
- Gas may be helped by regular abdominal massage.
- All other strokes and techniques are appropriate for this client.

---

chlorambucil (klor-AM-byoo-sil)

Leukeran

Drug Class: Antineoplastic

Drug Actions

Kills selected cancer cells

Use

- Chronic lymphocytic leukemia
- Malignant lymphomas, including lymphosarcoma, giant follicular lymphoma, non-Hodgkin's lymphoma, and Hodgkin's disease
- Autoimmune hemolytic anemia
- Nephrotic syndrome
- Polycythemia vera
- Ovarian neoplasms
- Macroglobulinemia
- Metastatic trophoblastic neoplasia
- Idiopathic uveitis
- Rheumatoid arthritis

Side Effects

Gastrointestinal: nausea, vomiting, stomatitis.
Nervous System: seizures.
Urinary: absence of sperm in semen, infertility.
Skin: exfoliative dermatitis, rash, Stevens-Johnson syndrome.
Other: allergic febrile reaction, hepatotoxicity, hyperuricemia, interstitial pneumonitis, pulmonary fibrosis, abnormal blood profiles, bone marrow suppression.

Onset, Peak, and Duration

Route	Onset	Peak	Duration
Oral	3–4 wk	1 hr	Unknown

Massage Considerations

- This drug is toxic to cells and a poison in the body.
- Deep tissue massage is completely contraindicated.
- Circulatory massage with effleurage that moves fluids through the body should be limited or not used at all to avoid increasing the work of the already overtaxed liver and kidneys.
- Duration of action of the drug is unknown, but half is excreted within 2 to 2½ hours.
- Given that the drug is usually taken daily and peak effect of the drug occurs in 1 hour, massage would best be given at least 2 to 4 hours after the drug is taken.
- Rash would be a local contraindication for massage and should be reported to the physician immediately. If severe, massage should be withheld.
- The best strokes for this client will be the systemic reflex strokes of rocking and the mechanical strokes of gentle compression, friction, and pétrissage. Local reflex strokes such as stretching and myofascial techniques for tight and gluteated areas may be used.

---

chloramphenicol sodium succinate (klor-am-FEN-eh-kol SOH-dee-um SUK-seh-nayt)

Chloromycetin, Chloromycetin Sodium Succinate, Pentamycetin

Drug Class: Antibiotic

Drug Actions

Inhibits growth of susceptible bacteria

Use

- *Haemophilus influenzae* meningitis
- Acute *Salmonella typhi* infection
- Meningitis
- Bacteremia
- Other severe infection

Side Effects

Gastrointestinal: nausea, vomiting, stomatitis, diarrhea, enterocolitis.
Nervous System: headache, mild depression, confusion, delirium; peripheral neuropathy (with prolonged therapy).
Other: infection with nonsusceptible organisms, hypersensitivity reactions (fever, rash, urticaria, anaphylaxis), jaundice, gray syndrome in neonates, optic neuritis (in patients with cystic fibrosis), glossitis, decreased visual acuity, jaundice, abnormal blood profiles.

Onset, Peak, and Duration

Route	Onset	Peak	Duration
Oral	Unknown	1–3 hr	Unknown
I.V.	Immediate	Immediate	Unknown

Massage Considerations

- Although there are no contraindications or cautions to massage related to this drug, the client condition or severity of infection may require changes in application of massage or contraindicate it completely.
- Side effects of peripheral neuropathy locally mean deep tissue massage must be used with caution, and if severe may contraindicate deep tissue massage completely.
- All strokes and techniques may be used for this client depending on the condition of the client.

---

chlordiazepoxide (klor-digh-eh-zuh-POKS-ighd)

Libritabs

chlordiazepoxide hydrochloride

Apo-Chlordiazepoxide, Librium, Novo-Poxide

Drug Class: Benzodiazepine anxiolytic, sedative-hypnotic

Drug Actions

Relieves anxiety and promotes sleep and calmness

Use

- Mild to moderate anxiety
- Severe anxiety
- Withdrawal symptoms of acute alcoholism
- Preoperative apprehension and anxiety

Side Effects

Cardiovascular: thrombophlebitis, transient hypotension.
Gastrointestinal: nausea, vomiting, constipation, abdominal discomfort.
Nervous System: drowsiness, lethargy, hangover, fainting, restlessness, psychosis, confusion, suicidal tendencies.
Urinary: incontinence, urine retention, menstrual irregularities.
Hematologic: agranulocytosis.
Skin: swelling, pain at injection site.
Other: visual disturbances, agranulocytosis.

Onset, Peak, and Duration

Route	Onset	Peak	Duration
Oral, I.V., I.M.	Unknown	$^{1}/_{2}$–4 hr	Unknown

Massage Considerations

- The sedating effects of this drug in the central nervous system will increase the relaxing effects of massage. Deep tissue massage should be used with caution because the client perceptions may be slowed or dulled. Local reflex strokes such as stretching, traction, and compression may have less of an effect. Systemic reflex strokes such as rocking, effleurage, and friction may have increased effects.
- Side effects of drowsiness, lethargy, and hypotension along with the increased relaxation of massage will require care in getting the client on and off the table. Using rapid effleurage and pétrissage, as well as tapotement at the end of the session, may help. In many cases, using these more stimulating techniques throughout the massage will be needed to achieve relaxation with alertness.

- Constipation may be helped by regular abdominal massage.
- Problems at the injection site are a local contraindication to massage.
- Mechanical strokes will have the best effect for this client. Slightly more rapid effleurage, pétrissage, and friction will give good results.

---

chloroquine hydrochloride (KLOR-uh-qwin high-droh-KLOR-ighd)

Aralen HCl

chloroquine phosphate

Chloroquin

Drug Class: Antimalarial, amebicide

Drug Actions

Prevents or eradicates malarial infections; eradicates amebiasis, seems to slow the progression of certain autoimmune diseases.

Use

- Acute malarial attacks
- Malaria prophylaxis
- Extraintestinal amebiasis
- Rheumatoid arthritis
- Lupus erythematosus

Side Effects

Cardiovascular: hypotension, electrocardiogram changes.
Gastrointestinal: anorexia, abdominal cramps, diarrhea, nausea, vomiting, stomatitis.
Nervous System: mild and transient headache, neuromyopathy, psychic stimulation, fatigue, irritability, nightmares, seizures, dizziness.
Skin: itching, skin eruptions, skin and mucosal pigmentary changes.
Other: visual disturbances (blurred vision; difficulty in focusing; reversible corneal changes; typically irreversible, sometimes progressive or delayed retinal changes, such as narrowing of arterioles; macular lesions; pallor of optic disc; optic atrophy; patchy retinal pigmentation, typically leading to blindness), ototoxicity (nerve deafness, vertigo, tinnitus), abnormal blood profiles.

Onset, Peak, and Duration

Route	Onset	Peak	Duration
Oral	Unknown	1–3 hr	Unknown
I.M.	Unknown	30 min	Unknown

 Massage Considerations

- There are no cautions or contraindications to massage because the client is taking this medication. There may be cautions and contraindications related to the client condition.
- Side effects of dizziness and hypotension require care in getting the client on and off the table. Stimulating strokes such as rapid effleurage and tapotement at the end of the session may help.
- Skin itching and eruptions are a local contraindication to massage and should be reported to the physician immediately. If severe, massage should be withheld.

- Neuromyopathy causes pain in both muscles and nerves. Deep tissue massage would be contraindicated in its presence. If severe, massage may be completely contraindicated.
- Except as noted above, all massage strokes and techniques may be used.

---

chlorothiazide (klor-oh-THIGH-uh-zighd)

Chlotride, Diurigen, Diuril

chlorothiazide sodium

Drug Class: Diuretic, antihypertensive

Drug Actions

Promotes sodium and water excretion, lowers blood pressure

Use

- Edema
- Hypertension
- To promote excretion of fluid from the body

Side Effects

Cardiovascular: orthostatic hypotension.
Gastrointestinal: anorexia, nausea, pancreatitis.
Urinary: impotence, nocturia, frequent urination, renal impairment.
Skin: photosensitivity, rash.
Other: hypersensitivity reaction, blood abnormalities, hepatic encephalopathy, asymptomatic hyperuricemia; hypokalemia; hyperglycemia and impaired glucose tolerance; fluid and electrolyte imbalances, including dilutional hyponatremia and hypochloremia, metabolic alkalosis and hyperkalemia; gout.

Onset, Peak, and Duration

Route	Onset	Peak	Duration
Oral	≤2 hr	4 hr	6–12 hr
I.V.	≤15 min	30 min	6–12 hr

 Massage Considerations

- There are no cautions or contraindications to massage because the client is taking this drug. Client condition may warrant certain cautions and contraindications.
- Side effects of orthostatic hypotension require care in getting the client on and off the table. Using stimulating strokes such as rapid effleurage and tapotement at the end of the session may help prevent problems.
- Frequent urination may require that the client get up in the middle of the session. Provide privacy and quick access to the bathroom. Avoid using water fountains or water music, which may stimulate the need to urinate.
- Rash is a local contraindication to massage and should be reported to the physician. If severe, massage should be withheld.
- All strokes and techniques are appropriate for the client taking this drug.

chlorpromazine hydrochloride (klor-PROH-meh-zeen high-droh-KLOR-ighd)

Chlorpromanyl-20, Chlorpromanyl-40, Largactil, Novo-Chlorpromazine, Thorazine

Drug Class: Antipsychotic, antinausea

Drug Actions

Probably blocks postsynaptic dopamine receptors in brain and inhibits medullary chemoreceptor trigger zone. Relieves nausea and vomiting; hiccups; and signs and symptoms of psychosis, acute intermittent porphyria, and tetanus. Produces calmness and sleep preoperatively.

Use

- Psychosis
- Nausea and vomiting
- Intractable hiccups
- Acute intermittent porphyria
- Tetanus
- Relief of apprehension and nervousness before surgery

Side Effects

Cardiovascular: orthostatic hypotension, tachycardia, electrocardiogram changes.
Gastrointestinal: dry mouth, constipation.
Nervous System: extrapyramidal reactions, sedation, seizures, tardive dyskinesia, pseudoparkinsonism, dizziness, neuroleptic malignant syndrome.
Urinary: erectile dysfunction, urine retention, menstrual irregularities, inhibited ejaculation.
Skin: mild photosensitivity.
Other: gynecomastia, allergic reactions, intramuscular injection site pain, sterile abscess, ocular changes, blurred vision, cholestatic jaundice, abnormal blood profiles.

Onset, Peak, and Duration

Route	Onset	Peak	Duration
Oral	30–60 min	Unknown	4–6 hr
Oral controlled-release	30–60 min	Unknown	10–12 hr
I.V., I.M.	Unknown	Unknown	Unknown
Rectal	>1 hr	Unknown	3–4 hr

 Massage Considerations

- Although the actions of the drug on the body do not contraindicate massage, the use of this drug is for very serious conditions that many times will contraindicate massage.
- Consult with a physician in all cases before doing massage.
- Intramuscular injection sites for this drug should not be massaged because this may speed up the rate of absorption. Because peak and duration are unknown, err on the side of caution and do not massage the site for at least 6 hours.
- Side effects of sedation, dizziness, and orthostatic hypotension require care in getting the client on and off the table. Use stimulating strokes such as rapid effleurage and tapotement at the end of the session. If symptoms are severe, use a more rapid and stimulating massage throughout the session with rapid effleurage and pétrissage.
- Constipation may be helped by regular abdominal massage.

chlorzoxazone (klor-ZOKS-uh-zohn)

Paraflex, Parafon Forte, Remular-S

Drug Class: Skeletal muscle relaxant

Drug Actions

Appears to modify central perception of pain without modifying pain reflexes. Blocks interneuronal activity in descending reticular activating system and in spinal cord. Relaxes skeletal muscles.

Use

- Adjunct in acute, painful musculoskeletal conditions

Side Effects

Nervous System: drowsiness, dizziness, light-headedness, malaise, headache, overstimulation, tremor.
Gastrointestinal: anorexia, nausea, vomiting, heartburn, abdominal distress, constipation, diarrhea.
Urinary: urine discoloration (orange or purple-red).
Skin: hives, itching, petechiae, bruising, redness.
Other: anaphylaxis, anemia, agranulocytosis, liver dysfunction.

Onset, Peak, and Duration

Route	Onset	Peak	Duration
Oral	1 hr	1–2 hr	3–4 hr

 Massage Considerations

- The actions of this drug decrease pain perception; therefore, deep tissue massage should be used with great caution because the client will not be able to give accurate feedback.
- The decrease in nerve activity in the spinal cord may make local reflex strokes less effective. These include compression, stretching, and vibration. They may be used but may take longer to have an effect.
- Systemic reflex strokes may have a deeper and quicker effect, with the client going into relaxation quickly. This can be handled as described below for the side effects.
- Side effects of drowsiness, dizziness, and light-headedness require care in getting the client on and off the table.
- Use stimulating strokes such as rapid effleurage and tapotement at the end of the session, and if severe, use a more rapid and stimulating massage throughout the session.
- Constipation may be helped by regular abdominal massage.
- Hives and itching are a local contraindication to massage and should be reported to the physician immediately. If severe, massage should be withheld.
- Because of the actions of this drug on the nervous system, the best strokes and techniques to use are the mechanical strokes such as effleurage, pétrissage, and friction. Myofascial techniques may help with areas of tightness and gluteation.

cholestyramine (koh-leh-STIGH-ruh-meen)

LoCHOLEST, Prevalite, Questran, Questran Light, Questran Life

Drug Class: Antilipemic, bile acid sequestrant

Drug Actions

Lowers cholesterol levels and relieves itching caused by partial bile obstruction

Use

- Primary hyperlipidemia
- Pruritus caused by partial bile obstruction
- Adjunct for reduction of elevated cholesterol level in patients with primary hypercholesterolemia

Side Effects

Gastrointestinal: constipation, fecal impaction, hemorrhoids, abdominal discomfort, gas, nausea, vomiting, steatorrhea.
Skin: rash; irritation of skin, tongue, and perianal area.
Other: vitamin A, D, E, and K deficiency; hyperchloremic acidosis (with long-term use or very high dosage).

Onset, Peak, and Duration

Route	Onset	Peak	Duration
Oral	1–2 wk	Unknown	2–4 wk

 Massage Considerations

- There are no cautions or contraindications to massage related to taking this medication.
- The client condition, especially if the drug is taken for itching related to bile obstruction, may contraindicate massage completely. If not, care should be taken to not increase the itching by using rocking, shaking, and compression strokes.
- Wear gloves if bile acids are visible on the skin as a powdery substance.
- When the drug is taken to lower cholesterol, no such cautions or contraindications exist.
- Side effects of constipation and gas may be helped by regular abdominal massage.
- Rash is a local contraindication to massage and should be reported to the physician. If severe, massage should be withheld.

---

cidofovir (sigh-doh-FOH-veer)

Vistide

Drug Class: Antiviral

Drug Actions

Reduces cytomegalovirus replication

Use

- Cytomegalovirus retinitis in patients with AIDS

Side Effects

Cardiovascular: hypotension, orthostatic hypotension, pallor, syncope, tachycardia, vasodilation, facial edema.
Gastrointestinal: nausea, vomiting, diarrhea, anorexia, abdominal pain, dry mouth, taste perversion, colitis, constipation, tongue discoloration, painful digestion, difficulty swallowing, gas gastritis, melena, oral candidiasis, rectal disorders, stomatitis, aphthous stomatitis, mouth ulcerations.
Nervous System: fever, asthenia, headache, amnesia, anxiety, confusion, seizures, depression, dizziness, malaise, abnormal gait, hallucinations, insomnia, neuropathy, paresthesia, sleepiness.

Urinary: nephrotoxicity, proteinuria, glycosuria, hematuria, urinary incontinence, urinary tract infection.
Skin: rash, alopecia, acne, hives, itching, skin discoloration, dry skin, sweating.
Other: infections, chills, sarcoma, sepsis, allergic reactions, *Herpes simplex,* amblyopia, conjunctivitis, eye disorders, ocular hypotony, iritis, pharyngitis, retinal detachment, rhinitis, sinusitis, uveitis, abnormal vision, hepatomegaly, fluid imbalance, hyperglycemia, hyperlipemia, hypocalcemia, hypokalemia, weight loss, decreased bicarbonate level, arthralgia, myasthenia, myalgia; pain in back, chest, or neck; asthma, bronchitis, cough, shortness of breath, hiccups, increased sputum, lung disorders, pneumonia, abnormal blood profiles.

Onset, Peak, and Duration

Route	Onset	Peak	Duration
I.V.	Unknown	Unknown	Unknown

Massage Considerations

- Although the drug itself does not present any cautions or contraindications for massage, the client condition and the severity of infection may contraindicate massage. Consult with the physician before doing massage.
- Side effects of dizziness, sleepiness, and hypotension require care in getting the client on and off the table. Use stimulation with rapid effleurage and tapotement at the end of the session.
- Neuropathies and paresthesia require caution with deep tissue massage and if severe may contraindicate deep tissue massage completely.
- Constipation and gas may respond well to abdominal massage.
- Rash, hives, and itching are local contraindications to massage and should be reported to the physician immediately. If severe, massage should be withheld.
- Alopecia or hair loss will contraindicate scalp massage if the client is upset by the hair loss that can occur with scalp massage or the scalp is tender.

---

cilostazol (sil-OS-tah-zol)

Pletal

Drug Class: Antiplatelet drug

Drug Actions

Drug reversibly inhibits the aggregation of platelets induced by various stimuli. Drug also has a vasodilating effect that is greatest in the femoral vascular beds. Reduces symptoms of intermittent claudication.

Use

- Reduction of symptoms of intermittent claudication

Side Effects

Cardiovascular: palpitations, tachycardia, peripheral edema.
Gastrointestinal: abnormal stools, diarrhea, painful digestion, abdominal pain, gas, nausea.
Nervous System: headache, dizziness.
Other: infection, pharyngitis, rhinitis, back pain, myalgia, increased cough.

Onset, Peak, and Duration

Route	Onset	Peak	Duration
Oral	Unknown	2–4 hr	Unknown

 Massage Considerations

- This drug affects blood clotting, with easy bruising being common, and therefore deep tissue massage and tapotement should be used with caution throughout the body and not at all in the legs.
- Side effect of dizziness requires care in getting the client on and off the table. Stimulating strokes such as rapid effleurage should be used at the end of the session.
- Gas may respond well to gentle abdominal massage.

---

cimetidine (sih-MEH-tih-deen)

Tagamet, Tagamet HB

Drug Class: H_2-receptor antagonist antiulcer agent

Drug Actions

Competitively inhibits action of H_2 at receptor sites of parietal cells, decreasing gastric acid secretion.

Use

- Prevention of upper gastrointestinal bleeding in critically ill patients
- Duodenal ulcer (short-term therapy)
- Active benign gastric ulceration
- Pathologic hypersecretory conditions (such as Zollinger-Ellison syndrome, systemic mastocytosis, and multiple endocrine adenomas)
- Hospitalized patients with intractable ulcers or hypersecretory conditions or patients who cannot take oral medication
- Gastroesophageal reflux disease
- Heartburn
- Active upper gastrointestinal bleeding
- Peptic esophagitis
- Stress ulcers

Side Effects

Nervous System: confusion, dizziness, headaches, peripheral neuropathy.
Cardiovascular: bradycardia.
Gastrointestinal: mild and transient diarrhea.
Nervous System: confusion,dizziness, headaches, peripheral neuropathy.
Skin: acne-like rash, hives.
Other: hypersensitivity reactions, mild gynecomastia (if used longer than 1 month), jaundice, muscle pain, abnormal blood profiles.

Onset, Peak, and Duration

Route	Onset	Peak	Duration
Oral	Unknown	45–90 min	4–5 hr
I.V.	Unknown	Immediate	Unknown
I.M.	Unknown	Unknown	Unknown

Massage Considerations

- There are no cautions or contraindications to massage for the client taking this medication.
- Side effect of dizziness requires care in getting the client on and off the table. Use stimulating strokes such as rapid effleurage and tapotement at the end of the session.

- Gas may be helped by abdominal massage.
- All strokes and techniques are appropriate for this client.

ciprofloxacin (sih-proh-FLOKS-uh-sin)

Cipro, Cipro IV, Ciproxin, Cipro XR

Drug Class: Antibiotic

Drug Action

Kills susceptible bacteria

Use

- Urinary tract infection
- Bone and joint infections
- Respiratory tract infections
- Skin and skin-structure infections
- Infectious diarrhea
- Intra-abdominal infection
- Acute sinusitis
- Chronic bacterial prostatitis
- Febrile neutropenia
- Inhalation anthrax (postexposure)
- Acute uncomplicated cystitis
- Cutaneous anthrax
- Uncomplicated urethral, endocervical, rectal, or pharyngeal gonorrhea
- *Neisseria meningitidis* in nasal passages

Side Effects

Cardiovascular: thrombophlebitis.
Gastrointestinal: nausea, diarrhea, vomiting, abdominal pain or discomfort, oral candidiasis.
Nervous System: headache, restlessness, tremor, light-headedness, confusion, hallucinations, seizures, paresthesia.
Urinary: crystalluria, interstitial nephritis.
Skin: rash, itching, photosensitivity, Stevens-Johnson syndrome.
Other: burning, erythema, swelling with intravenous administration, blood profile abnormalities, arthralgia, joint or back pain, joint inflammation, joint stiffness, achiness, neck or chest pain.

Onset, Peak, and Duration

Route	Onset	Peak	Duration
Oral	Unknown	1–2 hr	Unknown
Oral extended-release	Unknown	1–4 hr	Unknown
I.V.	Immediate	Immediate	Unknown

 Massage Considerations

- There are no cautions or contraindications to massage related to taking this drug. The client condition and severity of infection may require cautions and contraindications.
- Side effect of light-headedness requires care in getting the client on and off the table. Use rapid effleurage and tapotement at the end of the session to stimulate the client.

- Paresthesia requires caution when using deep tissue massage and if severe may contraindicate it completely.
- Thrombophlebitis with the presence of a blood clot is an absolute contraindication to massage of any kind.
- Rash or itching are local contraindications to massage and should be reported to the physician immediately. If severe, massage should be withheld.

---

cisplatin (sis-PLAH-tin)

Platinol-AQ

Drug Class: Antineoplastic

Drug Actions

Kills selected cancer cells

Use

- Adjunct therapy in metastatic testicular cancer
- Adjunct therapy in metastatic ovarian cancer
- Advanced bladder cancer
- Head and neck cancer
- Cervical cancer
- Non–small cell lung cancer
- Brain tumor
- Osteogenic sarcoma
- Neuroblastoma
- Advanced esophageal cancer

Side Effects

Gastrointestinal: nausea and vomiting beginning 1 to 4 hours after dose and lasting 24 hours, diarrhea, loss of taste, metallic taste.
Nervous System: peripheral neuritis, seizures.
Urinary: more prolonged and severe renal toxicity with repeated courses of therapy.
Other: anaphylactoid reaction, ringing in the ears, hearing loss, hypomagnesemia, hypokalemia, hypocalcemia, abnormal blood profiles.

Onset, Peak, and Duration

Route	Onset	Peak	Duration
I.V.	Unknown	Unknown	Several days

Massage Considerations

- Because this drug is toxic to cells, deep tissue massage should be used minimally and with great caution, if at all.
- Circulatory massage that moves fluid in the body, such as effleurage, should also be limited so as not to overtax liver and kidneys as they try to eliminate the drug from the system.
- The peak and duration of action of this drug is unknown. Its half-life is up to 3 days. Because the drug is usually given once every 3 to 4 weeks, timing of the massage is best done before the dose is given and at least 3 to 6 days after it is given. Massage would best be done on the weeks the drug is not being taken. Consult closely with the physician.
- Side effects of peripheral neuritis or nerve inflammation would be a local contraindication to massage and if severe may contraindicate massage completely. In mild cases, massage may help. Use gentle compression, stretching, and firm, slow pétrissage.

- The best strokes to use are the systemic reflex and local reflex strokes such as rocking, gentle friction, compression, and stretching, and traction. Gentle compression may also be used.

---

citalopram hydrobromide (sih-TAL-oh-pram high-droh-BROH-mighd)

Celexa

Drug Class: Selective serotonin reuptake inhibitor (SSRI) antidepressant

Drug Actions

Probably enhances serotonergic activity in the central nervous system resulting from its inhibition of central nervous system neuronal reuptake of serotonin. Relieves depression.

Use

- Depression
- Panic disorder

Side Effects

Cardiovascular: tachycardia, orthostatic hypotension, hypotension.
Gastrointestinal: nausea, dry mouth, diarrhea, anorexia, dyspepsia, vomiting, abdominal pain, increased saliva, taste perversion, gas, weight changes, increased appetite.
Nervous System: fever, tremor, sleepiness, insomnia, anxiety, agitation, dizziness, paresthesia, migraine, impaired concentration, amnesia, depression, apathy, suicide attempt, confusion, fatigue.
Urinary: painful menstruation, lack of menstruation, ejaculation disorder, impotence, excessive urination.
Skin: rash, itching, increased sweating.
Other: yawning, decreased libido, rhinitis, sinusitis, abnormal accommodation, arthralgia, myalgia, upper respiratory tract infection, cough.

Onset, Peak, and Duration

Route	Onset	Peak	Duration
Oral	Unknown	4 hr	Unknown

 Massage Considerations

- There are no cautions or contraindications to massage because the client is taking this medication.
- The action of the drug in increasing serotonin will increase the relaxation effects of massage, especially of the systemic reflex strokes such as effleurage and rocking. The client may relax very quickly and deeply. Applying effleurage in a more stimulating manner and limiting or not using rocking will help prevent any problems with the client feeling too "out of it."
- Side effects of sleepiness, dizziness, and hypotension will require care in getting the client on and off the table. Using stimulating strokes at the end of the massage may help. In some cases, using a more stimulating massage throughout may be needed. Rapid effleurage, pétrissage, and tapotement are appropriate.
- Gas may be helped by regular abdominal massage.
- Rash and itching are local contraindications to massage and should be reported to the physician. If severe, massage should be withheld.

- Using more stimulating mechanical strokes, such as effleurage and pétrissage, and the local reflex strokes of friction, compression, and stretching, and traction, are the best strokes to use with this client.

---

clarithromycin (klah-rith-roh-MIGH-sin)

Biaxin, Biaxin XL

Drug Class: Antibiotic

Drug Actions

Hinders or kills susceptible bacteria

Use

- Pharyngitis
- Tonsillitis
- Acute maxillary sinusitis
- Acute exacerbations of chronic bronchitis
- Uncomplicated skin and skin-structure infections
- Prophylaxis and treatment of disseminated infection from *Mycobacterium avium complex*
- Acute otitis media
- *Helicobacter pylori* eradication to reduce risk of duodenal ulcer recurrence
- Community-acquired pneumonia

Side Effects

Cardiovascular: arrhythmias.
Gastrointestinal: pseudomembranous colitis, diarrhea, nausea, abnormal taste, painful digestion, abdominal pain or discomfort, vomiting (pediatric).
Nervous System: headache.
Skin: rash (pediatric).
Other: coagulation abnormalities, leukopenia.

Onset, Peak, and Duration

Route	Onset	Peak	Duration
Oral	Unknown	2–3 hr	Unknown
Oral extended-release	Unknown	5–6 hr	Unknown

Massage Considerations

- There are no cautions or contraindications to massage related to the client taking this drug. The client condition and severity of infection may require cautions and contraindications.
- The side effect of blood coagulation abnormalities will contraindicate deep tissue massage and may contraindicate massage completely. Consult with a physician.
- All strokes and techniques for massage may be used with this client.

---

clindamycin hydrochloride (klin-duh-MIGH-sin high-droh-KLOR-ighd)

Cleocin, Dalacin C

clindamycin palmitate hydrochloride

Cleocin Pediatric

clindamycin phosphate

Drug Class: Antibiotic

Drug Actions

Hinders or kills susceptible bacteria

Use

- Infections caused by sensitive bacteria
- Endocarditis prophylaxis for dental procedures in patients allergic to penicillin
- Acne vulgaris
- *Pneumocystis carinii* pneumonia
- Toxoplasmosis (cerebral or ocular) in immunocompromized patients

Side Effects

Cardiovascular: thrombophlebitis.
Gastrointestinal: unpleasant or bitter taste, nausea, vomiting, abdominal pain, diarrhea, pseudomembranous colitis, esophagitis, gas, anorexia, bloody or tarry stools, difficulty swallowing.
Skin: rash, hives.
Other: anaphylaxis; pain, induration, sterile abscess (intramuscular injection); erythema, pain (intravenous administration), abnormal blood profiles.

Onset, Peak, and Duration

Route	Onset	Peak	Duration
Oral	Unknown	45–60 min	Unknown
I.V.	Immediate	Immediate	Unknown
I.M.	Unknown	3 hr	Unknown

 Massage Considerations

- There are no cautions or contraindications to massage because a client is taking this drug.
- The client condition and severity of infection may caution or contraindicate massage in some cases.
- If the drug is given by intramuscular injection, the site of injection should not massaged for at least 3 hours or more so as not to increase the rate of absorption.
- Side effects of gas may be helped by abdominal massage.
- Rash or hives is a local contraindication to massage and should be reported to the physician immediately. If severe, massage should be withheld.
- If thrombophlebitis with blood clot is present, massage is completely contraindicated.

---

clobetasol propionate (kloh-BAY-tah-sol PRO-pee-uh-nayt)

Cormax, Dermovate, Embeline E, Temovate, Temovate Emollient, Olux

Drug Class: Topical adrenocorticoid anti-inflammatory

Drug Actions

Decreases inflammation and itching

Use

- Inflammation and itching from moderate to severe corticosteroid-responsive skin conditions
- Inflammation and itching from moderate to severe corticosteroid-responsive skin conditions of the scalp
- Short-term topical therapy for mild to moderate plaque-type psoriasis of nonscalp regions

Side Effects

Urinary: glucosuria.
Skin: burning and stinging sensation, itching, irritation, dryness and cracking, erythema, folliculitis, perioral dermatitis, allergic contact dermatitis, hypopigmentation, hypertrichosis, acneiform eruptions, skin atrophy, telangiectasia (dilatation of capillaries), striae.
Other: hypothalamic-pituitary-adrenal axis suppression, Cushing syndrome, numbness of fingers, hyperglycemia.

Onset, Peak, and Duration

Route	Onset	Peak	Duration
Topical	Unknown	Unknown	Unknown

 Massage Considerations

- Because this drug is used topically for severe skin inflammation, the local site of the problem and application of the drug is contraindicated for massage. If the condition is widespread, massage may be contraindicated completely.
- Side effects of skin problems with this drug are local contraindications to massage. If severe and widespread, massage should not be given at all.
- Numbness of the fingers requires caution in using deep tissue massage in this area. If the client is experiencing Cushing syndrome from long-term use of this drug, there will be changes in the connective tissue of the body as well as fatty deposits. In these cases, deep tissue massage is completely contraindicated.
- Myofascial techniques may be less effective and should be used with caution. Using mechanical strokes and systemic reflex strokes such as effleurage, pétrissage, rocking, and gentle friction will work best.
- If none of the above issues is present, all strokes and techniques of massage may be used in the areas not affected by the condition or the drug.

clomiphene citrate (KLOH-meh-feen SIGH-trayt)

Clomid, Milophene, Serophene

Drug Class: Ovulation stimulant

Drug Actions

Appears to stimulate release of pituitary gonadotropins, follicle-stimulating hormone, and luteinizing hormone. This results in maturation of ovarian follicle, ovulation, and development of corpus luteum.

Use

- Induction of ovulation
- Infertility

Side Effects

Cardiovascular: hypertension.
Gastrointestinal: nausea, vomiting, bloating, distention.

Nervous System: headache, restlessness, insomnia, dizziness, light-headedness, depression, fatigue, tension, vasomotor flushes.
Urinary: urinary frequency, ovarian enlargement, and cyst formation, which regress spontaneously when the drug is stopped.
Metabolic: hyperglycemia, increased appetite, weight gain.
Skin: reversible hair loss, hives, rash.
Other: breast discomfort, blurred vision, double vision, scotoma, photophobia.

Onset, Peak, and Duration

Route	Onset	Peak	Duration
Oral	Unknown	Unknown	Unknown

 Massage Considerations

- There are no cautions or contraindications to massage for the client taking this drug.
- Side effects of dizziness and light-headedness require care in positioning and getting the client on and off the table. Use stimulating strokes such as rapid effleurage and tapotement at the end of the session.
- Urinary frequency may cause the client to have to get up in the middle of the session.
- Provide privacy and quick access to the bathroom. Avoid the use of water fountains and water music, which may stimulate the need to urinate.
- Rash and hives are local contraindications to massage and should be reported to the physician. If severe, massage should be withheld.
- Hair loss is a contraindication to massage of the scalp.
- If the client experiences breast discomfort or tenderness, gentle breast massage may help. Use pillows when the client is facedown to relieve pressure on the chest and if the discomfort is severe, do not massage the area and try side-lying positioning.

---

clomipramine hydrochloride (kloh-MIH-pruh-meen high-droh-KLOR-ighd)

Anafranil

Drug Class: Tricyclic antidepressant (TCA)

Drug Actions

Selectively inhibits reuptake of serotonin. Reduces obsessive-compulsive behaviors and depression.

Use

- Obsessive-compulsive disorder

Side Effects

Cardiovascular: orthostatic hypotension, palpitations, tachycardia.
Gastrointestinal: dry mouth, constipation, nausea, painful digestion, diarrhea, anorexia, abdominal pain, belching.
Nervous System: sleepiness, tremors, dizziness, headache, insomnia, nervousness, myoclonus, fatigue, electroencephalogram changes, seizures, extrapyramidal reactions, loss of strength, aggressiveness.
Urinary: urinary hesitancy, urinary tract infections, painful menstruation, impaired ejaculation, impotence.
Skin: diaphoresis, rash, itching, photosensitivity, dry skin.
Other: altered libido, otitis media in children, abnormal vision, laryngitis, pharyngitis, rhinitis, anemia, bone marrow suppression, increased appetite, weight gain, myalgia.

Onset, Peak, and Duration

Route	Onset	Peak	Duration
Oral	≥2 wk	Unknown	Unknown

 Massage Considerations

- The action of the drug in increasing serotonin will increase the relaxing effects of massage, especially of the systemic reflex strokes. Applying these strokes in a slightly more stimulating manner by using more rapid effleurage and friction, limiting rocking, and using tapotement will allow relaxation without the client feeling too "out of it."
- Side effects of sleepiness, dizziness, and hypotension will be aided by the changes in massage application noted above.
- Constipation may respond well to abdominal massage.
- Rash or itching is a local contraindication to massage and should be reported to the physician. If severe, massage should be withheld.
- The best strokes for this client are the mechanical strokes and local reflex strokes of effleurage, pétrissage, friction, and compression and vibration.

clonazepam (kloh-NEH-zuh-pam)

Klonopin, Rivotril

Drug Class: Benzodiazepine anticonvulsant

Drug Actions

It probably acts by facilitating effects of inhibitory neurotransmitter GABA. Prevents or stops seizure activity.

Use

- Lennox-Gastaut syndrome
- Atypical absence seizures
- Akinetic and myoclonic seizures
- Status epilepticus
- Panic disorder
- Restless legs syndrome
- Adjunct in schizophrenia
- Parkinsonian dysarthria
- Acute manic episodes
- Multifocal tic disorders
- Neuralgia

Side Effects

Gastrointestinal: constipation, gastritis, nausea, abnormal thirst.
Nervous System: drowsiness, ataxia, behavioral disturbances (especially in children), slurred speech, tremor, confusion, psychosis, agitation.
Urinary: painful urination, lack of urination, nocturia, urine retention.
Skin: rash.
Other: increased salivation, double vision, nystagmus, abnormal eye movements, sore gums, change in appetite, muscle weakness or pain, respiratory depression, abnormal blood profiles.

Onset, Peak, and Duration

Route	Onset	Peak	Duration
Oral	Unknown	1–2 hr	Unknown
I.V.	Unknown	Unknown	Unknown

Massage Considerations

- The action of this drug increases sedating effects of Gamma-aminobutyric acid (GABA) on the nervous system and may decrease the perception of the sensory nervous system. Use deep tissue massage with caution. It will increase the relaxing effects of massage, especially the systemic reflex strokes of effleurage, rocking, and friction. Use these strokes less or in a more stimulating manner throughout the massage.
- In some cases, tapotement may stimulate seizure activity, so use with caution in clients whose seizure disorder is not well controlled.
- The client condition may require cautions and even contraindications to massage.
- Especially in its use for seizures and manic disorders, consult with the physician.
- Side effect of drowsiness requires care in getting the client on and off the table. Use the stimulation of rapid effleurage at the end of the session and even throughout the session if this symptom is severe.
- Constipation may respond well to abdominal massage.
- Rash is a local contraindication to massage and should be reported to the physician. If severe, massage should be withheld.
- Mechanical massage strokes of effleurage, pétrissage, and friction applied in a more stimulating manner will work best with this client as well as the local reflex strokes of compression, vibration, and stretching and traction.

---

clonidine hydrochloride (KLON-uh-deen high-droh-KLOR-ighd)

Catapres, Catapres-TTS, Dixarit, Duracion

Drug Class: Centrally acting sympatholytic antihypertensive

Drug Actions

Thought to inhibit central vasomotor centers, thereby decreasing sympathetic outflow to heart, kidneys, and peripheral vasculature; this results in decreased peripheral vascular resistance, decreased systolic and diastolic blood pressure, and decreased heart rate.

Use

- Essential, renal, and malignant hypertension
- Severe pain
- Prophylaxis for vascular headache
- Adjunctive therapy for nicotine withdrawal
- Adjunct in opiate withdrawal
- Adjunct in menopausal symptoms
- Dysmenorrhea
- Ulcerative colitis
- Diabetic diarrhea
- Neuralgia
- Growth delay in children
- Attention deficit hyperactivity disorder (ADHD)

Side Effects

Cardiovascular: orthostatic hypotension, hypotension, bradycardia, severe rebound hypertension.
Gastrointestinal: constipation, dry mouth, nausea, vomiting.
Nervous System: anxiety, sleepiness, confusion, drowsiness, dizziness, fatigue, sedation, nervousness, headache, vivid dreams.
Urinary: urine retention, impotence, urinary tract infections.
Skin: itching and rash with transdermal patch.
Other: transient glucose intolerance.

Onset, Peak, and Duration

Route	Onset	Peak	Duration
Oral	15–30 min	$1\,^1/_2$–$2\,^1/_2$ hr	6–8 hr
Epidural	Immediate	19 min	Unknown
Transdermal	2–3 days	2–3 days	Several days

 Massage Considerations

- This drug inhibits the actions of the sympathetic nervous system. The relaxing and parasympathetic nervous system effects of massage will be increased, especially the effects of the systemic reflex strokes of effleurage, rocking, and friction. Limit the use of rocking and apply massage more rapidly and in a stimulating manner to prevent the client from being too sedated.
- Side effects of sleepiness, drowsiness, dizziness, sedation, and hypotension should be addressed as noted above.
- Constipation may be helped by regular abdominal massage.
- The area of a transdermal patch should be avoided during the massage, and if rash or itching occurs at the site after removal, it is a local contraindication to massage until this clears up.
- The best strokes for this client are the mechanical strokes of effleurage, pétrissage, friction, and tapotement. Local reflex strokes of compression and stretching may be used as well as other techniques such as myofascial massage.

---

clopidogrel bisulfate (kloh-PIH-doh-grel bigh-SUL-fayt)

Plavix

Drug Class: Antiplatelet

Drug Actions

Prevents clot formation.

Use

- To reduce atherosclerotic events in patients with atherosclerosis documented by recent stroke, heart attack, or peripheral arterial disease
- To reduce atherosclerotic events in patients with acute coronary syndrome

Side Effects

Cardiovascular: chest pain, edema, hypertension.
Gastrointestinal: hemorrhage, abdominal pain, painful digestion, gastritis, constipation, diarrhea, ulcers.
Nervous System: headache, dizziness, fatigue, depression, pain.
Urinary: urinary tract infection

Skin: rash, itching.
Other: flulike symptoms, nosebleed, rhinitis, purpura, arthralgia, back pain, bronchitis, cough, shortness of breath, upper respiratory tract infection.

Onset, Peak, and Duration

Route	Onset	Peak	Duration
Oral	2 hr	Unknown	5 days

 Massage Considerations

- This drug effects the clotting action of the blood. Use caution with deep tissue massage until the client's response is determined. The client's condition may require cautions and contraindications for massage.
- Side effects of dizziness require care in getting the client off the table. Use stimulating strokes such as rapid effleurage at the end of the session.
- Constipation may respond well to regular abdominal massage.
- Rash and itching are local contraindications to massage and should be reported to the physician. If severe, massage should be withheld.

clorazepate dipotassium (klor-AYZ-eh-payt digh-po-TAH-see-um)

Apo-Clorazepate, ClorazeCaps, Gen-Xene, Novoclopate, Tranxene, Tranxene-SD, Tranxene T-Tab

Drug Class: Benzodiazepine anxiolytic, anticonvulsant, sedative-hypnotic agent

Drug Actions

May facilitate action of inhibitory neurotransmitter GABA. Depresses central nervous system at limbic and subcortical levels of brain and suppresses spread of seizure activity. Relieves anxiety, prevents seizure activity, and promotes sleep and calmness.

Use

- Acute alcohol withdrawal
- Anxiety
- Adjunct in partial seizure disorder

Side Effects

Cardiovascular: transient hypotension.
Gastrointestinal: nausea, vomiting, abdominal discomfort, dry mouth.
Nervous System: drowsiness, lethargy, hangover, fainting, restlessness, psychosis.
Urinary: urine retention, incontinence.
Other: visual disturbances.

Onset, Peak, and Duration

Route	Onset	Peak	Duration
Oral	Unknown	$^1/_2$–2 hr	Unknown

 Massage Considerations

- This drug depresses the central nervous system and may decrease sensory perception. Deep tissue massage should be used with caution. The action of the drug will increase the effects of the systemic reflex strokes in massage and increase the relaxation effects. Use effleurage and friction in a more rapid and stimulating manner and limit use of rocking to prevent the client from being too sedated.

- Side effects of drowsiness, lethargy, and hypotension require care in getting the client on and off the table. Use stimulating strokes of rapid effleurage and tapotement at the end of the session and if the side effects are severe, throughout the massage session.
- The use of mechanical strokes such as effleurage and pétrissage applied in a more stimulating manner throughout the session will work best with this client. Local reflex strokes may also be used, such as compression, vibration, and stretching/traction.

clozapine (KLOH-zuh-peen)

Clozaril

Drug Class: Antipsychotic

Drug Actions

Relieves psychotic signs and symptoms

Use

- Schizophrenia

Side Effects

Cardiovascular: tachycardia, hypotension, hypertension, chest pain, electrocardiogram changes, orthostatic hypotension, cardiomyopathy.
Gastrointestinal: dry mouth, constipation, nausea, vomiting, excessive salivation, heartburn.
Nervous System: fever, drowsiness, sedation, seizures, dizziness, syncope, headache, tremor, disturbed sleep or nightmares, restlessness, hypokinesia or akinesia, agitation, rigidity, akathisia, confusion, fatigue, insomnia, hyperkinesia, weakness, lethargy, ataxia, slurred speech, depression, myoclonus, anxiety.
Urinary: urinary frequency, urinary urgency, urine retention, incontinence, abnormal ejaculation.
Skin: rash.
Other: abnormal blood profiles, weight gain, severe hyperglycemia, muscle pain or spasm, muscle weakness.

Onset, Peak, and Duration

Route	Onset	Peak	Duration
Oral	Unknown	2 1/2 hr	4–12 hr

 Massage Considerations

- Although there are no cautions or contraindications to massage related to this drug, the client condition in most cases will have cautions and even contraindications to massage. Consult with the physician closely.
- Side effects of drowsiness, sedation, dizziness, and hypotension require care in getting the client on and off the table. Use stimulating strokes such as rapid effleurage and tapotement at the end of the session and even throughout the massage if this symptom is severe.
- Constipation may be helped by abdominal massage.
- Urinary frequency and urgency may cause the client to need to get up in the middle of the session. Provide privacy and quick access to the bathroom and avoid the use of water fountains or water music, which may stimulate the urge to urinate.
- Rash is a local contraindication to massage and should be reported to the physician. If severe, massage should be withheld.

codeine phosphate (KOH-deen FOS-fayt)

Paveral

codeine sulfate

Drug Class: Opioid analgesic, antitussive

Drug Actions

Binds with opiate receptors in central nervous system, altering both perception of and emotional response to pain through unknown mechanism. Also suppresses cough reflex by direct action on cough center in medulla.

Use

- Mild to moderate pain
- Nonproductive cough

Side Effects

Cardiovascular: hypotension, flushing, bradycardia.
Gastrointestinal: nausea, vomiting, constipation, dry mouth, ileus.
Nervous System: sedation, clouded sensorium, euphoria, dizziness, seizures.
Urinary: urine retention.
Skin: itching.
Other: physical dependence, respiratory depression.

Onset, Peak, and Duration

Route	Onset	Peak	Duration
Oral	30–45 min	1–2 hr	4–6 hr
I.V.	Immediate	Immediate	4–6 hr
I.M.	10–30 min	$^1/_2$–1 hr	4–6 hr
S.C.	10–30 min	Unknown	4–6 hr

 Massage Considerations

- This drug decreases the perception of pain. Deep tissue massage should be used with extreme caution. The sedating effects of this drug will significantly increase the relaxation effects of massage, especially the effect of the systemic reflex strokes such as effleurage, friction, and rocking. Limit use of rocking; apply effleurage and friction in a stimulating manner throughout the massage to avoid having the client feeling too sedated.
- Side effects of sedation, dizziness, and hypotension, as well as clouded senses, will respond well to the above suggestion. Care should be taken in getting the client on and off the table.
- Constipation may respond well to regular abdominal massage.
- Itching would be a local contraindication to massage and if severe may contraindicate it completely.
- The sedating effects of this drug on the central nervous system will decrease the effectiveness of the local reflex strokes. The best strokes for this client will be mechanical strokes of effleurage, pétrissage, friction, and tapotement as well as giving a more stimulating session throughout.

colchicine (KOHL-chih-seen)

Colgout

Drug Class: Antigout agent

Drug Actions

Decreases urate crystal deposits, reducing inflammation. Relieves gout signs and symptoms.

Use

- Prevention of acute gout attacks as prophylactic or maintenance therapy
- Prevention of gout attacks in patients undergoing surgery
- Acute gout, acute gouty arthritis
- Familial Mediterranean fever
- Hepatic cirrhosis

Side Effects

Gastrointestinal: nausea, vomiting, abdominal pain, diarrhea.
Nervous System: peripheral neuritis.
Skin: hair loss, rash, hives.
Other: severe local irritation (if extravasation occurs), hypersensitivity reactions, anaphylaxis, hepatic necrosis, abnormal blood profiles.

Onset, Peak, and Duration

Route	Onset	Peak	Duration
Oral	≤12 hr	$^1/_2$–2 hr	Unknown
I.V.	6–12 hr	$^1/_2$–2 hr	Unknown

 Massage Considerations

- There are no cautions or contraindications to massage related to the client taking this drug; however, client condition may require cautions and contraindications.
- Side effects of peripheral neuritis may be aided by gentle, calming massage. Use slow and firm effleurage, gentle compression, and rocking. If severe, neuritis may be a local or even a complete contraindication to massage.
- Rash and hives are local contraindications to massage and should be reported to the physician. If severe, massage should be withheld.
- Hair loss is a contraindication to massage of the scalp, especially if the client is disturbed by the hair loss during massage or the scalp is tender.

colesevelam hydrochloride (koh-leh-SEV-eh-lam high-droh-KLOR-ighd)

Welchol

Drug Class: Antilipemic

Drug Actions

Lowers low-density lipoprotein (LDL) and total cholesterol levels

Use

- Reduction of elevated LDL cholesterol in patients with primary hypercholesterolemia

Side Effects

Gastrointestinal: abdominal pain, constipation, diarrhea, painful digestion, gas, nausea.
Nervous System: headache, pain, muscle weakness.
Other: accidental injury, infection, flulike syndrome, pharyngitis, rhinitis, sinusitis, myalgia, back pain, increased cough.

Onset, Peak, and Duration

Route	Onset	Peak	Duration
Oral	Unknown	2 wk	Unknown

Massage Considerations

- There are no cautions or contraindications to massage for the client related to taking this drug.
- Side effects of constipation and gas may be helped by regular abdominal massage.

corticotropin (adrenocorticotropic hormone, ACTH)

(kor-teh-koh-TROH-pin)

ACTH, Acthar

repository corticotropin

Drug Class: Anterior pituitary hormone

Drug Actions

By replacing the body's own tropic hormone, drug stimulates secretion of adrenal cortex hormones.

Use

- Diagnostic test of adrenocortical function
- Inflammation

Side Effects

Cardiovascular: hypertension, heart failure, shock.
Gastrointestinal: peptic ulceration (with perforation and hemorrhage), pancreatitis, abdominal distension, ulcerative esophagitis, nausea, vomiting.
Nervous System: seizures, dizziness, papilledema, headache, euphoria, insomnia, mood swings, personality changes, depression, psychosis, increased intracranial pressure.
Urinary: menstrual irregularities.
Skin: impaired wound healing, thin and fragile skin, petechiae, ecchymoses, facial erythema, diaphoresis, acne, hyperpigmentation, allergic skin reactions, hirsutism.
Other: cushingoid symptoms, progressive increase in antibodies, loss of corticotropin stimulatory effect, hypersensitivity reactions (rash, bronchospasm), activation of latent diabetes mellitus, suppression of growth in children, sodium and fluid retention, calcium and potassium loss, hypokalemic alkalosis, negative nitrogen balance, cataracts, glaucoma, muscle weakness, steroid myopathy, loss of muscle mass, osteoporosis, vertebral compression fractures.

Onset, Peak, and Duration

Route	Onset	Peak	Duration
I.V., I.M., S.C.			
Aqueous	Rapid	Varies	2 hr
Repository	Rapid	Varies	≤3 days

Massage Considerations

- This drug treats serious hormonal problems and can cause changes in the connective tissue of the body as well as immunosuppression. Consult with the physician before doing massage.
- Deep tissue massage is contraindicated.
- Traction and stretching should be used with caution because of changes in muscle and connective tissue.
- Myofascial massage may not be effective and should be used with caution.
- Care should be taken with infection control to avoid exposing the client. Schedule the appointment as the first of the day so there is less exposure to other clients. If you have any infection, do not work with the client.
- Side effect of dizziness requires care in getting the client off the table. Use more rapid effleurage at the end of the session to stimulate and awaken the client.
- Thin and fragile skin, if severe, may contraindicate massage. Pressure may need to be very light and effleurage may not be able to be used. Gentle compression, rocking, and warming holds may be the only manipulation the client can handle if this symptom is severe.
- Cushing symptoms, osteoporosis, and fractures may be addressed as above.
- For the client taking this drug, gentle mechanical strokes will work best. Gentle effleurage, pétrissage, and rocking with gentle compression will relax without manipulating the tissues that may be weak and easily damaged. Variations in depth and pressure and techniques will depend on the individual client condition.

---

cortisone acetate (KOR-tih-sohn AS-ih-tayt)

Cortone Acetate

Drug Class: Glucocorticoid, mineralocorticoid anti-inflammatory

Drug Actions

Decreases inflammation, suppresses immune response; stimulates bone marrow; and influences protein, fat, and carbohydrate metabolism.

Use

- Adrenal insufficiency
- Allergy
- Inflammation

Side Effects

Cardiovascular: arrhythmias, heart failure, thromboembolism, hypertension, edema.
Gastrointestinal: peptic ulceration, gastrointestinal irritation, increased appetite, pancreatitis.
Nervous System: euphoria, insomnia, psychotic behavior, pseudotumor cerebri, seizures.
Skin: hirsutism, delayed wound healing, acne, various skin eruptions.
Other: susceptibility to infections, acute adrenal insufficiency following increased stress (infection, surgery, or trauma) or abrupt withdrawal after long-term therapy, atrophy at intramuscular injection site, cataracts, glaucoma, possible hypokalemia, growth suppression in children, hyperglycemia, and carbohydrate intolerance, muscle weakness, osteoporosis.

Onset, Peak, and Duration

Route	Onset	Peak	Duration
Oral	Rapid	2 hr	30–36 hr
I.M.	Slow	20–48 hr	Varies

Massage Considerations

- Consult with the physician before giving massage of any kind.
- This drug works as a steroid and if used long-term changes connective tissue in the body. In these cases, deep tissue massage is contraindicated and myofascial massage may not be effective and should be used with caution.
- Immunosuppression requires care in infection control. Schedule the client for the first session of the day to avoid contact with other clients. If the massage therapist has an infection, no massage should be given.
- If the drug is used short term (2 weeks or less) for allergy or inflammation, the above cautions are not generally needed.
- When the drug is given intramuscularly, no massage should be applied to the site for at least 48 hours to avoid increasing the rate of absorption.
- Side effects of thromboembolus contraindicates massage completely.
- Acne and skin eruptions are local contraindications to massage.
- Osteoporosis requires caution in depth and pressure and if severe may contraindicate massage completely.
- The best strokes for this client, if on long-term treatment with this drug, would be the mechanical strokes of gentle effleurage, pétrissage, and systemic reflex stroke of rocking. Gentle compression may also be used.

---

co-trimoxazole (sulfamethoxazole-trimethoprim)

(koh-trigh-MOX-uh-zohl)

Apo-Sulfatrim, Apo-Sulfatrim DS, Bactrim, Bacrim DS, Bactrim IV, Cotrim, Cotrim DS, Novo-Trimel, Novo-Trimel D.S., Resprim, Roubac, Septra, Septra DS, Septra-IV, Septrin, SMZ-TMP

Drug Class: Antibiotic

Drug Actions

Inhibits susceptible bacteria

Use

- Urinary tract infection
- Shigellosis
- Otitis media in patients with penicillin allergy or penicillin-resistant infections
- *Pneumocystis carinii* pneumonia
- Chronic bronchitis
- Traveler's diarrhea
- Urinary tract infections in men with prostatitis
- Chronic urinary tract infections
- Septic agranulocytosis
- *Nocardia* infection
- Pharyngeal gonococcal infections
- Chancroid
- Pertussis
- Cholera

Side Effects

Cardiovascular: thrombophlebitis.
Gastrointestinal: nausea, vomiting, diarrhea, abdominal pain, anorexia, stomatitis.
Nervous System: headache, mental depression, seizures, hallucinations, ataxia, nervousness, fatigue, vertigo, insomnia.
Urinary: toxic nephrosis with oliguria and anuria, crystalluria, hematuria.
Skin: erythema multiforme, Stevens-Johnson syndrome, generalized skin eruption, epidermal necrolysis, exfoliative dermatitis, photosensitivity, hives, itching.
Other: hypersensitivity reactions (serum sickness, drug fever, anaphylaxis), jaundice, hepatic necrosis, muscle weakness, abnormal blood profiles.

Onset, Peak, and Duration

Route	Onset	Peak	Duration
Oral	Unknown	1–4 hr	Unknown
I.V.	Immediate	Immediate	Unknown

 Massage Considerations

- There are no cautions or contraindications to massage because the client is taking this drug. There may be cautions and contraindications related to the client condition and the severity of the infection.
- Side effects of thrombophlebitis are a complete contraindication to massage.
- Any of the skin problems will locally contraindicate massage and if severe may contraindicate massage completely.

---

cyanocobalamin (vitamin B_{12}) (sigh-an-oh-koh-BAH-luh-meen)

Anacobin, Bedoz, Crystamine, Crysti 1000, Cyanocobalamin, Cyanoject, Cyomin

hydroxocobalamin (vitamin B_{12})

Hydro-Cobex, LA-12

Drug Class: Vitamin, nutrition supplement

Drug Actions

Increases vitamin B_{12} level

Use

- Vitamin B_{12} deficiency caused by inadequate diet, subtotal gastrectomy, or any other condition, disorder, or disease except malabsorption related to pernicious anemia or other gastrointestinal disease
- Pernicious anemia or vitamin B_{12} malabsorption
- Methylmalonic aciduria
- Schilling test flushing dose

Side Effects

Cardiovascular: peripheral vascular thrombosis, pulmonary edema, heart failure.
Gastrointestinal: transient diarrhea.
Skin: itching, rash, hives.
Other: anaphylaxis, anaphylactoid reactions (with parenteral administration); pain, burning (at subcutaneous or intramuscular injection sites).

Onset, Peak, and Duration

Route	Onset	Peak	Duration
Oral	Unknown	8–12 hr	Unknown
I.M.	Unknown	60 min	Unknown
S.C.	Unknown	Unknown	Unknown

 Massage Considerations

- There are no cautions or contraindications to massage for the client taking this medication.
- Because the onset, peak, and duration of the drug is unknown, when it is given intramuscularly or subcutaneously, the site of injection should not be massaged for 24 hours.
- Side effects of thrombosis contraindicate massage completely.
- Rash, hives, or itching is a local contraindication to massage.

cyclobenzaprine hydrochloride (sigh-kloh-BEN-zah-preen high-droh-KLOR-ighd)

Flexeril

Drug Class: Skeletal muscle relaxant

Drug Actions

Relieves muscle spasms

Use

- Adjunct to rest and physical therapy for relief of muscle spasm associated with acute, painful musculoskeletal conditions
- Fibrositis

Side Effects

Cardiovascular: tachycardia, arrhythmias.
Gastrointestinal: dry mouth, abdominal pain, painful digestion, abnormal taste, constipation.
Nervous System: drowsiness, euphoria, weakness, headache, insomnia, nightmares, paresthesia, dizziness, depression, visual disturbances, seizures.
Urinary: urine retention.
Skin: rash, hives, itching.
Other: blurred vision.

Onset, Peak, and Duration

Route	Onset	Peak	Duration
Oral	≤1 hr	3–8 hr	12–24 hr

 Massage Considerations

- Although the action of this drug is unclear, it does decrease the perception of sensations and pain; therefore, deep tissue massage should be used with caution.
- The effects of local reflex strokes such as compression, vibration, and stretching and traction may not be as effective. Systemic reflex strokes such as effleurage, friction, and rocking will be more effective, because massage will increase the sedating effects of this drug.
- Side effects of drowsiness require care in getting the client on and off the table. Use rapid effleurage and tapotement to stimulate the client.

- Constipation may respond well to abdominal massage.
- Rash, hives, or itching are local contraindications to massage and should be reported to the physician. If severe, massage should be withheld.
- The best strokes to use with this client are the mechanical strokes of effleurage, pétrissage, friction, and tapotement applied in a slightly more stimulating manner. The client will be relaxed but alert.

---

cyclophosphamide (sigh-kloh-FOS-fuh-mighd)

Cycloblastin, Cytoxan, Cytoxan Lyophilized, Endoxan-Asta, Neosar, Procytox

Drug Class: Antineoplastic

Drug Actions

Kills specific types of cancer cells; improves renal function in mild nephrotic syndrome in children.

Use

- Breast, head, neck, prostate, lung, and ovarian cancers
- Hodgkin's disease
- Chronic lymphocytic leukemia
- Chronic myelocytic leukemia
- Acute lymphoblastic leukemia
- Acute myelocytic leukemia
- Neuroblastoma
- Retinoblastoma
- Non-Hodgkin's lymphoma
- Multiple myeloma
- Mycosis fungoides
- Sarcoma
- "Minimal change" nephrotic syndrome in children
- Polymyositis
- Rheumatoid arthritis
- Wegener granulomatosis

Side Effects

Cardiovascular: cardiotoxicity (with very high doses and with doxorubicin).
Gastrointestinal: anorexia, nausea and vomiting beginning within 6 hours, stomatitis, mucositis.
Urinary: gonadal suppression (may be irreversible), sterile hemorrhagic cystitis, bladder fibrosis.
Skin: reversible hair loss in 50% of patients, especially with high doses.
Other: secondary malignancies, anaphylaxis, syndrome of inappropriate antidiuretic hormone (with high doses), sterility, gonadal suppression, hyperuricemia, abnormal blood profiles, pulmonary fibrosis (with high doses).

Onset, Peak, and Duration

Route	Onset	Peak	Duration
Oral, I.V.	Unknown	Unknown	Unknown

Massage Considerations

- This drug is toxic to cells; therefore, deep tissue massage should be used with great caution, if at all. Always consult with the physician before giving massage to this client.
- Circulatory massage that moves fluid through the body, such as effleurage, should be minimized to avoid overtaxing the liver and kidneys as they try to eliminate the drug from the body.
- Side effects of hair loss will contraindicate massage of the scalp, especially if the client is upset by massage causing hair loss or if scalp is tender.
- The best strokes to use with this client are the mechanical strokes of pétrissage and friction and the local reflex strokes of gentle compression, vibration, and stretching and traction. Rocking may also be used as well as myofascial techniques.

---

cycloserine (sigh-kloh-SER-een)

Seromycin

Drug Class: Antituberculotic

Drug Actions

Aids in eradicating tuberculosis

Use

- Adjunct in pulmonary or extrapulmonary tuberculosis

Side Effects

Nervous System: seizures, drowsiness, headache, tremor, dysarthria, confusion, loss of memory, possible suicidal tendencies and other psychotic symptoms, nervousness, hallucinations, depression, hyperirritability, paresthesia, paresis, hyperreflexia, coma.
Other: hypersensitivity reactions (allergic dermatitis).

Onset, Peak, and Duration

Route	Onset	Peak	Duration
Oral	Unknown	3–4 hr	Unknown

Massage Considerations

- Although the drug itself does not have any cautions or contraindications to massage, the client condition will have. Consult with the physician to see if massage will be appropriate for this client.
- Side effects of drowsiness require care in getting the client on and off the table. Stimulate the client with gentle, rapid effleurage at the end of the session.

---

cyclosporine (cyclosporin) (sigh-kloh-SPOOR-een)

Neoral, Sandimmun, Sandimmune

cyclosporine, modified

Gengraf

Drug Class: Immunosuppressant

Drug Actions

Prevents organ rejection

Use

- Prevention of organ rejection in kidney, liver, or heart transplantation
- Severe, active rheumatoid arthritis that has not adequately responded to methotrexate
- Recalcitrant, plaque psoriasis that is not adequately responsive to at least one systemic therapy or in patients for whom other systemic therapy is contraindicated or is not tolerated

Side Effects

Cardiovascular: flushing, hypertension.
Gastrointestinal: gum hyperplasia, oral thrush, nausea, vomiting, diarrhea.
Nervous System: tremor, headache, seizures.
Urinary: nephrotoxicity.
Skin: hirsutism, acne.
Other: infections, anaphylaxis, abnormal blood profiles, hepatotoxicity, sinusitis.

Onset, Peak, and Duration

Route	Onset	Peak	Duration
Oral	Unknown	$1\,^1/_2$–3 hr	Unknown
I.V.	Unknown	Unknown	Unknown

 Massage Considerations

- This drug itself does not affect how the body receives massage, however, the client condition will require cautions and contraindications for massage. Consult with the physician before doing any massage.
- This is an immunosuppressant, so take care with infection control. Schedule the client as the first session of the day to limit the client's contact with other clients. Do not massage if the massage therapist has any infection.

---

cyproheptadine hydrochloride (sigh-proh-HEP-tah-deen high-droh-KLOR-ighd)

Periactin

Drug Class: Antihistamine (H_1-receptor antagonist), antipruritic

Drug Actions

Relieves allergy symptoms and itching

Use

- Allergy symptoms
- Itching
- Cushing syndrome

Side Effects

Gastrointestinal: nausea, vomiting, epigastric distress, dry mouth.
Nervous System: drowsiness, dizziness, headache, fatigue, seizures (especially in older adult patients).
Urinary: urine retention.
Skin: rash.
Other: anaphylaxis, abnormal blood profiles, weight gain.

Onset, Peak, and Duration

Route	Onset	Peak	Duration
Oral	15–60 min	6–9 hr	8 hr

Massage Considerations

- Although the drug itself does not have any cautions or contraindications to massage, the client condition may. If the allergic response or itching is severe, massage may be completely contraindicated.
- Side effects of drowsiness require care in getting the client on and off the table. Use stimulating massage such as rapid effleurage and tapotement at the end of the session.
- Rash is a local contraindication for massage.

cytarabine (ara-C, cytosine arabinoside) (sigh-TAR-uh-been)

Cytosar, Cytosar-U

Drug Class: Antineoplastic

Drug Actions

Kills selected cancer cells

Use

- Acute nonlymphocytic leukemia
- Acute lymphocytic leukemia
- Blast phase of chronic myelocytic leukemia
- Meningeal leukemia

Side Effects

Gastrointestinal: nausea, vomiting, diarrhea, constipation, anorexia, anal ulceration, difficulty swallowing; reddened area at juncture of lips, followed by sore mouth and oral ulcers in 5 to 10 days; high dose given by rapid intravenous injection may cause projectile vomiting.
Nervous System: neurotoxicity, including ataxia and cerebellar dysfunction (with high doses).
Urinary: urate nephropathy.
Skin: rash.
Other: flu syndrome, anaphylaxis, hepatotoxicity (usually mild and reversible), hyperuricemia, keratitis, nystagmus, abnormal blood profiles.

Onset, Peak, and Duration

Route	Onset	Peak	Duration
I.V., intrathecal	Unknown	Unknown	Unknown
S.C.	Unknown	20–60 min	Unknown

Massage Considerations

- This drug is toxic to cells; therefore, deep tissue massage is contraindicated. Circulatory massages such as effleurage that move fluid through the body should be limited so as not to overtax the liver and kidneys as they try to eliminate the drug from the body.
- The physician should be consulted before giving any massage. Because the drug has a short half-life, of up to 3 hours, massage is probably best given no sooner than the next day.
- Side effects of constipation may respond well to abdominal massage. Rash is a local contraindication to massage and should be reported to the physician immediately. If severe, massage should be withheld.

- The best massage strokes for this client are the systemic reflex strokes of rocking, mechanical strokes of pétrissage and friction, and the local reflex strokes of compression, vibration, and stretching/traction. Myofascial massage may also be helpful for areas of tightness and gluteation.

---

cytomegalovirus immune globulin, intravenous (CMV-IGIV) (sigh-toh-meh-GEH-loh-VIGH-rus ih-MYOON GLOH-byoo-lin)

DTTC, DTTC-DOME

CytoGam

Drug Class: Immune globulin

Drug Actions

Provides passive immunity to cytomegalovirus (CMV)

Use

- To attenuate primary CMV disease in seronegative kidney transplant recipients who receive a kidney from a CMV-seropositive donor
- Prophylaxis of CMV disease related to lung, liver, pancreas, and heart transplants

Side Effects

Cardiovascular: flushing, hypotension.
Gastrointestinal: nausea, vomiting.
Nervous System: fever.
Other: anaphylaxis, chills, muscle cramps, back pain, wheezing.

Onset, Peak, and Duration

Route	Onset	Peak	Duration
I.V.	Unknown	Unknown	Unknown

Massage Considerations

- Although the drug itself does not have cautions or contraindications for massage, the client condition will have serious implications and may even contraindicate massage completely. Always consult the physician before doing any massage.
- Side effects of hypotension require care in getting the client on and off the table. Use stimulation at the end of the session with gentle tapotement.

D

---

dacarbazine (DTIC) (deh-KAR-buh-zeen)

DTIC, DTIC-DOME

Drug Class: Antineoplastic

Drug Actions

Kills selected cancer cells

Use

- Metastatic malignant melanoma
- Hodgkin's disease

Side Effects

Gastrointestinal: severe nausea and vomiting, anorexia
Skin: hair loss, phototoxicity.
Other: flulike syndrome (fever, malaise, myalgia beginning 7 days after treatment and possibly lasting 7 to 21 days), anaphylaxis, severe pain with concentrated solution or extravasation, tissue damage, leukopenia, thrombocytopenia, hyperuricemia.

Onset, Peak, and Duration

Route	Onset	Peak	Duration
I.V.	Unknown	Unknown	Unknown

Massage Considerations

- As a result of the toxic nature of this drug, deep tissue massage would be contraindicated.
- Other cautions will depend on the client's condition. Close contact and coordination of care with the physician are essential.
- Although onset, peak, and duration of action are not clearly known, half-life takes about 5 hours. The drug is often given daily initially then every 4 weeks. In order not to tax the kidneys and liver as they try to rid the body of this drug, circulatory massage should not be given on the days the client is receiving the drug.
- The side effect of hair loss would contraindicate scalp massage, if the client is upset by hair coming out during massage or if the scalp is tender.
- The best strokes and types of massage would be systemic reflex strokes such as rocking and gentle friction. Mechanical strokes such as pétrissage and local reflex strokes such as gentle compression and vibration also may be used. Myofascial techniques may be helpful for areas of gluteation and muscle knotting.

---

daclizumab (da-KLIZ-yoo-mab)

Zenapax

Drug Class: Immunosuppressant

Drug Actions

Prevents organ rejection

Use

- Prevention of acute organ rejection in patients receiving renal transplants with an immunosuppressive regimen that includes cyclosporine and corticosteroids

Side Effects

Cardiovascular: tachycardia, hypertension, hypotension, aggravated hypertension, edema, fluid overload, chest pain.
Gastrointestinal: constipation, nausea, diarrhea, vomiting, abdominal pain, painful digestion, heartburn, abdominal distention, epigastric pain, gas, gastritis, hemorrhoids.
Nervous System: tremors, headache, dizziness, insomnia, generalized weakness, prickly sensation, fever, pain, fatigue, depression, anxiety.
Skin: acne, impaired wound healing without infection, itching, abnormal hair growth, rash, night sweats, increased sweating.

Urinary: lack of urination, painful urination, renal tubular necrosis, renal damage, urine retention, hydronephrosis, urinary tract bleeding, urinary tract disorder, renal insufficiency. *Other:* lymphocele, bleeding, diabetes mellitus, dehydration, musculoskeletal or back pain, joint pain, muscle pain, leg cramps, shortness of breath, coughing, atelectasis, congestion, hypoxia, rales, abnormal breath sounds, pleural effusion, pulmonary edema.

Onset, Peak, and Duration

Route	Onset	Peak	Duration
I.V.	Unknown	Unknown	Unknown

Massage Considerations

- Because this drug suppresses the immune system, it does not affect how the body receives and reacts to massage. Any cautions or contraindications will depend on the client condition. Close contact and coordination with the physician will be essential.
- If massage is approved by the physician, it is important to limit the exposure of the client to others. Scheduling as the first client of the day and not doing massage if the massage therapist has any infection will help.
- Side effects of concern are hypotension and dizziness. Using rapid effleurage and tapotement at the end of the session and taking care in getting the client on and off the table will help prevent problems. Constipation and gas may respond well to regular abdominal massage. Itching or rash are local contraindications to massage and should be reported to the physician immediately. If severe, they may contraindicate massage completely.
- All strokes and types of massage may be utilized for this client as long as the client condition does not contraindicate it and the physician is in agreement.

dalteparin sodium (dal-TEH-peh-rin SOH-dee-um)

Fragmin

Drug Class: Anticoagulant

Drug Actions

Prevents blood clotting and deep vein thrombosis

Use

- Prevention of deep vein thrombosis (DVT) in patients undergoing abdominal or hip replacement surgery who are at risk for thromboembolism
- To decrease risk of thromboembolism in patients with severely restricted mobility
- Unstable angina
- Non-Q wave heart attack

Side Effects

Nervous System: fever.
Skin: itching, bruising, rash.
Other: anaphylaxis, hematoma at injection site (when given with heparin), pain at injection site, hemorrhage, bleeding complications, thrombocytopenia.

Onset, Peak, and Duration

Route	Onset	Peak	Duration
S.C.	Unknown	4 hr	Unknown

Massage Considerations

- In the presence of an actual blood clot, massage would be contraindicated completely. When the drug is used for prevention, deep tissue massage is contraindicated and circulatory massage with effleurage should be limited or not used at all. Physician approval for massage should be obtained and the client condition may require other cautions and contraindications.
- The site of injection of the drug should not be massaged for at least 4 hours after the drug is given to avoid speeding up the absorption of the drug.
- The side effects of itching, bruising, and rash are local contraindications to massage and should be reported to the physician immediately. If severe, massage may be completely contraindicated.
- The best strokes to use will be the mechanical strokes of gentle pétrissage, local reflex strokes of stretching, vibration, and gentle friction and systemic reflex strokes of rocking and shaking.

---

dantrolene sodium (DAN-troh-leen SOH-dee-um)

Dantrium, Dantrium Intravenous

Drug Class: Skeletal muscle relaxant

Drug Actions

Acts directly on skeletal muscle to interfere with intracellular calcium movement. Relieves muscle spasms.

Use

- Spasticity from severe chronic disorders (such as multiple sclerosis, cerebral palsy, spinal cord injury, stroke)
- Management of malignant hyperthermic crisis
- Prevention or attenuation of malignant hyperthermia in susceptible patients who need surgery
- Prevention of recurrence of malignant hyperthermia
- To reduce succinylcholine-induced muscle fasciculations and postoperative muscle pain

Side Effects

Cardiovascular: tachycardia, blood pressure changes.
Gastrointestinal: anorexia, constipation, cramping, difficulty swallowing, metallic taste, severe diarrhea, drooling, bleeding.
Nervous System: muscle weakness, drowsiness, dizziness, light-headedness, malaise, headache, confusion, nervousness, insomnia, hallucinations, seizures, fever.
Urinary: urinary frequency, hematuria, incontinence, increased urination at night, painful urination, crystalluria, difficulty achieving erection.
Skin: sweating, abnormal hair growth, rash, itching, hives photosensitivity.
Other: chills, excessive tearing, auditory or visual disturbances, hepatitis, painful muscles, pleural effusion.

Onset, Peak, and Duration

Route	Onset	Peak	Duration
oral	≤1 week	5 hr	Unknown
I.V.	Unknown	Unknown	Unknown

Massage Considerations

- Although there are no cautions or contraindications to massage for the client taking this drug, the action of the drug on the muscle tonus may make the local reflex strokes such as stretching, traction, and vibration less effective.
- The side effects of blood pressure changes, dizziness, drowsiness and light-headedness require care in getting the client on and off the table. Rapid effleurage and tapotement may be used at the end of the session to stimulate the client. If these side effects are severe, giving a more stimulating massage throughout the session may be helpful.
- Constipation may be helped by regular abdominal massage. Frequent urination may require the client to get up during the massage. Allowing privacy and quick access to the bathroom and avoiding use of water fountains and music that could stimulate the need to urinate is the best way to approach this concern. Rash, itching, or hives are local contraindications to massage and should be reported to the physician immediately. If severe, they may contraindicate massage completely.
- The best strokes to use with this client are the mechanical strokes of effleurage, pétrissage and friction. Myofascial massage may be helpful for areas of tightness. Deep tissue massage may not be as effective but can be utilized if the client condition warrants it. Trigger point massage also may not be as effective but may be utilized.

---

dapsone (DDS) (DAP-sohn)

Avlosulfon, Dapsone 100

Drug Class: Antileprotic, antimalarial

Drug Actions

Hinders or kills selected bacteria

Use

- Multibacillary leprosy
- Paucibacillary leprosy
- Dermatitis herpetiformis.
- Malaria suppression or prophylaxis
- *Pneumocystis carinii* pneumonia
- Prophylaxis of *P. carinii* pneumonia
- Prophylaxis of toxoplasmosis in HIV-infected patients

Side Effects

Cardiovascular: tachycardia.
Gastrointestinal: anorexia, abdominal pain, pancreatitis, nausea, vomiting.
Nervous System: fever, insomnia, psychosis, headache, dizziness, lethargy, severe malaise, paresthesia, peripheral neuropathy, vertigo.
Urinary: albuminuria, nephrotic syndrome, renal papillary necrosis, male infertility.
Skin: lupus erythematosus, phototoxicity, variety of skin rashes, hives.
Other: infectious mononucleosis-like syndrome, sulfone syndrome, lymphadenopathy, ringing in the ears, blurred vision, allergic rhinitis, abnormal blood profiles, hepatitis, cholestatic jaundice, pulmonary eosinophilia.

Onset, Peak, and Duration

Route	Onset	Peak	Duration
Oral	Unknown	4–8 hr	Unknown

Massage Considerations

- The drug itself does not have any cautions or contraindications for massage. The client condition and severity of infection may contraindicate massage.
- Side effects of dizziness, lethargy, and vertigo require care in getting the client on and off the table. Using rapid effleurage and tapotement at the end of the session may prevent problems. Rash or hives of any kind should be reported to the physician and massage should be withheld.
- All strokes and massage techniques may be used with this client depending on the client condition.

---

daptomycin (dap-toh-MY-sin)

Cubicin

Drug Class: Antibiotic

Drug Actions

Kills bacteria in susceptible organisms

Use

- Complicated skin and skin structure infections

Side Effects

Cardiovascular: heart failure, chest pain, edema, hypertension, hypotension.
Gastrointestinal: abdominal pain, constipation, decreased appetite, diarrhea, nausea, pseudomembranous colitis, vomiting.
Nervous System: anxiety, confusion, dizziness, fever, headache, insomnia.
Urinary: renal failure, urinary tract infection.
Skin: cellulitis, itching, rash.
Other: injection site reactions, fungal infections, anemia, hyperglycemia, hypoglycemia, hypokalemia, limb and back pain, cough, shortness of breath.

Onset, Peak, and Duration

Route	Onset	Peak	Duration
I.V.	Rapid	<1 hr	Unknown

Massage Considerations

- Although the drug does not have any cautions or contraindications for massage, the client condition in most cases will contraindicate massage because of the severity of the infection and in all cases, the area of infection is contraindicated for massage at the site and above and below it.
- Side effects of dizziness and hypotension require care in moving and positioning the client. Using effleurage and tapotement at the end of the session may help. Constipation may be helped by regular abdominal massage. Any itching or rash will locally contraindicate massage and if severe, no massage should be given.
- The best strokes to utilize with this client will be systemic reflex and local reflex strokes such as rocking, gentle compression, vibration, and gentle friction. Effleurage may be used in areas not affected by infection but should be limited in use.

darbepoetin alfa (dar-be-POE-e-tin AL-fa)

Aranesp

Drug Class: Hematopoietic

Drug Actions

Increases RBC production and corrects anemia in patients with chronic renal impairment.

Use

- Anemia related to chronic renal failure (CRF) for patient on or off dialysis
- Anemia related to chemotherapy in patients with nonmyeloid malignancies

Side Effects

Cardiovascular: hypertension, hypotension, cardiac arrhythmia, cardiac arrest, angina, heart failure, thrombosis, edema, chest pain, fluid overload, acute heart attack.
Gastrointestinal: diarrhea, vomiting, nausea, abdominal pain, constipation.
Nervous System: headache, dizziness, fatigue, fever, asthenia, seizures.
Skin: hemorrhage at access site, itching, rash.
Other: infection, flulike symptoms, dehydration, muscle pain, joint pain, limb pain, back pain, upper respiratory tract infection, shortness of breath, cough, bronchitis, pneumonia, pulmonary embolism.

Onset, Peak, and Duration

Route	Onset	Peak	Duration
I.V.	Unknown	Unknown	21 hr
S.C.	Unknown	34 hr	49 hr

Massage Considerations

- Deep tissue massage is contraindicated for the client taking this drug. There may be other cautions and contraindications related to the client condition and the physician should be consulted before any massage is given.
- The site of S.C. (subcutaneous) injection should not be massaged for at least 2 days to avoid increasing the rate of absorption. Because the drug is usually given once weekly, scheduling the massage between injections will take care of this problem.
- Side effects of hypotension and dizziness require care in getting the client on and off the table. Using rapid effleurage at the end of the session will help. Tapotement should be used with caution. Constipation may be helped by regular abdominal massage. Itching and rash are local contraindications for massge and should be reported to the physician immediately. If severe, massage should be withheld.

daunorubicin citrate liposomal (daw-noh-roo-BYE-sin SIH-trayt li-po-SOE-mul)

DaunoXome

Drug Class: Antineoplastic

Drug Actions

Decreases tumor growth for advanced HIV-related Kaposi's sarcoma

Use

- First-line cytotoxic therapy for advanced HIV-related Kaposi's sarcoma

Side Effects

Cardiovascular: cardiomyopathy, chest pain, hypertension, palpitations, arrhythmias, pericardial effusion, cardiac tamponade, cardiac arrest, angina pectoris, pulmonary hypertension, flushing, edema, tachycardia, MI.
EENT: rhinitis, sinusitis, abnormal vision, conjunctivitis, tinnitus, eye pain, deafness, taste disturbances, earache, gingival bleeding, tooth caries, dry mouth.
Gastrointestinal: nausea, diarrhea, abdominal pain, vomiting, anorexia, constipation, GI hemorrhage, gastritis, dysphagia, stomatitis, increased appetite, melena, hemorrhoids, tenesmus.
Nervous System: fever, headache, neuropathy, depression, dizziness, insomnia, amnesia, anxiety, ataxia, confusion, seizures, hallucinations, tremor, hypertonia, meningitis, fatigue, malaise, emotional lability, abnormal gait, hyperkinesia, somnolence, abnormal thinking, syncope.
Urinary: painful urination, increased urination at night, frequent urination.
Skin: hair loss, itching, increased sweating, dry skin, seborrhea, folliculitis.
Other: opportunistic infections, allergic reactions, flulike symptoms, thirst, injection site inflammation, rhinitis, sinusitis, abnormal vision, conjunctivitis, tinnitus, eye pain, deafness, taste disturbances, earache, gingival bleeding, tooth caries, dry mouth, neutropenia, splenomegaly, lymphadenopathy, hepatomegaly, dehydration, rigors, back pain, joint pain, muscle pain, cough, shortness of breath, rhinitis, hemoptysis, hiccups, pulmonary infiltration, increased sputum.

Onset, Peak, and Duration

Route	Onset	Peak	Duration
I.V.	Unknown	Unknown	Unknown

Massage Considerations

- This drug is used for Kaposi's sarcoma, a cancer of the blood vessel walls. This condition is a complete contraindication to massage. No manipulation of soft tissue should be performed.

daunorubicin hydrochloride (daw-noh-ROO-buh-sin high-droh-KLOR-ighd)

Cerubidine

Drug Class: Antineoplastic

Drug Actions

Kills selected cancer cells

Use

- Remission induction in acute nonlymphocytic (myelogenous, monocytic, erythroid) leukemia
- Remission induction in acute lymphocytic leukemia

Side Effects

Cardiovascular: irreversible cardiomyopathy, electrocardiogram changes, arrhythmias, pericarditis, myocarditis.
Gastrointestinal: nausea, vomiting, stomatitis, esophagitis, anorexia, diarrhea.
Nervous System: fever.
Urinary: red urine.

Skin: rash, pigmentation of fingernails and toenails, generalized hair loss, tissue sloughing with extravasation.
Other: severe cellulitis, chills, anaphylaxis, bone marrow suppression, hepatotoxicity, hyperuricemia.

Onset, Peak, and Duration

Route	Onset	Peak	Duration
I.V.	Unknown	Unknown	Unknown

 Massage Considerations

- Because of the toxic effects of this drug, deep tissue massage is contraindicated.
- Circulatory massage with effleurage should be used with caution. The physician approval should be obtained prior to massage being given and close collaboration is essential.
- This drug is given anywhere from daily to weekly and peak duration of action is unknown. The half-life is over 18 hours. If would be best to not give massage on the day the drug is given. If given daily and massage is given, limit or do not use circulatory massage to avoid overtaxing the liver and kidneys as they work to clear the drug from the body.
- Side effects of rash are a local contraindication to massage and should be reported to the physician immediately. If severe, massage should be withheld. Hair loss will contraindicate scalp massage and may contraindicate massage completely in the male when hair loss is widespread in the body especially if the client is disturbed by it or there is tenderness with the hair loss.
- The best strokes to utilize for this client are the systemic reflex strokes of rocking, local reflex strokes of stretching, traction and gentle friction and compression, and the mechanical strokes of pétrissage. Myofascial massage may be used for areas of tightness.

delavirdine mesylate (deh-luh-VEER-deen MES-ih-layt)

Rescriptor

Drug Class: Antiviral

Drug Actions

Inhibits HIV replication

Use

- HIV-1 infection

Side Effects

Gastrointestinal: nausea, vomiting, diarrhea, abdominal pain (generalized or localized).
Nervous System: weakness, fatigue, headache, anxiety, depression, insomnia, fever, localized pain.
Skin: rash.
Other: flu syndrome, pharyngitis, sinusitis, upper respiratory tract infection, bronchitis, cough.

Onset, Peak, and Duration

Route	Onset	Peak	Duration
Oral	Unknown	1 hr	Unknown

Massage Considerations

- There are no cautions or contraindications to massage related to this drug. There may be cautions or contraindications to massage related to the client condition.
- The side effect of rash is a local contraindication to massage and should be reported to the physician immediately. If severe, massage should be withheld.

---

desipramine hydrochloride (deh-SIP-rah-meen high-droh-KLOR-ighd)

Norpramin

Drug Class: Dibenzazepine tricyclic antidepressant (TCA)

Drug Actions

May increase amount of norepinephrine, serotonin, or both in the CNS by blocking their reuptake by neurons. Relieves depression.

Use

- Depression

Side Effects

Cardiovascular: orthostatic hypotension, tachycardia, ECG changes, hypertension.
Gastrointestinal: dry mouth, constipation, nausea, vomiting, anorexia, paralytic ileus.
Nervous System: drowsiness, dizziness, excitation, tremors, weakness, confusion, headache, nervousness, EEG changes, seizures, extrapyramidal reactions.
Urinary: urine retention.
Skin: rash, hives, sweating, photosensitivity.
Other: sudden death, hypersensitivity reaction,blurred vision, ringing in the ears, dilated pupils.

Onset, Peak, and Duration

Route	Onset	Peak	Duration
Oral	2–4 wk	4–6 hr	Unknown

Massage Considerations

- There are no cautions or contraindications to massage related to this drug. The client condition may warrant cautions or contraindications.
- Side effects of dizziness, drowsiness or hypotension require care in getting the client on and off the table. Using rapid effleurage and tapotement at the end of the session may help. If the side effect is severe, using more rapid strokes and a more stimulating massage throughout the session may alleviate any problems. Constipation may be helped by regular abdominal massage. Rash or hives are a local contraindication to massage and should be reported to the physician immediately. If severe, massage should be withheld.

---

desloratadine (des-lor-AT-a-deen)

Clarinex, Clarinex Reditabs

Drug Class: Antihistamine

Drug Actions

Relieves allergy symptoms

Use

- Relief of nasal and nonnasal symptoms of allergic rhinitis (seasonal and perennial)
- Symptomatic relief of itching and reduction in the number and size of hives in patients with chronic idiopathic hives

Side Effects

Cardiovascular: tachycardia.
Gastrointestinal: nausea, dry mouth, painful digestion.
Nervous System: headache, sleepiness, fatigue, dizziness.
Other: flulike symptoms, hypersensitivity reaction (including rash, edema, or anaphylaxis), painful menstruation, pharyngitis, muscle pain.

Onset, Peak, and Duration

Route	Onset	Peak	Duration
Oral	Unknown	3 hr	Unknown
Orally disintegrating	Unknown	2.5–4 hours	Unknown

 Massage Considerations

- There are no cautions or contraindications to massage for the client taking this medication.
- Side effects of sleepiness and dizziness require care in getting the client on and off the table. Using rapid effleurage and tapotement at the end of the session will help prevent problems.

---

desmopressin acetate (dez-moh-PREH-sin AS-ih-tayt)

DDAVP, Stimate

Drug Class: Posterior pituitary hormone

Drug Actions

Decreases urination and promotes clotting

Use

- Nonnephrogenic diabetes insipidus
- Temporary polyuria, and polydipsia from pituitary trauma
- Hemophilia A
- Von Willebrand's disease
- Primary nocturnal enuresis (bedwetting)

Side Effects

Cardiovascular: slight rise in blood pressure.
Gastrointestinal: nausea, abdominal cramps.
Nervous System: headache.
Urinary: vulvar pain.
Other: flushing, local redness, swelling or burning after injection, nasal congestion, rhinitis, epistaxis, sore throat, cough.

Onset, Peak, and Duration

Route	Onset	Peak	Duration
Oral	1 hr	4–7 hr	8–12 hr
I.V.	15–30 min	1.5–2 hr	4–12 hr
Subcutaneous injection	Unknown	Unknown	Unknown
Nasal spray	≤1 hr	1–5 hr	8–12 hr

 Massage Considerations

- Circulatory massage with effleurage should be used with caution and limited in use for clients taking this drug for diabetes insipidus or polyuria. There are no cautions or contraindications to massage otherwise.
- The site of subcutaneous injection should be avoided and no massage given to the area for at least 24 hours.
- Side effects of redness at the site of injection is a local contraindication to massage until it is resolved. If severe, the physician should be notified and massage withheld.
- All massage strokes and techniques may be used except as noted earlier.

dexamethasone (deks-ah-METH-uh-sohn)

Decadron, DexaMeth, Dexamethasone Intensol, Dexasone, Dexone 0.5, Dexone 0.75, Dexone 1.5, Dexone 4, Hexadrol, Mymethasone, Oradexon

dexamethasone acetate

Cortostat LA, Dalalone D.P., Decaject-L.A., Dexasone-L.A., Dexone L.A., Solurex-LA

dexamethasone sodium phosphate

AK-Dex, Cortastat, Cortastat 10, Dalalone, Decadrol, Decadron Phosphate, Decaject, Dexacen-4, Dexacorten, Dexone, Hexadrol Phosphate, Primethasone, Solurex

Drug Class: Glucocorticoid anti-inflammatory, immunosuppressant

Drug Actions

Relieves cerebral edema, reduces inflammation and immune response, and reverses shock

Use

- Cerebral edema
- Inflammatory conditions
- Allergic reactions
- Neoplasias
- Shock
- Dexamethasone suppression test for Cushing's syndrome
- Prevention of hyaline membrane disease in premature infants
- Prevention of chemotherapy-induced nausea and vomiting

Side Effects

Cardiovascular: heart failure, hypertension, edema, arrhythmias, thromboembolism.
Gastrointestinal: peptic ulceration, GI irritation, increased appetite, pancreatitis.
Nervous System: euphoria, insomnia, psychotic behavior, pseudotumor cerebri, seizures.

Skin: abnormal hair growth, delayed wound healing, acne, skin eruptions, atrophy at I.M. injection sites.
Other: cushingoid state (moonface, buffalo hump, central obesity), susceptibility to infections, acute adrenal insufficiency may follow increased stress (infection, surgery, or trauma) or abrupt withdrawal after long-term therapy, menstrual irregularities, hypokalemia, hyperglycemia, carbohydrate intolerance,muscle weakness, osteoporosis, growth suppression in children, cataracts, glaucoma.

Onset, Peak, and Duration

Route	Onset	Peak	Duration
Oral	1–2 hr	1–2 hr	2.5 days
I.V., I.M.	≤1 hr	1 hr	2 days–3 wk

 Massage Considerations

- Clients taking this drug for longer than two weeks will have changes in metabolism and in connective tissue. Deep tissue massage is contraindicated. The changes in connective tissue may make mysofascial massage techniques less effective. They should be used with caution until client response is determined. Further cautions and contraindications may be indicated by the client condition.
- Side effect of thromboembolism contraindicates massage completely. If redness, swelling, heat, or pain is present especially in the lower extremities, massage should be withheld until the physician can evaluate the client. The side effect of osteoporosis, if severe, may contraindicate massage completely. Consult with the physician to determine safety. The side effect of acne or skin eruptions is a local contraindication to massage. If the condition is severe and the client still wishes massage, using gloves during the massage will protect the massage therapist and client from possible contact with blood and body fluids.
- This drug may prevent the client from relaxing into the massage easily. The best approach is to utilize the systemic reflex strokes of gentle rocking and slow and rhythmic effleurage. These may need to be applied for a longer period of time than usual to achieve the desired relaxation. The mechanical strokes of pétrissage and local reflex stroke of vibration may also be effective.

dexmedetomidine hydrochloride (DEX-meh-dih-TOE-mih-deen high-droh-KLOR-ighd)

Precedex

Drug Class: Sedative

Drug Actions

Produces sedation of initially intubated and mechanically ventilated patients

Use

- Sedation of initially intubated and mechanically ventilated patients in ICU setting

Side Effects

Cardiovascular: hypotension, bradycardia, arrhythmias.
Gastrointestinal: nausea, thirst.
Nervous System: pain.
Urinary: oliguria.
Other: infection, anemia, leukocytosis, hypoxia, pleural effusion, pulmonary edema.

Onset, Peak, and Duration

Route	Onset	Peak	Duration
I.V.	Unknown	Unknown	Unknown

 Massage Considerations

- The sedation of this drug and the severity of the client condition contraindicates massage completely.
- If the client is intubated for a long period for chronic disorders and massage is desired, deep tissue massage would be contraindicated.
- Gentle, rythmic effleurage, and pétrissage would be the best strokes to apply.

dexmethylphenidate hydrochloride (dex-meth-il-FEN-uh-date high-droh-KLOR-ighd)

Focalin

Drug Class: CNS stimulant

Drug Actions

May block presynaptic reuptake of norepinephrine and dopamine and increase the release of these neurotransmitters. Increases attention span and decreases hyperactivity and impulsiveness related to ADHD.

Use

- Attention deficit hyperactivity disorder (ADHD)

Side Effects

Cardiovascular: tachycardia, hypertension.
Gastrointestinal: anorexia, abdominal pain, nausea.
Nervous System: fever, insomnia, nervousness, growth suppression, psychosis, blurred vision.
Other: leukopenia, anemia, weight loss, twitching (motor or vocal tics), joint pain.

Onset, Peak, and Duration

Route	Onset	Peak	Duration
Oral	Unknown	1–1.5 hr	Unknown

Massage Considerations

- There are no cautions or contraindications for massage related to the client taking this drug.
- The action of the drug in stimulating the CNS may make systemic reflex strokes less effective and it may take more time to relax the client. Applying rocking for longer periods of time especially at the beginning of the massage and using slow, rythmic effleurage will help to ameliorate this effect. The mechanical strokes of pétrissage, and friction may also be effective. Deep tissue massage and local reflex strokes such as compression, and stretching may not be as effective. Myofascial massage may be helpful for areas of tightness and gluteation.

dextroamphetamine sulfate (deks-troh-am-FET-uh-meen SUL-fayt)

Dexedrine, Dexedrine Spansule, Dextrostat, Ferndex, Osydess II, Spancap #1

Drug Class: Amphetamine CNS stimulant

Drug Actions

Helps prevent sleep and calms hyperactive children

Use

- Narcolepsy
- Attention deficit hyperactivity disorder (ADHD)
- Short-term adjunct in exogenous obesity

Side Effects

Cardiovascular: tachycardia, palpitations, hypertension, arrhythmias.
Gastrointestinal: dry mouth, unpleasant taste, diarrhea, constipation, anorexia, weight loss, and other G.I. disturbances.
Nervous System: restlessness, tremors, insomnia, dizziness, headache, overstimulation, dysphoria.
Urinary: impotence.
Skin: hives.
Other: altered libido, chills.

Onset, Peak, and Duration

Route	Onset	Peak	Duration
Oral	Unknown	Unknown	Unknown

Massage Considerations

- There are no cautions or contraindication to massage for the client taking this drug.
- The action of the drug in stimulating the CNS may make the systemic reflex strokes such as rocking and effleurage less effective. The relaxation effect of massage may be more difficult to achieve. The local reflex strokes of stretching, compression, and vibration as well as deep tissue massage may be less effective.
- Side effects of dizziness require care in getting the client on and off the table. Because the CNS is already stimulated, tapotement should be avoided. Talking with the client and stimulating the lower extremities with friction may be helpful. Rash is a local contraindication to massage and should be reported to the physician immediately. If severe, massage should be withheld.
- The best approach to massage is to use the systemic reflex strokes for longer periods at the beginning of the massage. Rocking and rythmic effleurage may be applied. Using mechanical strokes such as pétrissage, and friction and applying local reflex strokes of compression for longer periods will help to relax the muscles. Myofascial massage techniques may be helpful for areas of tightness and gluteation.

---

dextromethorphan hydrobromide (deks-troh-meth-OR-fan high-droh-BROH-mighd)

Balminil D.M., Benylin DM, Broncho-Grippol-DM, Children's Hold, DexAlone, Hold, Koffex, Pertussin Cough Suppressant, Pertussin CS, Pertussin ES, Robitussin Pediatric, St. Joseph Cough Suppressant for Children, Sucrets Cough Control Formula, Trocal, Vicks Formula 44 Pediatric Formula
More commonly available in combination products such as: Anti-Tuss DM Expectorant, Cheracol D Cough, Extra Action Cough, Glycotuss DM, Guiamid D.M. Liquid, Guiatuss-DM, Halotussin-DM Expectorant, Kolephrin GG/DM, Mytussin DM,

Naldecon Senior DX, Pertussin All-Night CS, Rhinosyn-DMX Expectorant, Robitussin-DM, Silexin Cough, Tolu-Sed DM, Tuss-DM, Unproco, Vicks Children's Cough Syrup, Vicks Dayquill Liquicaps

Drug Class: Antitussive (nonnarcotic)

Drug Actions

Suppresses cough reflex by direct action on cough center in medulla.

Use

- Nonproductive cough

Side Effects

Gastrointestinal: nausea, vomiting, stomach pain.
Nervous System: drowsiness, dizziness.

Onset, Peak, and Duration

Route	Onset	Peak	Duration
Oral	≤30 min	Unknown	3–12 hr

Massage Considerations

- There are no cautions or contraindications to massage for the client taking this drug.
- Side effects of dizziness and drowsiness require care in getting the client on and off the table. Using rapid effleurage and tapotement at the end of the session may help.
- All strokes and massage techniques may be used with this client.

diazepam (digh-AZ-uh-pam)

Diastat, Apo-Diazepam, Diazemuls, Diazepam Intensol, Novo-Dipam, PMS-Diazepam, Valium, Vivol

Drug Class: Benzodiazepine anxiolytic, skeletal muscle relaxant, anticonvulsant, sedative-hypnotic

Drug Actions

Probably depresses CNS at limbic and subcortical levels of brain. Relieves anxiety, muscle spasms, and seizures (parenteral form); promotes calmness and sleep.

Use

- Anxiety
- Acute alcohol withdrawal
- Before endoscopic procedures
- Muscle spasm
- Preoperative sedation
- Cardioversion
- Adjunct in seizure disorders
- Status epilepticus
- Control of acute repetitive seizure activity in patients already taking anticonvulsants

Side Effects

Cardiovascular: transient hypotension, bradycardia, cardiovascular collapse.
Gastrointestinal: nausea, vomiting, abdominal discomfort, constipation.

Nervous System: pain, drowsiness, lethargy, hangover, ataxia, fainting, depression, restlessness, anterograde amnesia, psychosis, slurred speech, tremors, headache, insomnia.
Urinary: incontinence, urine retention.
Skin: rash, hives, peeling.
Other: physical or psychological dependence, acute withdrawal syndrome after sudden discontinuation in physically dependent people, phlebitis at injection site, double vision, blurred vision, nystagmus, respiratory depression.

Onset, Peak, and Duration

Route	Onset	Peak	Duration
Oral	30 min	.5–2 hr	3–8 hr
I.V.	1–5 min	≤15 min	15–60 min
I.M.	Unknown	2 hr	Unknown
Rectal	Unknown	1–5 hr	Unknown

 Massage Considerations

- Because this drug suppresses the CNS, deep tissue massage is contraindicated. Local reflex strokes such as compression, stretching and vibration may be less effective as well.
- Systemic reflex strokes such as rocking and effleurage may be more effective, putting the client quickly in a relaxed state.
- Other cautions or contraindications may exist related to the client condition.
- Side effects of hypotension, drowsiness, and dizziness require care in getting the client on and off the table. Using rapid effleurage, more stimulating application of massage and tapotement either at the end of the massage or throughout the session will help prevent problems. Constipation may be helped by regular abdominal massage. Rash, hives, or peeling are a local contraindication to massage and should be reported to the physician immediately. If severe, massage should be withheld.

diazoxide (digh-uz-OKS-ighd)

Hyperstat IV, Proglycem

Drug Class: Antihypertensive

Drug Actions

Directly relaxes arteriolar smooth muscle and decreases peripheral vascular resistance. Increases glucose levels by inhibiting pancreatic release of insulin, stimulating catecholamine release or increasing hepatic release of glucose. Lowers blood pressure; increases blood sugar.

Use

- Hypertensive crisis
- Hypoglycemia from hyperinsulinism

Side Effects

Cardiovascular: orthostatic hypotension, flushing, warmth, angina, myocardial ischemia, arrhythmias, ECG changes, shock, heart attack.
Gastrointestinal: nausea, vomiting, abdominal discomfort, dry mouth, constipation, diarrhea.
Nervous System: headache, dizziness, light-headedness, euphoria, cerebral ischemia, paralysis.

Skin: sweating.
Other: inflammation, pain (with extravasation), thrombocytopenia, sodium and water retention, hyperglycemia, hyperuricemia.

Onset, Peak, and Duration

Route	Onset	Peak	Duration
Oral	≤1 hr	Unknown	<8 hr
I.V.	≤1 min	2–5 min	2–12 hr

 Massage Considerations

- There are no cautions or contraindication to massage just because the client taking this medication. The client condition, in many cases, will contraindicate massage. Consult the physician before any massage is given.
- Side effects of dizziness, lightheadedness, and hypotension may be strong as massage may increase the effects of the medication. Using a more stimulating massage throughout the session with rapid effleurage and pétrissage as well as tapotement is indicated.
- Constipation may be helped by regular abdominal massage.

---

diclofenac potassium (digh-KLOH-fen-ek poh-TAH-see-um)

Cataflam

diclofenac sodium

Solaraze, Voltaren, Voltaren SR, Voltaren-XR

Drug Class: Nonsteroidal anti-inflammatory drug (NSAID) antiarthritic, anti-inflammatory

Drug Actions

Produces anti-inflammatory, analgesic, and antipyretic effects, possibly by inhibiting prostaglandin synthesis.

Use

- Ankylosing spondylitis
- Osteoarthritis
- Rheumatoid arthritis
- Analgesia and primary dysmenorrhea
- Actinic keratosis

Side Effects

Cardiovascular: heart failure, hypertension, edema, fluid retention.
Gastrointestinal: taste disorder, abdominal pain or cramps, constipation, diarrhea, indigestion, nausea, abdominal distention, gas, peptic ulceration, bleeding, melena, bloody diarrhea, appetite change, colitis.
Nervous System: anxiety, depression, dizziness, drowsiness, insomnia, irritability, myoclonus, migraine, headache.
Urinary: azotemia, proteinuria, acute renal failure, oliguria, interstitial nephritis, papillary necrosis, nephrotic syndrome, fluid retention.
Skin: rash, itching, hives, eczema, dermatitis, hair loss, photosensitivity, bullous eruption, Stevens-Johnson syndrome, allergic purpura.

Other: anaphylaxis, angioedema, ringing in the ears, laryngeal edema, swelling of lips and tongue, blurred vision, eye pain, night blindness, epistaxis, reversible hearing loss, jaundice, hepatitis, hepatotoxicity, hypoglycemia, hyperglycemia, back, leg, or joint pain, asthma.

Onset, Peak, and Duration

Route	Onset	Peak	Duration
Oral or rectal	30 min	Unknown	8 hr
Oral enteric-coated	30 min	2–3 hr	8 hr

 Massage Considerations

- This drug decreases the perception of pain; therefore, deep tissue massage should be used with caution. There are no other cautions or contraindications to massage related to the client taking this drug. There may, however, be cautions or contraindications related to the client condition.
- Side effects of dizziness and drowsiness require care in getting the client on and off the table. Using rapid effleurage and tapotement at the end of the session will help.
- Constipation and gas may be helped by regular abdominal massage. Rash, hives, or itching of any kind is a local contraindication for massage and should be reported to the physician immediately. If severe, massage should be withheld.

---

dicyclomine hydrochloride (digh-SIGH-kloh-meen high-droh-KLOR-ighd)

Antispas, Bemote, Bentyl, Bentylol, Byclomine, Dibent, Dilomine, Di-Spaz, Formulex, Lomine, Merbentyl, Or-Tyl, Spasmoban

Drug Class: Anticholinergic GI antispasmodic

Drug Actions

Appears to exert nonspecific, indirect spasmolytic action on smooth muscle. Dicyclomine also possesses local anesthetic properties that may be partly responsible for spasmolysis. Relieves GI spasms.

Use

- Irritable bowel syndrome and other functional GI disorders
- Infant colic

Side Effects

Cardiovascular: palpitations, tachycardia.
Gastrointestinal: nausea, vomiting, constipation, dry mouth, abdominal distention, heartburn, paralytic ileus.
Nervous System: fever, headache, dizziness, drowsiness, insomnia, nervousness, confusion, excitement (in elderly patients).
Urinary: urinary hesitancy, urine retention, impotence.
Skin: hives, decreased sweating or possibly anhidrosis, other dermal changes.
Other: allergic reactions, blurred vision, increased intraocular pressure, dilated pupils.

Onset, Peak, and Duration

Route	Onset	Peak	Duration
Oral	Unknown	1–1.5 hr	Unknown
I.M.	Unknown	Unknown	Unknown

 Massage Considerations

- There are no cautions or contraindications to massage for the client taking this medication.
- The action of the drug as an anticholinergic may block the parasympathetic nervous system (PNS) and make it harder for the client to relax. Systemic reflex strokes such as rocking, effleurage, and friction may require a longer application time to achieve the desired effect.
- Side effects of dizziness or drowsiness require care in getting the client on and off the table. Using more stimulation with rapid effleurage and tapotement at the end of the session may help. Constipation may be helped by regular abdominal massage. Hives are a local contraindication to massage and should be reported to the physician. If severe, massage should be withheld.

---

didanosine (ddl) (digh-DAN-uh-zeen)

Videx, Videx EC

Drug Class: Antiviral

Drug Actions

Inhibits replication of HIV

Use

- HIV infection when antiretroviral therapy is warranted
- CNS: headache, fever, insomnia, dizziness, seizures, confusion, anxiety, nervousness, hypertonia, abnormal thinking, twitching, depression, asthenia, pain, peripheral neuropathy.

Side Effects

Cardiovascular: hypertension, edema, hyperlipemia, heart failure.
Gastrointestinal: diarrhea, nausea, vomiting, abdominal pain, pancreatitis, dry mouth, painful digestion, gas.
Skin: rash, itching, hair loss.
Other: infection, sarcoma, anaphylactoid reaction, chills, thrombocytopenia, leukopenia, granulocytosis, anemia, liver abnormalities, hepatic failure, severe hepatomegaly, lactic acidosis, muscle pain arthritis, myopathy, cough, shortness of muscle, pneumonia.

Onset, Peak, and Duration

Route	Onset	Peak	Duration
Oral	Unknown	30 min–1 hr	Unknown

 Massage Considerations

- There are no cautions or contraindications to massage related to the client taking this medication. There may be cautions and contraindications related to the client's condition.

- Side effects of dizziness require care in getting the client on and off the table. Using rapid effleurage and tapotement at the end of the massage may help. Peripheral neuropathy contraindicates deep tissue massage. Gas may respond well to regular abdominal massage. Rash or itching are a local contraindication to massage and should be reported to the physician immediately. If severe, massage should be withheld. Hair loss may be a local contraindication if the client is upset by losing hair during massage or the scalp is tender.

---

diflunisal (digh-FLOO-neh-sol)

Dolobid

Drug Class: Salicylic acid derivative nonopioid analgesic, antipyretic, anti-inflammatory

Drug Actions

May inhibit prostaglandin synthesis. Relieves inflammation and pain; reduces body temperature

Use

- Mild to moderate pain
- Osteoarthritis
- Rheumatoid arthritis

Side Effects

Gastrointestinal: nausea, painful digestion, GI pain, diarrhea, vomiting, constipation, gas.
Nervous System: dizziness, sleepiness, insomnia, headache, fatigue.
Urinary: renal impairment, hematuria, interstitial nephritis.
Skin: rash, itching, sweating, stomatitis, erythema multiforme, Stevens-Johnson syndrome.
Other: dry mucous membranes, ringing in the ears, visual disturbances.

Onset, Peak, and Duration

Route	Onset	Peak	Duration
Oral	1 hr	2–3 hr	8–12 hr

Massage Considerations

- This drug decreases the perception of pain; therefore, deep tissue massage should be used with cautions. There are no other cautions or contraindications to massage related to the client taking this drug.
- Side effects of dizziness and sleepiness require care in getting the client on and off the table. Using rapid effleurage and tapotement at the end of the session may help.
- Constipation and gas may be helped by regular abdominal massage. Rash and itching are a local contraindication to massage and should be reported to the physician. If severe, massage should be withheld.

---

digoxin (dih-JOKS-in)

Digitek, Digoxin, Lanoxicaps, Lanoxin

Drug Class: Cardiac glycoside antiarrhythmic, inotropic

Drug Actions

Strengthens myocardial contractions and slows conduction through SA and AV nodes.

Use

- Heart failure
- Atrial fibrillation and flutter
- Paroxysmal atrial tachycardia

Side Effects

Cardiovascular: arrhythmias, heart failure, hypotension.
Gastrointestinal: anorexia, nausea, vomiting, diarrhea.
Nervous System: fatigue, generalized muscle weakness, agitation, hallucinations, headache, malaise, dizziness, stupor, paresthesia.
Other: yellow-green halos around visual images, blurred vision, light flashes, photophobia, double vision.

Onset, Peak, and Duration

Route	Onset	Peak	Duration
Oral	30 min–2 hr	2–6 hr	3–4 days
I.V.	5–30 min	1–4 hr	3–4 days

Massage Considerations

- There are no cautions or contraindications to massage related to the client taking this drug. There may be cautions and contraindications related to the client condition.
- Side effects of hypotension and dizziness require care in getting on and off the table.
- Using rapid effleurage or tapotement at the end of the session may help. Paresthesia contraindicates deep tissue massage.

---

diltiazem hydrochloride (dil-TIGH-uh-zem high-droh-KLOR-ighd)

Cardizem, Cardizem CD, Cardizem LA, Cardizem SR, Cartia XT, Dilacor XR, Diltia XT, Tiazac

Drug Class: Calcium channel blocker antianginal

Drug Actions

Inhibits calcium ion influx across cardiac and smooth muscle cells, decreasing myocardial contractility and oxygen demand; also dilates coronary arteries and arterioles. Relieves anginal pain, lowers blood pressure, and restores normal sinus rhythm.

Use

- Vasospastic angina (Prinzmetal's [variant] angina),
- Classic chronic stable angina pectoris
- Hypertension
- Atrial fibrillation or flutter
- Paroxysmal supraventricular tachycardia

Side Effects

Cardiovascular: edema, arrhythmias, flushing, bradycardia, hypotension, conduction abnormalities, heart failure, AV block, abnormal ECG.
Gastrointestinal: nausea, constipation, vomiting, diarrhea, abdominal discomfort.
Nervous System: headache, sleepiness, dizziness, insomnia, weakness.
Urinary: increased urination at night, frequent urination.
Skin: rash, itching, photosensitivity.

Onset, Peak, and Duration

Route	Onset	Peak	Duration
Oral	30 min–4 hr	2–18 hr	6–24 hr
I.V.			
Bolus	3 min	Immediate	1–3 hr
Infusion	3 min	Immediate	<10 hr

Massage Considerations

- There are no cautions or contraindications to massage related to the client taking this medication. There may be cautions and contraindications related to the client condition.
- Side effects of hypotension, sleepiness, or dizziness require care in getting the client on and off the table. Using rapid effleurage or tapotement at the end of the session may help prevent problems. Constipation may be helped by regular abdominal massage. Rash or itching is a local contraindication to massage and should be reported to the physician. If severe, massage should be withheld.

---

diphenhydramine hydrochloride (digh-fen-HIGH-drah-meen high-droh-KLOR-ighd)

Allerdryl, AllerMax Caplets, Allermed, Banophen, Banophen Caplets, Beldin, Belix, Benadryl, Benadryl 25, Benadryl Kapseals, Benylin Cough, Bydramine Cough, Compoz, Diphenadryl, Diphen Cough, Diphenhist, Diphenhist Captabs, Genahist, Hyrexin-50, Nytol Maximum Strength, Nytol with DPH, Sleep-Eze 3, Sominex Formula 2, Tusstat, Twilite Caplets, Uni-Bent Cough

Drug Class: Antihistamine (H_1-receptor antagonist), antiemetic, antivertigo agent, antitussive, sedative-hypnotic, antidyskinetic (anticholinergic)

Drug Actions

Relieves allergy symptoms, motion sickness, and cough; improves voluntary movement; and promotes sleep and calmness.

Use

- Rhinitis
- Allergy symptoms
- Motion sickness
- Parkinson's disease
- Sedation
- Nighttime sleep aid
- Nonproductive cough

Side Effects

Cardiovascular: palpitations, hypotension, tachycardia.
Gastrointestinal: nausea, vomiting, diarrhea, dry mouth, constipation, epigastric distress, anorexia.
Nervous System: drowsiness, confusion, insomnia, headache, vertigo, sedation, sleepiness, dizziness, incoordination, fatigue, restlessness, tremor, nervousness, seizures.
Urinary: painful urination, urine retention, urinary frequency.
Skin: hives, photosensitivity, rash.

Other: anaphylactic shock, double vision, blurred vision, nasal congestion, ringing in the ears, hemolytic anemia, thrombocytopenia, agranulocytosis, thickening of bronchial secretions.

Onset, Peak, and Duration

Route	Onset	Peak	Duration
Oral	≤15 min	1–4 hr	6–8 hr
I.V.	Immediate	1–4 hr	6–8 hr
I.M.	Unknown	1–4 hr	6–8 hr

Massage Considerations

- There are no contraindications to massage for the client taking this medication. Deep tissue massage should be used with caution because of the sedating effects of this drug.
- Because this drug can interrupt nerve transmissions, in some cases local reflex strokes such as compression, vibration, and stretching may not be as effective.
- The site of I.M. injection should not be massaged for at least 4–6 hours so as not to speed up the absorption of the drug.
- Side effects of hypotension, drowsiness, vertigo, sleepiness, and sedation require care in positioning the client and getting on and off the table. Using rapid effleurage and tapotement at the end of the session may help. Staying with the client until they are sitting up may be necessary. If side effects are severe or worsened with massage, using a more rapid and stimulating massage technique throughout the session may help. Constipation may be helped by regular abdominal massage. Urinary frequency may require that the client get up in the middle of the session. Providing privacy and quick access to the bathroom is appropriate. Water fountains or music that may stimulate the need to urinate should be avoided. Rash or hives are a local contraindication to massage and should be reported to the physician. If severe, massage should be withheld.

---

diphenoxylate hydrochloride and atropine sulfate

(digh-fen-OKS-ul-ayt high-droh-KLOR-ighd and AH-troh-peen SUL-fayt)

Logen, Lomanate, Lomotil, Lonox

Drug Class: Opioid antidiarrheal

Drug Actions

Probably increases smooth-muscle tone in GI tract, inhibits motility and propulsion, and diminishes secretions. Relieves diarrhea.

Use

- Acute, nonspecific diarrhea

Side Effects

Cardiovascular: tachycardia.
Gastrointestinal: dry mouth, nausea, vomiting, abdominal discomfort or distention, paralytic ileus, anorexia, fluid retention in bowel, pancreatitis.
Nervous System: sedation, dizziness, headache, drowsiness, lethargy, restlessness, depression, euphoria, malaise, confusion, numbness in limbs.
Urinary: urine retention.
Skin: itching, rash.
Other: angioedema, anaphylaxis, possible physical dependence with long-term use, dilated pupils, respiratory depression.

Onset, Peak, and Duration

Route	Onset	Peak	Duration
Oral	45–60 min	3 hr	3–4 hr

Massage Considerations

- For the client with acute diarrhea, massage would be contraindicated until the condition clears. For the client taking this drug regularly for chronic problems, abdominal massage should be done with caution and may be contraindicated in severe conditions.
- This drug is an opiate and may decrease perception of pain. Deep tissue massage should be done with great caution.
- Side effects of sedation, dizziness, lethargy, and drowsiness require care in getting the client on and off the table. Using rapid effleurage and tapotement at the end of the session may help. If severe, more stimulating massage throughout the session is indicated to prevent problems. Rash or itching is a local contraindication to massage and should be reported to the physician. If severe, massage should be withheld.

dipyridamole (digh-peer-IH-duh-mohl)

Apo-Dipyridamole, Novo-Dipiradol, Persantin, Persantin 100, Persantine

Drug Class: Coronary vasodilator, platelet aggregation inhibitor

Drug Actions

Dilates coronary arteries and helps prevent clotting

Use

- Inhibition of platelet adhesion in prosthetic heart valves
- Chronic angina pectoris
- Prevention of thromboembolic complications in patients with various thromboembolic disorders other than prosthetic heart valves

Side Effects

Cardiovascular: flushing, fainting, hypotension, chest pain, ECG abnormalities, blood pressure lability, hypertension (with I.V. infusion).
Gastrointestinal: nausea, vomiting, diarrhea, abdominal distress.
Nervous System: headache, dizziness, weakness.
Skin: rash, irritation (with undiluted injection), itching.

Onset, Peak, and Duration

Route	Onset	Peak	Duration
Oral	Unknown	45–150 min	Unknown
I.V.	Unknown	2 min after	Unknown therapy stops
I.M.	Unknown	Unknown	Unknown

Massage Considerations

- Because of this drug's effects on blood clotting, deep tissue massage should be used with caution and in many cases will be contraindicated. Consult with the physician before doing any massage. Circulatory massage with effleurage should be used with caution and limited. Further cautions and contraindications may exist related to the client's condition.
- Side effects of dizziness and hypotension require care in getting the client on and off the table. Using light tapotement or friction to lower legs may help. Rash or itching is a local contraindication to massage and should be reported to the physician. If severe, massage should be withheld.
- The best strokes to utilize are the systemic reflex strokes of rocking and gentle friction and local reflex strokes of stretching, traction, and vibration. Myofascial massage techniques also may be used.

---

disulfiram (digh-SUL-fih-ram)

Antabuse

Drug Class: Alcohol deterrent

Drug Actions

Blocks oxidation of ethanol at acetaldehyde stage. Excess acetaldehyde produces highly unpleasant reaction in presence of even small amounts of ethanol. Deters alcohol consumption.

Use

- Adjunct in management of chronic alcoholism

Side Effects

Gastrointestinal: metallic or garlic aftertaste.
Nervous System: drowsiness, headache, fatigue, delirium, depression, neuritis, peripheral neuritis, polyneuritis, restlessness, and psychotic reactions.
Urinary: impotence.
Skin: acneiform or allergic dermatitis.
Other: disulfiram reaction, optic neuritis.

Onset, Peak, and Duration

Route	Onset	Peak	Duration
Oral	1–2 hr	Unknown	<14 days

Massage Considerations

- There are no cautions or contraindications to massage for the client taking this drug.
- Side effects of drowsiness require care in getting the client on and off the table. Rapid effleurage or tapotement at the end of the session should help prevent problems. Neuritis is a local contraindication to deep tissue massage and if severe may contraindicate massage completely. Skin problems are a local contraindication to massage and should be reported to the physician. If severe, withhold massage until the client has been cleared by the physician. If the client continues on the drug and wishes to receive massage, the massage therapist should wear gloves to massage the affected areas.

docetaxel (doks-uh-TAKX-ul)

Taxotere

Drug Class: Antineoplastic

Drug Actions

Inhibits cancer cells from reproducing, producing antineoplastic effect

Use

- Locally advanced or metastatic breast cancer for which prior chemotherapy has failed.
- Locally advanced or metastatic non–small-cell lung cancer after failure of platinum-based chemotherapy.
- Unresectable, locally advanced, or metastatic non–small-cell lung cancer in patient who has not previously received chemotherapy for this condition, with cisplatin

Side Effects

Cardiovascular: fluid retention, hypotension.
Gastrointestinal: stomatitis, nausea, vomiting, diarrhea.
Nervous System: pain, weakness, paresthesia, painful sensations of the skin, weakness.
Skin: hair loss, skin eruptions, peeling, nail pigmentation alterations, nail pain, flushing, rash.
Other: hypersensitivity reactions, infection, chest tightness, drug fever, chills, anemia, abnormal blood profiles, myelosuppression, septic and nonseptic death, back pain, muscle pain, joint pain, shortness of breath.

Onset, Peak, and Duration

Route	Onset	Peak	Duration
I.V.	Immediate	Unknown	Unknown

Massage Considerations

- Because of the toxic effects of this drug, deep tissue massage therapy is to be used with caution if at all. Circulatory massage with effleurage should be used with caution and limited to avoid taxing the liver and kidney as they try to rid the body of this drug. Further cautions or contraindications to massage will depend on the client condition.
- The peak and duration of action of this drug are unknown, but the half-life is 12 hours.
- Because the drug is most often given once every three weeks, time the massage for prior to the administration of at least 24–48 hours after administration of the drug.
- Side effects of hypotension require care in getting the client on and off the table. Gentle friction to the lower extremities at the end of the session may help. Light tapotement may also be used. Paresthesia or painful sensation are a local contraindication to deep tissue massage and, if severe, may contraindicate massage completely. Hair loss contraindicates scalp massage if the client is disturbed by hair coming out during the massage or if the scalp is tender. Skin problems, peeling, and rash are local contraindications to massage and should be reported to the physician immediately. If severe, massage should be withheld.
- The best strokes for this client are the systemic and local reflex strokes of rocking, stretching, traction, and vibration and the mechanical stroke of pétrissage. Myofascial massage techniques may be used for areas of tightness and gluteation.

docosanol (doe-KOE-san-ole)

Abreva

Drug Class: Antiviral

Drug Actions

Shortens healing time and relieves pain from the herpes simplex lesions

Use

- Recurrent oral-facial herpes simplex (cold sores)

Side Effects

Nervous System: headache.
Other: reaction at application site.

Onset, Peak, and Duration

Route	Onset	Peak	Duration
Topical	Unknown	Unknown	Unknown

Massage Considerations

- There are no cautions or contraindications to massage for a client taking this medication.
- The area of outbreak and application of the drug should not be massaged.

docusate calcium (dioctyl calcium sulfosuccinate)

(DOK-yoo-sayt KAL-see-um)

DC Softgels, Pro-Cal-Sof , Surfak

docusate potassium (dioctyl potassium sulfosuccinate)

Diocto-K, Kasof

docusate sodium (dioctyl sodium sulfosuccinate)

Colace, Coloxyl, Coloxyl Enema Concentrate, Dialose, Diocto, Dioeze, Disonate, DOK, DOS Softgels, Doxinate, D-S-S, Modane Soft, Pro-Sof, Regulax SS, Regulux, Regutol, Therevac Plus, Therevac-SB

Drug Class: Emollient laxative

Drug Actions

Reduces surface tension of interfacing liquid contents of bowel. This detergent activity promotes incorporation of additional liquid into stool, thus forming softer mass.

Use

- Stool softener

Side Effects

Gastrointestinal: bitter taste, mild abdominal cramping, diarrhea, laxative dependence with long-term or excessive use.
Other: throat irritation.

Onset, Peak, and Duration

Route	Onset	Peak	Duration
Oral	Varies	Varies	24–72 hr
Rectal	Unknown	Unknown	Unknown

 Massage Considerations

- There are no cautions or contraindications to massage for the client taking this medication.

---

dofetilide (doh-FET-eh-lighd)

Tikosyn

Drug Actions: Antiarrhythmic

Drug Actions

Maintains normal sinus rhythm in patients with symptomatic atrial fibrillation or atrial flutter who have been converted to normal sinus rhythm; converts atrial fibrillation and atrial flutter to normal sinus rhythm.

Use

- Maintenance of normal sinus rhythm in patients with symptomatic atrial fibrillation or atrial flutter for longer than 1 week who have been converted to normal sinus rhythm.
- Conversion of atrial fibrillation and atrial flutter to normal sinus rhythm.

Side Effects

Cardiovascular: ventricular fibrillation, ventricular tachycardia, torsades de pointes, AV block, bundle branch block, heart block, chest pain, angina, atrial fibrillation, peripheral edema, hypertension, palpitations, bradycardia, edema, cardiac arrest, heart attack.
Gastrointestinal: nausea, diarrhea, abdominal pain.
Nervous System: headache, dizziness, insomnia, anxiety, migraine, cerebral ischemia, stroke, weakness, paresthesia, syncope.
Urinary: urinary tract infection.
Skin: rash, sweating.
Other: flulike syndrome, angioedema, liver damage, back pain, joint pain, respiratory tract infection, shortness of breath, increased cough, facial paralysis.

Onset, Peak, and Duration

Route	Onset	Peak	Duration
Oral	Unknown	2–3 hr	Unknown

 Massage Considerations

- There are no cautions or contraindications to massage related to this drug. However, there may be cautions and contraindications related to the client condition. The physician should be consulted before any massage being given.
- Side effects of dizziness require care in getting the client on and off the table. Stimulation at the end of the session with effleurage or tapotement may help. Paresthesia is a local contraindication to deep tissue massage. Rash is a local contraindication to massage and should be reported to the physician. If severe, massage should be withheld.

dolasetron mesylate (doh-LEH-seh-trohn MES-ih layt)

Anzemet

Drug Class: Antiemetic

Drug Actions

Blocks the action of serotonin, thereby preventing serotonin from stimulating the vomiting reflex. Prevents nausea and vomiting.

Use

- Prevention of nausea and vomiting from cancer chemotherapy
- Prevention of postoperative nausea and vomiting
- Postoperative nausea and vomiting

Side Effects

Cardiovascular: arrhythmias, bradycardia, ECG changes, hypotension, hypertension, tachycardia.
Gastrointestinal: diarrhea, painful digestion, abdominal pain, constipation, anorexia.
Nervous System: fever, headache, dizziness, drowsiness, fatigue.
Urinary: absence of urination, urine retention.
Skin: itching, rash.
Other: chills, pain at injection site.

Onset, Peak, and Duration

Route	Onset	Peak	Duration
Oral	Rapid	1 hr	8 hr
I.V.	Rapid	36 min	7 hr

Massage Considerations

- There are no cautions or contraindications to massage related to a client taking this drug.
- There may be cautions or contraindications to massage related to the client condition.
- Side effects of hypotension, dizziness, and drowsiness require care in getting the client on and off the table. Using rapid effleurage and tapotement at the end of the session will help prevent problems. Constipation may be helped by regular abdominal massage. Rash or itching are local contraindications to massage and should be reported to the physician. If severe, massage should be withheld.

donepezil hydrochloride (doh-NEH-peh-zil high-droh-KLOR-ighd)

Aricept

Drug Class: Psychotherapeutic agent for Alzheimer's disease

Drug Actions

Reversibly inhibits acetylcholinesterase in the CNS, thereby increasing the acetylcholine level. Temporarily improves cognitive function in patients with Alzheimer's disease.

Use

- Mild to moderate dementia of the Alzheimer's type

Side Effects

Cardiovascular: chest pain, hypertension, vasodilation, atrial fibrillation, hypotension.
Gastrointestinal: nausea, diarrhea, vomiting, anorexia, fecal incontinence, GI bleeding, bloating, epigastric pain.
Nervous System: syncope, pain, headache, insomnia, dizziness, depression, abnormal dreams, sleepiness, seizures, tremor, irritability, paresthesia, aggression, ataxia, restlessness, abnormal crying, fatigue, nervousness, aphasia.
Urinary: frequent urination.
Skin: itching, hives, sweating, bruising.
Other: hot flushes, increased libido, accident, influenza, cataracts, sore throat, weight decrease, dehydration, muscle cramps, arthritis, toothache, bone fracture, shortness of breath, bronchitis, blurred vision, eye irritation.

Onset, Peak, and Duration

Route	Onset	Peak	Duration
Oral	Unknown	3–4 hr	Unknown

Massage Considerations

- There are no cautions or contraindications to massage for the client taking this drug.
- There may be cautions or contraindications to massage related to the client condition.
- Side effects of hypotension, dizziness, and sleepiness require care in getting the client on and off the table. Stimulating the client with effleurage and tapotement at the end of the session may help. Paresthesia is a local contraindication to deep tissue massage.
- Frequent urination may require the client to get up in the middle of the session. Providing privacy and quick access to the bathroom is appropriate. Water fountains or music that may stimulate the need to urinate should not be used. Rash or hives are a local contraindication to massage and should be reported to the physician. If severe, massage should be withheld. If bruising is a problem, deep tissue massage should be used with great caution or not at all.

dorzolamide hydrochloride (dor-ZOLE-uh-mighd high-droh-KLOR-ighd)

Trusopt

Drug Class: Antiglaucoma agent

Drug Actions

Reduces Intraocular Pressure in glaucoma

Use

- Increased intraocular pressure (IOP) in patients with ocular hypertension or open-angle glaucoma.

Side Effects

Gastrointestinal: bitter taste, nausea.
Urinary: kidney stones,
Nervous System: weakness, fatigue, headache, dizziness, paresthesia.

Skin: rash, itching, hives, contact dermatitis.
Other: angioedema, ocular burning, stinging, discomfort; superficial punctate keratitis; ocular allergic reactions (including conjunctivitis, itching, and lid reactions), bronchospasm, shortness of breath, blurred vision; lacrimation; dryness; photophobia; iridocyclitis; redness; transient myopia; eyelid crusting; ocular pain; throat irritation.

Onset, Peak, and Duration

Route	Onset	Peak	Duration
Ophthalmic	1–2 hr	2–3 hr	8 hr

Massage Considerations

- There are no cautions or contraindications to massage related to the client taking this drug.
- Side effects of dizziness require care in getting the client on and off the table. Using stimulating strokes at the end of the massage will help prevent problems. Paresthesia is a local contraindication to deep tissue massage. Rash, itching, or hives are a local contraindication to massage and should be reported to the physician. If severe, massage should be withheld.

doxazosin mesylate (doks-AY-zoh-sin MES-ih-layt)

Cardura

Drug Class: Alpha-adrenergic blocker antihypertensive

Drug Actions

Acts on peripheral vasculature to produce vasodilation. Lowers blood pressure.

Use

- Essential hypertension.
- Benign prostatic hypertrophy

Side Effects

Cardiovascular: orthostatic hypotension, hypotension, edema, palpitations, arrhythmias, tachycardia.
Gastrointestinal: nausea, vomiting, diarrhea, constipation.
Nervous System: dizziness, weakness, headache, drowsiness, pain.
Skin: rash, itching.
Other: rhinitis, pharyngitis, abnormal vision, joint pain, muscle pain, shortness of breath.

Onset, Peak, and Duration

Route	Onset	Peak	Duration
Oral	1–2 hr	5–6 hr	24 hr

Massage Considerations

- There are no contraindications to massage for the client taking this medication. There may be cautions or contraindications to massage related to the client condition.
- The action of the drug in dilating peripheral blood vessels may increase this effect of massage and drop blood pressure. Using rapid effleurage and tapotement at the end of the massage may help. If severe, stimulating massage throughout the session should be used.
- Side effects of hypotension, dizziness, and drowsiness should be handled as noted earlier.
- Constipation may respond well to regular abdominal massage. Rash or itching is a local contraindication to massage and should be reported to the physician. If severe, massage should be withheld.

doxepin hydrochloride (DOKS-eh-pin high-droh-KLOR-ighd)

Novo-Doxepin, Sinequan, Triadapin

Drug Class: Tricyclic antidepressant antidepressant

Drug Actions

Increases amount of norepinephrine, serotonin, or both in CNS by blocking their reuptake by presynaptic neurons. Relieves depression and anxiety.

Use

- Depression
- Anxiety

Side Effects

Cardiovascular: orthostatic hypotension, tachycardia, ECG changes, hypertension.
Gastrointestinal: dry mouth, glossitis, constipation, nausea, vomiting, anorexia.
Nervous System: drowsiness, dizziness, excitation, tremors, weakness, confusion, headache, nervousness, EEG changes, seizures, extrapyramidal reactions, ataxia, paresthesia, hallucinations.
Urinary: urine retention.
Skin: sweating, rash, hives, photosensitivity.
Other: hypersensitivity reaction, blurred vision, ringing in the ears, dilated pupils, abnormal blood profiles, bone marrow suppression.

Onset, Peak, and Duration

Route	Onset	Peak	Duration
Oral	Unknown	$\leq$2 hr	Unknown

Massage Considerations

- There are no cautions or contraindications to massage for the client taking this medication. There may be cautions and contraindications related to the client condition.
- Side effects of hypotension, drowsiness or dizziness require care in getting the client on and off the table. Using stimulating strokes such as rapid effleurage or tapotement at the end of the session may help. Constipation may be helped by regular abdominal massage.
- Rash or hives are a local contraindication to massage and should be reported to the physician. If severe, massage should be withheld.

doxercalciferol (dox-er-kal-SIF-eh-rol)

Hectorol

Drug Class: Parathyroid hormone antagonist

Drug Actions

Reduces elevated intact parathyroid hormone levels

Use

- Reduction of elevated intact parathyroid hormone (PTH) levels in the management of secondary hyperparathyroidism in patients undergoing long-term renal dialysis.

Side Effects

Cardiovascular: bradycardia, edema.
Gastrointestinal: anorexia, painful digestion, nausea, vomiting, constipation.
Nervous System: dizziness, headache, malaise, sleep disorder.
Skin: itching.
Other: abscess, weight gain or loss, joint pain, shortness of breath.

Onset, Peak, and Duration

Route	Onset	Peak	Duration
Oral	Unknown	11–12 hr	Unknown

 Massage Considerations

- Although there are no cautions or contraindications to massage related to the client taking this drug, in most cases, the client condition will have cautions and contraindications. Consult the physician before giving any massage.
- Side effects of dizziness require care in getting the client on and off the table. Stimulating the client with rapid effleurage or tapotement at the end of the session may help prevent problems. Constipation may be helped by regular abdominal massage. Itching is a local contraindication to massage and should be reported to the physician. If widespread and the client is still taking the drug, massage may be given if the itching is not worsened by the massage.

---

doxorubicin hydrochloride (doks-oh-ROO-bih-sin high-droh-KLOR-ighd)

Adriamycin, Adriamycin PFS, Adriamycin RDF, Rudex

Drug Class: Antineoplastic

Drug Actions

Hinders or kills certain cancer cells

Use

- Bladder, breast, lung, ovarian, stomach, testicular, and thyroid cancers
- Hodgkin's disease
- Acute lymphoblastic
- Myeloblastic leukemia
- Wilms' tumor
- Neuroblastoma
- Lymphoma
- Sarcoma

Side Effects

Cardiovascular: cardiac depression, seen in such ECG changes as sinus tachycardia, T-wave flattening, ST-segment depression, voltage reduction; arrhythmias; irreversible cardiomyopathy.
Gastrointestinal: nausea, vomiting, diarrhea, stomatitis, esophagitis, anorexia.
Urinary: transient red urine.
Skin: complete hair loss, hives; facial flushing; hyperpigmentation of nails, dermal creases, or skin (especially in previously irradiated areas).
Other: severe cellulitis or tissue sloughing if drug extravasates, hyperuricemia, conjunctivitis, blood abnormalities, myelosuppression, anaphylaxis.

Onset, Peak, and Duration

Route	Onset	Peak	Duration
I.V.	Unknown	Unknown	Unknown

 Massage Considerations

- Because of the toxicity of this drug, deep tissue massage is contraindicated. Circulatory massage with effleurage should be used with caution to prevent overtaxing the liver and kidneys as they try to rid the body of the drug. There may be other cautions or contraindications to massage related to the client condition. Close collaboration with the physician is essential.
- Although peak and duration of the action of the drug is unknown, half-life is 16.5 hours. Because the drug is most often given every 3–4 weeks, massage is best done on the weeks that the client is not receiving the drug. At minimum, no massage should be given for at least 24–48 hours after the drug is given.
- Side effects of hair loss contraindicate scalp massage if the client is disturbed by hair coming out during the massage or if the scalp is tender. Hives are a local contraindication to massage and should be reported to the physician. If severe, massage should be withheld.
- The best strokes for this client will be systemic and local reflex strokes of rocking, friction, stretching, traction, and vibration. Pétrissage and myofascial massage techniques may also be used.

---

doxorubicin hydrochloride liposomal (doks-oh-ROO-bih-sin high-droh-KLOR-ighd li-po-SOE-mal)

Doxil

Drug Class: Antineoplastic

Drug Actions

Hinders or kills certain cancer cells in patients with ovarian cancer or AIDS-related Kaposi's sarcoma.

Use

- Metastatic carcinoma of the ovary
- AIDS-related Kaposi's sarcoma

Side Effects

Cardiovascular: chest pain, hypotension, tachycardia, peripheral edema, cardiomyopathy, heart failure, arrhythmias, pericardial effusion.
Gastrointestinal: nausea, vomiting, constipation, anorexia, diarrhea, abdominal pain, taste perversion, painful digestion, oral candidiasis, enlarged abdomen, esophagitis, difficulty swallowing, stomatitis, glossitis.
Nervous System: fever, weakness, paresthesia, headache, sleepiness, dizziness, depression, insomnia, anxiety, malaise, emotional lability, fatigue.
Urinary: albuminuria.
Skin: rash, hair loss, dry skin, itching, skin discoloration, skin disorder, exfoliative dermatitis, herpes zoster, sweating, palmar-plantar erythrodysesthesia.
Other: allergic reaction, chills, infection, sepsis, infusion-related reactions, mucous membrane disorder, mouth ulceration, pharyngitis, rhinitis, conjunctivitis, retinitis, optic neuritis, abnormal blood profiles, hyperbilirubinemia, dehydration, weight loss, hypocalcemia, hyperglycemia, muscle pain, back pain, shortness of breath, increased cough, pneumonia.

Onset, Peak, and Duration

Route	Onset	Peak	Duration
I.V.	Unknown	Unknown	Unknown

Massage Considerations

- Because of the toxicity of this drug, deep tissue massage is contraindicated. Circulatory massage with effleurage should be used with caution to prevent overtaxing the liver and kidneys as they try to rid the body of the drug. There may be other cautions or contraindications to massage related to the client condition. Close collaboration with the physician is essential.
- Although peak and duration of the action of the drug is unknown, half-life is 16.5 hours.
- Because the drug is most often given every 3–4 weeks, massage is best done on the weeks that the client is not receiving the drug. At minimum, no massage should be given for at least 24–48 hours after the drug is given.
- Dizziness, sleepiness, and hypotension require care in getting the client on and off the table. Gentle friction to the lower leg at the end of the session may help prevent problems. Constipation may be helped by regular abdominal massage. Side effects of hair loss contraindicate scalp massage if the client is disturbed by hair coming out during the massage or if the scalp is tender. Paresthesia is a local contraindication to deep tissue massage. Hives are a local contraindication to massage and should be reported to the physician. If severe, massage should be withheld.
- The best strokes for this client will be systemic and local reflex strokes of rocking, friction, stretching, traction, and vibration. Pétrissage and myofascial massage techniques also may be used.

doxycycline (doks-e-sigh-kleen)

doxycycline hyclate

Apo-Doxy, Doryx, Doxy-100, Doxy-200, Doxycin, Doxytec, Novo-Doxylin, Nu-Doxycycline, Periostat, Vibramycin, Vibra-Tabs

doxycycline hydrochloride

Doryx, Doxsig, Doxylin, Doxy Tablets, Vibramycin, Vibra-Tabs

doxycycline monohydrate

Adoxa, Monodox, Vibramycin

Drug Class: Tetracycline antibiotic

Drug Actions

Hinders bacterial growth

Use

- Infections caused by sensitive gram-negative and gram-positive organisms
- Chlamydia
- Mycoplasma
- Rickettsia
- Organisms that cause trachoma
- Gonorrhea in patients allergic to penicillin
- Primary or secondary syphilis in patients allergic to penicillin
- Uncomplicated urethral, endocervical, or rectal infection
- Prevention of malaria

- Adjunct to scaling and root planing to promote attachment level gain and to reduce pocket depth in patients with adult periodontitis
- Adjunct to other antibiotics for inhalation, GI, and oropharyngeal anthrax
- Cutaneous anthrax
- Adjunct to severe acne
- Prevention of traveler's diarrhea commonly caused by enterotoxigenic *E. coli*
- Prophylaxis for rape victims
- Lyme disease
- Pleural effusions related to cancer

Side Effects

Cardiovascular: pericarditis, thrombophlebitis.
Gastrointestinal: anorexia, epigastric distress, nausea, vomiting, diarrhea, oral candidiasis, enterocolitis, anogenital inflammation.
Nervous System: intracranial hypertension (pseudotumor cerebri).
Skin: maculopapular and erythematous rash, photosensitivity, increased pigmentation, hives.
Other: hypersensitivity reactions, anaphylaxis, superinfection, permanent discoloration of teeth, enamel defects, glossitis, difficulty swallowing, blood abnormalities, bone growth retardation if used in children under age 8.

Onset, Peak, and Duration

Route	Onset	Peak	Duration
Oral	Unknown	1.5–4 hr	Unknown
I.V.	Immediate	Unknown	Unknown

 Massage Considerations

- Although there are no cautions or contraindications to massage related to this drug, the client condition and severity of infection may be a source of cautions and contraindications. Consult with the physician as needed.
- Side effects of thrombophlebitis are a complete contraindication to massage. Rash or hives are a local contraindication to massage and should be reported to the physician immediately. If severe, massage should be withheld.

dronabinol (delta-9-tetrahydrocannabinol) (droh-NAB-eh-nohl)

Marinol

Drug Class: Cannabinoid antiemetic, appetite stimulant

Drug Actions

Relieves nausea and vomiting caused by chemotherapy and stimulates appetite

Use

- Nausea and vomiting from chemotherapy
- Anorexia and weight loss in patients with AIDS

Side Effects

Cardiovascular: tachycardia, orthostatic hypotension, palpitations, vasodilation.
Gastrointestinal: dry mouth, nausea, vomiting, abdominal pain, diarrhea.

Nervous System: dizziness, drowsiness, euphoria, ataxia, depersonalization, disorientation, hallucinations, sleepiness, headache, muddled thinking, weakness, amnesia, confusion, paranoia.
Other: visual disturbances.

Onset, Peak, and Duration

Route	Onset	Peak	Duration
Oral	Unknown	2–4 hr	4–6 hr

 Massage Considerations

- This drug effects the CNS and may decrease the perception of pain and interfere with thought processes. Deep tissue massage is contraindicated. Other cautions and contraindications to massage may exist related to the client condition.
- Side effects of hypotension, vasodilation, drowsiness, and dizziness require care in getting the client on and off the table. Stimulating strokes such as rapid effleurage and tapotement at the end of the session may help. If symptoms are severe or worsened by massage, using a more stimulating massage technique throughout the session may help.

---

dutasteride (doo-TAS-teer-ighd)

Avodart

Drug Class: Benign Prostatic Hypertrophy (BPH) drug

Drug Actions

Inhibits the conversion of testosterone to dihydrotestosterone (DHT), the androgen primarily responsible for the initial development and subsequent enlargement of the prostate gland.

Use

- Benign prostatic hypertrophy

Side Effects

Urinary: impotence, decreased libido, ejaculation disorder.
Other: abnormal growth of breast tissue.

Onset, Peak, and Duration

Route	Onset	Peak	Duration
Oral	Unknown	2–3 hr	Unknown

Massage Considerations

- There are no cautions or contraindications to massage for the client taking this drug.
- Side effects of abnormal breast tissue growth may make the chest area tender. Using caution with depth and avoiding the area if tenderness are severe are appropriate.

E

efalizumab (eh-fah-LEE-zoo-mab)

Raptiva

Drug Class: Immunosuppressant antipsoriatic

Drug Actions

Decreases inflammation of psoriatic skin

Use

- Chronic moderate to severe plaque psoriasis

Side Effects

Gastrointestinal: nausea.
Nervous System: stroke, fever, headache, pain.
Skin: acne.
Other: chills, flu syndrome, hypersensitivity reaction, infection, back pain, muscle pain.

Onset, Peak, and Duration

Route	Onset	Peak	Duration
S.C.	1–2 days	Unknown	25 days

Massage Considerations

- No cautions or contraindications to massage are indicated because a client is taking this drug. Cautions and contraindications to massage may be related to the client condition.
- Side effects of acne are a local contraindication to massage. If the acne is severe or widespread and the client needs to continue taking this drug, massage may be given with the massage therapist wearing gloves when massaging the affected areas.

efavirenz (eh-fah-VEER-enz)

Sustiva

Drug Class: Antiretroviral agent

Drug Actions

Lowers amount of HIV in the blood (viral load) and increases CD4 lymphocytes

Use

- HIV-1 infection

Side Effects

Gastrointestinal: abdominal pain, anorexia, diarrhea, painful digestion, gas, nausea, vomiting.
Nervous System: abnormal dreams or thinking, agitation, amnesia, confusion, depersonalization, depression, dizziness, euphoria, fatigue, hallucinations, headache, hypesthesia, impaired concentration, insomnia, sleepiness, nervousness, fever.
Urinary: hematuria, renal calculi.

Skin: increased sweating, erythema multiforme, Stevens-Johnson syndrome, toxic epidermal necrolysis, rash, itching.

Onset, Peak, and Duration

Route	Onset	Peak	Duration
Oral	Unknown	3–5 hr	Unknown

Massage Considerations

- No cautions or contraindications to massage are indicated because a client is taking this drug. Cautions and contraindications to massage may be related to the client condition.
- Side effects of dizziness and sleepiness require care in getting the client on and off the table. Using rapid effleurage and tapotement at the end of the session may help.
- Hypesthesia, or a decrease in sensation, is a contraindication to deep tissue massage.
- Gas may respond well to regular abdominal massage.
- Rash or itching is a local contraindication to massage and should be reported to the physician immediately. If severe, massage should be withheld.

---

eflornithine hydrochloride (ee-FLOR-ni-theen high-droh-KLOR-ighd)

Vaniqua

Drug Class: Hair growth retardant

Drug Actions

Decreases facial hair growth rate

Use

- To reduce unwanted facial hair

Side Effects

Cardiovascular: facial edema.
Gastrointestinal: painful digestion, anorexia, nausea.
Nervous System: headache, dizziness, asthenia, numbness.
Skin: acne; pseudofolliculitis barbae; dry skin; itching; erythema; skin irritation; rash; hair loss; folliculitis; ingrown hair; bleeding; cheilitis; contact dermatitis; swollen lips; herpes simplex; rosacea; stinging, tingling, or burning sensation.

Onset, Peak, and Duration

Route	Onset	Peak	Duration
Topical	Unknown	8 hr	Unknown

Massage Considerations

- No cautions or contraindications to massage are indicated because a client is taking this drug.
- Side effects of dizziness require care in getting the client on and off the table. Using stimulating strokes at the end of the massage may help. Any skin problems are usually localized, and the area should not be massaged.

eletriptan hydrobromide (el-eh-TRIP-tan high-dro-BRO-mighd)

Relpax

Drug Class: Antimigraine drug

Drug Actions

Binds to 5-HT_1 receptors and may constrict intracranial blood vessels and inhibit pro-inflammatory neuropeptide release. Relieves migraine symptoms.

Use

- Acute migraine with or without aura

Side Effects

Cardiovascular: chest tightness, pain, and pressure; flushing; palpitations.
Gastrointestinal: abdominal pain, discomfort, or cramps; dry mouth; painful digestion; difficulty swallowing; nausea.
Nervous System: weakness, dizziness, headache, hypertonia, hyperesthesia, paresthesia, sleepiness, pain.
Skin: increased sweating.
Other: chills, back pain, pharyngitis.

Onset, Peak, and Duration

Route	Onset	Peak	Duration
Oral	$^1/_2$ hr	1 $^1/_2$–2 hr	Unknown

Massage Considerations

- No cautions or contraindications to massage are indicated because a client is taking this drug. The client condition may warrant some cautions and even contraidicate massage.
- Side effects of dizziness and sleepiness require care in getting the client on and off the table. Using rapid effleurage or tapotement at the end of the session may help.
- Paresthesia or hyperesthesia contraindicate deep tissue massage in the local area.

emtricitabine (em-trih-SIGH-tah-been)

Emtriva

Drug Class: Antiretroviral

Drug Actions

Helps block HIV replication

Use

- HIV-1 infection

Side Effects

Gastrointestinal: diarrhea, nausea, abdominal pain, painful digestion, vomiting.
Nervous System: headache, weakness, nightmares, depression, insomnia, peripheral neuropathy, neuritis, paresthesia.
Skin: rash, hives, itching.
Other: rhinitis, severe hepatomegaly, steatosis, lactic acidosis, joint pain, muscle pain, cough.

Onset, Peak, and Duration

Route	Onset	Peak	Duration
Oral	Unknown	1–2 hr	Unknown

Massage Considerations

- No cautions or contraindications to massage are indicated because a client is taking this drug. Cautions and contraindications to massage may be related to the client condition.
- Side effects of peripheral neuropathy, neuritis, or paresthesia contraindicate deep tissue massage in those areas affected.
- Rash or itching is a local contraindication to massage and should be reported to the physician immediately. If severe, massage should be withheld.

enalaprilat (eh-NAH-leh-prel-at)

enalapril maleate

Amprace, Renitec, Vasotec

Drug Class: Angiotensin-converting enzyme (ACE) inhibitor antihypertensive

Drug Actions

Inhibits ACE. Lowers blood pressure.

Use

- Hypertension
- Heart failure
- Asymptomatic left ventricular dysfunction

Side Effects

Cardiovascular: hypotension, chest pain.
Gastrointestinal: diarrhea, nausea, abdominal pain, vomiting.
Nervous System: headache, dizziness, fatigue, weakness, fainting.
Urinary: decreased renal function (in patients with bilateral renal artery stenosis or heart failure).
Skin: rash.
Other: angioedema; abnormal blood profiles; hyperkalemia; dry, persistent, tickling, nonproductive cough; shortness of breath.

Onset, Peak, and Duration

Route	Onset	Peak	Duration
Oral	1 hr	4–6 hr	24 hr
I.V.	15 min	1–4 hr	6 hr

Massage Considerations

- No cautions or contraindications to massage are indicated because a client is taking this drug. Cautions and contraindications to massage may be related to the client condition.
- The vasodilating effects of the drug may be increased by massage and cause drops in blood pressure. Using stimulating massage at the end of the session with effleurage and tapotement may help.
- Side effects of hypotension and dizziness may be approached as above.
- Rash is a local contraindication for massage and should be reported to the physician. If severe, massage should be withheld.

enfuvirtide (ehn-FOO-ver-tighd)

Fuzeon

Drug Class: Anti-HIV drug, antiviral

Drug Actions

Controls symptoms of HIV infection

Use

- HIV-1 infection

Side Effects

Gastrointestinal: abdominal pain, constipation, diarrhea, nausea, pancreatitis.
Nervous System: anxiety, weakness, depression, insomnia, peripheral neuropathy.
Skin: itching, skin papilloma, bruising.
Other: herpes simplex, influenza, flulike illness, injection site reactions, conjunctivitis, sinusitis, taste disturbance, lymphadenopathy, anorexia, weight decrease, muscle pain, bacterial pneumonia, cough.

Onset, Peak, and Duration

Route	Onset	Peak	Duration
S.C.	Unknown	4–8 hr	Unknown

Massage Considerations

- No cautions or contraindications to massage are indicated because a client is taking this drug. Cautions and contraindications to massage may be related to the client condition.
- The side effect of peripheral neuropathy is a contraindication to deep tissue massage.
- Constipation may be helped by regular abdominal massage.
- Itching or skin eruptions are local contraindications to massage and should be reported to the physician. If severe, massage should be withheld.
- If bruising is a problem, deep tissue massage is contraindicated.

enoxaparin sodium (eh-NOKS-uh-pah-rin SOH-dee-um)

Lovenox

Drug Class: Anticoagulant

Drug Actions

Prevents pulmonary embolism and deep vein thrombosis

Use

- Prevention of deep vein thrombosis (DVT), which may lead to pulmonary embolism, following hip or knee replacement surgery
- Prevention of DVT, which may lead to pulmonary embolism, following abdominal surgery
- Prevention of ischemic complications of unstable angina and non–Q-wave heart attack
- In inpatients with acute DVT with or without pulmonary embolism
- In outpatients with acute DVT without pulmonary embolism
- In patients during acute illness who are at risk of embolism because of decreased mobility

Side Effects

Cardiovascular: edema, peripheral edema, cardiovascular toxicity.
Gastrointestinal: nausea.
Nervous System: fever, pain, confusion, neurologic injury (when used with spinal or epidural puncture).
Skin: irritation, pain, hematoma, or erythema at injection site; rash, hives, bruising.
Other: angioedema, abnormal blood profiles, hemorrhage, bleeding complications.

Onset, Peak, and Duration

Route	Onset	Peak	Duration
S.C.	Unknown	3–5 hr	<24 hr

 Massage Considerations

- In most cases, clients taking this drug may have a blood clot. If there is a blood clot, massage is completely contraindicated. If the client is taking this drug to prevent blood clots, massage may be given once physician approval has been obtained.
- Because of the action of the drug in decreasing blood clotting, deep tissue massage is contraindicated and circulatory massage with effleurage should be limited and used with caution.
- The site of injection of the drug should not be massaged for at least 5 hours or more to avoid speeding up the rate of absorption into the body.
- Side effects of rash or hives are a local contraindication to massage and should be reported to the physician immediately. If severe, massage should be withheld.
- If bruising is a problem, lightening up on pressure and depth is appropriate. If severe, the physician should be notified.

---

entacapone (en-TAK-uh-pohn)

Comtan

Drug Class: Antiparkinsonian

Drug Actions

Controls idiopathic Parkinson's disease signs and symptoms

Use

- Adjunct to levodopa and carbidopa in idiopathic Parkinson's disease

Side Effects

Gastrointestinal: nausea, diarrhea, abdominal pain, constipation, vomiting, dry mouth, painful digestion, gas, gastritis, taste perversion.
Nervous System: dyskinesia, hyperkinesia, hypokinesia, dizziness, anxiety, sleepiness, agitation, fatigue, weakness, hallucinations.
Urinary: urine discoloration.
Skin: sweating.
Other: bacterial infection, purpura, back pain, shortness of breath.

Onset, Peak, and Duration

Route	Onset	Peak	Duration
Oral	1 hr	1 hr	6 hr

Massage Considerations

- No cautions or contraindications to massage are indicated because a client is taking this drug. Cautions and contraindications to massage may be related to the client condition.
- Massage has been shown to increase levels of dopamine in the body. This will work with the desired effect of this drug. Using systemic reflex strokes such as rocking, rhythmic effleurage, and gentle friction will work well with this client.
- Side effects of dizziness and sleepiness require care in getting the client on and off the table. Using rapid effleurage and tapotement at the end of the session may help.
- Constipation may be helped by regular abdominal massage.
- The best strokes to use with this client are described above. Using mechanical strokes such as pétrissage is also appropriate. The local reflex strokes of stretching, traction, vibration, and compression may be less effective. Myofascial massage techniques may also be less effective, but this will vary depending on the client condition.

---

ephedrine sulfate (eh-FED-rin SUL-fayt)

Kondon's Nasal, Pretz-D

Drug Class: Adrenergic bronchodilator, vasopressor (parenteral form), nasal decongestant

Drug Actions

Stimulates alpha-adrenergic and beta-blocker receptors; direct- and indirect-acting sympathomimetic. Raises blood pressure, causes bronchodilation, and relieves nasal congestion.

Use

- Hypotension
- Bronchodilation
- Nasal decongestion

Side Effects

Cardiovascular: palpitations, tachycardia, hypertension, precordial pain.
Gastrointestinal: nausea, vomiting, anorexia.
Nervous System: insomnia, nervousness, dizziness, headache, euphoria, confusion, delirium.
Urinary: urine retention, painful urination from visceral sphincter spasm.
Skin: sweating.
Other: dryness of nose and throat, muscle weakness.

Onset, Peak, and Duration

Route	Onset	Peak	Duration
Oral	15–60 min	Unknown	3–5 hr
I.V.	≤5 min	Unknown	Unknown
I.M.	10–20 min	Unknown	30 min–1 hr
S.C.	Unknown	Unknown	30 min–1 hr
Intranasal	Unknown	Unknown	Unknown

Massage Considerations

- No cautions or contraindications to massage are indicated because a client is taking this drug. Cautions and contraindications to massage may be related to the client condition.
- This drug mimics the sympathetic nervous system (SNS) in the body. This may make the systemic reflex strokes of effleurage, rocking, and friction less effective, and it may take a

longer time for the client to feel the relaxing effects of massage. Using this strokes for longer periods than usual and throughout the session may help.
- The site of intramuscular or subcutaneous injection of the drug should not be massaged for at least 1 hour to avoid increasing the rate of absorption into the body.
- Side effects of dizziness require care in getting the client on and off the table. Stimulating the client at the end of the session with gentle friction to the lower legs will work best. Tapotement, which also turns on the SNS, should be used with caution.

---

epinastine hydrochloride (eh-pin-AH-stein high-droh-KLOR-ighd)

Elestat

Drug Class: Ophthalmic antihistamine

Drug Actions

Temporarily prevents eye itching

Use

- To prevent itching in allergic conjunctivitis

Side Effects

Nervous System: headache.
Other: infection (cold symptoms), burning eyes, hyperemia, increased lymph nodes near eyes, pharyngitis, itching of the eyes, rhinitis, sinusitis, increased cough, upper respiratory tract infection.

Onset, Peak, and Duration

Route	Onset	Peak	Duration
Eyedrops	Immediate	Unknown	8 hr

Massage Considerations

- No cautions or contraindications to massage are indicated because a client is taking this drug.

---

epinephrine (adrenaline) (eh-pih-NEF-rin)

Adrenalin, Bronkaid Mist, Bronkaid Mistometer, Primatene Mist

epinephrine bitartrate

AsthmaHaler Mist, Bronitin Mist, Bronkaid Mist Suspension, Medihaler-Epi, Primatene Mist Suspension

epinephrine hydrochloride

Adrenalin Chloride, Ana-Guard, EpiPen Auto-Injector, EpiPen Jr. Auto-Injector, Sus-Phrine

Drug Class: Adrenergic bronchodilator, vasopressor, cardiac stimulant, local anesthetic, topical antihemorrhagic

Drug Actions

Stimulates alpha-adrenergic and beta-blocker receptors in the SNS, causing a sympathomimetic response. Relaxes bronchial smooth muscle, causes cardiac stimulation, relieves allergic signs and symptoms, stops local bleeding, and decreases pain sensation.

Use

- Bronchospasm
- Hypersensitivity reactions
- Anaphylaxis
- Hemostasis
- Acute asthma attacks
- Prolonging local anesthetic effect
- Restoring cardiac rhythm in cardiac arrest

Side Effects

Cardiovascular: palpitations, widened pulse pressure, hypertension, tachycardia, ventricular fibrillation, shock, anginal pain, electrocardiogram changes (including decreased T-wave amplitude).
Gastrointestinal: nausea, vomiting.
Nervous System: nervousness, tremors, euphoria, anxiety, cold limbs, dizziness, headache, drowsiness, sweating, disorientation, agitation, fear, weakness, cerebral hemorrhage, stroke, increased rigidity and tremors (in patients with Parkinson's disease).
Skin: hives, pain.
Other: pallor, hemorrhage at injection site, hyperglycemia, glycosuria, shortness of breath.

Onset, Peak, and Duration

Route	Onset	Peak	Duration
I.V.	Immediate	≤5 min	1–4 hr
I.M.	Varies	Unknown	1–4 hr
S.C.	6–15 min	≤30 min	1–4 hr
Inhalation	3–5 min	Unknown	1–3 hr

 Massage Considerations

- In many cases, this drug is used for emergency situations and severe allergic reactions. Massage is completely contraindicated until the situation has resolved and the physician indicates massage is appropriate.
- In cases in which this drug is used regularly for control of asthma symptoms, massage may be given as long as the symptoms have resolved.
- The action of the drug mimics the sympathetic nervous system (SNS). The systemic reflex strokes of effleurage, rocking, and friction may not be as effective, and it may take longer for the client to feel the relaxation effects of massage. Using rocking and slow rythmic effleurage and applying them for longer periods of time throughout the session may help.
- The site of injection of the drug should not be massaged for up to 4 hours.
- Side effects of dizziness and drowsiness require care in getting the client on and off the table. Using gentle friction to the lower extremities will work best. Tapotement, because it also stimulates the SNS, should not be used.
- Hives are a local contraindication to massage and should be reported to the physician immediately. If severe, massage should be withheld until the condition resolves.

epirubicin hydrochloride (ep-uh-ROO-bih-sin high-droh-KLOR-ighd)

Ellence

Drug Class: Antineoplastic

Drug Actions

Kills certain cancer cells

Use

- Adjuvant therapy in patients with evidence of axillary node tumor involvement following resection of primary breast cancer

Side Effects

Cardiovascular: cardiomyopathy, heart failure.
Gastrointestinal: nausea, vomiting, diarrhea, anorexia, mucositis.
Nervous System: lethargy, fever.
Skin: hair loss, rash, itch, skin changes.
Other: infection, local toxicity, hot flushes, conjunctivitis, keratitis, lack of menstruation, abnormal blood profiles.

Onset, Peak, and Duration

Route	Onset	Peak	Duration
I.V.	Unknown	Unknown	Unknown

Massage Considerations

- Because of the toxic effects of this drug, deep tissue massage is contraindicated and circulatory massage with effleurage should be limited and used with caution. Other cautions and contraindications to massage may be related to the client condition. Close collaboration with the physician is essential.
- Because the drug is given every 3 to 4 weeks, it would be best to massage on weeks that the drug is not being given. The duration of action is unknown, but the half-life is 35 hours. If you are giving the massage after the drug is given, wait at least 2 days so as not to overtax the liver and kidneys as they try to rid the body of the drug.
- Side effects of rash or itching are local contraindications to massage and should be reported to the physician immediately. If severe, massage should be withheld.
- Hair loss is a contraindication to massage of the scalp if the client is disturbed by the loss of hair during the massage or if the scalp is tender.
- The best strokes to use are the systemic reflex strokes of rocking and gentle friction, mechanical strokes of pétrissage, and local reflex strokes of stretching, traction, and vibration. Myofascial massage techniques may be used for areas of tightness and gluteation.

eplerenone (eh-PLAIR-eh-nown)

Inspra

Drug Class: Antihypertensive

Drug Actions

Lowers blood pressure.

Use

- Hypertension
- Heart failure after heart attack

Side Effects

Gastrointestinal: diarrhea, abdominal pain.
Nervous System: dizziness, fatigue.
Urinary: albuminuria.
Other: flu syndrome, abnormal growth of breast tissue, abnormal vaginal bleeding, hyperkalemia, cough.

Onset, Peak, and Duration

Route	Onset	Peak	Duration
Oral	Unknown	$1\,^1/_2$ hr	Unknown

Massage Considerations

- No cautions or contraindications to massage are indicated because a client is taking this drug. Cautions and contraindications to massage may be related to the client condition.
- Side effects of dizziness require care in getting the client on and off the table. Using rapid effleurage or tapotement to stimulate the client at the end of the session may help.
- Abnormal growth of breast tissue may make the chest tender; using caution when massaging this area is indicated. If tenderness is severe, avoid massaging the chest area completely.

---

epoetin alfa (erythropoietin) (ee-POH-eh-tin AL-fah)

Epogen, Eprex, Procrit

Drug Class: Hematopoietic

Drug Actions

Mimics effects of erythropoietin, a naturally occurring hormone produced by the kidneys. Drug acts on erythroid tissues in bone marrow, enhancing rate of red blood cell production.

Use

- Anemia from reduced production of endogenous erythropoietin caused by end-stage renal disease
- Anemia in children with chronic renal impairment who are undergoing dialysis
- Adjunct treatment for HIV-infected patients with anemia secondary to zidovudine therapy
- Anemia secondary to chemotherapy
- Anemia related to rheumatoid arthritis and rheumatic disease
- Anemia related to prematurity

Side Effects

Cardiovascular: increased clotting of arteriovenous grafts, hypertension, edema.
Gastrointestinal: nausea, vomiting, diarrhea.
Nervous System: headache, seizures, paresthesia, fatigue, fever, dizziness, weakness.
Skin: rash, hives.
Other: injection site reaction, iron deficiency, thrombocytosis, joint pain, cough, shortness of breath.

Onset, Peak, and Duration

Route	Onset	Peak	Duration
I.V.	1–6 wk	Immediate	Unknown
S.C.	1–6 wk	5–24 hr	Unknown

 Massage Considerations

- The physician should be consulted before any massage is given. Deep tissue massage should be used with great caution or not at all.
- The site of injection should not be massaged for at least 24 hours to avoid increasing the rate of absorption of the drug into the body.
- Side effects of dizziness require care in getting the client on and off the table. Using stimulating strokes such as rapid effleurage at the end of the session may help.
- Paresthesia is a local caution related to depth; no deep tissue massage should be given.
- Rash or hives are local contraindications to massage and should be reported to the physician immediately. If severe, massage should be withheld.

eprosartan mesylate (eh-proh-SAR-ten MEH-sih-layt)

Teveten

Drug Class: Antihypertensive

Drug Actions

Lowers blood pressure

Use

- Hypertension

Side Effects

Cardiovascular: chest pain, dependent edema, hypertriglyceridemia.
Gastrointestinal: abdominal pain, painful digestion, diarrhea.
Nervous System: depression, fatigue, headache, dizziness.
Urinary: urinary tract infection.
Other: injury, viral infection, pharyngitis, rhinitis, sinusitis, neutropenia, joint pain, muscle pain, cough, upper respiratory tract infection, bronchitis.

Onset, Peak, and Duration

Route	Onset	Peak	Duration
Oral	1–2 hr	1–3 hr	24 hr

 Massage Considerations

- No cautions or contraindications to massage are indicated because a client is taking this drug. There may be cautions or contradictions to massage related to the client condition.
- Side effects of dizziness require care in getting the client on and off the table. Using stimulating strokes such as rapid effeurage or tapotement at the end of the session may help.

ertapenem sodium (er-ta-PEN-uhm SOH-dee-um)

Invanz

Drug Class: Anti-infective

Drug Actions

Kills susceptible bacteria

Use

- Complicated intra-abdominal infections
- Complicated skin and skin-structure infections
- Community-acquired pneumonia
- Complicated urinary tract infections, including pyelonephritis
- Acute pelvic infections including postpartum endomyometritis, septic abortion, and post-surgical gynecologic infections

Side Effects

Cardiovascular: edema, swelling, chest pain, hypertension, hypotension, tachycardia.
Gastrointestinal: abdominal pain, acid regurgitation, oral candidiasis, constipation, diarrhea, painful digestion, nausea, vomiting, abdominal distension, *Clostridium difficile* infection, pseudomembranous colitis.
Nervous System: weakness, fatigue, anxiety, altered mental status, dizziness, headache, insomnia, seizures, fever, pain.
Urinary: vaginitis, renal dysfunction, hematuria, urinary retention.
Skin: redness, itching, rash, extravasation, infused vein complication, phlebitis, thrombophlebitis.
Other: septicemia, death, chills, hypersensitivity reactions, coagulation abnormalities, abnormal blood profiles, thrombocytosis, jaundice, hyperglycemia, hyperkalemia, hypernatremia, leg pain, cough, shortness of breath, rales, rhonchi, respiratory distress.

Onset, Peak, and Duration

Route	Onset	Peak	Duration
I.V.	Immediate	30 min	24 hr
I.M.	Unknown	2 hr	24 hr

Massage Considerations

- Although there are no cautions or contraindications to massage related to the action of this drug, cautions and contraindications to massage may exist related to the client's condition and severity of infection. The physician should be consulted prior to any massage.
- The site of intramuscular injection should not be massaged for at least 24 hours so as not to increase the rate of absorption of the drug into the body.
- Side effects of hypotension and dizziness require care in getting the client on and off the table. Using stimulation at the end of the massage with tapotement and effleurage may help.
- Constipation may be helped by abdominal massage.
- Rash or itching is a local contraindication to massage and should be reported to the physician immediately. If severe, massage should be withheld.
- Thrombophlebitis is a complete contraindication to massage.

---

erythromycin base (eh-rith-roh-MIGH-sin bays)

Apo-Erythro, E-Base, E-Mycin, Erybid, ERYC, Ery-Tab, Erythromycin Base Filmtab, Erythromycin Delayed-Release, PCE Dispertab

erythromycin estolate

Ilosone, Ilosone Pulvules

erythromycin ethylsuccinate

Apo-Erythro-ES, EES, EES Granules, EryPed, EryPed 200, EryPed 400

erythromycin lactobionate

Erythrocin

erythromycin stearate

Apo-Erythro-S, Erythrocin Stearate

Drug Class: Antibiotic

Drug Actions

Inhibits bacterial growth

Use

- Acute pelvic inflammatory disease
- Endocarditis prophylaxis for dental procedures in patients allergic to penicillin
- Intestinal amebiasis
- Mild to moderately severe respiratory tract, skin, and soft tissue infections
- Syphilis
- Legionnaires' disease
- Uncomplicated urethral, endocervical, or rectal infections when tetracyclines are contraindicated
- Urogenital *Chlamydia trachomatis* infections during pregnancy
- Conjunctivitis caused by *C. trachomatis* in neonates
- Pneumonia of infancy caused by *C. trachomatis*
- Early form of Lyme disease in persons allergic to penicillins and cephalosporins and in whom tetracyclines are contraindicated
- Early Lyme disease manifested as erythema migrans

Side Effects

Cardiovascular: ventricular arrhythmias, venous irritation or thrombophlebitis after intravenous injection.
Gastrointestinal: abdominal pain and cramping, nausea, vomiting, diarrhea.
Nervous System: fever.
Skin: hives, rash, eczema.
Other: overgrowth of nonsusceptible bacteria or fungi, anaphylaxis, hearing loss with high intravenous doses.

Onset, Peak, and Duration

Route	Onset	Peak	Duration
Oral	Unknown	1–4 hr	Unknown
I.V.	Immediate	Immediate	Unknown

 Massage Considerations

- No cautions or contraindications to massage are indicated because a client is taking this drug. Cautions and contraindications to massage may be related to the client condition.
- Side effects of thrombophlebitis are a complete contraindication to massage.
- Hives and rash are a local contraindication to massage and should be reported to the physician immediately. If severe, massage should be withheld.

escitalopram oxalate (ES-sigh-TAL-uh-pram ocks-UH-layt)

Lexapro

Drug Class: Selective serotonin reuptake inhibitor (SSRI) antidepressant

Drug Actions

May increase serotonergic activity in the central nervous system resulting from inhibition of neuronal reuptake of serotonin. Relieves depressive symptoms and anxiety.

Use

- Major depressive disorder

Side Effects

Cardiovascular: palpitations, hypertension, flushing, chest pain.
Gastrointestinal: nausea, diarrhea, constipation, indigestion, abdominal pain, vomiting, increased or decreased appetite, dry mouth, gas, heartburn, cramps, gastroesophageal reflux.
Nervous System: fever, headache, insomnia, dizziness, sleepiness, paresthesia, light-headedness, migraine, tremor, abnormal dreams, irritability, impaired concentration, fatigue, lethargy.
Urinary: ejaculation disorder, impotence, anorgasmia, menstrual cramps, urinary tract infection, urinary frequency.
Skin: rash, increased sweating.
Other: decreased libido, yawning, flulike symptoms, toothache, rhinitis, sinusitis, blurred vision, ringing in the ears, earache, weight gain or loss, joint pain, muscle pain, muscle cramps, extremity pain, bronchitis, cough.

Onset, Peak, and Duration

Route	Onset	Peak	Duration
Oral	Unknown	5 hr	Unknown

Massage Considerations

- No cautions or contraindications to massage are indicated because a client is taking this drug. Cautions and contraindications to massage may be related to the client condition.
- Side effects of dizziness, sleepiness, or light-headedness require care in getting the client on and off the table. Using rapid effleurage and tapotement at the end of the session may help.
- Constipation and gas may be helped by regular abdominal massage.
- Urinary frequency may require the client to get up during the session. Privacy and quick access to the bathroom should be provided. Water fountains or water music, which may stimulate the need to urinate, should be avoided.
- Rash is a local contraindication to massage and should be reported to the physician. If severe, massage should be withheld.

esomeprazole magnesium (e-soh-MEP-rah-zohl mag-NEEZ-ee-uhm)

Nexium

Drug Class: Proton pump inhibitor gastroesophageal drug

Drug Actions

Suppresses gastric secretion through proton pump inhibition. Decreases gastric acid.

Use

- Gastroesophageal reflux disease (GERD)
- Healing of erosive esophagitis
- Long-term maintenance of healing in erosive esophagitis
- Eradication of *Helicobacter pylori* to reduce duodenal ulcer recurrence

Side Effects

Gastrointestinal: diarrhea, abdominal pain, nausea, gas, dry mouth, vomiting, constipation.
Nervous System: headache.

Onset, Peak, and Duration

Route	Onset	Peak	Duration
Oral	Unknown	1 1/2 hr	13–17 hr

 Massage Considerations

- No cautions or contraindications to massage are indicated because a client is taking this drug.
- Side effects of gas and constipation may be helped by regular abdominal massage.

---

estazolam (eh-STAZ-uh-lam)

ProSom

Drug Class: Benzodiazepine hypnotic

Drug Actions

May act on limbic system and thalamus of central nervous system by binding to specific benzodiazepine receptors, resulting in sedation.

Use

- Insomnia

Side Effects

Gastrointestinal: painful digestion, abdominal pain.
Nervous System: fatigue, dizziness, daytime drowsiness, weakness, hypokinesia, headache, abnormal thinking.
Other: back pain, stiffness.

Onset, Peak, and Duration

Route	Onset	Peak	Duration
Oral	Unknown	1–3 hr	Unknown

 Massage Considerations

- The sedative effects of this drug may interfere with perception of pain and sensations. Deep tissue massage should be used with caution.
- The action of the drug may increase the effects of systemic reflex strokes such as rocking and effleurage and increase the relaxing effects of massage. It may also decrease the effectiveness of local reflex strokes such as stretching, compression, and vibration. Using

a more stimulating massage throughout the session and applying the local reflex strokes for a longer period of time will help.

- Side effects of dizziness and drowsiness require care in getting the client on and off the table. Using more stimulating massage as noted above may help.

---

estradiol (oestradiol) (eh-struh-DIGH-ol)

Alora, Climara, Dermestril, Esclim, Estrace, Estrace Vaginal Cream, Estraderm, Estraderm MX, Estring, FemPatch, Femtran, Gynodiol, Menorest, Oesclim, Vivelle, Vivelle-Dot

estradiol acetate

Femring Vaginal Ring

estradiol cypionate

Depo-Estradiol

estradiol hemihydrate

Estrasorb, Vagifem

estradiol valerate (oestradiol valerate)

Delestrogen

Drug Class: Estrogen replacement, antineoplastic

Drug Actions

Relieves vasomotor menopausal symptoms, provides estrogen replacement, relieves vaginal dryness, and palliates advanced prostate or breast cancer.

Use

- Vasomotor symptoms
- Vulvar and vaginal atrophy
- Hypoestrogenism from hypogonadism, castration, or primary ovarian failure
- Atrophic vaginitis
- Kraurosis vulvae
- Palliative treatment for advanced, inoperable breast cancer
- Palliative treatment for advanced, inoperable prostate cancer
- Prevention of postmenopausal osteoporosis in high-risk patients

Side Effects

Cardiovascular: thrombophlebitis, thromboembolism, hypertension, edema.
Gastrointestinal: nausea, vomiting, abdominal cramps, bloating, diarrhea, constipation, pancreatitis.
Nervous System: headache, dizziness, chorea, depression, seizures.
Skin: skin discoloration, hives, rash, dermatitis, hair loss.
Other: possibility of increased risk of breast cancer, breast changes (tenderness, enlargement, secretion), abnormal growth of breast tissue, worsening of myopia or astigmatism, intolerance of contact lenses, breakthrough bleeding, altered menstrual flow, dysmenorrhea, amenorrhea, increased risk of endometrial cancer, cervical erosion, altered cervical secretions, enlargement of uterine fibromas, vaginal candidiasis, testicular atrophy, impotence, cholestatic jaundice, gallbladder disease, hepatic adenoma, increased appetite, weight changes, hyperglycemia, hypercalcemia.

Onset, Peak, and Duration

Route	Onset	Peak	Duration
Oral, I.M. intravaginal	Unknown	Unknown	Unknown
Transdermal Esclim	Unknown	27–30 hr	Unknown

Massage Considerations

- No cautions or contraindications to massage are indicated because a client is taking this drug. Cautions and contraindications to massage may be related to the client condition.
- The site of intramuscular injection should not be massaged for 2 to 4 weeks, until the next injection is given. Do not massage the site of the transdermal patch.
- Side effects of thrombophlebitis or embolism are a complete contraindication to massage. If the client is having pain, redness, swelling, or heat, especially in the lower extremities, do not massage and refer to the physician for evaluation of possible blood clot immediately.
- Dizziness requires care in getting the client on and off the table. Using stimulation at the end of the session with effleurage and tapotement may help.
- Constipation may be helped by regular abdominal massage.
- Rash or dermatitis is a local contraindication to massage and should be reported to the physician. If severe, massage should be withheld.
- Hair loss contraindicates scalp massage because it may increase the hair loss.
- Breast changes or abnormal growth of breast tissue may cause tenderness. Caution should be used in massaging this area and if tenderness is severe, massage of the area should be avoided.

---

estrogens, conjugated (estrogenic substances, conjugated; oestrogens, conjugated) (ES-troh-jenz, KAHN-jih-gayt-ed)

C.E.S., Cenestin, Premarin, Premarin Intravenous

Drug Class: Estrogen replacement, antineoplastic, antiosteoporotic

Drug Actions

Provides estrogen replacement, relieves vasomotor menopausal symptoms and vaginal dryness, helps prevent severity of osteoporosis, and provides palliative action for prostate and breast cancer.

Use

- Abnormal uterine bleeding caused by hormonal imbalance
- Vulvar or vaginal atrophy
- Castration
- Primary ovarian failure
- Hypogonadism
- Moderate to severe vasomotor symptoms with or without moderate to severe symptoms of vulvar and vaginal atrophy related to menopause
- Palliative treatment for inoperable prostatic cancer
- Palliative treatment for breast cancer
- Prevention of osteoporosis

Side Effects

Cardiovascular: thrombophlebitis; thromboembolism; hypertension; edema; increased risk of stroke, pulmonary embolism, and heart attack.
Gastrointestinal: nausea, vomiting, abdominal cramps, bloating, diarrhea, constipation, anorexia, pancreatitis.
Nervous System: headache, dizziness, chorea, depression, lethargy, seizures.
Skin: skin discoloration, hives, rash, dermatitis, flushing (with rapid intravenous administration), abnormal hair growth, hair loss.
Other: breast changes (tenderness, enlargement, secretion), possibility of increased risk of breast cancer, abnormal growth of breast tissue, worsening of myopia or astigmatism, intolerance of contact lenses, breakthrough bleeding, altered menstrual flow, dysmenorrhea, amenorrhea, increased risk of endometrial cancer, cervical erosion, altered cervical secretions, enlargement of uterine fibromas, vaginal candidiasis, testicular atrophy, impotence, gallbladder disease, cholestatic jaundice, hepatic adenoma, increased appetite, weight changes, hyperglycemia, hypercalcemia.

Onset, Peak, and Duration

Route	Onset	Peak	Duration
All routes	Unknown	Unknown	Unknown

Massage Considerations

- No cautions or contraindications to massage are indicated because a client is taking this drug. Cautions and contraindications to massage may be related to the client condition.
- The site of intramuscular injection should not be massaged for at least 24 hours.
- Side effects of thrombophlebitis or embolism are a complete contraindication to massage. If the client is having pain, redness, swelling, or heat, especially in the lower extremities, do not massage and refer to the physician for evaluation of possible blood clot immediately.
- Dizziness requires care in getting the client on and off the table. Using stimulation at the end of the session with effleurage and tapotement may help.
- Constipation may be helped by regular abdominal massage.
- Rash or dermatitis is a local contraindication to massage and should be reported to the physician. If severe, massage should be withheld.
- Hair loss contraindicates scalp massage because it may increase the hair loss.
- Breast changes or abnormal growth of breast tissue may cause tenderness. Caution should be used in massaging this area and if tenderness is severe, massage of the area should be avoided.

---

estrogens, esterified (ES-troh-jenz, ES-ter-eh-fighd)

Estratab, Menest, Neo-Estronel

Drug Class: Estrogen replacement, antineoplastic

Drug Actions

Provides estrogen replacement, hinders prostate and breast cancer cell growth, and relieves vasomotor menopausal symptoms and vaginal dryness.

Use

- Inoperable prostate cancer
- Breast cancer
- Hypogonadism

- Castration
- Primary ovarian failure
- Vasomotor menopausal symptoms
- Atrophic vaginitis or urethritis
- Prevention of osteoporosis

Side Effects

Cardiovascular: thrombophlebitis; thromboembolism; hypertension; edema; increased risk of stroke, pulmonary embolism, and heart attack.
Gastrointestinal: nausea, vomiting, abdominal cramps, bloating, diarrhea, constipation, anorexia, pancreatitis.
Nervous System: headache, dizziness, chorea, depression, lethargy, seizures.
Skin: skin discoloration, rash, dermatitis, abnormal hair growth, hair loss.
Other: abnormal growth of breast tissue, breast changes (tenderness, enlargement, secretion), worsening of myopia or astigmatism, intolerance of contact lenses. breakthrough bleeding, altered menstrual flow, dysmenorrhea, amenorrhea, possibility of increased risk of breast cancer, increased risk of endometrial cancer, cervical erosion, altered cervical secretions, enlargement of uterine fibromas, vaginal candidiasis, testicular atrophy, impotence, cholestatic jaundice, hepatic adenoma, gallbladder disease, increased appetite, weight changes, hypercalcemia.

Onset, Peak, and Duration

Route	Onset	Peak	Duration
Oral	Unknown	Unknown	Unknown

Massage Considerations

- No cautions or contraindications to massage are indicated because a client is taking this drug. Cautions and contraindications to massage may be related to the client condition.
- Side effects of thrombophlebitis or embolism are a complete contraindication to massage. If the client is having pain, redness, swelling, or heat, especially in the lower extremities, do not massage and refer to the physician for evaluation of possible blood clot immediately.
- Dizziness requires care in getting the client on and off the table. Using stimulation at the end of the session with effleurage and tapotement may help.
- Constipation may be helped by regular abdominal massage.
- Rash or dermatitis is a local contraindication to massage and should be reported to the physician. If severe, massage should be withheld.
- Hair loss contraindicates scalp massage because it may increase the hair loss.
- Breast changes or abnormal growth of breast tissue may cause tenderness. Caution should be used in massaging this area and if tenderness is severe, massage of the area should be avoided.

---

estropipate (piperazine estrone sulfate) (es-troh-PIH-payt)

Ogen, Ortho-Est

Drug Class: Estrogen replacement

Drug Actions

Provides estrogen replacement, relieves vasomotor menopausal symptoms, and helps reduce severity of osteoporosis.

Use

- Management of moderate to severe vasomotor symptoms
- Vulvar and vaginal atrophy
- Primary ovarian failure
- Castration
- Hypogonadism
- Prevention of osteoporosis

Side Effects

Cardiovascular: edema; thrombophlebitis; increased risk of stroke, pulmonary embolism, thromboembolism, and heart attack.
Gastrointestinal: nausea, vomiting, abdominal cramps, bloating.
Nervous System: depression, headache, dizziness, migraine, seizures.
Skin: hemorrhagic eruption, rash, abnormal hair growth, skin discoloration, hair loss.
Other: breast engorgement or enlargement, libido changes, aggravation of porphyria, increased size of uterine fibromas, increased risk of endometrial cancer, possibility of increased risk of breast cancer, vaginal candidiasis, cystitis-like syndrome, dysmenorrhea, amenorrhea, breakthrough bleeding, cholestatic jaundice, hypercalcemia, weight changes.

Onset, Peak, and Duration

Route	Onset	Peak	Duration
Oral, intravaginal	Unknown	Unknown	Unknown

Massage Considerations

- No cautions or contraindications to massage are indicated because a client is taking this drug. Cautions and contraindications to massage may be related to the client condition.
- Side effects of thrombophlebitis or embolism are a complete contraindication to massage. If the client is having pain, redness, swelling, or heat, especially in the lower extremities, do not massage and refer to the physician for evaluation of possible blood clot immediately.
- Dizziness requires care in getting the client on and off the table. Using stimulation at the end of the session with effleurage and tapotement may help.
- Rash or dermatitis is a local contraindication to massage and should be reported to the physician. If severe, massage should be withheld.
- Hair loss contraindicates scalp massage because it may increase the hair loss.
- Breast changes may cause tenderness. Caution should be used in massaging this area and if tenderness is severe, massage of the area should be avoided.

---

etanercept (ee-TAN-er-sept)

Enbrel

Drug Class: Antirheumatic

Drug Actions

Reduces signs and symptoms of rheumatoid arthritis

Use

- Psoriatic arthritis
- Ankylosing spondylitis
- Reducing signs and symptoms and delaying structural damage in patients with moderately to severely active rheumatoid arthritis
- Reducing signs and symptoms of moderately to severely active polyarticular-course juvenile rheumatoid arthritis

Side Effects

Gastrointestinal: abdominal pain, painful digestion.
Nervous System: weakness, headache, dizziness.
Skin: rash.
Other: infections, malignancies, injection site reaction, rhinitis, pharyngitis, sinusitis, upper respiratory tract infections, cough, respiratory disorder.

Onset, Peak, and Duration

Route	Onset	Peak	Duration
S.C.	Unknown	72 hr	Unknown

 Massage Considerations

- No cautions or contraindications to massage are indicated because a client is taking this drug. Cautions and contraindications to massage may be related to the client condition.
- The site of injection of the drug should not be massaged for 3 days (72 hours) after injection to avoid increasing the rate of absorption of the drug into the body.
- Side effects of dizziness require care in getting the client on and off the table. Using rapid effleurage or tapotement at the end of the session to stimulate the client may help.
- Rash is a local contraindication to massage and should be reported to the physician. If severe or widespread, massage should be withheld.

---

ethacrynate sodium (eth-uh-KRIH-nayt SOH-dee-um)

Sodium Edecrin

ethacrynic acid

Edecril, Edecrin

Drug Class: Diuretic

Drug Actions

Promotes sodium and water excretion

Use

- Acute pulmonary edema
- Edema
- Hypertension

Side Effects

Cardiovascular: volume depletion and dehydration, orthostatic hypotension.
Gastrointestinal: cramping, diarrhea, anorexia, nausea, vomiting, gastrointestinal bleeding, pancreatitis.
Nervous System: fever, malaise, confusion, fatigue, dizziness, headache, nervousness.
Urinary: increase urination at night, frequent urination, lack of urination, hematuria.
Skin: dermatitis, rash.
Other: chills, transient deafness (with too-rapid intravenous injection), blurred vision, ringing in the ears, hearing loss, abnormal blood profiles, asymptomatic hyperuricemia; hypochloremic alkalosis; fluid and electrolyte imbalances, including dilutional hyponatremia, hypokalemia, hypocalcemia, hypomagnesemia; hyperglycemia and impairment of glucose tolerance.

Onset, Peak, and Duration

Route	Onset	Peak	Duration
Oral	30 min	2 hr	6–8 hr
I.V.	5 min	15–30 min	2 hr

Massage Considerations

- No cautions or contraindications to massage are indicated because a client is taking this drug. Cautions and contraindications to massage may be related to the client condition.
- Side effects of hypotension or dizziness require care in getting the client on and off the table. Using tapotement at the end of the massage or gentle friction to the legs may help.
- Frequent urination may require the client to get up during the session. Privacy and quick access to the bathroom are needed. Water fountains or water music, which may stimulate the need to urinate, should not be used. Limiting circulatory massage with effleurage may also help. Rash is a local contraindication to massage and should be reported to the physician. If severe, massage should be withheld.

---

ethambutol hydrochloride (ee-THAM-byoo-tol high-droh-KLOR-ighd)

Etibi, Myambutol

Drug Class: Antituberculotic

Drug Actions

Hinders bacterial growth.

Use

- Adjunct therapy for pulmonary tuberculosis
- Adjunct therapy for pulmonary *Mycobacterium avium* complex (MAC) infections in patients without HIV
- Adjunct therapy for disseminated MAC complex infections

Side Effects

Gastrointestinal: anorexia, nausea, vomiting, abdominal pain.
Nervous System: fever, malaise, headache, dizziness, confusion, possibly hallucinations, peripheral neuritis.
Skin: dermatitis, itching, toxic epidermal necrolysis.
Other: anaphylactoid reactions, precipitation of gout, dose-related optic neuritis (vision loss and loss of color discrimination, especially red and green), thrombocytopenia, bloody sputum.

Onset, Peak, and Duration

Route	Onset	Peak	Duration
Oral	Unknown	2–4 hr	Unknown

Massage Considerations

- No cautions or contraindications to massage are indicated because a client is taking this drug. Cautions and contraindications to massage may be related to the client condition.
- Side effects of dizziness require care in getting the client on and off the table. Stimulation at the end of the massge with effleurage or tapotement may help.
- Peripheral neuritis is a contraindication to deep tissue massage and if severe, may contraindicate massage completely.

- Rash or itching are local contraindications to massage and should be reported to the physician immediately. If severe, massage should be withheld.

---

ethinyl estradiol and desogestrel (ETH-uh-nil es-truh-DIGH-ol and DAY-so-jest-rul)

monophasic

Apri, Desogen, Ortho-Cept

biphasic

Mircette, Kariva

triphasic

Cyclessa

ethinyl estradiol and ethynodiol diacetate

monophasic

Demulen 1/35, Demulen 1/50, Zovia 1/35E, Zovia 1/50E

ethinyl estradiol and levonorgestrel

emergency

Preven

monophasic

Levlen, Nordette, Alesse, Aviane, Lessina, Portia

triphasic

Tri-Levlen, Triphasil, Trivora, Enpresse

ethinyl estradiol and norethindrone

monophasic

Brevicon, Genora 0.5/35, Genora 1/35, ModiCon, NEE 1/35, Norethin 1/35E, Norinyl 1 + 35, Ortho-Novum 1/35, Ovcon-35, Ovcon-50

biphasic

Necon 10/11, Nortrel, Ortho-Novum 10/11

triphasic

Necon 7/7/7, Nortrel 7/7/7, Ortho-Novum 7/7/7, Tri-Norinyl

ethinyl estradiol and norethindrone acetate

monophasic

Junel 21-1/20, Junel 21-1.5/30, Loestrin 21 1/20, Loestrin 21 1.5/30

triphasic

Estrostep

ethinyl estradiol and norgestimate

monophasic

MonoNessa, Ortho-Cyclen, Sprintec

triphasic

Ortho Tri-Cyclen, Ortho Tri-Cyclen Lo, Tri-Sprintec

ethinyl estradiol and norgestrel

monophasic

Cryselle, Lo/Ovral, Ovral, Ogestrel

ethinyl estradiol, norethindrone acetate, and ferrous fumarate

monophasic

Loestrin Fe 1/20, Loestrin Fe 1.5/30, Microgestin Fe 1/20, Microgestin Fe 1.5/30

mestranol and norethindrone

monophasic

Necon, Norinyl 1 + 50, Ortho-Novum 1/50

triphasic

Estrostep Fe, Estrostep 21

Drug Class: Estrogen with progestin hormonal contraceptive

Drug Actions

Chemical effect: Inhibits ovulation through negative feedback mechanism directed at hypothalamus. Estrogen suppresses secretion of follicle-stimulating hormone, blocking follicle development and ovulation. Progestin suppresses secretion of luteinizing hormone so ovulation cannot occur. Progestin thickens cervical mucus, which interferes with sperm migration and prevents implantation. Prevents pregnancy and relieves signs and symptoms of endometriosis.

Use

- Contraception
- Moderate acne vulgaris in women and girls age 15 and older

Side Effects

Cardiovascular: thromboembolism, hypertension, edema, pulmonary embolism, stroke.
Gastrointestinal: granulomatous colitis, nausea, vomiting, abdominal cramps, bloating, diarrhea, constipation, anorexia, pancreatitis.
Nervous System: headache, dizziness, depression, lethargy, migraine.
Skin: rash, acne.
Other: breast changes (tenderness, enlargement, secretion), worsening of myopia or astigmatism, intolerance of contact lenses, exophthalmos, diplopia. breakthrough bleeding, dysmenorrhea, amenorrhea, cervical erosion or abnormal secretions, enlargement of uterine fibromas, vaginal candidiasis, gallbladder disease, cholestatic jaundice, liver tumors, changes in appetite, weight gain, hyperglycemia, hypercalcemia.

Onset, Peak, and Duration

Route	Onset	Peak	Duration
Oral	Unknown	Varies	Unknown

Massage Considerations

- No cautions or contraindications to massage are indicated because a client is taking thisdrug. There may be cautions or contradictions to massage related to the client condition.
- Side effects of thromboembolism are a complete contraindication to massage. If the client has pain, redness, heat, or swelling, especially of the lower extremities, do not massage and refer to the physician immediately to evaluate for possible blood clots.

- Dizziness requires care in getting the client on and off the table. Using stimulation at the end of the session with effleurage and tapotement may help.
- Constipation may be helped by regular abdominal massage.
- Rash or acne is a local contraindication to massage and should be reported to the physician. If the acne is widespread and the client still desires massage, wearing gloves when massaging the affected areas is appropriate to prevent contact with blood and body fluids.
- Breast changes may cause tenderness. Caution should be used when massaging the chest. If tenderness is severe, massage of the chest should be avoided.

ethinyl estradiol (EE) and drospirenone (DRSP)

(ETH-in-il es-tra-DIE-ol and droh-SPEER-ih-nohn)

Yasmin

Drug Class: Hormonal contraceptive

Drug Actions

Suppresses gonadotropins, follicle-stimulating hormone, and luteinizing hormone, thereby preventing ovulation, changing the cervical mucus to increase the difficulty of the sperm to penetrate, and changing the endometrium to increase the difficulty of implantation. Reduces the opportunity for conception.

Use

- Contraception

Side Effects

Cardiovascular: arterial thromboembolism, hypertension, edema, mesenteric thrombosis, heart attack, thrombophlebitis.
Gastrointestinal: abdominal pain, abdominal cramping, bloating, changes in appetite, colitis, diarrhea, gastroenteritis, nausea, vomiting.
Nervous System: weakness, cerebral hemorrhage, cerebral thrombosis, depression, dizziness, emotional lability, headache, migraine nervousness.
Skin: acne, rash, hemorrhagic eruption, abnormal growth of hair, loss of scalp hair, skin discoloration, itching.
Other: changes in libido, breast changes, decreased lactation, cataracts, change in corneal curvature (steepening), intolerance to contact lenses, pharyngitis, retinal thrombosis, sinusitis, amenorrhea, breakthrough bleeding, change in cervical erosion and secretion, change in menstrual flow, cystitis, cystitis-like syndrome, dysmenorrhea, hemolytic uremic syndrome, renal impairment, leukorrhea, menstrual disorder, premenstrual syndrome, spotting, temporary infertility after discontinuing treatment, urinary tract infection, vaginal candidiasis, vaginitis, Budd-Chiari syndrome, cholestatic jaundice, gallbladder disease, hepatic adenomas, benign liver tumors, reduced tolerance to carbohydrates, porphyria, weight gain, back pain, bronchitis, pulmonary embolism, upper respiratory tract infection.

Onset, Peak, and Duration

Route	Onset	Peak	Duration
Oral	Unknown	1–3 hr	Unknown

Massage Considerations

- There are no cautions or contraindications to massage because the client is taking this medication. There may be cautions or contraindications to massage related to the client condition.
- Side effects of thromboembolism are a complete contraindication to massage. If the client has pain, redness, heat, or swelling, especially of the lower extremities, do not massage and refer to the physician immediately to evaluate for possible blood clots.

- Dizziness requires care in getting the client on and off the table. Using stimulation at the end of the session with effleurage and tapotement may help.
- Rash, itching, or acne are local contraindications to massage and should be reported to the physician. If the acne is widespread and the client still desires massage, wearing gloves when massaging the affected areas is appropriate to prevent contact with blood and body fluids.
- Breast changes may cause tenderness. Caution should be used when massaging the chest. If tenderness is severe, massage of the chest should be avoided.

ethinyl estradiol and etonogestrel vaginal ring

(ETH-ih-nil es-tra-DYE-ole and et-oh-noe-JES-trel)

NuvaRing

Drug Class: Progestin/estrogen intravaginal contraceptive

Drug Actions

Suppresses gonadotropins, which inhibits ovulation, increases the viscosity of cervical mucus (decreasing the ability of sperm to enter the uterus), and alters the endometrial lining (reducing potential for implantation). Decreases risk of pregnancy.

Use

- Contraception

Side Effects

Gastrointestinal: nausea.
Nervous System: headache, emotional lability.
Other: vaginitis, leukorrhea, device-related events (such as foreign body sensation, coital difficulties, device expulsion), vaginal discomfort, weight gain, upper respiratory tract infection.

Onset, Peak, and Duration

Route	Onset	Peak	Duration
Vaginal	Immediate	Unknown	Unknown

 Massage Considerations

- There are no cautions or contraindications to massage related to this drug.

ethinyl estradiol and norelgestromin transdermal system (ETH-ih-nil es-tra-DYE-ole and nor-el-GES-tro-min)

Ortho-Evra

Drug Class: Transdermal contraceptive patch

Drug Actions

Suppresses gonadotropins and inhibits ovulation. Changes cervical mucus, complicating entry of sperm into the uterus and changes endometrium, decreasing the likelihood of implantation. Reduces risk of pregnancy.

Use

- Contraception

Side Effects

Cardiovascular: thromboembolic events, heart attack, hypertension, edema, cerebral hemorrhage.
Gastrointestinal: nausea, abdominal pain, vomiting.
Nervous System: headache, emotional lability.
Skin: application site reaction.
Other: breast tenderness, enlargement, or secretion; contact lens intolerance; menstrual cramps; changes in menstrual flow; vaginal candidiasis; hepatic adenomas; benign liver tumors; gallbladder disease; weight changes; upper respiratory tract infection.

Onset, Peak, and Duration

Route	Onset	Peak	Duration
Transdermal	Rapid	2 days	Unknown

Massage Considerations

- There are no cautions or contraindications to massage because the client is taking this medication. There may be cautions or contraindications to massage related to the client condition.
- Side effects of thromboembolism are a complete contraindication to massage. If the client has pain, redness, heat, or swelling, especially of the lower extremities, do not massage and refer to the physician immediately to evaluate for possible blood clots.
- Breast changes may cause tenderness. Caution should be used when massaging the chest. If tenderness is severe, massage of the chest should be avoided.

---

etodolac (ultradol) (eh-toh-DOH-lak)

Lodine, Lodine XL

Drug Class: Nonsteroidal anti-inflammatory drug (NSAID) antiarthritic

Drug Actions

May inhibit prostaglandin synthesis. Relieves inflammation and pain.

Use

- Acute pain
- Acute or long-term management of osteoarthritis or rheumatoid arthritis

Side Effects

Cardiovascular: hypertension, heart failure, flushing, palpitations, edema, fluid retention.
Gastrointestinal: painful digestion, gas, abdominal pain, diarrhea, nausea, constipation, gastritis, melena, vomiting, anorexia, peptic ulceration with or without gastrointestinal bleeding or perforation, ulcerative stomatitis, thirst.
Nervous System: weakness, malaise, dizziness, depression, drowsiness, nervousness, insomnia, headache, fever, syncope.
Urinary: painful urination, urinary frequency, renal impairment.
Skin: itching, rash, photosensitivity, Stevens-Johnson syndrome.
Other: chills, blurred vision, tinnitus, photophobia, dry mouth, hemolytic anemia, abnormal blood profiles, hepatitis, weight gain, asthma.

Onset, Peak, and Duration

Route	Onset	Peak	Duration
Oral	≤30 min	1–2 hr	4–12 hr

Massage Considerations

- This drug may decrease the perception of pain; therefore, deep tissue massage should be used with caution. Other cautions and contraindications to massage may be related to the client condition.
- Side effects of dizziness and drowsiness require care in getting the client on and off the table. Using rapid effleurage and tapotement at the end of the massage may help.
- Gas and constipation may be helped by regular abdominal massage.
- Urinary frequency may require the client to get up during the session. Providing privacy and quick access to the bathroom is needed. Water fountains or water music, which may stimulate the need to urinate, should not be used.
- Itching or rash are local contraindications to massge and should be reported to the physician. If severe, the massage should be withheld.

etoposide (VP-16) (eh-toh-POH-sighd)

Etopophos, Toposar, VePesid

Drug Class: Antineoplastic

Drug Actions

Inhibits selected cancer cell growth

Use

- Testicular cancer
- Small cell carcinoma of lung
- AIDS-related Kaposi sarcoma

Side Effects

Cardiovascular: hypotension.
Gastrointestinal: nausea, vomiting, anorexia, diarrhea, abdominal pain, stomatitis.
Nervous System: peripheral neuropathy.
Skin: reversible hair loss, rash.
Other: anaphylaxis, abnormal blood profiles, myelosuppression.

Onset, Peak, and Duration

Route	Onset	Peak	Duration
Oral, I.V.	Unknown	Unknown	Unknown

Massage Considerations

- Because of the toxic effects of this drug, deep tissue massage is contraindicated and circulatory massage with effleurage should be limited. Further cautions or contraindications to massage may be related to the client condition. Close collaboration with the physician is essential.
- This drug is usually given for several days every 2 to 4 weeks and has a half-life of up to 11 hours. It would be best to give massage on the weeks when the client is not receiving the drug. No massage should be given for at least 24 hours.

- Side effects of hypotension require care in getting the client on and off the table. Using tapotement or gentle friction to stimulate the client at the end of the massage may help.
- Peripheral neuropathy requires caution in depth of massage.
- Hair loss is a contraindication to scalp massage if the client is disturbed by hair loss during the massage or if the scalp is tender.
- Rash is a local contraindication to massage and should be reported to the physician immediately. If severe, massage should be withheld.

---

exemestane (ecks-eh-MES-tayn)

Aromasin

Drug Class: Antineoplastic

Drug Actions

Hinders function of breast cancer cells.

Use

- Advanced breast cancer in postmenopausal women whose disease has progressed after tamoxifen therapy.

Side Effects

Cardiovascular: hot flushes, hypertension, edema, chest pain.
Gastrointestinal: nausea, vomiting, abdominal pain, anorexia, constipation, diarrhea, painful digestion.
Nervous System: fever, depression, insomnia, anxiety, fatigue, pain, dizziness, headache, paresthesia, generalized weakness, confusion, hypesthesia.
Urinary: urinary tract infection.
Skin: rash, increased sweating, hair loss, itching.
Other: infection, flulike syndrome, lymphedema, sinusitis, rhinitis, pharyngitis, increased appetite, pathologic fractures, joint pain, back pain, skeletal pain, shortness of breath, bronchitis, coughing, upper respiratory tract infection.

Onset, Peak, and Duration

Route	Onset	Peak	Duration
Oral	Unknown	1–2 hr	Unknown

Massage Considerations

- No cautions or contraindications to massage are indicated because a client is taking this drug. In most cases, cautions or contraindications to massage will be related to the client condition. Close collaboration with the physician is essential, and contact with the physician should be made before starting massage therapy.
- Side effects of dizziness require care in getting the client on and off the table. Using stimulation at the end of the massage with effleurage or tapotement may help.
- Paresthesia or hypesthesia (decrease in sensation) contraindicates deep tissue massage.
- Constipation may be helped by regular abdominal massage.
- Rash or itching is a local contraindication to massage and should be reported to the physician immediately. If severe, massage should be withheld.
- Hair loss is a contraindication to massage if the client is disturbed by loss of hair during the massage or if the scalp is tender.

ezetimibe (eh-ZET-eh-mighb)

Zetia

Drug Class: Antilipemic

Drug Actions

Lowers cholesterol levels

Use

- Primary hypercholesterolemia, alone or with HMG-CoA reductase inhibitors
- Adjunct to atorvastatin or simvastatin in patients with homozygous familial hypercholesterolemia
- Homozygous sitosterolemia to reduce sitosterol and campesterol levels

Side Effects

Cardiovascular: chest pain.
Gastrointestinal: abdominal pain, diarrhea.
Nervous System: dizziness, headache, fatigue.
Other: viral infection, pharyngitis, sinusitis, back pain, joint pain, muscle pain, cough, upper respiratory tract infection.

Onset, Peak, and Duration

Route	Onset	Peak	Duration
Oral	Unknown	4–12 hr	Unknown

 Massage Considerations

- No cautions or contraindications to massage are indicated because a client is taking this drug.
- Side effects of dizziness require care in getting the client on and off the table. Using rapid effleurage or tapotement at the end of the session may help.

F

factor IX complex (FAK-tor nighn KOM-pleks)

Bebulin VH Immuno, Benefix, Konyne 80, Profilnine SD, Proplex T

factor IX (human)

AlphaNine SD, Mononine

Drug Class: Blood derivative

Drug Actions

Directly replaces deficient clotting factor

Use

- Factor IX deficiency (hemophilia B or Christmas disease)
- Anticoagulant overdosage

Side Effects

Cardiovascular: thromboembolic reactions, heart attack, disseminated intravascular coagulation, pulmonary embolism, flushing, changes in blood pressure.
Gastrointestinal: nausea, vomiting.
Nervous System: transient fever, headache.
Skin: hives.
Other: chills, tingling, hypersensitivity reactions (anaphylaxis, hives, chest tightening, hypotension).

Onset, Peak, and Duration

Route	Onset	Peak	Duration
I.V.	Immediate	10–30 min	Unknown

Massage Considerations

- Because this drug has to do with blood clotting, serious cautions and contraindications may exist related to the client condition. Massage should not be given without first consulting with the physician. If massage is given, deep tissue massage and tapotement are contraindicated and myofascial techniques must be used with caution until the client response to the technique is determined.
- Side effect of thromboembolism is a complete contraindication to massage. Changes in blood pressure may cause dizziness and require care in getting the client on and off the table. Using more stimulating effleurage at the end of the session may help. Hives are a local contraindication to massage and should be reported to the physician immediately. If severe, massage should be withheld.
- The best strokes to use with this client are systemic and local reflex strokes of rocking, effleurage, gentle stretching, vibration and the mechanical stroke of pétrissage.

---

famciclovir (fam-SIGH-kloh-veer)

Famvir

Drug Class: Antiviral

Drug Actions

Inhibits viral replication. Spectrum of activity includes herpes simplex types 1 and 2 and varicella-zoster viruses.

Use

- Acute herpes zoster
- Recurrent episodes of genital herpes
- Recurrent herpes simplex virus infections in HIV-infected patients
- Long-term suppressive therapy of recurrent episodes of genital herpes

Side Effects

Gastrointestinal: diarrhea, nausea, vomiting, constipation, anorexia, abdominal pain.
Nervous System: headache, fatigue, dizziness, paresthesia, sleepiness.
Skin: itching, zoster-related signs, symptoms, complications.
Other: pharyngitis, sinusitis, back pain, joint pain.

Onset, Peak, and Duration

Route	Onset	Peak	Duration
Oral	Unknown	≤1 hr	Unknown

Massage Considerations

- There are no cautions or contraindications to massage related solely to the client taking this medication. There may be cautions and contraindications to massage related to the client condition.
- Side effects of sleepiness require care in getting the client off the table. Using stimulation at the end of the session with effleurage and tapotement may help. Paresthesia is a contraindication to deep tissue massage. Constipation may be helped by regular abdominal massage. Itching is a local contraindication to massage and should be reported to the physician. If severe, or if massage worsens the symptoms, massage should be withheld.

famotidine (fam-OH-tih-deen)

Pepcid, Pepcid AC, Pepcid RPD, Pepcidine

Drug Class: Antiulcer agent

Drug Actions

Competitively inhibits action of H_2 at receptor sites of parietal cells, decreasing gastric acid secretion. Decreases gastric acid levels and prevents heartburn.

Use

- Duodenal ulcer (short-term treatment)
- Benign gastric ulcer (short-term treatment)
- Pathologic hypersecretory conditions (such as Zollinger-Ellison syndrome)
- Gastroesophageal reflux disease (GERD)
- Peptic ulcer in children
- Heartburn, prevention of heartburn
- Hospitalized patients with intractable ulcerations or hypersecretory conditions or patients who can't take oral medication

Side Effects

Cardiovascular: palpitations, flushing.
Gastrointestinal: constipation, anorexia, taste disorder, dry mouth.
Nervous System: headache, dizziness, malaise, paresthesia, fever.
Skin: acne, dry skin.
Other: transient irritation at I.V. site, ringing in the ears, orbital edema, musculoskeletal pain.

Onset, Peak, and Duration

Route	Onset	Peak	Duration
Oral	≤1 hr	1–3 hr	10–12 hr
I.V.	≤1 hr	20 min	10–12 hr

Massage Considerations

- There are no cautions or contraindications to massage related to this drug.
- Side effects of dizziness require care in getting the client on and off the table. Using rapid effleurage or tapotement at the end of the session may help. Paresthesia is a contraindication to deep tissue massage. Constipation may be helped by regular abdominal massage.

---

felodipine (feh-LOH-dih-peen)

Agon, Agon SR, Plendil, Plendil ER, Renedil

Drug Class: Calcium-channel blocker antihypertensive

Drug Actions

Lowers blood pressure

Use

- Hypertension

Side Effects

Cardiovascular: flushing, peripheral edema, chest pain, palpitations.
Gastrointestinal: abdominal pain, nausea, constipation, diarrhea.
Nervous System: headache, dizziness, paresthesia, weakness.
Skin: rash.
Other: rhinorrhea, pharyngitis, gingival hyperplasia, muscle cramps, back pain, upper respiratory infection, cough.

Onset, Peak, and Duration

Route	Onset	Peak	Duration
Oral	2–5 hr	2 ½–5 hr	24 hr

Massage Considerations

- There are no cautions or contraindications to massage because the client is taking this drug. There may be cautions and contraindications to massage related to the client condition.
- The action of the drug in lowering blood pressure may be increased by massage. Using stimulation at the end of the session or even a more stimulating massage throughout the session may be used to help with any problems.
- Side effects of dizziness may be addressed as noted earlier. Paresthesia is a contraindication to deep tissue massage. Constipation may be helped by regular abdominal massage. Rash is a local contraindication to massage and should be reported to the physician. If severe, massage should be withheld.

---

fenofibrate (feh-noh-FIGH-brayt)

Tricor, Lofibra

Drug Class: Antilipemic

Drug Actions

Decreases triglyceride levels

Use

- Adjunct to diet for patients with very high triglyceride levels (type IV and V hyperlipidemia)
- Adjunct to diet for the reduction of LDL cholesterol, total cholesterol, triglycerides, and apolipoprotein B, and to increase HDL in patients with primary hypercholesterolemia or mixed dyslipidemia

Side Effects

Cardiovascular: arrhythmias.
Gastrointestinal: painful digestion, belching, gas nausea, vomiting, abdominal pain, constipation, diarrhea, pancreatitis, increased appetite.
Nervous System: dizziness, pain, weakness, fatigue, paresthesia, insomnia, headache.
Urinary: polyuria, vaginitis.
Skin: itching, rash.
Other: hypersensitivity reaction, infection, flulike syndrome, decreased libido, eye irritation, eye floaters, earache, conjunctivitis, blurred vision, rhinitis, sinusitis, cholelithiasis, joint pain, cough.

Onset, Peak, and Duration

Route	Onset	Peak	Duration
Oral	Unknown	6–8 hr	Unknown

 Massage Considerations

- There are no cautions or contraindications to massage related to the client taking this drug. There may be cautions and contraindications related to the client condition.
- Side effects of dizziness require care in getting the client on and off the table. Using stimulation at the end of the massage with effleurage and tapotement may help. Paresthesia is a contraindication to deep tissue massage. Gas and constipation may be helped by regular abdominal massage. Rash or itching are a local contraindication to massage and should be reported to the physician. If severe, massage should be withheld.

---

fentanyl citrate (FEN-tuh-nihl SIGH-trayt)

Sublimaze

fentanyl transdermal system

Duragesic-25, Duragesic-50, Duragesic-75, Duragesic-100

fentanyl transmucosal

Actiq

Drug Class: Opioid analgesic, adjunct to anesthesia, anesthetic

Drug Actions

May bind with opioid receptors in CNS, altering both perception of and emotional response to pain

Use

- Adjunct to general anesthetic
- Adjunct to regional anesthesia
- Postoperative pain
- Management of chronic pain
- Breakthrough cancer pain in opioid-tolerant patients

Side Effects

Cardiovascular: hypotension, hypertension, arrhythmias, chest pain, bradycardia.
Gastrointestinal: nausea, vomiting, constipation, ileus, abdominal pain.
Nervous System: sedation, sleepiness, clouded sensorium, euphoria, dizziness, headache, confusion, weakness, nervousness, hallucinations, anxiety, depression.
Urinary: urine retention.
Skin: itching, sweating.
Other: physical dependence, reaction at application site (erythema, papules, edema), respiratory depression, hypoventilation, shortness of breath, apnea.

Onset, Peak, and Duration

Route	Onset	Peak	Duration
I.V.	1–2 min	3–5 min	30 min–1 hr
I.M.	7–15 min	20–30 min	1–2 hr
Transmucosal	15 min	20–30 min	Unknown
Transdermal	12–24 hr	1–3 days	Varies

Massage Considerations

- This drug alters sensation and the perceptions of pain; therefore, deep tissue massage is contraindicated. There may be other cautions or contraindications to massage related to the client condition.
- The sedating effect on the CNS may increase the relaxing effects of massage and the systemic reflex strokes of effleurage, pétrissage, and friction. These may be applied in a more stimulating manner by increasing speed. It also may decrease the effectiveness of local reflex strokes such as compression, stretching, traction, and vibration. These may need to be applied for longer than usual periods to have effect.
- The site of I.M. injection should not be massaged for at least an hour to prevent increasing the rate of absorption. The site of transdermal patches should not be massaged.
- The side effects of sedation, dizziness, sleepiness, and hypotension may require stimulation at the end of the massage with rapid effleurage and tapotement. If severe or worsened by massage, a more stimulating massage throughout the session is indicated. Stay with the client as they sit up after the massage until certain they are not dizzy and are able to get up safely. Constipation may be helped by regular abdominal massage. Itching is a local contraindication to massage and should be reported to the physician immediately. If severe or worsened by massage, massage should be withheld.
- The best strokes to use with this client are the mechanical strokes of effluerage, pétrissage, and friction. Other strokes and techniques may be used as noted earlier.

---

ferous fumarate (FEH-rus FYOO-muh-rayt)

Femiron, Feostat, Feostat Drops, Ferretts , Fumasorb, Fumerin, Hemocyte, Ircon, Maniron , Neo-Fer, Nephro-Fer, Novofumar, Palafer, Palafer Pediatric Drops, Span-FF

ferrous gluconate

Fergon, Fertinic, Novoferrogluc

ferrous sulfate

Apo-Ferrous Sulfate, Feosol, Feratab, Fer-Gen-Sol Drops, Fer-In-Sol, Fer-Iron Drops, Fero-Grad, Fero-Gradumet, Irospan, Mol-Iron

ferrous sulfate, dried

Feosol, Fer-In-Sol, Fe 50, Slow-Fe

Drug Class: Oral iron supplement

Drug Actions

Provides elemental iron, relieves iron deficiency and anemia

Use

- Iron deficiency anemia

Side Effects

Gastrointestinal: nausea, epigastric pain, vomiting, constipation, diarrhea, black stools, anorexia.
Other: suspension and drops may temporarily stain teeth.

Onset, Peak, and Duration

Route	Onset	Peak	Duration
Oral	≤4 days	7–10 days	2–4 mo

Massage Considerations

- There are no cautions or contraindications to massage related to this drug
- Side effects of constipation may be helped by regular abdominal massage

fexofenadine hydrochloride (feks-oh-FEN-uh-deen high-droh-KLOR-ighd)

Allegra, Telfast

Drug Class: Antihistamine

Drug Actions

Selectively inhibits peripheral H_1-receptors. Relieves symptoms of seasonal allergies.

Use

- Seasonal allergic rhinitis
- Chronic idiopathic hives

Side Effects

Gastrointestinal: nausea, painful digestion.
Nervous System: fatigue, drowsiness.
Other: viral infection, painful menstruation.

Onset, Peak, and Duration

Route	Onset	Peak	Duration
Oral	Unknown	3 hr	14 hr

Massage Considerations

- There are no cautions or contraindications to massage related to the client taking this drug.
- Side effects of drowsiness may be helped by stimulating the client at the end of the session with effleurage or tapotement.

filgrastim (granulocyte colony-stimulating factor; G-CSF) (fil-GRAH-stem)

Neupogen

Drug Class: Biologic response modifier, colony-stimulating factor, hematopoietic

Drug Actions

Stimulates proliferation and differentiation of hematopoietic cells. Drug is specific for neutrophils. Raises White blood cell (WBC) levels.

Use

- Agranulocytosis
- Pancytopenia with colchine overdose
- Acute leukemia
- Hematologic toxicity with zidovudine therapy
- Decrease risk of infection in patients with nonmyeloid cancers receiving myelosuppressive antineoplastics
- To decrease risk of infection in patients with nonmyeloid cancers receiving myelosuppressive antineoplastics followed by bone marrow transplant
- Congenital neutropenia
- Idiopathic or cyclic neutropenia
- Peripheral blood progenitor cell collection
- Myelodysplasia
- Neutropenia from HIV infection

Side Effects

Cardiovascular: heart attack, arrhythmias, chest pain.
Gastrointestinal: nausea, vomiting, diarrhea, mucositis, stomatitis, constipation.
Nervous System: fever, fatigue, headache, weakness.
Urinary: hematuria, proteinuria.
Skin: hair loss, rash, cutaneous vasculitis.
Other: hypersensitivity reactions, thrombocytopenia, leukocytosis, skeletal pain, shortness of breath, cough.

Onset, Peak, and Duration

Route	Onset	Peak	Duration
I.V.	5–60 min	24 hr	1–7 days
Subcutaneous Injection	5–60 min	2–8 hr	1–7 days

 Massage Considerations

- This drug is indicative of a client who is immunosuppressed. The physician should be consulted before massage is given. Care should be taken to not expose the client to infection by scheduling them as the first client of the day. The massage therapist should not give massage if they have any signs of infection.
- The site of subcutaneous injection should not be massaged for at least 8 hours and preferably not for at least 24 hours.

- Side effects of contipation may be helped by regular abdominal massage. Rash is a local contraindication to massage and should be reported to the physician immediately. If severe, no massage should be given. Hair loss is a contraindication to scalp massage if the client is upset by loss of hair occuring during the massage or if the scalp is tender.

finasteride (fin-ES-teh-righd)

Propecia, Proscar

Drug Class: Steroid derivative, androgen synthesis inhibitor

Drug Actions

Relieves symptoms of BPH, reduces hair loss, and promotes hair growth

Use

- Adjunct therapy after radical prostatectomy
- First-stage prostate cancer
- Acne
- Hirsutism
- To reduce risk of acute urinary retention and need for surgery, including prostatectomy and transurethral resection of prostate in symptomatic benign prostatic hypertrophy
- Male pattern baldness

Side Effects

Urinary: impotence, decreased volume of ejaculate.
Other: decreased libido.

Onset, Peak, and Duration

Route	Onset	Peak	Duration
Oral	Unknown	1–2 hr	About 2 wk

Massage Considerations

- There are no cautions or contraindications to massage related to the client taking this medication. There may be cautions and contraindications to massage related to the client condition.

fluconazole (floo-KON-uh-zohl)

Diflucan

Drug Class: Antifungal

Drug Actions

Hinders fungal growth

Use

- Oropharyngeal and esophageal candidiasis
- Vulvovaginal candidiasis
- Systemic candidiasis
- Cryptococcal meningitis
- Prevention of candidiasis in bone marrow transplant
- Suppression of relapse of cryptococcal meningitis in patients with AIDS

- Candidal infection, long-term suppression in patients with HIV infection
- Prevention of mucocutaneous *candidiasis, cryptococcosis,* coccidioidomycosis, or histoplasmosis in patients with HIV infection

Side Effects

Gastrointestinal: nausea, vomiting, abdominal pain, diarrhea.
Nervous System: headache.
Skin: rash, Stevens-Johnson syndrome.
Other: anaphylaxis, hepatotoxicity.

Onset, Peak, and Duration

Route	Onset	Peak	Duration
Oral	Unknown	1–2 hr	Unknown
I.V.	Immediate	Immediate	Unknown

 Massage Considerations

- There are no cautions or contraindications to massage related to this drug itself. There may be cautions and contraindications to massage related to the client condition.
- The side effect of rash is a local contraindication to massage and should be reported to the physician immediately. If severe, massage should be withheld.

---

flucytosine (5-fluorocytosine, 5-FC) (floo-SIGH-toh-seen)

Ancobon, Ancotil

Drug Class: Antifungal

Drug Actions

Hinders fungal growth, including some strains of Cryptococcus and Candida

Use

- Severe fungal infections caused by susceptible strains of *Candida* (including septicemia, endocarditis, urinary tract and pulmonary infections) and *Cryptococcus* (meningitis, pulmonary infection, and possible urinary tract infections)
- Chromomycosis

Side Effects

Cardiovascular: chest pain, cardiac arrest.
Gastrointestinal: nausea, vomiting, diarrhea, abdominal pain, dry mouth, duodenal ulcer, hemorrhage, ulcerative colitis.
Nervous System: dizziness, confusion, headache, sedation, fatigue, weakness, hallucinations, psychosis, ataxia, paresthesia, parkinsonism, peripheral neuropathy.
Urinary: azotemia, crystalluria, renal impairment.
Skin: occasional rash, itching, hives photosensitivity.
Other: hypoglycemia, hypokalemia, abnormal blood profiles, bone marrow suppression, hearing loss, jaundice, respiratory arrest, shortness of breath.

Onset, Peak, and Duration

Route	Onset	Peak	Duration
Oral	Unknown	1–2 hr	Unknown

 Massage Considerations

- There are no cautions and contraindications to massage related to the action of the drug. However, the client condition will have cautions and contraindications to massage and the physician should be consulted before any massage is given.
- Side effects of dizziness and sedation requires care in getting the client on and off the table. Using stimulation at the end of the session such as friction to the lower legs may help. Paresthesia is a contraindication to deep tissue massage. Rash, itching, and hives are local contraindications to massage and should be reported to the physician immediately. If severe, massage should be withheld.

---

fludarabine phosphate (floo-DAR-uh-been FOS-fayt)

Fludara

Drug Class: Antineoplastic

Drug Actions

Kills susceptible cancer cells

Use

- B-cell chronic lymphocytic leukemia
- Mycosis fungoides
- Hairy cell leukemia
- Hodgkin's and malignant lymphoma
- CNS: fever, fatigue, malaise, weakness, paresthesia, headache, peripheral neuropathy, sleep disorder, depression, pain, cerebellar syndrome, CVA, transient ischemic attack, agitation, confusion, coma

Side Effects

Cardiovascular: edema, angina, phlebitis, arrhythmias, heart failure, heart attack, supraventricular tachycardia, deep venous thrombosis, aneurysm, hemorrhage.
Gastrointestinal: nausea, vomiting, diarrhea, constipation, anorexia, stomatitis, GI bleeding, esophagitis, mucositis.
Urinary: painful urination, urinary tract infection, urinary hesitancy, proteinuria, hematuria, renal impairment.
Skin: hair loss, sweating, rash, itching.
Other: chills, infection, tumor lysis syndrome, anaphylaxis, visual disturbances, hearing loss, delayed blindness (with high doses), sinusitis, pharyngitis, epistaxis, anemia, myelosuppression, neutropenia, thrombocytopenia, liver failure, cholelithiasis, hyperglycemia, dehydration, hyperuricemia, hyperphosphatemia, muscle pain, cough, pneumonia, dyspnea, upper respiratory infection, allergic pneumonitis, hemoptysis, hypoxia, bronchitis.

Onset, Peak, and Duration

Route	Onset	Peak	Duration
I.V.	7–21 hr	Unknown	Unknown

 Massage Considerations

- Because of the toxic nature of this drug, deep tissue massage in contraindicated.
- Circulatory massage with effleurage should be done with caution and limited.
- Close collaboration with the physician is essential as there may be further cautions and contraindications to massage related to the client condition.

- This drug is usually given for several days in a row, one time a month. With an unknown duration of action and a half-life of about 10 hours, massage would best be given on weeks that the drug is not given. If given in the same week, massage at least 24 hours after the drug was last given.
- Side effects of paresthesia requires care in depth of massage. Deep vein thrombosis is a complete contraindication to massage. Constipation may be helped by regular abdominal massage. Rash and itching are a local contraindication to massage and should be reported to the physician immediately. If severe, massage should be withheld. Hair loss is a contraindication to scalp massage if the client is disturbed by hair coming out during the massage or if the scalp is tender.
- The best strokes to use are the systemic and local reflex strokes of rocking, friction, stretching, traction, and vibration. Pétrissage and myofascial massage techniques also may be used.

fludrocortisone acetate (floo-droh-KOR-tuh-sohn AS-ih-tayt)

Forinef

Drug Class: Mineralocorticoid, glucocorticoid

Drug Actions

Increases sodium levels and decreases potassium and hydrogen levels

Use

- Adrenal insufficiency (partial replacement)
- Adrenogenital syndrome
- Orthostatic hypotension

Side Effects

Cardiovascular: sodium and water retention, hypertension, cardiac hypertrophy, edema, heart failure.
Skin: bruising, sweating, urticaria, allergic rash.
Other: hypokalemia.

Onset, Peak, and Duration

Route	Onset	Peak	Duration
Oral	Varies	Varies	1–2 days

Massage Considerations

- Although this drug is used for replacement therapy, it is difficult to regulate and each client's condition will require different approaches. Close consultation with the physician is required. Deep tissue massage should be use with great caution and in many cases will be contraindicated.
- Side effects of bruising require care with depth and if deep tissue massage is being used it should no longer be applied. Hives or rash are a local contraindication to massage and should be reported to the physician immediately. If severe, massage should be withheld.

fluorouracil (5-fluorouracil, 5-FU) (floo-roh-YOOR-uh-sil)

Adrucil, Carac, Efudex, Fluoroplex

Drug Class: Antineoplastic

Drug Actions

Inhibits cell growth of selected cancers

Use

- Colon, rectal, breast, stomach, and pancreatic cancers
- Palliative treatment of advanced colorectal cancer
- Multiple actinic (solar) keratoses
- Superficial basal cell carcinoma
- Multiple actinic or solar keratosis of the face and anterior scalp

Side Effects

Cardiovascular: thrombophlebitis, myocardial ischemia, angina.
Gastrointestinal: stomatitis, GI ulcer (may precede leukopenia), nausea and vomiting, diarrhea, anorexia, GI bleeding.
Nervous System: acute cerebellar syndrome, ataxia, confusion, disorientation, euphoria, headache, nystagmus, weakness, malaise.
Skin: reversible hair loss, rash, itching, nail changes; pigmented palmar creases; erythematous, desquamative rash of hands and feet with long-term use ("hand-foot syndrome"); photosensitivity; pain, burning, soreness, suppuration, and swelling with topical use.
Other: anaphylaxis, nose bleeds, photophobia, lacrimation, lacrimal duct stenosis, visual changes, abnormal blood profiles.

Onset, Peak, and Duration

Route	Onset	Peak	Duration
I.V. Topical	Unknown	Unknown	Unknown

Massage Considerations

- Because of the toxic effects of this drug when taken orally, deep tissue massage is contraindicated and circulatory massage with effleurage should be used with caution and limited. Topical use of the drug does not have these cautions but the site of application should not be massaged.
- Close collaboration with the physician is essential. There may be other cautions and contraindications to massage related to the client condition.
- The I.V. drug is usually given several days in a row and then repeated every 2–4 weeks. It has a short half-life of 20 minutes. Massage would be best given on weeks when the drug is not being administered or at minimum 24 hours after administration.
- Side effects of thrombophlebitis are a complete contraindication to massage. Rash or itching are a local contraindication to massage and should be reported to the physician. If severe, no massage should be given. Hair loss is a contraindication to scalp massage if the client is disturbed by hair loss during the massage or if the scalp is tender.
- The best strokes for this client include the systemic and reflex strokes of rocking, friction, stretching, traction, and vibration, and the mechanical stroke of pétrissage. Myofascial massage techniques may be used for areas of tightness and gluteation.

fluoxetine hydrochloride (floo-OKS-eh-teen high-droh-KLOR-ighd)

Prozac, Prozac-20, Prozac Weekly, Sarafem

Drug Class: Selective Serotonin Reuptake Inhibitor (SSRI) antidepressant

Drug Actions

May inhibit CNS neuronal uptake of serotonin. Relieves depression and obsessive-compulsive behaviors.

Use

- Depression
- Obsessive-compulsive disorder
- Maintenance therapy for depression in stabilized patients
- Binge eating and vomiting behaviors in patients with moderate-to-severe bulimia nervosa
- Premenstrual dysphoric disorder (PMDD)
- Anorexia nervosa
- Depression linked to bipolar disorder
- Panic disorder with or without agoraphobia
- Cataplexy
- Alcohol dependence

Side Effects

Cardiovascular: palpitations.
Gastrointestinal: nausea, diarrhea, dry mouth, anorexia, painful digestion, constipation, abdominal pain, vomiting, gas, increased appetite.
Nervous System: fever, nervousness, anxiety, insomnia, sleepiness, headache, drowsiness, fatigue, tremor, dizziness, weakness.
Skin: rash, itching, hives.
Other: flulike syndrome, hot flushes, sexual dysfunction, nasal congestion, pharyngitis, sinusitis, weight loss, muscle pain, cough, upper respiratory infection, respiratory distress.

Onset, Peak, and Duration

Route	Onset	Peak	Duration
Oral	1–4 wk	6–8 hr	Unknown

 Massage Considerations

- There are no cautions or contraindications to massage related to this drug. There may be cautions and contraindications to massage related to the client condition.
- Side effects of dizziness, sleepiness, and drowsiness require care in getting the client on and off the table. Using rapid effleurage and tapotement at the end of the session may help. If severe, more stimulating and rapid massage techniques throughout the session may be useful. Constipation may be helped by regular abdominal massage. Rash, itching, or hives are local contraindications to massage and should be reported to the physician. If severe or worsened by massage, no massage should be given.

fluphenazine decanoate (floo-FEN-uh-zeen deh-kuh-NOH-ayt)

Modecate, Modecate Concentrate, Prolixin Decanoate

fluphenazine enanthate

Moditen Enanthate, Prolixin Enanthate

fluphenazine hydrochloride

Anatensol, Apo-Fluphenazine, Modecate Concentrate, Moditen HCL, Permitil, Permitil Concentrate, Prolixin, Prolixin Concentrate

Drug Class: Antipsychotic

Drug Actions

May block dopamine receptors in brain. Relieves psychotic signs and symptoms.

Use

- Psychotic disorders

Side Effects

Cardiovascular: orthostatic hypotension, tachycardia, ECG changes.
EENT: dry mouth, ocular changes, blurred vision, nasal congestion.
Gastrointestinal: constipation.
Nervous System: extrapyramidal reactions, tardive dyskinesia, sedation, pseudoparkinsonism, EEG changes, drowsiness, seizures, dizziness, neuroleptic malignant syndrome.
Urinary: urine retention, dark urine, menstrual irregularities, abnormal growth of breast tissue, inhibited ejaculation.
Skin: mild photosensitivity.
Other: allergic reactions, dry mouth, ocular changes, blurred vision, nasal congestion, abnormal blood profiles, cholestatic jaundice, weight gain, increased appetite.

Onset, Peak, and Duration

Route	Onset	Peak	Duration
Oral	≤1 hr	30 min	6–8 hr
I.M., Subcutaneous Injection.	1–3 days	Unknown	1–6 wk

 Massage Considerations

- The actions of this drug on the CNS are unknown, but because of the sedative effects deep tissue massage is contraindicated.
- The physician should be consulted before any massage is given, and close collaboration with the physician is essential.
- The site of I.M. of subcutaneous injection should not be massaged for at least 2 weeks.
- The side effects of sedation, drowsiness, dizziness, and hypotension requires care in positioning and getting the client on and off the table. Using rapid effleurage or friction to the lower legs may help. If severe, more stimulating and rapid massage techniques used throughout the session would be appropriate. Constipation may be helped by regular abdominal massage. Abnormal growth of breast tissue in men or women may cause tenderness. Massage of the area should be done with caution and, if severe, the area should be avoided.

---

flurazepam hydrochloride (floo-RAH-zuh-pam high-droh-KLOR-ighd)

Apo-Flurazepam, Dalmane, Novo-Flupam, Somnol

Drug Class: Benzodiazepine sedative-hypnotic

Drug Actions

May act on limbic system, thalamus, and hypothalamus of CNS to produce hypnotic effects. Promotes sleep and calmness.

Use

- Insomnia

Side Effects

Gastrointestinal: nausea, vomiting, heartburn, diarrhea, abdominal pain.
Nervous System: daytime sedation, dizziness, drowsiness, disturbed coordination, lethargy, confusion, headache, nervousness, hallucinations, staggering, ataxia, disorientation, coma.
Other: physical or psychological dependence.

Onset, Peak, and Duration

Route	Onset	Peak	Duration
Oral	Unknown	30 min–1 hr	Unknown

 Massage Considerations

- The sedative and CNS depressant effects of this drug require that deep tissue massage be used with caution.
- Side effects of dizziness, sedation, and drowsiness require care in getting the client on and off the table. Using rapid effleurage and tapotement at the end of the session may help. If severe, more stimulating massage throughout the session may be required.

flutamide (FLOO-tuh-mighd)

Euflex, Eulexin

Drug Class: Antineoplastic

Drug Actions

Hinders prostatic cancer cell activity

Use

- Locally advanced (stage B2) or metastatic (stage D2) prostatic carcinoma

Side Effects

Cardiovascular: peripheral edema, hypertension.
Gastrointestinal: diarrhea, nausea, vomiting, anorexia.
Nervous System: drowsiness, confusion, depression, anxiety, nervousness, paresthesia.
Urinary: impotence.
Skin: rash, photosensitivity.
Other: hot flushes, loss of libido, abnormal growth of breast tissue, hepatitis, hepatic encephalopathy, abnormal blood profiles.

Onset, Peak, and Duration

Route	Onset	Peak	Duration
Oral	Unknown	2 hr	Unknown

 Massage Considerations

- Although this drug itself does not have cautions or contraindications to massage or affect how the body reacts to massage, there may be cautions and contraindications related to the client condition. The physician should be consulted before giving massage.
- Side effects of drowsiness may require care in getting the client on and off the table.
- Using stimulation with effleurage or friction to the lower legs may help. Rash is a local contraindication to massage and should be reported to the physician immediately. If severe, massage should be withheld.

fluticasone propionate (FLU-tih-ka-sohn proh-PIGH-oh-nayt)

Flonase, Flovent Inhalation Aerosol, Flovent Rotadisk

Drug Class: Corticosteroid topical and inhalation anti-inflammatory

Drug Actions

Synthetic glucocorticoid improves breathing ability by reducing inflammation

Use

- Asthma prevention and chronic asthma
- Management of nasal symptoms of seasonal and perennial allergic and nonallergic rhinitis

Side Effects

Gastrointestinal: diarrhea, abdominal pain, viral gastroenteritis, colitis, abdominal discomfort, nausea, vomiting.
Nervous System: fever, headache, dizziness, migraine, nervousness.
Skin: rash, hives.
Other: dental problems, influenza, mouth irritation, oral candidiasis, pharyngitis, acute nasopharyngitis, nasal congestion, sinusitis, dysphonia, rhinitis, otitis media, tonsillitis, nasal discharge, earache, laryngitis, epistaxis, sneezing, hoarseness, conjunctivitis, eye irritation, dysmenorrhea, candidiasis of vagina, pelvic inflammatory disease, vaginitis, vulvovaginitis, irregular menstrual cycle, cushingoid features, weight gain, growth retardation in children, pain in joints, aches and pains, disorder or symptoms of neck sprain or strain, sore muscles, upper respiratory tract infection, bronchitis, chest congestion, shortness of breath, irritation from inhalant.

Onset, Peak, and Duration

Route	Onset	Peak	Duration
Inhalation	24 hr	1–2 wk	Several days
Nasal	12 hr–3 days	4–7 days	Several days

 Massage Considerations

- This drug causes changes in the metabolism of the body and in the connective tissue of the body when used long-term (longer than 2 weeks). Deep tissue massage is contraindicated. Myofascial massage techniques may not be as effective and should be used with caution. Stretching and traction should be used with caution.
- Side effects of dizziness may require care in getting the client on and off the table. Using rapid effleurage at the end of the session may help. Rash or hives are a local contraindication to massage and should be reported to the physician. If severe, massage should be withheld.
- The best strokes are the mechanical strokes of effleurage and pétrissage and the local reflex strokes of gentle compression and vibration.

fluticasone propionate and salmeterol inhalation powder (FLU-tih-ka-sohn proh-PIGH-oh-nayt and sal-MEH-teh-rohl)

Advair Diskus 100/50, Advair Diskus 250/50, Advair Diskus 500/50

Drug Class: Corticosteroid, long-acting beta$_2$-adrenergic agonist anti-inflammatory, bronchodilator

Drug Actions

Reduces inflammation in the lungs and opens airways to improve pulmonary function

Use

- Chronic asthma
- Maintenance therapy for airflow obstruction in patients with Chronic obstructive pulmonary disease (COPD) from chronic bronchitis

Side Effects

Cardiovascular: palpitations, chest pains, fluid retention, rapid heart rate, arrhythmias.
Gastrointestinal: nausea, vomiting, abdominal pain and discomfort, diarrhea, gastroenteritis, oral discomfort and pain, constipation, oral ulcerations, oral erythema and rashes, appendicitis, dental discomfort and pain, unusual taste.
Nervous System: pain, sleep disorder, tremor, hypnagogic effects, fever, compressed nerve syndromes, headache, agitation, nervousness.
Skin: viral skin infections, hives, skin flakiness, disorders of sweat and sebum, sweating.
Other: bacterial infections, allergies, allergic reactions, influenza, pharyngitis, sinusitis, hoarseness/dysphonia, oral candidiasis, rhinorrhea, rhinitis, sneezing, nasal irritation, blood in nasal mucosa, keratitis, conjunctivitis, eye redness, viral eye infections, congestion., muscle pain, joint pain, articular rheumatism, muscle stiffness, tightness, rigidity, bone and cartilage disorders, back pain, upper respiratory tract infection, lower viral respiratory infections, bronchitis, cough, pneumonia, paradoxical bronchospasms, severe asthma or asthma-related deaths (especially in African Americans).

Onset, Peak, and Duration

Route	Onset	Peak	Duration
Inhalation			
Salmeterol	Unknown	5 min	Unknown
Fluticasone	Unknown	1–2 hr	Unknown

 Massage Considerations

- This drug causes changes in the metabolism of the body and in the connective tissue of the body when used long-term (longer than 2 weeks). Deep tissue massage is contraindicated. Myofascial massage techniques may not be as effective and should be used with caution. Stretching and traction should be used with caution.
- Side effects of constipation may be helped by regular abdominal massage. Hives are a local contraindication to massage and should be reported to the physician. If severe, massage should be withheld.
- The best strokes are the mechanical strokes of effleurage and pétrissage and the local reflex strokes of gentle compression and vibration.

---

fluvastatin sodium (floo-vuh-STAH-tin SOH-dee-um)

Lescol, Lescol XL

Drug Class: Cholesterol inhibitor

Drug Actions

Lowers blood LDL and cholesterol levels

Use

- Reduction of LDL and total cholesterol levels in patients with primary hypercholesterolemia
- To slow progression of coronary atherosclerosis in patients with coronary artery disease
- Elevated triglyceride and apolipoprotein B levels in patients with primary hypercholesterolemia and mixed dyslipidemia
- To reduce the risk of undergoing coronary revascularization procedures

Side Effects

Gastrointestinal: painful digestion, diarrhea, nausea, vomiting, abdominal pain, constipation, gas.
Nervous System: headache, fatigue, dizziness, insomnia.
Skin: rash.
Other: tooth disorder, hypersensitivity reactions (thrombocytopenia, leukopenia, hemolytic anemia), sinusitis, rhinitis, pharyngitis, joint problems, joint pain, muscle pain, upper respiratory infection, cough, bronchitis.

Onset, Peak, and Duration

Route	Onset	Peak	Duration
Oral	Unknown	30–45 min	Unknown

 Massage Considerations

- There are no cautions or contraindications to massage related to the client taking this drug.
- Side effects of dizziness require care in getting the client on and off the table and may be helped by using stimulating effleurage at the end of the session. Constipation may be helped by regular abdominal massage. Rash is a local contraindication to massage and should be reported to the physician. If severe, massage should be withheld. Reports of ongoing or worsening pain in muscles and joints should be reported to the physician, as they may indicate a need to stop the medication or adjust the dose.

---

fluvoxamine maleate (floo-VOKS-uh-meen MAL-ee-ayt)

Luvox

Drug Class: Selective Serotonin Reuptake Inhibitor (SSRI) antidepressant

Drug Actions

May selectively inhibit neuronal uptake of serotonin, which is thought to reduce obsessive-compulsive behavior.

Use

- Depression
- Obsessive-compulsive disorder

Side Effects

Cardiovascular: palpitations, vasodilation.
Gastrointestinal: nausea, diarrhea, constipation, painful digestion, anorexia, vomiting, gas, swallowing difficulties, taste perversion, dry mouth.
Nervous System: headache, weakness, sleepiness, insomnia, nervousness, dizziness, tremor, anxiety, hypertonia, agitation, depression, CNS stimulation.
Urinary: abnormal ejaculation, urinary frequency, impotence, anorgasmia, urine retention.
Skin: sweating.
Other: decreased libido, flulike syndrome, chills, tooth disorder, upper respiratory tract infection, shortness of breath, yawning, reduced vision.

Onset, Peak, and Duration

Route	Onset	Peak	Duration
Oral	3–10 wk	3–8 hr	Unknown

Massage Considerations

- There are no cautions or contraindications to massage because the client is taking this drug. There may be cautions or contraindications to massage related to the client condition.
- Side effects of sleepiness, dizziness, and vasodilation may require care in getting the client on and off the table. Stimulation at the end of the session with rapid effleurage and tapotement may help. Constipation and gas may be helped by regular abdominal massage. Frequent urination may mean the client has to get up in the middle of the session. Privacy and quick access to the bathroom are essential. Water fountains or music that may stimulate the need to urinate should be avoided.

---

folic acid (vitamin B) (FOH-lek AS-id)

Apo-Folic, Folvite, Novo-Folacid

Drug Class: Vitamin supplement

Drug Actions

Stimulates normal erythropoiesis and nucleoprotein synthesis

Use

- To maintain health
- Megaloblastic or macrocytic anemia caused by folic acid or other nutritional deficiency, hepatic disease, alcoholism, intestinal obstruction, excessive hemolysis
- Prevention of megaloblastic anemia in pregnancy and fetal damage
- Nutritional supplement
- To test folic acid deficiency in patients with megaloblastic anemia without masking pernicious anemia
- Tropical sprue

Side Effects

Gastrointestinal: bitter taste, anorexia, nausea, gas.
Nervous System: general malaise.
Other: allergic reactions (rash, itching, redness), bronchospasm.

Onset, Peak, and Duration

Route	Onset	Peak	Duration
Oral, I.M., or Subcutaneous Injection	Unknown	30–60 min	Unknown

Massage Considerations

- There are no cautions or contraindications to massage related to this drug.
- Side effects of gas may be helped by abdominal massage. Rash, itching, or redness are a local contraindication to massage and should be reported to the physician. If severe, massage should not be given.

fondaparinux sodium (fon-duh-PAIR-in-ux SOH-dee-uhm)

Arixtra

Drug Class: Anticoagulant

Drug Action

Prevents the formation of blood clots

Use

- To prevent deep vein thrombosis, which may lead to pulmonary embolism in patients undergoing surgery for hip fracture, hip replacement, or knee replacement.

Side Effects

Cardiovascular: hypotension, edema.
Gastrointestinal: nausea, constipation, vomiting, diarrhea, painful digestion.
Nervous System: insomnia, dizziness, confusion, pain, headache, fever, spinal and epidural hematomas.
Urinary: urinary tract infections, urinary retention.
Skin: mild local irritation (injection site bleeding, rash, itching), bullous eruption, purpura increased wound drainage, rash.
Other: hemorrhage, anemia, hematoma, postoperative hemorrhage, thrombocytopenia, hypokalemia.

Onset, Peak, and Duration

Route	Onset	Peak	Duration
Subcutaneous Injection	Unknown	2–3 hr	Unknown

 Massage Considerations

- This drug affects blood clotting; therefore, deep tissue massage is contraindicated. The presence of any blood clot would contraindicate massage completely.
- The physician should be consulted before any massage is given. There may be further cautions or contraindications to massage related to the client condition.
- The site of injection should not be massaged for at least 3 hours.
- Side effects of dizziness and hypotension require care in positioning the client.
- Stimulation at the end of the session with rapid effleurage may help. Constipation may be helped by abdominal massage. Rash or irritation of the skin are a local contraindication to massage and should be reported to the physician. If severe, no massage should be given.

formoterol fumarate, inhalation powder (for-MOE-tur-all FOO-muh-rayt)

Foradil Aerolizer

Drug Class: Long-acting selective beta$_2$-adrenergic agonist bronchodilator

Drug Actions

Relaxes bronchial and cardiac smooth muscle by acting on beta$_2$-adrenergic receptors. Prevents and controls bronchospasm.

Use

- Prevention and maintenance treatment of bronchospasm in patients with reversible obstructive airway disease or nocturnal asthma who usually need short-acting inhaled $beta_2$-adrenergic agonists
- Prevention of exercise-induced bronchospasm
- Maintenance of chronic obstructive pulmonary disease (COPD)

Side Effects

Cardiovascular: chest pain, angina, hypertension, hypotension, tachycardia, arrhythmias, palpitations.
Gastrointestinal: nausea.
Nervous System: tremor, dizziness, insomnia, nervousness, headache, fatigue, malaise.
Skin: rash.
Other: viral infection, dry mouth, tonsillitis, dysphonia, hypokalemia, hyperglycemia, metabolic acidosis, muscle cramps, bronchitis, chest infection, shortness of breath.

Onset, Peak, and Duration

Route	Onset	Peak	Duration
Oral Inhalation	1–3 min	$\frac{1}{2}$–1 $\frac{1}{2}$ hr	12 hr

 Massage Considerations

- There are no cautions or contraindications to massage related to this drug. There may be cautions or contraindications to massage related to the client condition.
- This drug stimulates specific receptors in the sympathetic nervous system (SNS) and may make it more difficult to achieve the relaxing effects of massage. Systemic reflex strokes such as rocking, effleurage, and friction may take longer to have their desired effect.
- Side effects of hypotension or dizziness may require care in getting the client on and off the table. Using tapotement to stimulate the client at the end of the session may help. Rash is a local contraindication to massage and should be reported to the physician. If severe, massage should be withheld.

---

fosamprenavir calcium (foss-am-PREH-nuh-veer CAL-see-um)

Lexiva

Drug Class: Antiretroviral

Drug Actions

Hinders HIV activity

Use

- HIV infection with other antiretrovirals

Side Effects

Gastrointestinal: abdominal pain, diarrhea, nausea, vomiting.
Nervous System: depression, fatigue, headache, oral paresthesia.
Skin: itching, rash.

Onset, Peak, and Duration

Route	Onset	Peak	Duration
Oral	Unknown	1 $\frac{1}{2}$–4 hr	Unknown

Massage Considerations

- There are no cautions or contraindications to massage because the client is taking this medication. There may be cautions or contraindications to massage related to the client condition.
- Side effects of rash or itching are a local contraindication to massage and should be reported to the physician immediately . If severe or widespread, massage should not be given.

---

foscarnet sodium (fos-KAR-net SOH-dee-um)

Foscavir

Drug Class: Antiviral

Drug Actions

Kills viruses

Use

- Cytomegalovirus retinitis in patients with AIDS
- Mucocutaneous acyclovir-resistant herpes simplex virus (HSV) infections
- Varicella zoster infection

Side Effects

Cardiovascular: hypertension, palpitations, ECG abnormalities, sinus tachycardia, cerebrovascular disorder, first-degree AV block, hypotension, flushing, edema, facial edema.
Gastrointestinal: taste perversion, dry mouth, nausea, diarrhea, vomiting, abdominal pain, anorexia, constipation, difficulty swallowing, rectal hemorrhage, black and tarry feces, gas, ulcerative stomatitis, pancreatitis.
Nervous System: fever, pain, headache, seizures, fatigue, malaise, weakness, paresthesia, dizziness, hypesthesia, neuropathy, tremor, ataxia, generalized spasms, dementia, stupor, sensory disturbances, meningitis, aphasia, abnormal coordination, EEG abnormalities, depression, confusion, anxiety, insomnia, sleepiness, nervousness, amnesia, agitation, aggressive reaction.
Urinary: abnormal renal function, albuminuria, painful urination, frequent urination, urethral disorder, urine retention, urinary tract infections, acute renal impairment, nephrotoxicity, candidiasis.
Skin: rash, increased sweating, itching, skin ulceration, erythematous rash, seborrhea, skin discoloration.
Other: sepsis, rigors, inflammation, pain at infusion site, lymphoma-like disorder, sarcoma, back or chest pain, bacterial or fungal infections, abscess, flulike symptoms, visual disturbances, eye pain, conjunctivitis, sinusitis, pharyngitis, rhinitis, leg cramps, joint pain, muscle pain, cough, shortness of breath, pneumonic respiratory insufficiency, pulmonary infiltration, stridor, pneumothorax, bronchospasm, hemoptysis, anemia, bone marrow suppression, thrombosis, lymphadenopathy, abnormal blood profiles, abnormal hepatic function, hypokalemia, hypomagnesemia, hypophosphatemia or hyperphosphatemia, hypocalcemia, hyponatremia.

Onset, Peak, and Duration

Route	Onset	Peak	Duration
I.V.	Immediate	Immediate	Unknown

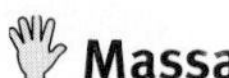 Massage Considerations

- There are no cautions or contraindications to massage related to this drug. There may be cautions or contraindications to massage related to the client condition.
- The physician should be consulted before any massage is given.
- Side effects of hypotension or dizziness require care in getting the client on and off the table. Stimulating the client at the end of the session with rapid effleurage or tapotement may help. Paresthesia, hypesthesia, or neuropathies are local contraindications to deep tissue massage. Constipation and gas may respond well to abdominal massage.
- Frequency of urination may mean the client has to get up in the middle of the session. Privacy and quick access to the bathroom are essential. Water fountains or music that could stimulate the need to urinate should be avoided. Thrombosis is a complete contraindication to massage. Rash or itching is a local contraindication to massage and should be reported to the physician immediately. If severe or widespread, massage should not be given.

---

fosinopril (foh-SIN-oh-pril SOH-dee-um)

Monopril

Drug Class: Angiotensin Converting Enzyme (ACE) Inhibitor antihypertensive

Drug Actions

Lowers blood pressure

Use

- Hypertension
- Adjunct therapy for heart failure

Side Effects

Cardiovascular: chest pain, angina, heart attack, rhythm disturbances, palpitations, hypotension, orthostatic hypotension.
Gastrointestinal: dry mouth, nausea, vomiting, diarrhea, pancreatitis, abdominal distention, abdominal pain, constipation.
Nervous System: headache, dizziness, fatigue, fainting, paresthesia, sleep disturbance, stroke.
Urinary: renal insufficiency.
Skin: hives, rash, photosensitivity, itching
Other: decreased libido, sexual dysfunction, gout, angioedema, hepatitis, hyperkalemia, joint pain, musculoskeletal pain, muscle pain, dry, persistent, tickling, nonproductive cough; bronchospasm, ringing in the ears, sinusitis.

Onset, Peak, and Duration

Route	Onset	Peak	Duration
Oral	≤1 hr	2–6 hr	24 hr

Massage Considerations

- There are no cautions or contraindications to massage related to this drug. There may be cautions or contraindications to massage related to the client condition.
- Side effects of hypotension or dizziness require care in getting the client on and off the table. Stimulation with rapid effleurage or tapotement at the end of the session may help. If severe, using more stimulating and rapid strokes throughout the session may be needed. Constipation may be helped by regular abdominal massage. Rash, hives, or itching are local contraindications to massage and should be reported to the physician immediately. If severe, no massage should be given.

fosphenytoin sodium (fahs-FEN-eh-toyn SOH-dee-um)

Cerebyx

Drug Class: Anticonvulsant

Drug Actions

Because fosphenytoin is a prodrug of phenytoin, its anticonvulsant action is the same. Phenytoin is thought to stabilize neuronal membranes and limit seizure activity.

Use

- Status epilepticus
- Prevention and treatment of seizures during neurosurgery
- Short-term substitution for oral phenytoin therapy

Side Effects

Cardiovascular: hypotension, hypertension, tachycardia, tremor, facial edema, vasodilatation, severe CV reactions (such as ventricular fibrillation).
Gastrointestinal: constipation, dry mouth, nausea, taste perversion, tongue disorder, vomiting.
Nervous System: abnormal thinking, agitation, weakness, ataxia, brain edema, decreased reflexes, dizziness, dysarthria, headache, extrapyramidal syndrome, fever, hypesthesia, increased reflexes, incoordination, intracranial hypertension, nervousness, paresthesia, speech disorder, sleepiness, stupor, dizziness.
Skin: bruising, itching, rash.
Other: accidental injury, chills, infection, injection-site reaction and pain, decreased vision, deafness, double vision, nystagmus, ringing in the ears, hepatotoxicity, hypokalemia, back pain, myasthenia, pelvic pain, pneumonia.

Onset, Peak, and Duration

Route	Onset	Peak	Duration
I.V.	Unknown	Immediate	Unknown
I.M.	Unknown	30 min	Unknown

Massage Considerations

- This drug calms the CNS and may potentially decrease perceptions. Deep tissue massage should be used with caution. There may be further cautions and contraindications to massage related to the client condition.
- The physician should be consulted before any massage is given.
- The effects of systemic reflex strokes of rocking, effleurgae, and friction, and the relaxation effect of massage may be increased with this drug. Local reflex strokes such as compression, stretching, and vibration may be less effective or take longer to have the desired effects.
- Side effects of dizziness, sleepiness, or hypotension require care in getting the client on and off the table. Using a more stimulating massage throughout the session with rapid effleurage and tapotement may be helpful. Constipation may be helped by abdominal massage. Bruising requires extra care; therefore, in-depth and deep tissue massage should not be given. Rash and itching are local contraindications to massage and should be reported to the physician immediately. If severe, massage should be withheld.

frovatriptan succinate (froh-vah-TRIP-tan SUK-seh-nayt)

Frova

Drug Class: Antimigraine drug

Drug Actions

May inhibit excessive dilation of extracerebral, intracranial arteries in migraine headaches

Use

- Migraine attacks with or without aura

Side Effects

Cardiovascular: flushing, palpitations, chest pain.
Gastrointestinal: dry mouth, painful digestion, vomiting, abdominal pain, diarrhea, nausea.
Nervous System: dizziness, headache, fatigue, pain, paresthesia, insomnia, anxiety, sleepiness, abnormal sensations, hypesthesia.
Skin: increased sweating.
Other: hot or cold sensation, abnormal vision, ringing in the ears, sinusitis, rhinitis, skeletal pain.

Onset, Peak, and Duration

Route	Onset	Peak	Duration
Oral	Unknown	2–4 hr	Unknown

Massage Considerations

- There are no cautions or contraindications to massage related to this drug.
- Side effects of dizziness or sleepiness require care in getting the client on and off the table. Stimulation with rapid effleurage and tapotement at the end of the session may help. Paresthesia, abnormal sensations, or hypesthesia are contraindications to deep tissue massage. If severe, massage may be completely contraindicated.

fulvestrant (ful-VES-trant)

Faslodex

Drug Class: Antineoplastic

Drug Actions

Competitively binds estrogen receptors and down-regulates estrogen-receptor protein in breast cancer cells. Fights cancer cells.

Use

- Hormone-receptor–positive metastatic breast cancer in postmenopausal women with disease progression following antiestrogen therapy

Side Effects

Cardiovascular: vasodilation (hot flashes), chest pain, peripheral edema.
Gastrointestinal: nausea, vomiting, constipation, abdominal pain, diarrhea, anorexia.
Nervous System: pain, dizziness, weakness, headache, insomnia, fever, paresthesia, depression, anxiety.
Urinary: urinary tract infections.

Skin: rash, sweating.
Other: accidental injury, flulike syndrome, injection site pain, anemia, bone pain, back pain, pelvic pain, arthritis, shortness of breath, cough.

Onset, Peak, and Duration

Route	Onset	Peak	Duration
I.M.	Unknown	7 days	1 month

Massage Considerations

- Although there are no cautions or contraindications to massage related to this drug, there will be cautions and contraindications to massage related to the client condition.
- The physician should be consulted before any massage is given, and close collaboration is essential.
- Side effects of dizziness require care in getting the client on and off the table. Gentle friction to the legs at the end of the session may help, as will rapid effleurage.
- Constipation may be helped by abdominal massage. Rash is a local contraindication to massage and should be reported to the physician immediately. If severe, massage should not be given.

---

furosemide (frusemide) (fyoo-ROH-seh-mighd)

Apo-Furosemide, Furoside, Lasix, Lasix Special, Myrosemide, Novosemide, Uritol

Drug Actions: Diuretic, antihypertensive

Drug Actions

Promotes water and sodium excretion

Use

- Acute pulmonary edema
- Edema
- Heart failure
- Chronic renal impairment
- Hypertension
- Hypercalcemia

Side Effects

Cardiovascular: volume depletion and dehydration, orthostatic hypotension, thrombophlebitis (with I.V. use).
Gastrointestinal: abdominal discomfort and pain, diarrhea, anorexia, nausea, vomiting, constipation, pancreatitis.
Nervous System: fever, headache, dizziness, paresthesia, restlessness, weakness.
Urinary: azotemia, increased urination at night, frequent urination, lack of urination.
Skin: dermatitis, purpura, photosensitivity.
Other: gout, transient pain at I.M. injection site, transient deafness (with too-rapid I.V. injection), blurred or yellow vision, hepatic dysfunction, hypokalemia, hypochloremic alkalosis, asymptomatic hyperuricemia, hyperglycemia and glucose intolerance, fluid and electrolyte imbalances, including dilutional hyponatremia, hypocalcemia, and hypomagnesemia, muscle spasm.

Onset, Peak, and Duration

Route	Onset	Peak	Duration
Oral	20–60 min	1–2 hr	6–8 hr
I.V.	5 min	30 min	2 hr
I.M.	Unknown	Unknown	Unknown

Massage Considerations

- There are no cautions or contraindications to massage related to this drug. There may be cautions or contraindications to massage related to the client condition.
- Side effects of dizziness and hypotension require care in getting the client on and off the table. Using stimulation with rapid effleurage and tapotement at the end of the session may help. Paresthesia is a contraindication to deep tissue massage. Thrombophlebitis is a complete contraindication to massage. Constipation may be helped by abdominal massage. Frequency of urination may require the client to get up in the middle of the session. Providing privacy and quick access to the bathroom as well as avoiding water fountains or music that may stimulate the need to urinate are appropriate.

G

gabapentin (geh-buh-PEN-tin)

Neurontin

Drug Class: Anticonvulsant

Drug Actions

Prevents and treats partial seizures and treats postherpetic neuralgia

Use

- Adjunct treatment of partial seizures with and without secondary generalization in patients with epilepsy
- Postherpetic neuralgia

Side Effects

Cardiovascular: peripheral edema, vasodilation.
Gastrointestinal: nausea, vomiting, painful digestion, dry mouth, constipation.
Nervous System: sleepiness, dizziness, ataxia, fatigue, nystagmus, tremor, nervousness, dysarthria, amnesia, depression, abnormal thinking, twitching, abnormal coordination.
Urinary: impotence.
Skin: itching, abrasion.
Other: dental abnormalities, double vision, rhinitis, pharyngitis, dry throat, decreased vision, leukopenia, increased appetite, weight gain, back pain, muscle pain, fractures, cough.

Onset, Peak, and Duration

Route	Onset	Peak	Duration
Oral	Unknown	2–4 hr	Unknown

Massage Considerations

- No cautions or contraindications to massage are indicated because a client is taking this drug. Cautions and contraindications to massage may be related to the client condition.
- The sedating effect of this drug on the central nervous system (CNS) may increase the effects of the systemic reflex strokes of rocking, effleurage, and friction and the relaxing effects of massage. A decrease in the effectiveness of the local reflex strokes of compression, stretching, and vibration may also occur.
- Side effects of dizziness, sleepiness, and vasodilation may require care in getting the client on and off the table. Stimulation at the end of the session with tapotement and rapid effleurage may help. If side effects are severe, stimulating massage throughout the session may be needed.
- Constipation may be helped by regular abdominal massage.
- Itching or skin abrasions are local contraindications to massage and should be reported to the physician. If severe, no massage should be given.
- The best strokes for this client will be the mechanical strokes of pétrissage and effleurage. Local reflex strokes may need to be applied for a longer period of time to be effective, and systemic reflex strokes may need to be applied in a more stimulating manner to avoid sedation. Myofascial massage techniques may be helpful as well.

---

galantamine hydrobromide (gah-LAN-tah-meen high-droh-BROH-mide)

Reminyl

Drug Class: Reversible, competitive acetylcholinesterase inhibitor, cholinomimetic

Drug Actions

May enhance cholinergic function by increasing the level of acetylcholine in the brain. Improves cognition in patients with Alzheimer disease.

Use

- Mild to moderate dementia of Alzheimer type

Side Effects

Cardiovascular: bradycardia.
Gastrointestinal: nausea, vomiting, anorexia, diarrhea, abdominal pain, painful digestion.
Nervous System: dizziness, headache, tremor, depression, insomnia, sleepiness, fatigue, syncope.
Urinary: urinary tract infection, hematuria.
Other: anemia, weight loss, rhinitis.

Onset, Peak, and Durations

Route	Onset	Peak	Duration
Oral	Unknown	1 hr	Unknown

Massage Considerations

- No cautions or contraindications to massage are indicated because a client is taking this drug. Cautions and contraindications to massage may be related to the client condition.
- Side effects of dizziness and sleepiness may be helped by stimulating the client with effleurage or tapotement at the end of the session. Care should be taken in getting the client on and off the table.

ganciclovir (jan-SIGH-kloh-veer)

Cytovene, Cytovene-IV

Drug Class: Antiviral

Drug Actions

Inhibits cytomegalovirus (CMV).

Use

- Cytomegalovirus retinitis in immunocompromised patients, including those with AIDS Prevention of CMV disease in transplant recipients at risk for CMV disease
- Prevention of CMV disease in patients with advanced HIV infection at risk for development of CMV disease
- Other CMV infections

Side Effects

Cardiovascular: arrhythmias, hypotension, hypertension.
Gastrointestinal: nausea, vomiting, diarrhea, anorexia.
Nervous System: pain, altered dreams, confusion, ataxia, dizziness, headache, seizures, coma, behavioral changes.
Urinary: hematuria.
Other: inflammation, phlebitis at injection site, retinal detachment in CMV retinitis patients, abnormal blood profiles.

Onset, Peak, and Duration

Route	Onset	Peak	Duration
Oral fasting	Unknown	1 3/4 hr	Unknown
Oral with food	Unknown	3 hr	Unknown
I.V.	Immediate	Immediate	Unknown

Massage Considerations

- No cautions or contraindications to massage are indicated because a client is taking this drug. Cautions and contraindications to massage may be related to the client condition.
- Side effects of dizziness or hypotension require care in getting the client on and off the table. Using stimulation with effleurage or tapotement at the end of the session may help.

ganirelix acetate (gan-eh-REL-iks AS-ih-tayt)

Antagon

Drug Class: Gonadotropin-releasing hormone (GnRH) antagonist fertility drug

Drug Actions

Increases fertility

Use

- Inhibition of premature luteinizing hormone surges in women undergoing medically supervised, controlled ovarian hyperstimulation

Side Effects

Gastrointestinal: abdominal pain, nausea.
Nervous System: headache.
Other: injection site reaction, vaginal bleeding, gynecologic abdominal pain, ovarian hyperstimulation syndrome, miscarriage.

Onset, Peak, and Duration

Route	Onset	Peak	Duration
Subcutaneous Injection	Unknown	1 hr	Unknown

 Massage Considerations

- Although no cautions or contraindications to massage are related to the actions of this drug, the client condition and efforts for fertility may have cautions and contraindications to massage. Consultation with the physician during this process is recommended before any massage is given.

gatifloxacin (ga-tih-FLOCKS-ah-sin)

Tequin

Drug Class: Antibiotic

Drug Actions

Kills susceptible bacteria

Use

- Acute bacterial exacerbation of chronic bronchitis
- Complicated urinary tract infections
- Acute sinusitis
- Community-acquired pneumonia
- Inhalation anthrax
- Postexposure to inhalation anthrax, prevention or treatment when parenteral regimen is not available
- Uncomplicated urethral gonorrhea in men and cervical gonorrhea or acute uncomplicated rectal infections in women
- Uncomplicated urinary tract infection
- Uncomplicated skin and skin-structure infections

Side Effects

Cardiovascular: palpitations, chest pain, peripheral edema.
Gastrointestinal: nausea, diarrhea, abdominal pain, constipation, painful digestion, oral candidiasis, pseudomembranous colitis, glossitis, stomatitis, mouth ulcer, vomiting, disturbed taste.
Nervous System: headache, dizziness, abnormal dreams, insomnia, paresthesia, tremor, fever.
Urinary: painful urination, hematuria, vaginitis.
Skin: rash, sweating.
Other: anaphylaxis, chills, redness at injection site, ringing in the ears, abnormal vision, pharyngitis, joint pain, muscle pain, back pain, shortness of breath.

Onset, Peak, and Duration

Route	Onset	Peak	Duration
Oral	Unknown	1–2 hr	Unknown
I.V.	Unknown	Unknown	Unknown

Massage Considerations

- No cautions or contraindications to massage are indicated because a client is taking this drug. Cautions and contraindications to massage may be related to the client condition or severity of infection.
- Side effects of dizziness require care in getting the client on and off the table. Using stimulating effleurage or tapotement at the end of the session may help.
- Constipation may be helped by abdominal massage.
- Rash is a local contraindication to massage and should be reported to the physician immediately. If severe, massage should be withheld.

gatifloxacin ophthalmic solution (gah-ti-FLOCKS-ah-sin off-THAL-mick suh-LOO-shun)

Zymar

Drug Class: Antibiotic

Drug Actions

Clears eye infection from susceptible bacteria

Use

- Bacterial conjunctivitis

Side Effects

Gastrointestinal: taste disturbance.
Nervous System: headache.
Other: chemosis, conjunctival hemorrhage, conjunctival irritation, discharge, dry eyes, eye irritation, eyelid edema, increased lacrimation, keratitis, pain, papillary conjunctivitis, red eyes, reduced visual acuity.

Onset, Peak, and Duration

Route	Onset	Peak	Duration
Ophthalmic	Unknown	Unknown	Unknown

Massage Considerations

- No cautions or contraindications to massage are indicated because a client is taking this drug.
- The site of administration, the eyes, and surrounding tissue should not be massaged until the infection is completely cleared.

gefitinib (geh-FIT-eye-nib)

Iressa

Drug Class: Antineoplastic

Drug Actions

Kills cancer cells

Use

- Locally advanced or metastatic non–small-cell lung cancer after platinum-based and docetaxel chemotherapies have failed.

Side Effects

Cardiovascular: peripheral edema.
Gastrointestinal: anorexia, diarrhea, mouth ulcers, nausea, vomiting.
Nervous System: weakness.
Skin: acne, dry skin, itching, rash.
Other: decreased vision, conjunctivitis, weight loss, shortness of breath, interstitial lung disease.

Onset, Peak, and Duration

Route	Onset	Peak	Duration
Oral	Unknown	3–7 hr	48 hr

Massage Considerations

- Because of the toxic effects of this drug, deep tissue massage should be used with caution. Circulatory massage with effleurage should be used with caution and limited so as not to tax the liver and kidneys as they try to rid the body of the drug.
- Other cautions and contraindications to massage may be related to the client condition. Close contact and collaboration with the physician is essential.
- Side effects of acne, rash, or itching are local contraindications to massage and should be reported to the physician immediately. If severe, massage should not be given. If acne is widespread and the client still desires massage, wearing gloves during the session is appropriate.
- The best strokes to use with this client are the mechanical strokes of pétrissage, local reflex strokes of gentle compression, stretching, and vibration, and the systemic reflex strokes of rocking and gentle friction. Myofascial massage techniques may be used for areas of tightness or gluteation.

---

gemfibrozil (jem-FIGH-broh-zil)

Apo-Gemfibrozil, Gen-Fibro, Lopid, Novo-Gemfibrozil, Nu-Gemfibrozil

Drug Class: Antilipemic

Drug Actions

Lowers triglyceride levels and raises high density lipoprotein levels

Use

- Type IV and V hyperlipidemia unresponsive to diet and other drugs
- Reduction of risk of coronary heart disease in patients with type IIb hyperlipidemia who cannot tolerate or who are refractory to treatment with bile acid sequestrants or niacin

Side Effects

Gastrointestinal: abdominal and epigastric pain, diarrhea, nausea, vomiting, gas, painful digestion.
Nervous System: blurred vision, headache, dizziness.
Skin: rash, dermatitis, itching.
Other: abnormal blood profiles, bone marrow hypoplasia, bile duct obstruction, gallstones, painful limbs, rhabdomyolysis.

Onset, Peak, and Duration

Route	Onset	Peak	Duration
Oral	2–5 days	>4 wk	Unknown

 **Massage Considerations**

- No cautions or contraindications to massage are indicated because a client is taking this drug.
- Side effects of dizziness require care in getting the client on and off the table. Stimulating massage with effleurage or tapotement at the end of the session may help.
- Gas may be helped by abdominal massage.
- Rash or itching is a local contraindication to massage and the physician should be notified. If severe, no massage should be given.
- A serious side effect of this drug is rhabdomyolysis. It may present as muscle pain with no clear cause. Always immediately refer the patient to the physician if muscle pain starts without cause and continues to worsen, because this can be a life-threatening symptom. Massage should not be given until the client has been evaluated.

---

gemifloxacin mesylate (geh-mih-FLOCKS-a-sin MESS-ih-late)

Factive

Drug Class: Antibacterial

Drug Actions

Kills susceptible bacteria

Use

- Acute bacterial exacerbation of chronic bronchitis
- Mild to moderate community-acquired pneumonia

Side Effects

Gastrointestinal: abdominal pain, diarrhea, nausea, pseudomembranous colitis, vomiting.
Nervous System: headache.
Skin: rash.
Other: hypersensitivity reactions, ruptured tendons.

Onset, Peak, and Duration

Route	Onset	Peak	Duration
Oral	Unknown	$^1/_2$–2 hr	Unknown

 **Massage Considerations**

- No cautions or contraindications to massage are indicated because of this drug's actions. Cautions and contraindications to massage may be related to the client condition and severity of infection.
- The side effect of rash is a local contraindication to massage and should be reported to the physician immediately. If severe, no massage should be given.

---

gemtuzumab ozogamicin (gem-TOO-zuh-mab oh-zoh-GAM-ih-sin)

Mylotarg

Drug Class: Chemotherapeutic drug

Drug Actions

Kills cancer cells

Use

- Patients with CD33-positive acute myeloid leukemia in first relapse who are not considered candidates for cytotoxic chemotherapy.

Side Effects

Cardiovascular: hypertension, hypotension, tachycardia.
Gastrointestinal: enlarged abdomen, abdominal pain, anorexia, constipation, diarrhea, painful digestion, nausea, stomatitis, vomiting.
Nervous System: weakness, depression, dizziness, headache, insomnia, pain, fever.
Urinary: hematuria, vaginal hemorrhage.
Skin: rash.
Other: herpes simplex, chills, sepsis, nosebleed, pharyngitis, rhinitis, abnormal blood profiles, myelosuppression, hepatotoxicity, hyperbilirubinemia, hyperglycemia, hypokalemia, hypomagnesemia, joint pain, back pain, increased cough, shortness of breath, hypoxia, pneumonia.

Onset, Peak, and Duration

Route	Onset	Peak	Duration
I.V.	Unknown	Unknown	Unknown

Massage Considerations

- Because of the toxic effects of this drug, deep tissue massage is contraindicated. Circulatory massage with effleurage should be limited and used with caution.
- The physician should be consulted and close collaboration maintained.
- This drug has a half-life of up to 100 hours. It is usually given every other week. Massage would best be given on the week the drug is not received and before the administration of the drug in the week it is received.
- Side effects of hypotension or dizziness require care in getting the client on and off the table. Stimulation with gentle friction to the legs or tapotement at the end of the session may help.
- Constipation may be helped by regular abdominal massage.
- Rash is a local contraindication to massage and should be reported to the physician immediately. If severe, massage should not be given.
- The best strokes to use with this client are the mechanical stroke of pétrissage and the local reflex strokes of gentle compression, stretching, and vibration. Rocking may be used for relaxation effects, and myofascial massage techniques may be used as well.

---

gentamicin sulfate (jen-tuh-MIGH-sin SUL-fayt)

Cidomycin, Garamycin, Gentamicin Sulfate ADD-Vantage, Jenamicin

Drug Class: Antibiotic

Drug Actions

Kills susceptible bacteria (many aerobic gram-negative organisms and some aerobic gram-positive organisms). Drug may act against some aminoglycoside-resistant bacteria.

Use

- Serious infections caused by sensitive strains of *Pseudomonas aeruginosa, Escherichia coli, Proteus, Klebsiella, Serratia, Enterobacter, Citrobacter, Staphylococcus*

- Meningitis
- Endocarditis prophylaxis for gastrointestinal or genitourinary procedure or surgery
- Posthemodialysis to maintain therapeutic level

Side Effects

Nervous System: headache, lethargy, numbness, paresthesias, twitching, peripheral neuropathy, seizures, neurotoxicity.
Urinary: nephrotoxicity.
Other: hypersensitivity reactions, abnormal blood profiles, ototoxicity.

Onset, Peak, and Duration

Route	Onset	Peak	Duration
I.V.	Immediate	15–30 min	Unknown
I.M.	Unknown	30–90 min	Unknown
Intrathecal	Unknown	Unknown	Unknown

Massage Considerations

- Although the drug action itself does not have any cautions or contraindications to massage, the client condition most likely will require cautions or contraindications to massage.
- The physician should be consulted before any massage is given.
- Side effects of numbness, paresthesia, or peripheral neuropathy are contraindications to deep tissue massage.

---

glimepiride (gligh-MEH-peh-righd)

Amaryl

Drug Class: Antidiabetic

Drug Actions

Stimulates release of insulin from pancreatic beta cells; increases sensitivity of peripheral tissues to insulin. Lowers glucose levels.

Use

- Adjunct to diet and exercise to lower glucose level in patients with type 2 (non–insulin-dependent) diabetes mellitus
- Adjunct to insulin therapy in patients with type 2 (non–insulin-dependent) diabetes mellitus

Side Effects

Gastrointestinal: nausea.
Nervous System: dizziness, weakness, headache.
Skin: allergic skin reactions (itching, redness, hives, rash).
Other: abnormal blood profiles, cholestatic jaundice, hypoglycemia, changes in accommodation.

Onset, Peak, and Duration

Route	Onset	Peak	Duration
Oral	$\leq$1 hr	2–3 hr	24 hr

Massage Considerations

- No cautions or contraindications to massage are indicated because a client is taking this drug. Cautions and contraindications to massage may be related to the client condition.
- The side effects of dizziness require care in getting the client on and off the table. Using stimulation with effleurage or tapotement at the end of the session may help.
- Skin reactions of rash, itching, or hives are local contraindications to massage and should be reported to the physician immediately. If severe or widespread, massage should be withheld.

---

glipizide (GLIGH-peh-zighd)

Glucotrol, Glucotrol XL, Minidiab

Drug Class: Antidiabetic

Drug Actions

May stimulate insulin release from pancreas, reduce glucose output by liver, and increase peripheral sensitivity to insulin. Lowers glucose levels.

Use

- Adjunct to diet to lower glucose level in patients with type 2 (non–insulin-dependent) diabetes mellitus
- To replace insulin therapy

Side Effects

Cardiovascular: facial flushing.
Gastrointestinal: nausea, vomiting, constipation.
Nervous System: dizziness.
Skin: rash, itching.
Other: abnormal blood profile, cholestatic jaundice, hypoglycemia.

Onset, Peak, and Duration

Route	Onset	Peak	Duration
Oral	15–30 min	1–3 hr	10–24 hr

Massage Considerations

- No cautions or contraindications to massage are related to the actions of this drug. Cautions and contraindications to massage may be related to the client condition.
- Side effects of dizziness require care in getting the client on and off the table. Stimulation with effleurage or tapotement at the end of the session may help.
- Constipation may be helped by regular abdominal massage.
- Rash or itching is a local contraindication to massage and should be reported to the physician immediately. If severe, massage should be withheld.

---

glipizide and metformin hydrochloride (GLIP-uh-zighd and met-FOR-min high-droh-KLOR-ighd)

Metaglip

Drug Class: Antidiabetic

Drug Actions

Glipizide appears to lower glucose levels by stimulating the pancreas to release insulin. Metformin decreases hepatic glucose production and intestinal absorption of glucose, improves insulin sensitivity, and lowers glucose levels.

Use

- First-line therapy, as adjunct to diet and exercise, to improve glycemic control in patients with type 2 (non–insulin-dependent) diabetes
- Second-line therapy in type 2 diabetes when diet, exercise, and initial treatment with a sulfonylurea or metformin cannot provide adequate glycemic control

Side Effects

Cardiovascular: hypertension.
Gastrointestinal: nausea, diarrhea, vomiting, abdominal pain.
Nervous System: headache, dizziness.
Urinary: urinary tract infections.
Other: hypoglycemia, lactic acidosis, muscle pain, upper respiratory tract infection.

Onset, Peak, and Duration

Route	Onset	Peak	Duration
Oral			
Glipizide	15–30 min	1–3 hr	Unknown
Metformin	Unknown	Unknown	Unknown

Massage Considerations

- No cautions or contraindications to massage are related to the actions of this drug. Cautions and contraindications to massage may be related to the client condition.
- Side effects of dizziness require care in getting the client on and off the table. Stimulation with effleurage or tapotement at the end of the session may help.

---

glyburide (glibenclamide) (GLIGH-byoo-righd)

Albert Glyburide, Apo-Glyburide, DiaBeta, Euglucon, Gen-Glybe, Glynase PresTab, Micronase, Novo-Glyburide, Nu-Glyburide

Drug Class: Antidiabetic

Drug Actions

May stimulate insulin release from pancreas, reduce glucose output by liver, increase peripheral sensitivity to insulin, and cause mild diuresis. Lowers glucose levels.

Use

- Adjunct to diet to lower glucose level in patients with type 2 (non–insulin-dependent) diabetes mellitus
- To replace insulin therapy

Side Effects

Cardiovascular: facial flushing.
Gastrointestinal: nausea, epigastric fullness, heartburn.
Skin: rash, itching.
Other: abnormal blood profiles, cholestatic jaundice, hypoglycemia.

Onset, Peak, and Duration

Route	Onset	Peak	Duration
Oral	45–60 min	2–4 hr	24 hr

Massage Considerations

- No cautions or contraindications to massage are related to the actions of this drug. Cautions and contraindications to massage may be related to the client condition.
- Side effects of rash or itching are local contraindications to massage and should be reported to the physician immediately. If severe or widespread, massage should be withheld.

glyburide and metformin hydrochloride (GLIGH-byoo-righd and met-FOR-min high-droh-KLOR-ighd)

Glucovance

Drug Class: Antidiabetic

Drug Actions

Glyburide stimulates the release of insulin from the pancreas. Metformin decreases hepatic glucose production and intestinal absorption of glucose and improves insulin sensitivity. Lowers glucose level.

Use

- Adjunct to diet and exercise to improve glycemic control in patients with type 2 (non–insulin-dependent) diabetes
- Second-line therapy in patients with type 2 diabetes when diet, exercise, and initial treatment with a sulfonylurea or metformin do not provide adequate glycemic control

Side Effects

Gastrointestinal: diarrhea, nausea, vomiting, abdominal pain.
Nervous System: headache, dizziness.
Other: hypoglycemia, upper respiratory infection.

Onset, Peak, and Duration

Route	Onset	Peak	Duration
Oral			
Glyburide	1 hr	4 hr	24 hr
Metformin	Unknown	Unknown	Unknown

 Massage Considerations

- No cautions or contraindications to massage are related to the actions of this drug. Cautions and contraindications to massage may be related to the client condition.
- Side effects of dizziness require care in getting the client on and off the table. Stimulation with effleurage or tapotement at the end of the session may help.

goserelin acetate (GOH-seh-reh-lin AS-ih-tayt)

Zoladex, Zoladex 3-month

Drug Class: Antineoplastic

Drug Actions

Decreases effects of sex hormones on tumor growth in prostate gland and tissue growth in uterus.

Use

- Endometriosis
- Advanced breast cancer
- Palliative treatment of advanced carcinoma of the prostate
- Endometrial thinning before endometrial ablation for dysfunctional uterine bleeding

Side Effects

Cardiovascular: edema, heart failure, arrhythmias, hypertension, heart attack, peripheral vascular disorder, chest pain.
Gastrointestinal: nausea, vomiting, diarrhea, constipation, ulcer.
Nervous System: stroke, lethargy, pain (worsened in first 30 days), dizziness, insomnia, anxiety, depression, headache, emotional lability, fever.
Urinary: impotence, lower urinary tract symptoms, renal insufficiency, urinary obstruction, urinary tract infection, amenorrhea, vaginal dryness.
Skin: rash, sweating.
Other: chills, hot flushes, breast swelling and tenderness, changes in breast size, sexual dysfunction, gout, anemia, hyperglycemia, weight increase, loss of bone mineral density, chronic obstructive pulmonary disease, upper respiratory tract infection.

Onset, Peak, and Duration

Route	Onset	Peak	Duration
Subcutaneous injection	2–4 wk	12–15 days	Throughout therapy

Massage Considerations

- No cautions or contraindications to massage are indicated because a client is taking this drug. Cautions and contraindications to massage may be related to the client condition.
- The physician should be consulted before any massage is given.
- This drug is implanted subcutaneously and left in place from 1 to 3 months. The site of implantation, which is usually the upper abdomen, is not to be massaged.
- Side effects of dizziness require care in getting the client on and off the table. Using stimulating massage with effleurage and tapotement at the end of the session may help.
- Constipation may be helped by general massage, but abdominal massage would be contraindicated.
- Rash is a local contraindication to massage and should be reported to the physician immediately. If severe, massage should be withheld.

---

granisetron hydrochloride (grah-NEEZ-eh-trohn high-droh-KLOR-ighd)

Kytril

Drug Class: Antiemetic, antinauseant

Drug Actions

Prevents nausea and vomiting from chemotherapy

Use

- Prevention of nausea and vomiting caused by emetogenic cancer chemotherapy
- Prevention of nausea and vomiting from radiation, including total body irradiation and fractionated abdominal radiation
- Postoperative nausea and vomiting

Side Effects

Cardiovascular: hypertension, hypotension, bradycardia.
Gastrointestinal: nausea, vomiting, diarrhea, constipation, taste disorder, abdominal pain, gas, painful digestion, decreased appetite.
Nervous System: headache, asthenia, sleepiness, agitation, anxiety, CNS stimulation, insomnia, fever, pain, dizziness.
Urinary: urinary tract infection, lack of urination.
Skin: rash, dermatitis, hair loss.
Other: hypersensitivity reactions (anaphylaxis, hives, shortness of breath, hypotension), infection, anemia, abnormal blood profiles, cough, increased sputum.

Onset, Peak, and Duration

Route	Onset	Peak	Duration
Oral, I.V.	Unknown	Unknown	Unknown

Massage Considerations

- No cautions or contraindications to massage are indicated because a client is taking this drug. Cautions and contraindications to massage may be related to the client condition.
- The physician should be consulted before any massage is given; close collaboration is essential.
- Side effects of hypotension, dizziness, and sleepiness require care in getting the client on and off the table. Using stimulation at the end of the massage with effleurage or tapotement may help.
- Constipation and gas may be helped by abdominal massage.
- Rash is a local contraindication to massage and should be reported to the physician immediately. If severe or widespread, no massage should be given.
- Hair loss is a contraindication to scalp massage if the client is disturbed by hair loss during the massage or the scalp is tender.

guaifenesin (glyceryl guaiacolate) (gwah-FEH-nih-sin)

Anti-Tuss, Balminil Expectorant, Breonesin, Diabetic Tussin EX, Fenesin, Ganidin NR, Gee-Gee, Genatuss, GG-Cen, Glyate, Glytuss, Guaifenex G, Guaifenex LA, Guiatuss, Halotussin, Humavent LA, Humibid LA, Humibid Pediatric, Humibid Sprinkle, Hytuss, Hytuss-2X, Mucinex, Muco-Fen LA, Mytussin AF, Neldecon Senior EX, Organidin NR, Respa-GF, Resyl, Robitussin, Touro EX

Drug Class: Expectorant

Drug Actions

Increases production of respiratory tract fluids to help liquefy and reduce viscosity of tenacious secretions. Thins respiratory secretions for easier removal.

Use

- Expectorant

Side Effects

Gastrointestinal: stomach pain, diarrhea, vomiting, nausea (with large doses).
Nervous System: drowsiness.
Skin: rash.

Onset, Peak, and Duration

Route	Onset	Peak	Duration
Oral	Unknown	Unknown	Unknown

Massage Consideration

- No cautions or contraindications to massage are indicated because a client is taking this drug.
- Side effects of drowsiness require care in getting the client on and off the table. Stimulation at the end of the session with effleurage or tapotement may help.
- Rash is a local contraindication to massage and should be reported to the physician. If severe, massage should be withheld.

---

guanfacine hydrochloride (GWAHN-fuh-seen high-droh-KLOR-ighd)

Tenex

Drug Class: Centrally acting sympatholytic antihypertensive

Drug Actions

May inhibit central vasomotor center, decreasing sympathetic outflow to heart, kidneys, and peripheral vasculature. Lowers blood pressure.

Use

- Hypertension

Side Effects

Cardiovascular: bradycardia, orthostatic hypotension, rebound hypertension.
Gastrointestinal: constipation, diarrhea, nausea, dry mouth.
Nervous System: drowsiness, dizziness, fatigue, headache, insomnia.
Skin: rash, itching.

Onset, Peak, and Duration

Route	Onset	Peak	Duration
Oral	Unknown	1–4 hr	24 hr

Massage Considerations

- No cautions or contraindications to massage are indicated because a client is taking this drug. Cautions and contraindications to massage may be related to the client condition.
- Side effects of drowsiness, dizziness, and hypotension require care in getting the client on and off the table. Using rapid effleurage and tapotement at the end of the session may help. If the symptoms are severe, more stimulating massage techniques used throughout the session may be needed.
- Constipation may be helped by abdominal massage.
- Rash or itching are local contraindications to massage and should be reported to the physician. If severe, massage should be withheld.

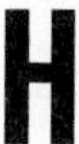

haloperidol (hal-oh-PER-uh-dol)

Apo-Haloperidol, Haldol, Novo-Peridol, Peridol, PMS- Haloperidol, Serenace

haloperidol decanoate

Haldol Decanoate, Haldol LA

haloperidol lactate

Haldol

Drug Class: Antipsychotic

Drug Actions

Decreases psychotic behaviors

Use

- Psychotic disorders
- Chronically psychotic patients who need prolonged therapy
- Nonpsychotic behavior disorders
- Tourette syndrome
- Delirium

Side Effects

Cardiovascular: tachycardia, ECG changes (including prolonged QT interval and torsades de pointes), hypotension, hypertension, bradycardia.
Nervous System: severe extrapyramidal reactions, tardive dyskinesia, sedation, seizures, neuroleptic malignant syndrome.
Urinary: urine retention, menstrual irregularities
Skin: rash.
Other: abnormal growth of breast tissue, transient leukopenia and leukocytosis, jaundice, blurred vision.

Onset, Peak, and Duration

Route	Onset	Peak	Duration
Oral	Unknown	3–6 hr	Unknown
I.M.			
Lactate	Unknown	10–20 min	Unknown
Decanoate	Unknown	3–9 days	Unknown

Massage Considerations

- The drug action does not caution or contraindicate massage, however, the client condition will have cautions and contraindications to massage. The physician should be consulted before any massage is given, and close collaboration is essential.

- Side effects of hypotension and sedation require care in getting the client on and off the table. Stimulating the client at the end of the session with rapid effleurage may help. If sedation is severe, stimulating massage techniques throughout the session may be needed.
- Rash is a local contraindication to massage and should be reported to the physician immediately. If severe, massage should not be given. Abnormal growth of breast tissue in men or women may cause tenderness in the area. Massage of the area should be done with caution and no deep tissue massage should be done. If tenderness is severe, no massage of the area should be done.

---

heparin sodium (HEH-puh-rin SOH-dee-um)

Hepalean, Heparin Leo, Heparin Lock Flush Solution (with Tubex), Hep-Lock, Liquaemin Sodium, Uniparin

Drug Class: Anticoagulant

Drug Actions

Decreases ability of blood to clot

Use

- Deep vein thrombosis
- Pulmonary embolism
- Embolism prevention
- Open-heart surgery
- Disseminated intravascular coagulation
- Maintaining patency of I.V. indwelling catheters
- Unstable angina
- Post heart attack
- Cerebral thrombosis in evolving stroke
- Left ventricular thrombi
- Heart failure
- History of embolism
- Atrial fibrillation

Side Effects

Nervous System: fever.
Skin: irritation, mild pain, hematoma, ulceration, itching, hives, cutaneous or subcutaneous necrosis.
Other: white clot syndrome; hypersensitivity reactions, chills, burning of feet, anaphylaxis, rhinitis, conjunctivitis, lacrimation, hemorrhage (with excessive dosage), overly prolonged clotting time, thrombocytopenia.

Onset, Peak, and Duration

Route	Onset	Peak	Duration
I.V.	Immediate	Unknown	Unknown
Subcutaneous Injection	20–60 min	2–4 hr	Unknown

Massage Considerations

- This drug affects the blood clotting mechanism of the body. If there is any blood clot, thrombus or embolus, present in the body, massage is completely contraindicated. If the drug is used for prevention of clots, massage may be given but deep tissue massage is contraindicated. Circulatory massage with effleurage should be used with caution and limited.
- Physician must be consulted prior to any massage being given.

- There may be other cautions and contraindications to massage related to the client condition.
- The site of subcutaneous injection should not be massaged for at least 4 hours to avoid increasing the rate of absorption of the drug.
- Side effects of itching or hives are a local contraindication to massage and should be reported to the physician immediately. If severe, no massage should be given.
- The best strokes to use with this client are the systemic and local reflex strokes of rocking, gentle compression, stretching, traction, and vibration. Pétrissage also may be used. Myofascial massage techniques may be used with caution as long as bruising does not occur.

hydralazine hydrochloride (high-DRAL-uh-zeen high-droh-KLOR-ighd)

Alphapress, Apresoline, Novo-Hylazin

Drug Class: Peripheral vasodilator antihypertensive

Drug Actions

As a direct-acting vasodilator, its predominant effect relaxes arteriolar smooth muscle. Lowers blood pressure.

Use

- Essential hypertension (orally, alone or with other antihypertensives)
- Severe essential hypertension (parenterally, to lower blood pressure quickly)
- Management of severe heart failure
- Management of hypertensive emergencies related to pregnancy (preeclampsia, eclampsia)

Side Effects

Cardiovascular: orthostatic hypotension, tachycardia, arrhythmias, angina, palpitations.
Gastrointestinal: nausea, vomiting, diarrhea, anorexia.
Nervous System: peripheral neuritis, headache, dizziness.
Skin: rash.
Other: lupus-like syndrome (especially with high doses), abnormal blood profiles, weight gain, sodium retention.

Onset, Peak, and Duration

Route	Onset	Peak	Duration
Oral	20–30 min	1–2 hr	2–4 hr
I.V.	≤5 min	15–30 min	2–6 hr
I.M.	10–30 min	1 hr	2–6 hr

Massage Considerations

- This drug vasodilates; therefore, the effect of circulatory massage with effleurage and the relaxing effects of massage will be increased. Care should be taken with positioning and getting the client on and off the table. Stimulating rapid effleurage and tapotement at the end of the session may help. Stimulating massage techniques throughout the massage may be needed if symptoms are severe. It may be necessary to stay with the client at the end of the massage to help them sit up and ascertain that they are not dizzy.
- The client condition may require further cautions and contraindications to massage.
- The site of I.M. injection of the drug should not be massaged for at least 1 hour to avoid increasing the rate of absorption of the drug.

- Side effects of dizziness and hypotension may be addressed as above. Peripheral neuritis is a contraindication to deep tissue massage and if severe, may contraindicate massage completely. Rash is a local contraindication to massage and should be reported to the physician immediately. If severe, massage should be withheld.

---

hydrochlorothiazide (high-droh-klor-oh-THIGH-uh-zighd)

Apo-Hydro, Aquazide-25, Aquazide-H, Dichlotride, Diuchlor H, Esidrix, Ezide, HydroDIURIL, Hydro-Par, Microzide, Neo-Codema, Novo-Hydrazide, Oretic, Urozide

Drug Class: Thiazide diuretic antihypertensive

Drug Actions

Promotes sodium and water excretion and lowers blood pressure

Use

- Edema
- Hypertension

Side Effects

Cardiovascular: volume depletion and dehydration, orthostatic hypotension.
Gastrointestinal: anorexia, nausea, pancreatitis.
Urinary: increased urination at night, frequent urination, renal impairment.
Skin: photosensitivity, rash.
Other: gout, anaphylactic reactions, hypersensitivity reactions, such as pneumonitis and vasculitis, abnormal blood profiles, hepatic encephalopathy, hypokalemia, asymptomatic hyperuricemia, hyperglycemia and impairment of glucose tolerance, fluid and electrolyte imbalances, including dilutional hyponatremia and hypochloremia, metabolic alkalosis, and hypercalcemia.

Onset, Peak, and Duration

Route	Onset	Peak	Duration
Oral	2 hr	4–6 hr	6–12 hr

 Massage Considerations

- There are no cautions or contraindications to massage related to the action of this drug.
- There may be cautions and contraindications to massage related to the client condition.
- Side effects of hypotension require care in getting the client on and off the table.
- Stimulation with rapid effleurage or tapotement at the end of the session may help.
- Frequent urination may require the client to go to the bathroom in the middle of the session. It is important to provide privacy and quick access to the bathroom. Water fountains or music that may stimulate the need to urinate should be avoided. Rash is a local contraindication to massage and should be reported to the physician. If severe, massage should be withheld.

---

hydrocortisone (high-droh-KOR-tuh-sohn)

Cortef, Cortenema, Hydrocortone

hydrocortisone acetate

Cortifoam, Hydrocortone Acetate

hydrocortisone cypionate

Cortef

hydrocortisone sodium phosphate

Hydrocortone Phosphate

hydrocortisone sodium succinate

A-hydroCort, Solu-Cortef

Drug Class: Adrenocortical steroids; glucocorticoid

Drug Actions

Reduces inflammation, suppresses immune function, and raises adrenocorticoid hormonal levels

Use

- Severe inflammation
- Adrenal insufficiency
- Adjunct for ulcerative colitis and proctitis

Side Effects

Cardiovascular: heart failure, hypertension, edema, arrhythmias, thromboembolism.
Gastrointestinal: peptic ulceration, GI irritation, increased appetite, pancreatitis.
Nervous System: euphoria, insomnia, psychotic behavior, pseudotumor cerebri, seizures.
Skin: abnormal hair growth, delayed wound healing, acne, various skin eruptions, easy bruising.
Other: susceptibility to infections, acute adrenal insufficiency with increased stress (infection, surgery, or trauma) or abrupt withdrawal after long-term therapy, cataracts, glaucoma, hypokalemia, hyperglycemia, carbohydrate intolerance, muscle weakness, growth suppression in children, osteoporosis.

Onset, Peak, and Duration

Route	Onset	Peak	Duration
Oral., I.V., Rectal I.M.,	Varies	Varies	Varies

Massage Considerations

- This drug affects metabolism and, with long-term use (longer than 2 weeks) will effect changes in muscle and connective tissues in the body. In these cases, deep tissue massage is contraindicated. As a result of changes in connective tissues, myofascial massage techniques may be less effective and should be used with caution.
- There may be other cautions and contraindications to massage related to the client conditon.
- Side effects of thromboembolism are a complete contraindication to massage. Redness, heat, swelling, and pain, especially in the extremities, should be evaluated by the physician immediately and massage withheld until evaluation is complete. Acne or skin eruptions are local contraindications to massage and should be reported to the physician.
  If the client still wishes massage but cannot stop taking the medication, massage may still be given but the massage therapist should wear gloves to work on the affected areas. The client will often be susceptible to infections. The massage therapist should not work on the client if they have any symptoms of infection and trying to schedule the client at the beginning of the day to decrease the exposure to others may help. Osteoporosis requires extra care in depth of masssage and if severe, massage may be contraindicated.
- The best approaches to this client are mechanical and local reflex strokes, such as pétrissage, effleurage, gentle stretching, and vibration. Rocking also may be helpful.

hydromorphone hydrochloride (dihydromorphinone hydrochloride) (high-droh-MOR-fohn high-droh-KLOR-ighd)

Dilaudid, Dilaudid-HP

Drug Class: Opioid analgesic, antitussive

Drug Actions

Binds with opioid receptors in CNS, altering perception of and emotional response to pain. Suppresses cough reflex by direct action on cough center in medulla.

Use

- Moderate to severe pain
- Cough

Side Effects

Cardiovascular: hypotension, bradycardia.
Gastrointestinal: nausea, vomiting, constipation, ileus.
Nervous System: sedation, sleepiness, clouded sensorium, dizziness, euphoria, seizures.
Urinary: urine retention.
Other: induration with repeated subcutaneous injections, physical dependence, blurred vision, double vision, nystagmus, respiratory depression, bronchospasm.

Onset, Peak, and Duration

Route	Onset	Peak	Duration
Oral	30 min	30 min–2 hr	4–5 hr
I.V.	10–15 min	15–30 min	2–3 hr
I.M.	15 min	30–60 min	4–5 hr
Subcutaneous Injection	15 min	30–90 min	4 hr
Rectal	Unknown	Unknown	4 hr

Massage Considerations

- This drug alters perception of pain; therefore, deep tissue massage should be used with great caution, if at all.
- There may be further cautions or contraindications to massage related to the client condition.
- The drug depresses the CNS; therefore, the relaxing effects of massage and the systemic reflex strokes or rocking and effleurage may be increased. Using stimulation at the end of the session or even a more stimulating massage technique throughout the session may be needed. The local reflex strokes of compression, vibration, stretching, and traction may be less effective or take a longer application time to have effect.
- The site of I.M. or subcutaneous injection should not be massaged for at least 90 minutes in order to avoid increasing the rate of absorption of the drug.
- Side effects of hypotension, sedation, sleepiness, and dizziness may be approached as described above. Constipation may be helped by regular abdominal massage.
- The best strokes to use with this patient are the mechanical strokes of effleurage and pétrissage. Myofascial massage techniques also may be effective for areas of tightness and gluteation.

hydroxychloroquine sulfate (high-droks-ee-KLOR-oh-kwin SUL-fayt)

Plaquenil

Drug Class: Antimalarial, anti-inflammatory

Drug Actions

Prevents or hinders growth of *Plasmodium malariae, Plasmodium ovale, Plasmodium vivax,* and *Plasmodium falciparum.* Relieves inflammation.

Use

- Suppressive prophylaxis of malaria attacks
- Acute malarial attacks
- Lupus erythematosus (chronic discoid and systemic)
- Rheumatoid arthritis

Side Effects

Gastrointestinal: anorexia, abdominal cramps, diarrhea, nausea, vomiting.
Nervous System: irritability, nightmares, ataxia, seizures, psychic stimulation, toxic psychosis, nystagmus, lassitude, fatigue, dizziness, hypoactive deep tendon reflexes.
Skin: itching, skin and mucosal pigmentary changes, skin eruptions, loss of hair, bleaching of hair.
Other: visual disturbances (blurred vision; difficulty in focusing; reversible corneal changes; typically irreversible, sometimes progressive or delayed retinal changes, such as narrowing of arterioles; macular lesions; pallor of optic disk; optic atrophy; visual field defects; patchy retinal pigmentation, commonly leading to blindness), ototoxicity (irreversible nerve deafness, ringing in the ears, labyrinthitis), abnormal blood profiles; hemolysis (in patients with G6PD deficiency), weight loss, skeletal muscle weakness.

Onset, Peak, and Duration

Route	Onset	Peak	Duration
Oral	Unknown	2–4.5 hr	Unknown

 Massage Considerations

- Although the action of this drug does not require cautions or contraindications to massage, the client condition may require cautions and contraindications.
- The physician should be consulted before any massage is given.
- Side effects of dizziness require care in getting the client on and off the table. Stimulation with rapid effleurage or tapotement at the end of the session may help. Hypoactive deep tendon reflexes may mean that the local reflex strokes such as compression, stretching and vibration may be less effective or require longer application to have effect. Itching or skin eruptions are a local contraindication to massage and should be reported to the physician immediately. If severe or widespread, no massage should be given.

hydroxyurea (high-droks-ee-yoo-REE-uh)

Droxia, Hydrea

Drug Class: Antineoplastic; antisickling drug

Drug Actions

Hinders growth of certain cancer cells

Use

- Solid tumors
- Head and neck cancers, excluding the lip
- Resistant chronic myelocytic leukemia
- To reduce the frequency of painful crises and to reduce the need for blood transfusions in patients with sickle cell anemia with recurrent moderate-to-severe painful crises (generally at least three during the preceding 12 months)

Side Effects

Gastrointestinal: anorexia, nausea, vomiting, diarrhea, stomatitis.
Nervous System: drowsiness, hallucinations, seizures.
Skin: rash, itching.
Other: abnormal blood profiles, megaloblastosis, bone marrow suppression (dose-limiting and dose-related, with rapid recovery), hyperuricemia.

Onset, Peak, and Duration

Route	Onset	Peak	Duration
Oral	Unknown	2 hr	Unknown

 Massage Considerations

- As a result of the toxic effects of this drug, deep tissue massage should be used with caution and circulatory massage with effleurage also should be used with caution and limited.
- There may be further cautions and contraindications to massage related to the client's condition.
- The physician should be consulted before any massage is given.
- Side effects of drowsiness require care in getting the client on and off the table. Using stimulation with gentle friction to the legs or tapotement at the end of the session may help. Rash or itching is a local contraindication to massage and should be reported to the physician immediately. If severe, massage should not be given.
- The best strokes for this client are pétrissage, gentle compression, vibration, and stretching. Myofascial massage techniques also may be helpful.

---

hydroxyzine embonate (high-DROKS-ih-zeen EM-boh-nayt)

Atarax

hydroxyzine hydrochloride

Anx, Apo-Hydroxyzine, Atarax, Hydroxacen, Hyzine-50, Multipax, Neucalm, Novo-Hydroxyzin, QYS, Vistacon-50, Vistaject-50, Vistaril

hydroxyzine pamoate

Vistaril

Drug Class: Antihistamine (piperazine derivative) anxiolytic, sedative, antipruritic, antiemetic, antispasmodic

Drug Actions

May suppress activity in key regions of subcortical area of CNS. Relieves anxiety and itching, promotes calmness and alleviates nausea and vomiting.

Use

- Anxiety
- Preoperative and postoperative adjunct therapy
- Itching from allergies
- Psychiatric and emotional emergencies, including acute alcoholism
- Nausea and vomiting (excluding nausea and vomiting of pregnancy)
- Prepartum and postpartum adjunct therapy

Side Effects

Gastrointestinal: dry mouth.
Nervous System: drowsiness, involuntary motor activity.
Other: marked discomfort at I.M. injection site, hypersensitivity reactions (wheezing, shortness of breath, chest tightness).

Onset, Peak, and Duration

Route	Onset	Peak	Duration
Oral	15–30 min	2 hr	4–6 hr
I.M.	Unknown	Unknown	4–6 hr

 Massage Considerations

- Because of the suppressive effects of this drug on the CNS, deep tissue massage should be used with great caution.
- There may be other cautions and contraindications to massage related to the client condition.
- The sedating effect of the drug may increase the relaxation effects of massage and the effects of the systemic reflex strokes of effleurage, rocking, and friction. Using more rapid strokes throughout the session may be helpful or stimulating the client at the end of the session with friction, effleurage, or tapotement may be used. The effects of local reflex strokes such as stretching, compression, and vibration may be less effective or require longer application to have the desired effect.
- The site of I.M. injection of the drug should not be massaged for at least 6 hours to avoid increasing the rate of absorption of the drug into the body.
- Side effects of drowsiness may be approached as described above.
- The best strokes to use with this client are the mechanical strokes of pétrissage and effleurage. Myofascial massage techniques also may be helpful.

I-J

ibuprofen (igh-byoo-PROH-fen)

ACT-3, Advil, Advil Children's, Advil Infants' Drops, Advil Liqui-Gels, Advil Migraine, Apo-Ibuprofen, Brufen, Genpril Caplets, Genpril Tablets, Haltran, IBU, Ibu-Tab, Junior Strength Motrin, Menadol, Midol Cramp, Midol IB, Motrin, Motrin Children's, Motrin Drops, Motrin IB Caplets, Motrin IB Gelcaps, Motrin IB Tablets, Motrin Infants' Drops, Motrin Migraine Pain Caplets, Novo-Profen, Nurofen, Rafen, Saleto-200

Drug Class: NSAID (nonsteroidal anti-inflammatory drug) nonopioid analgesic, antipyretic, anti-inflammatory

Drug Actions

Produces anti-inflammatory, analgesic, and antipyretic effects, possibly by inhibiting prostaglandin synthesis.

Use

- Rheumatoid arthritis
- Osteoarthritis
- Mild to moderate pain
- Dysmenorrhea
- Fever

Side Effects

Cardiovascular: peripheral edema, edema, hypertension, heart failure.
Gastrointestinal: epigastric distress, nausea, occult blood loss, peptic ulceration.
Nervous System: headache, drowsiness, dizziness, cognitive dysfunction, aseptic meningitis.
Urinary: reversible renal failure.
Skin: itching, rash, hives, photosensitivity reactions, Stevens-Johnson syndrome.
Other: visual disturbances, ringing in the ears, prolonged bleeding time, abnormal blood profiles, bronchospasm.

Onset, Peak, and Duration

Route	Onset	Peak	Duration
Oral	≤30 min	2–4 hr	≥4 hr

Massage Considerations

- This drug reduces the perception of pain; therefore, deep tissue massage should be used with caution. Other cautions or contraindications to massage may be related to the client condition.
- Side effects of drowsiness and dizziness require care in getting the client on and off the table. Using stimulation with rapid effleurage and tapotement at the end of the session may help.
- Itching, rash, or hives are local contraindications to massage and should be reported to the physician. If severe or widespread, no massage should be given.

---

idarubicin hydrochloride (igh-duh-ROO-bih-sin high-droh-KLOR-ighd)

Idamycin, Idamycin PFS

Drug Class: Antibiotic antineoplastic

Drug Actions

Hinders growth of susceptible cancer cells

Use

- Acute myeloid leukemia

Side Effects

Cardiovascular: heart failure, atrial fibrillation, chest pain, heart attack, myocardial insufficiency, arrhythmias, hemorrhage, myocardial toxicity.

Gastrointestinal: nausea, vomiting, cramps, diarrhea, mucositis, severe enterocolitis with perforation.
Nervous System: fever, headache, changed mental status, peripheral neuropathy, seizures.
Skin: hair loss, rash, hives, bullous erythrodermatous rash on palms and soles, hives at injection site, erythema at previously irradiated sites, tissue necrosis at injection site if extravasation occurs.
Other: infection, myelosuppression.

Onset, Peak, and Duration

Route	Onset	Peak	Duration
I.V.	Unknown	≤3 min	Unknown

 Massage Considerations

- Because of the toxic effects of this drug, deep tissue massage should be used with great caution if at all, and circulatory massage with effleurage should be used with great caution and limited.
- Further cautions and contraindications to massage may be related to the client condition.
- The physician should be consulted before any massage is given, and close collaboration is essential.
- The drug is usually given for 3 to 7 days in a row and has a half-life of 22 hours. It would be best to give massage on a week when the drug is not being given or at least 24 hours after the last dose, so as not to overtax the liver and kidneys as they try to rid the body of the drug.
- Side effects of peripheral neuropathy are local contraindications to deep tissue massage.
- Rash or skin eruptions of any kind are local contraindications to massage and should be reported to the physician immediately. If severe or widespread, massage should not be given.
- Hair loss is a contraindication to scalp massage if the client is disturbed when hair is lost during the massage or if the scalp is tender.
- The best strokes to use with this client are the mechanical strokes of pétrissage and the local and systemic reflex strokes of rocking, stretching, gentle compression, and vibration. Myofascial massage techniques may be used for areas of tightness or gluteation.

---

ifosfamide (igh-FOHS-fuh-mighd)

IFEX

Drug Class: Antineoplastic

Drug Actions

Kills cancer cells

Use

- Testicular cancer
- Lung cancer
- Hodgkins's and malignant lymphoma
- Breast cancer
- Acute lymphocytic leukemia
- Ovarian cancer
- Gastric cancer
- Pancreatic cancer
- Sarcomas
- Cervical cancer
- Uterine cancer

Side Effects

Gastrointestinal: nausea, vomiting.
Nervous System: lethargy, sleepiness, confusion, depressive psychosis, coma, seizures, ataxia.
Urinary: hemorrhagic cystitis (dose-limiting, occurring in up to 50% of patients), hematuria, nephrotoxicity.
Skin: hair loss.
Other: abnormal blood profiles, myelosuppression.

Onset, Peak, and Duration

Route	Onset	Peak	Duration
I.V.	Unknown	Unknown	Unknown

Massage Considerations

- Because of the toxic effects of this drug, deep tissue massage is contraindicated and circulatory massage with effleurage should be used with caution and limited. Further cautions and contraindications to massage may be related to the client condition.
- The physician should be consulted before any massage is given, and close collaboration is essential.
- The drug is usually given for 3 to 5 days in a row and has a half-life of 14 hours. It would be best to give massage on the weeks when the drug is not being given or at least not until 24 hours after the drug has been administered, so as not to tax the liver and kidneys as they try to rid the body of the drug.
- Side effects of sleepiness require care in getting the client on and off the table.
- Stimulating the client at the end of the session with gentle friction to the legs or light tapotement may help.
- Hair loss is a contraindication to massage, if the client is disturbed by hair coming out during the massage or if the scalp is tender.
- The best strokes to use with this client are the mechanical stroke of pétrissage and the systemic and local reflex strokes of rocking, stretching, and vibration. Myofascial techniques may also be used.

---

imatinib mesylate (i-MAH-tin-nib MES-uh-late)

Gleevec

Drug Class: Antineoplastic

Drug Actions

Stops tumor growth

Use

- Chronic myeloid leukemia (CML)
- Philadelphia chromosome–positive chronic-phase CML
- Patients with Kit (CD117)-positive unresectable or metastatic malignant GI stromal tumors (GIST)
- Philadelphia chromosome–positive chronic-phase CML

Side Effects

Cardiovascular: edema.
Gastrointestinal: anorexia, nausea, diarrhea, abdominal pain, constipation, vomiting, painful digestion, GI hemorrhage.

Nervous System: headache, cerebral hemorrhage, fatigue, weakness, fever.
Skin: rash, itching, petechiae.
Other: night sweats, nasopharyngitis, nosebleeds, hemorrhage, abnormal blood profiles, hypokalemia, weight increase, muscle pain, muscle cramps, musculoskeletal pain, joint pain, cough, shortness of breath, pneumonia.

Onset, Peak, and Duration

Route	Onset	Peak	Duration
Oral	Unknown	2–4 hr	Unknown

Massage Considerations

- Because of the toxic effects of this drug, deep tissue massage should be used with great caution, if at all. Further cautions and contraindications to massage may be related to the client condition.
- The physician should be consulted before any massage is given, and close, ongoing collaboration is essential.
- Side effects of constipation may be helped by abdominal massage.
- Rash or itching is a local contraindication to massage and should be reported to the physician immediately. If severe or widespread, massage should be withheld.
- The presence of petechiae, small red hemorrhagic spots on the skin, is a contraindication to deep tissue massage and if severe or worsened by massage, may contraindicate massage completely.

---

imipenem and cilastatin sodium (im-ih-PEN-em and sigh-luh-STAT-in SO-dee-um)

Primaxin IM, Primaxin IV

Drug Class: Antibiotic

Drug Actions

Kills susceptible organisms, including many Gram-positive, Gram-negative, and anaerobic bacteria.

Use

- Mild to moderate lower respiratory tract, skin, skin-structure, intra-abdominal, and gynecologic infections
- Serious lower respiratory and urinary tract, intra-abdominal, and gynecologic infections
- Bacterial septicemia
- Bone and joint infections
- Serious soft tissue infections
- Endocarditis
- Polymicrobic infections

Side Effects

Cardiovascular: hypotension, thrombophlebitis.
Gastrointestinal: nausea, vomiting, diarrhea, pseudomembranous colitis.
Nervous System: seizures, dizziness, sleepiness, fever.
Skin: rash, hives, itching.
Other: hypersensitivity reactions (anaphylaxis), pain at injection site.

Onset, Peak, and Duration

Route	Onset	Peak	Duration
I.V.	Unknown	Immediate	Unknown
I.M.	Unknown	1–2 hr	Unknown

Massage Considerations

- No cautions or contraindications to massage are related to the action of this drug in the body. Cautions and contraindications to massage may be related to the client condition and severity of the infection.
- The site of intramuscular injection of the drug should not be massaged for at least 2 hours to avoid increasing the rate of absorption of the drug into the body.
- Side effects of dizziness, sleepiness, or hypotension require care in positioning the client and getting the client on and off the table. Using stimulation at the end of the session with rapid effleurage or tapotement may help.
- Thrombophlebitis is a complete contraindication to massage.
- Rash, hives, or itching are local contraindications to massage and should be reported to the physician immediately. If severe, no massage should be given.

---

imipramine hydrochloride (ih-MIP-ruh-meen high-droh-KLOR-ighd)

Apo-Imipramine, Impril, Melipramine, Norfranil, Novopramine, Tipramine, Tofranil

imipramine pamoate

Tofranil-PM

Drug Class: Tricyclic antidepressant

Drug Actions

Increases amount of norepinephrine, serotonin, or both in the central nervous system by blocking their reuptake by presynaptic neurons. Relieves depression and childhood bed-wetting (hydrochloride form).

Use

- Depression
- Bed-wetting
- Attention deficit hyperactivity disorder

Side Effects

Cardiovascular: orthostatic hypotension, tachycardia, electrocardiogram changes, hypertension, heart attack, stroke, arrhythmias, heart block.
Gastrointestinal: dry mouth, constipation, nausea, vomiting, anorexia, paralytic ileus.
Nervous System: drowsiness, dizziness, excitation, tremor, weakness, confusion, headache, nervousness, electroencephalogram changes, seizures, extrapyramidal reactions.
Urinary: urine retention, impotence, testicular swelling.
Skin: rash, hives, sweating, photosensitivity reactions.
Other: hypersensitivity reactions, abnormal mild production and breast enlargement, altered libido, syndrome of inappropriate antidiuretic hormone (SIADH), blurred vision, ringing in the ears, dilated pupils, hypoglycemia, hyperglycemia.

Onset, Peak, and Duration

Route	Onset	Peak	Duration
Oral	Unknown	1–2 hr	Unknown

Massage Considerations

- No cautions or contraindications to massage are indicated because a client is taking this drug. Cautions and contraindications to massage may be related to the client condition.
- Side effects of hypotension, drowsiness, or dizziness require care in getting the client on and off the table. Stimulating the client at the end of the session with rapid effleurage and tapotement may help. If side effects are severe, more rapid and stimulating massage techniques should be used throughout the session.
- Constipation may be helped by regular abdominal massage.
- Rash or hives are local contraindications to massage and should be reported to the physician. If severe or widespread, massage should be withheld.
- Abnormal breast milk or breast enlargement requires caution in chest massage. No deep tissue massage should be done and if very tender, no massage of the area should be done at all. If leakage of breast fluid occurs, extra padding on the table may be required.

immune globulin intramuscular (gamma globulin, IG, IGIM) (ih-MYOON GLOB-yoo-lin in-truh-MUS-kyoo-ler)

BayGam

immune globulin intravenous (IGIV)

Gaminume N, Gammagard S/D, Gammar-P IV, Iveegam EN, Panglobulin, Polygram S/D, Carimune, Venoglobulin-S

Drug Class: Immune serum

Drug Actions

Provides passive immunity by increasing antibody titer. The primary component is IgG. Helps prevent infections.

Use

- Primary humoral immunodeficiency (IGIV)
- Treatment of primary defective antibody synthesis such as agammaglobulinemia or hypogammaglobulinemia in patients who are at increased risk of infection
- Idiopathic thrombocytopenic purpura (IGIV)
- Bone marrow transplant (IGIV)
- B-cell chronic lymphocytic leukemia (IGIV)
- Pediatric HIV infection (IGIV)
- Kawasaki syndrome (IGIV)
- Hepatitis A exposure (IGIM)
- Measles exposure (IGIM)
- Measles postexposure prophylaxis (IGIM)
- Chickenpox exposure (IGIM)
- Rubella exposure in first trimester of pregnancy (IGIM)

Side Effects

Cardiovascular: chest pain, heart attack, heart failure (Gammagard S/D).
Gastrointestinal: nausea, vomiting.

Nervous System: severe headache requiring hospitalization.
Urinary: nephrotic syndrome, acute tubular necrosis, osmotic nephrosis, acute renal impairment.
Skin: hives, redness.
Other: anaphylaxis, muscle stiffness at injection site, pulmonary embolism, transfusion-related acute lung injury.

Onset, Peak, and Duration

Route	Onset	Peak	Duration
I.V.	Immediate	Immediate	Unknown
I.M.	Unknown	2–5 days	Unknown

Massage Considerations

- No cautions or contraindications to massage are related to the action of this drug.
- Cautions and contraindications to massage may be related to the client condition.
- The site of I.M. injections should not be massaged for at least 1 week to avoid increasing the rate of absorption of the drug, because peak effect takes that long.
- Side effects of hives or redness are local contraindications to massage and should be reported to the physician immediately. If severe or widespread, massage should be withheld.

---

indapamide (in-DAP-uh-mighd)

Lozide, Lozol, Natrilix

Drug Class: Diuretic, antihypertensive

Drug Actions

Promotes water and sodium excretion and lowers blood pressure.

Use

- Edema
- Hypertension

Side Effects

Cardiovascular: volume depletion and dehydration, orthostatic hypotension.
Gastrointestinal: nausea, pancreatitis.
Nervous System: headache, irritability, nervousness, dizziness, light-headedness, weakness.
Urinary: increased urination at night, excessive urination, frequent urination.
Skin: dermatitis, photosensitivity reactions, rash.
Other: gout, anorexia, hypokalemia, asymptomatic hyperuricemia, metabolic alkalosis, hyponatremia, hypochloremia, muscle cramps and spasms.

Onset, Peak, and Duration

Route	Onset	Peak	Duration
Oral	1–2 hr	≤2 hr	≤36 hr

Massage Considerations

- No cautions or contraindications to massage are related to the actions of this drug.
- Cautions and contraindications to massage may be related to the client condition.
- Side effects of hypotension, dizziness, and light-headedness require care in getting the client on and off the table. Stimulation with rapid effleurage and tapotement at the end of the session may help.

- Frequent urination may require that the client get up during a session. Providing privacy and quick access to the bathroom is important. Water fountains or water music, which may stimulate the need to urinate, should be avoided.
- Rash is a local contraindication to massage and should be reported to the physician. If severe, massage should be withheld.

indinavir sulfate (in-DIH-nuh-veer SUL-fayt)

Crixivan

Drug Class: Antiviral

Drug Action

Reduces symptoms of HIV

Use

- HIV

Side Effects

Gastrointestinal: abdominal pain, nausea, diarrhea, vomiting, acid regurgitation, anorexia, dry mouth, taste perversion.
Nervous System: headache, insomnia, dizziness, malaise, sleepiness, weakness, fatigue.
Urinary: nephrolithiasis.
Other: redistribution and accumulation of body fat, anemia, neutropenia, hyperbilirubinemia, flank pain, back pain.

Onset, Peak, and Duration

Route	Onset	Peak	Duration
Oral	Unknown	<1 hr	1–8 hr

Massage Considerations

- No cautions or contraindications to massage are indicated because a client is taking this drug. Cautions and contraindications to massage may be related to the client condition.
- Side effects of dizziness or sleepiness require care in getting the client on and off the table. Stimulation with rapid effleurage or tapotement at the end of the session may help.

indomethacin (in-doh-METH-uh-sin)

Apo-Indomethacin, Arthrexin, Indocid, Indocid SR, Indocin, Indocin SR, Novo-Methacin

indomethacin sodium trihydrate

Apo-Indomethacin, Indocid PDA, Indocin I.V., Novo-Methacin

Drug Class: NSAID (nonsteroidal anti-inflammatory drug) nonopioid analgesic, antipyretic, anti-inflammatory

Drug Actions

Produces anti-inflammatory, analgesic, and antipyretic effects, possibly by inhibiting prostaglandin synthesis.

Use

- Moderate to severe rheumatoid arthritis or osteoarthritis
- Ankylosing spondylitis

- Acute gouty arthritis
- Acute painful shoulders (bursitis or tendinitis)
- To close hemodynamically significant patent ductus arteriosus in premature infants
- Pericarditis
- Dysmenorrhea
- Bartter syndrome

Side Effects

Cardiovascular: hypertension, edema, heart failure.
Gastrointestinal: nausea, vomiting, anorexia, diarrhea, peptic ulceration, GI bleeding, vomiting.
Nervous System: headache, dizziness, depression, drowsiness, confusion, peripheral neuropathy, seizures, psychic disturbances, syncope.
Urinary: renal dysfunction, azotemia, hematuria, acute renal failure.
Skin: itching, hives, Stevens-Johnson syndrome.
Other: hypersensitivity reactions (rash, respiratory distress, anaphylaxis, angioedema), blurred vision, corneal and retinal damage, hearing loss, ringing in the ears, abnormal blood profiles, hyperkalemia, hyponatremia, hyperkalemia, hypoglycemia.

Onset, Peak, and Duration

Route	Onset	Peak	Duration
Oral	30 min	1–4 hr	4–6 hr
I.V.	Immediate	Immediate	Unknown
Rectal	2–4 hr	Unknown	4–6 hr

 Massage Considerations

- This drug potentially decreases the perception of pain. Deep tissue massage should be use with caution. Other cautions or contraindications to massage may be related to the client condition.
- Side effects of dizziness or drowsiness require care in getting the client on and off the table. Stimulation at the end of the massage with rapid effleurage and tapotement may help.
- Peripheral neuropathy is a local contraindication to deep tissue massage.
- Itching or rash are local contraindications to massage and should be reported to the physician immediately. If severe or widespread, no massage should be given.

---

infliximab (in-FLICKS-ih-mab)

Remicade

Drug Class: Monoclonal antibody anti-inflammatory

Drug Actions

Reduces the infiltration of inflammatory cells in inflamed areas of the intestine

Use

- To reduce signs and symptoms and induce and maintain remission in patients with moderate to severely active Crohn's disease who have had an inadequate response to conventional therapy
- To reduce the number of draining enterocutaneous and rectovaginal fistulas and maintain fistula closure in patients with fistulizing Crohn's disease
- With methotrexate, to reduce signs and symptoms, inhibit the progression of structural damage, and improve function in patients with moderate to severely active rheumatoid arthritis who have not responded adequately to methotrexate

Side Effects

Cardiovascular: hypertension, peripheral edema, hypotension, tachycardia, chest pain, flushing.
Gastrointestinal: nausea, abdominal pain, vomiting, constipation, painful digestion, diarrhea, gas, intestinal obstruction, mouth pain, ulcerative stomatitis.
Nervous System: pain, headache, fatigue, fever, depression, dizziness, malaise, insomnia.
Urinary: painful urination, increased urinary frequency, urinary tract infection.
Skin: rash, itching, candidiasis, acne, hair loss, eczema, dry skin, increased sweating, hives, bruising.
Other: chills, flulike syndrome, hot flushes, abscess, toothache, hypersensitivity reaction, allergic reaction, pharyngitis, rhinitis, sinusitis, conjunctivitis, anemia, hematoma, muscle pain, joint pain, arthritis, back pain, upper respiratory tract infections, bronchitis, coughing, shortness of breath.

Onset, Peak, and Duration

Route	Onset	Peak	Duration
I.V.	Unknown	Unknown	Unknown

Massage Considerations

- No cautions or contraindications to massage are related to the actions of this drug. Cautions and contraindications to massage may be related to the client condition.
- The physician should be consulted before any massage is given.
- Side effects of dizziness require care in getting the client on and off the table. Stimulation with rapid effleurage or tapotement at the end of the session may help.
- Constipation and gas may be helped by regular abdominal massage but should be done with caution in Crohn's disease.
- Increased urinary frequency may require the client to get up in the middle of the session. Providing privacy and quick access to the bathroom is important. Water fountains or water music, which may stimulate the need to urinate, should be avoided.
- Rash, itching, acne, or hives are local contraindications to massage and should be reported to the physician.
- Bruising is a contraindication to deep tissue massage.

insulin aspart (rDNA origin) injection (IN-suh-lin AS-part)

NovoLog

insulin aspart (rDNA origin) protamine suspension and insulin aspart (rDNA origin) injection

Novolog 70/30

Drug Class: Human insulin analog

Drug Actions

Binds to insulin receptors on muscle and fat cells, lowers glucose level, facilitates the cellular uptake of glucose, and inhibits the output of glucose from the liver.

Use

- Control of hyperglycemia in diabetes mellitus

Side Effects

Skin: lipodystrophy, itching, rash.
Other: allergic reactions, injection site reactions, hypoglycemia, hyperkalemia.

Onset, Peak, and Duration

Route	Onset	Peak	Duration
S.C.			
Novolog	15–30 min	1–3 hr	3–5 hr
Novolog 70/30	Rapid	1–4 hr	24 hr

 Massage Considerations

- No cautions or contraindications to massage are related to the actions of this drug. Cautions and contraindications to massage may be related to the client condition.
- The physician should be consulted before any massage is given.
- The site of subcutaneous injection of insulin aspart or Novolog should not be massaged for at least 3 hours to avoid increasing the rate of absorption of the drug. The site of insulin aspart protamine suspension or Novolog 70/30 should not be massaged for at least 24 hours. This form of the drug crystallizes in the tissues so as to allow for gradual absorption into the body, and massage may increase the breakdown of the crystals and the drug absorption.
- Side effects of rash ot itching are local contraindications to massage and should be reported to the physician immediately. If severe, no massage should be given.
- Clients who take insulin are more likely to have hypogycemia as a side effect than those who take oral hypoglycemic agents. Massage may increase the likelihood of a reaction because it has been shown to decrease blood sugar. Telling the client to be sure to have a good snack or light meal before coming for massage may help prevent this problem. If dizziness, weakness, sweating, confusion, or decrease in alertness occurs, giving the client a quick source of sugar (such as orange juice, candy, or a soft drink) is the best course of action. If this does not reverse the symptoms within 5 to 10 minutes, emergency help should be called immediately. The massage therapist is not licensed to do blood sugar testing or give insulin.

---

insulin glargine (rDNA) injection (IN-suh-lin GLAR-gene (rDNA) in-JEK-shun)

Lantus

Drug Class: Insulin analog

Drug Actions

Increases glucose transport across muscle and fat cell membranes to reduce glucose level. Promotes conversion of glucose to its storage form, glycogen. Triggers amino acid uptake and conversion to protein in muscle cells and inhibits protein degradation. Stimulates triglyceride formation and inhibits release of free fatty acids from adipose tissue. Stimulates lipoprotein lipase activity, which converts circulating lipoproteins to fatty acids.

Use

- Management of type 1 or type 2 diabetes mellitus in patients who need basal (long-acting) insulin for the control of hyperglycemia
- Management of type 2 diabetes mellitus in patients previously treated with oral antidiabetic agents

Side Effects

Skin: lipodystrophy, itching, rash.
Other: allergic reactions, pain at injection site, hypoglycemia.

Onset, Peak, and Duration

Route	Onset	Peak	Duration
S.C.	Slow	None	10.75–24 hr

Massage Considerations

- No cautions or contraindications to massage are related to the actions of this drug. Cautions and contraindications to massage may be related to the client condition.
- The physician should be consulted before any massage is given.
- The site of subcutaneous injection of insulin glargine should not be massaged for at least 24 hours.
- Side effects of rash or itching are local contraindications to massage and should be reported to the physician immediately. If severe, no massage should be given.
- Clients who take insulin are more likely to have hypoglycemia as a side effect than those who take oral hypoglycemic agents. Massage may increase the likelihood of a reaction because it has been shown to decrease blood sugar. Telling the client to be sure to have a good snack or light meal before coming for massage may help prevent this problem. If dizziness, weakness, sweating, confusion, or decrease in alertness occurs, giving the client a quick source of sugar (such as orange juice, candy, or a soft drink) is the best course of action. If this does not reverse the symptoms within 5 to 10 minutes, emergency help should be called immediately. The massage therapist is not licensed to do blood sugar testing or give insulin.

---

insulins (IN-suh-linz)

insulin analog injection (lispro)

Humalog, Humalog mix 75/25, Humalog mix 50/50

insulin injection (regular insulin, crystalline zinc insulin)

Actrapid HM, Actrapid HM Penfill, Actrapid MC, Actrapid MC Penfill, Humulin R, Hypurin Neutra, Insulin 2 Neutral, Novolin R, Novolin R PenFill, Pork Regular Iletin II, Regular (Concentrated) Iletin II, Regular Purified Pork Insulin, Velosulin Human, Velosulin Insuject

insulin zinc suspension (lente)

Humulin L, Lente Iletin II, Lente Insulin, Lente MC, Lente Purified Pork Insulin Monotard HM, Monotard M

insulin zinc suspension, extended (ultralente)

Humulin U, Ultralente Insulin, Ultratard HM, Ultratard MC

insulin zinc suspension, prompt (semilente)

Semilente MC

isophane insulin suspension (neutral protamine Hagedorn insulin, NPH)

Humulin N, Hypurin Isophane, Insulatard, Insulatard Human, Isotard MC, Novolin N, Novolin N PenFill, NPH Insulin, Pork NPH Iletin II, Protaphane HM, Protaphane HM Penfill, Protaphane MC

isophane insulin suspension with insulin injection

Actraphane HM, Actraphane HM Penfill, Actraphane MC, Humulin 50/50, Humulin 70/30, Novolin 70/30, Novolin 70/30 PenFill

protamine zinc suspension (PZI)

Protamine Zinc Insulin MC

Drug Class: Pancreatic hormone insulin

Drug Actions

Increases glucose transport across muscle and fat cell membranes to reduce glucose level. Promotes conversion of glucose to its storage form, glycogen; triggers amino acid uptake and conversion to protein in muscle cells and inhibits protein degradation; stimulates triglyceride formation and inhibits release of free fatty acids from adipose tissue; stimulates lipoprotein lipase activity, which converts circulating lipoproteins to fatty acids.

Use

- Diabetic ketoacidosis
- Type 1 diabetes mellitus (insulin-dependent)
- Adjunct to type 2 diabetes mellitus (non–insulin-dependent) inadequately controlled by diet and oral antidiabetics
- Control of hyperglycemia with longer-acting insulin in patients with type 1 diabetes mellitus and with sulfonylureas in patients with type 2 diabetes mellitus
- Control of hyperglycemia with Humalog and longer-acting insulin in patients with type 1 diabetes mellitus
- Control of hyperglycemia with Humalog and sulfonylureas in patients with type 2 diabetes mellitus

Side Effects

Skin: hives, itching, swelling, redness, stinging, warmth at injection site, rash.
Other: lipoatrophy, lipohypertrophy, hypersensitivity reactions, anaphylaxis, hypoglycemia, hyperglycemia (rebound, or Somogyi, effect).

Onset, Peak, and Duration

Type of Insulin	Onset	Peak	Duration
Regular: S.C.	30–60 min	2–3 hr	6–8hr
Regular: I.V.	<30 min	15–30min	30 min–1 hour
Semilente	1–1.5 hr	5–10 hr	12–16 hr
NPH	1–1.5 hr	4–12 hr	24 hr
Lente	1–2.5 hr	7–15 hr	24 hr
PZI	4–8 hr	14–24 hr	36 hr
Ultralente	4–8 hr	10–30 hr	>36 hr
Lispro	15 min	1 hour	3.5–4.5 hr

*Note: Only Regular insulin can be given S.C., I.M., or I.V.; all other insulins can only be given S.C.

Quick Guide to Combination Insulin Onset, Peak, and Duration

Insulin Mix	Onset	Peak	Duration
NPH and Regular: Actraphane, Humulin 50/50, Humulin 70/30, Novolin 70/30	Regular 30–60 min NPH: 1–2 hr	Regular 2–4 hr NPH: 6–12 hr	Regular 6–8 hr NPH: 18–24 hr
NPH and lispro: Humalog Mix 75/25, Humalog Mix 50/50	Lispro: 15 min NPH: 1–2 hr	Lispro: 1 hour NPH: 6–12 hr	Lispro: 3.5–4.5 hr NPH: 18–24 hr

Massage Considerations

- No cautions or contraindications to massage are related to the actions of this drug. Cautions and contraindications to massage may be related to the client condition.
- The physician should be consulted before any massage is given.
- Except for regular or lispro insulins that are short-acting, the longer-acting insulins are crystallized in the tissue and broken down and absorbed over time. For the site of regular and lispro injections, no massage should be given to the site until the peak action of the drug is attained. For all other longer-acting insulins, no massage should be given at the site of injection for the duration of action of the drug. The table gives those times. For insulin mixes, the site of injection should not be massaged for the duration of action of the drug. See the table.
- Side effects of rash, itching, or hives are local contraindications to massage and should be reported to the physician immediately. If severe, no massage should be given.
- Clients who take insulin are more likely to have hypoglycemia as a side effect than those who take oral hypoglycemic agents. Massage may increase the likelihood of a reaction because it has been shown to decrease blood sugar. Telling the client to be sure to have a good snack or light meal before coming for massage may help prevent this problem. If dizziness, weakness, sweating, confusion, or decrease in alertness occurs, giving the client a quick source of sugar (such as orange juice, candy, or a soft drink) is the best course of action. If this does not reverse the symptoms within 5 to 10 minutes, emergency help should be called immediately. The massage therapist is not licensed to do blood sugar testing or give insulin.

---

interferon alpha-2a, recombinant (rIFN-A) (in-ter-FEER-on AL-fuh too-ay ree-COM-bih-nent)

interferon alpha-2a, recombinant (rIFN-A)

Roferon-A

interferon alpha-2b, recombinant (IFN-a-2)

Intron-A

Drug Class: Antineoplastic

Drug Actions

Inhibits growth of certain tumor cells and viral cells.

Use

- Hairy cell leukemia
- Condylomata acuminata
- Kaposi sarcoma
- Chronic hepatitis C
- Chronic hepatitis B
- Chronic myelogenous leukemia
- Malignant melanoma
- Initial treatment of aggressive follicular non-Hodgkin lymphoma in conjunction with anthracycline-containing combination chemotherapy
- Metastatic renal cell carcinoma

Side Effects

Cardiovascular: hypotension, chest pain, arrhythmias, palpitations, heart failure, hypertension, edema, flushing, heart attack.

Gastrointestinal: anorexia, nausea, diarrhea, vomiting, abdominal fullness, abdominal pain, gas, constipation, hypermotility, gastric distress, altered taste.
Nervous System: dizziness, confusion, paresthesia, numbness, lethargy, depression, nervousness, difficulty in thinking or concentrating, insomnia, sedation, apathy, anxiety, irritability, syncope, fatigue, vertigo, gait disturbances, poor coordination.
Urinary: transient impotence.
Skin: rash, dryness, itching, partial hair loss, hives, sweating.
Other: flulike syndrome (fever, fatigue, myalgia, headache, chills, arthralgia), hot flushes, excessive salivation, visual disturbances, dry or inflamed oropharynx, rhinorrhea, sinusitis, conjunctivitis, ear ache, eye irritation, rhinitis, abnormal blood profiles, hepatitis, coughing, shortnesss of breath, rapid respirations, cyanosis.

Onset, Peak, and Duration

Route	Onset	Peak	Duration
I.M.	Unknown	3.75 hr	Unknown
Subcutaneous Injection	Unknown	7.25 hr	Unknown
Intralesional	Unknown	Unknown	Unknown

 Massage Considerations

- No cautions or contraindications to massage are related to the actions of this drug. In most cases, cautions and contraindications to massage may be related to the client condition.
- The physician should be consulted before any massage is given.
- The site of subcutaneous injection of the drug should not be massaged for at least 8 hours.
- Side effects of hypotension, dizziness, or sedation require care in getting the client on and off the table. Stimulation with rapid effleurage and tapotement at the end of the session may help. If symptoms are severe, using more rapid and stimulating massage techniques throughout the session may be required.
- Paresthesia or numbness is a contraindication to deep tissue massage.
- Gas or constipation may be helped by abdominal massage.
- Rash, itching, or hives are local contraindications to massage and should be reported to the physician immediately. If severe, massage should be withheld.
- Hair loss is a contraindication to scalp massage if the client is disturbed by hair loss during the massage.

---

interferon beta-1b, recombinant (in-ter-FEER-on BAY-tuh wun bee ree-COM-bih-nent)

Betaseron

Drug Class: Antiviral, immunoregulator

Drug Actions

Attaches to membrane receptors and causes cellular changes, including increased protein synthesis. Decreases exacerbations in multiple sclerosis (MS).

Use

- To reduce frequency of exacerbations in patients with relapsing forms of MS

Side Effects

Cardiovascular: hemorrhage.
Gastrointestinal: nausea, diarrhea, constipation.

Nervous System: depression, anxiety, emotional lability, depersonalization, malaise, suicidal tendencies, confusion, seizures, headache, sleepiness, dizziness.
Other: flulike symptoms (fever, chills, myalgia, diaphoresis); breast pain; pelvic pain; lymphadenopathy; hypersensitivity reaction, inflammation, pain, and necrosis at injection site; menstrual disorders (bleeding or spotting, early or delayed menses, decreased days of menstrual flow, menorrhagia); abnormal blood profiles; shortness of breath; laryngitis.

Onset, Peak, and Duration

Route	Onset	Peak	Duration
Subcutaneous Injection	Unknown	1–8 hr	Unknown

Massage Considerations

- This drug affects cell membranes and changes cells; therefore, deep tissue massage and myofascial massage techniques should be used with caution.
- Further cautions and contraindications to massage may be related to the client condition.
- The physician should be consulted before any massage is given.
- The site of subcutaneous injection of the drug should not be massaged for at least 8 hours.
- Side effects of sleepiness or dizziness require care in getting the client on and off the table. Stimulation with effleurage or tapotement at the end of the session may help.
- Constipation may be helped by regular abdominal massage.

interferon gamma-1b (in-ter-FEER-on GAH-muh wun bee)

Actimmune

Drug Class: Immunomodulator; antineoplastic

Drug Actions

Acts as interleukin-type lymphokine. Drug has potent phagocyte-activating properties and enhances oxidative metabolism of tissue macrophages. Promotes phagocyte activity.

Use

- To delay disease progression in patients with severe, malignant osteopetrosis
- Chronic granulomatous disease

Side Effects

Gastrointestinal: nausea, vomiting, diarrhea.
Nervous System: fatigue, decreased mental status, gait disturbance.
Skin: rash.
Other: flulike syndrome, redness and tenderness at injection site, abnormal blood profiles.

Onset, Peak, and Duration

Route	Onset	Peak	Duration
Subcutaneous Injection	Unknown	≤7 hr	Unknown

Massage Considerations

- No cautions or contraindications to massage are related to the actions of this drug. In most cases, cautions and contraindications to massage may be related to the client condition.
- The physician should be consulted before any massage is given.
- The site of subcutaneous injection of the drug should not be massaged for at least 7 hours.
- Side effects of rash are a local contraindication to massage and should be reported to the physician immediately. If severe, no massage should be given.

ipratropium bromide (ip-ruh-TROH-pee-um BROH-mighd)

Atrovent

Drug Class: Anticholinergic bronchodilator

Drug Actions

Relieves bronchospasms and symptoms of seasonal allergic rhinitis

Use

- Bronchospasm caused by chronic obstructive pulmonary disease
- Rhinorrhea linked to allergic and nonallergic perennial rhinitis
- Rhinorrhea caused by the common cold
- Rhinorrhea linked to seasonal allergic rhinitis

Side Effects

Cardiovascular: palpitations.
Gastrointestinal: nausea, GI distress, dry mouth.
Nervous System: nervousness, dizziness, headache.
Skin: rash.
Other: blurred vision, nosebleeds, cough, upper respiratory tract infection, bronchitis, bronchospasm.

Onset, Peak, and Duration

Route	Onset	Peak	Duration
Inhalation	5–15 min	1–2 hr	3–6 hr

Massage Considerations

- This drug acts on receptors of the sympathetic nervous system (SNS) in the lung. Some generalized stimulation of the SNS may occur with long-term use. This may make the relaxation effects of massage and the effects of the systemic reflex strokes such as effleurage and rocking to be less effective. Applying rocking at the beginning of the session for longer periods may help the client to relax, and using slow, rhythmic effleurage throughout the session may counteract these effects.
- Other cautions and contraindications to massage may be related to the client condition.
- Side effects of dizziness require care in getting the client on and off table. Staying with the client as he or she sits up and until safety is ascertained may be necessary.
- Rash is a local contraindication to massage and should be reported to the physician. If severe, no massage should be given.

irbesartan (ir-buh-SAR-tun)

Avapro

Drug Class: Angiotensin II receptor antagonist antihypertensive

Drug Actions

Inhibits the vasoconstricting and aldosterone-secreting effects of angiotensin II and lowers blood pressure.

Use

- Hypertension
- Nephropathy in patients with type 2 diabetes

Side Effects

Cardiovascular: chest pain, edema, tachycardia.
Gastrointestinal: diarrhea, painful digestion, abdominal pain, nausea, vomiting.
Nervous System: fatigue, anxiety, dizziness, headache.
Urinary: urinary tract infection.
Skin: rash.
Other: pharyngitis, rhinitis, sinus abnormality, hyperkalemia, musculoskeletal trauma or pain, upper respiratory tract infection.

Onset, Peak, and Duration

Route	Onset	Peak	Duration
Oral	Unknown	1.5–2 hr	24 hr

 Massage Considerations

- No cautions or contraindications to massage are related to the actions of this drug. Cautions and contraindications to massage may be related to the client condition.
- Side effects of dizziness require care in getting the client on and off the table. Stimulation with rapid effleurage or tapotement at the end of the session may help.
- Rash is a local contraindication to massage and should be reported to the physician. If severe, massage should be withheld.

---

iron dextran (IGH-ern DEKS-tran)

DexFerrum, Dexiron, InFeD

Drug Class: Parenteral iron supplement

Drug Actions

Increases level of iron, an essential component of hemoglobin

Use

- Iron-deficiency anemia

Side Effects

Cardiovascular: chest pain, chest tightness, shock, hypertension, arrhythmias, hypotensive reaction, peripheral vascular flushing with overly rapid intravenous administration, tachycardia.
Gastrointestinal: nausea, vomiting, metallic taste, transient loss of taste, abdominal pain, diarrhea.
Nervous System: headache, transitory paresthesia, dizziness, malaise, syncope.
Skin: rash, hives, brown discoloration at IM injection site.
Other: soreness, inflammation, and local phlebitis at IV injection site; sterile abscess; necrosis; atrophy; fibrosis; anaphylaxis; delayed sensitivity reactions; bronchospasm; joint pain; muscle pain.

Onset, Peak, and Duration

Route	Onset	Peak	Duration
I.V., I.M.,	72 hr	Unknown	3–4 wk

 Massage Considerations

- No cautions and contraindications to massage are indicated because a client is taking this drug.
- The site of injection of the drug should not be massaged for the duration of action, which is 3 to 4 weeks.

- Side effects of dizziness require care in getting the client on and off the table. Stimulating with effleurage or tapotement at the end of the session may help.
- Paresthesia is a local contraindication to deep tissue massage.
- Rash or hives are local contraindications to massage and should be reported to the physician. If severe, no massage should be given.

---

isoniazid (isonicotinic acid hydride INH) (igh-soh-NIGH-uh-sid)

Isotamine, Laniazid, Nydrazid, PMS Isoniazid

Drug Class: Antituberculotic

Drug Actions

Kills susceptible bacteria, such as *Mycobacterium tuberculosis, Mycobacterium bovis,* and some strains of *Mycobacterium kansasii.*

Use

- Actively growing tubercle bacilli
- Prevention of tubercle bacilli in those closely exposed to tuberculosis or those with positive results on skin tests whose chest radiographs and bacteriologic studies are consistent with nonprogressive tuberculosis

Side Effects

Gastrointestinal: nausea, vomiting, epigastric distress, constipation, dry mouth.
Nervous System: peripheral neuropathy (especially in patients who are malnourished, alcoholic, diabetic, or slow acetylators), usually preceded by paresthesia of hands and feet; psychosis; seizures.
Other: rheumatic syndrome and lupuslike syndrome, hypersensitivity reactions (fever, rash, lymphadenopathy, vasculitis), irritation at I.M. injection site, abnormal blood profiles, hepatitis (occasionally severe and sometimes fatal, especially in older adult patients), hyperglycemia, metabolic acidosis.

Onset, Peak, and Duration

Route	Onset	Peak	Duration
Oral, I.M.	Unknown	1–2 hr	Unknown

 Massage Considerations

- No cautions or contraindications to massage are indicated because a client is taking this drug. Cautions and contraindications to massage may be related to the client condition.
- The site of I.M. injection of the drug should not be massaged for at least 2 hours.
- Side effects of paresthesia or peripheral neuropathy are local contraindications to deep tissue massage.
- Constipation may be helped by regular abdominal massage.

---

isoproterenol (isoprenaline) (igh-soh-proh-TEER-uh-nol)

Isuprel

isoproterenol hydrochloride
isoproterenol sulfate

Medihaler-Iso

Drug Class: Adrenergic bronchodilator, cardiac stimulant

Drug Actions

Relaxes bronchial smooth muscle by acting on β_2-adrenergic receptors. As cardiac stimulant, acts on β_1-adrenergic receptors in heart. Relieves bronchospasms and heart block and restores normal sinus rhythm after ventricular arrhythmia.

Use

- Bronchospasm
- Bronchospasm in chronic obstructive pulmonary disease
- Heart block and ventricular arrhythmias
- Shock
- Postoperative cardiac patients with bradycardia
- As an aid in diagnosing the cause of mitral regurgitation
- As an aid in diagnosing coronary artery disease or lesions

Side Effects

Cardiovascular: palpitations, tachycardia, angina, flushing of face, cardiac arrest, blood pressure that rises and then falls, arrhythmias.
Gastrointestinal: nausea, vomiting.
Nervous System: headache, mild tremor, weakness, dizziness, nervousness, insomnia, Stokes-Adams seizures.
Skin: sweating.
Other: hyperglycemia, bronchospasm.

Onset, Peak, and Duration

Route	Onset	Peak	Duration
I.V.	Immediate	Unknown	<1 hr
Inhalation	2–5 min	Unknown	0.5–2 hr

 Massage Considerations

- This drug stimulates the sympathetic nervous system (SNS) and may make systemic reflex strokes such as effleurage and rocking less effective and make it harder to achieve relaxation during the massage. Using rocking for a longer period at the beginning of the session and using slow, rhythmic effleurage throughout the session may help.
- Cautions and contraindications to massage may be related to the client condition.
- Side effects of dizziness require care in getting the client on and off the table. Stimulation with a little friction to the legs at the end of the session may help.

isosorbide dinitrate (igh-soh-SOR-bighd digh-NIGH-trayt)

Apo-ISDN, Cedocard SR, Coronex, Dilatrate-SR, Isordil, Isordil Titradose, Isotrate, Sorbitrate

isosorbide mononitrate

IMDUR, ISMO, Isotrate ER, Monoket

Drug Class: Nitrate antianginal, vasodilator

Drug Actions

Relieves angina

Use

- Acute angina
- Prophylaxis in situations likely to cause angina
- Adjunctive treatment of heart failure
- Diffuse esophageal spasm without gastroesophageal reflux

Side Effects

Cardiovascular: orthostatic hypotension, tachycardia, palpitations, ankle edema, fainting, flushing.
Gastrointestinal: nausea, vomiting.
Nervous System: headache, sometimes with throbbing; dizziness; weakness.
Skin: cutaneous vasodilation.
Other: hypersensitivity reactions, sublingual burning.

Onset, Peak, and Duration

Route	Onset	Peak	Duration
Oral	2–60 min	2–60 min	1–12 hr
Sublingual	2–5 min	2–5 min	1–2 hr

 Massage Considerations

- No cautions or contraindications to massage are indicated because a client is taking this drug. Cautions and contraindications to massage may be related to the client condition.
- Side effects of dizziness and hypotension require care in getting the client on and off the table. Stimulation with rapid effleurage and tapotement at the end of the session may help. If the symptoms are severe, more rapid and stimulating massage techniques may be needed throughout the session.

---

isotretinoin (igh-soh-TREH-tih-noyn)

Accutane, Accutane Roche, Amnesteem, Claravis, Roaccutane, Sotret

Drug Class: Antiacne drug

Drug Actions

May normalize keratinization, reversibly decrease size of sebaceous glands, and alter composition of sebum to less viscous form that is less likely to plug follicles. Improves skin integrity.

Use

- Severe recalcitrant nodular acne unresponsive to conventional therapy
- Keratinization disorders resistant to conventional therapy
- Prevention of skin cancer
- Squamous cell cancer of the head and neck

Side Effects

Cardiovascular: hypertriglyceridemia.
Gastrointestinal: nonspecific GI symptoms, gum bleeding and inflammation, nausea, vomiting, acute pancreatitis, inflammatory bowel disease.
Nervous System: headache, fatigue, depression, psychosis, suicide, depression, psychosis, aggressive and violent behavior, emotional instability, pseudotumor cerebri (benign intracranial hypertension).

Skin: cracked lips, rash, dry skin, peeling of palms and toes, skin infection, thinning of hair, photosensitivity.
Other: conjunctivitis, corneal deposits, dry eyes, visual disturbances, hearing impairment, decreased night vision, hepatitis, anemia, hyperglycemia, skeletal hyperostosis, calcification of tendons and ligaments, premature epiphyseal closure, decreases in bone mineral density, musculoskeletal symptoms (sometimes severe) including back pain and joint pain, arthritis, tendinitis, other types of bone abnormalities, rhabdomyolysis.

Onset, Peak, and Duration

Route	Onset	Peak	Duration
Oral	Unknown	3 hr	Unknown

 Massage Considerations

- No cautions or contraindications to massage are related to the actions of this drug. Cautions and contraindications to massage may be related to the client condition.
- The side effect of rash is a local contraindication to massage and should be reported to the physician immediately. If severe, massage should be withheld.
- Peeling is a local caution to massage; if the condition is severe or worsens with massage, massage may be locally contraindicated.
- Rhabdomyolysis is a serious and at times life-threatening disorder that presents as muscle pain and stiffness that worsens without cause. It should be referred to the physician for immediate evaluation and massage should be withheld until that evaluation is complete and the client is cleared by the physician.

itraconazole (ih-truh-KAHN-uh-zohl)

Sporanox

Drug Class: Antifungal

Drug Actions

Hinders fungi, including *Aspergillus* sp. and *Blastomyces dermatitidis.*

Use

- Pulmonary and extrapulmonary blastomycosis
- Histoplasmosis
- Aspergillosis
- Fungal infections of toenails with or without fingernail involvement
- Fungal infections of fingernails
- Esophageal candidiasis
- Oropharyngeal candidiasis

Side Effects

Cardiovascular: edema, hypertension, orthostatic hypotension, heart failure, hypertriglyceridemia.
Gastrointestinal: nausea, vomiting, diarrhea, abdominal pain, anorexia, painful digestion, gas, increased appetite, constipation, gastritis, gastroenteritis, ulcerative stomatitis, gingivitis.
Nervous System: malaise, fatigue, headache, dizziness, sleepiness, fever, weakness, pain, tremor, abnormal dreaming, anxiety, depression.
Urinary: albuminuria, impotence, cystitis, urinary tract infection.
Skin: rash, itching.

Other: decreased libido, injury, herpes zoster, hypersensitivity reactions (urticaria, angioedema, Stevens-Johnson syndrome), rhinitis, sinusitis, pharyngitis, neutropenia, impaired hepatic function, hepatotoxicity, liver failure (fatal), hypokalemia, muscle pain, upper respiratory tract infection, pulmonary edema.

Onset, Peak, and Duration

Route	Onset	Peak	Duration
Oral:			
Fasting	Unknown	2 hr	Unknown
Not fasting	Unknown	5 hr	Unknown
I.V.	Unknown	Unknown	Unknown

Massage Considerations

- No cautions or contraindications to massage are related to the actions of this drug. Cautions and contraindications to massage may be related to the client condition.
- Side effects of dizziness, sleepiness, or hypotension require care in getting the client on and off the table. Stimulating the client with rapid effleurage or tapotement at the end of the session may help.
- Gas or constipation may be helped by regular abdominal massage.
- Rash or itching are local contraindications to massage and should be reported to the physician immediately. If severe or widespread, massage should be withheld.

K

kaolin and pectin mixtures (KAY-oh-lin and PEK-tin MIX-cherz)

K-Pek, Kaodene Non-Narcotic, Kaolin, w/Pectin, Kao-Spen, Kapectolin

Drug Class: Antidiarrheal

Drug Actions

Decreases fluid content of feces and alleviates diarrhea

Use

- Mild, nonspecific diarrhea

Side Effects

Gastrointestinal: constipation; fecal impaction or ulceration (in infants and elderly or debilitated patients after long-term use).

Onset, Peak, and Duration

Route	Onset	Peak	Duration
Oral	Unknown	Unknown	Unknown

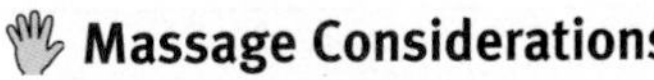

Massage Considerations

- There are no cautions or contraindications to massage related to the actions of this drug.
- There may be cautions or contraindications to massage related to the client condition.
- Because this drug is generally taken for acute episodes of diarrhea, it would be best to wait for the condition to resolve before giving massage. If the drug is being taken regularly, massage may be given. Providing quick access to the bathroom and privacy may be necessary.
- Constipation may be helped by abdominal massage.

---

ketoconazole (kee-toh-KAHN-uh-zohl)

Nizoral, Nozoral A-D

Drug Class: Antifungal

Drug Actions

Kills or hinders growth of susceptible fungi, including most pathogenic fungi

Use

- Systemic candidiasis
- Chronic mucocandidiasis
- Oral thrush
- Candiduria
- Coccidioidomycosis
- Histoplasmosis
- Chromomycosis
- Paracoccidioidomycosis
- Severe cutaneous dermatophyte infection resistant to therapy with topical or oral griseofulvin

Side Effects

Gastrointestinal: nausea, vomiting, abdominal pain, diarrhea, constipation.
Nervous System: headache, nervousness, dizziness, suicidal tendencies.
Skin: itching.
Other: abnormal growth of breast tissue with tenderness, thrombocytopenia, hepatotoxicity.

Onset, Peak, and Duration

Route	Onset	Peak	Duration
Oral	Unknown	1–2 hr	Unknown

Massage Considerations

- There are no cautions or contraindications to massage related to the action of this drug.
- There may be cautions or contraindications to massage related to the client condition or severity of infection.
- Side effects of dizziness require care in getting the client on and off the table. Using stimulation at the end of the massage with effleurage or tapotement may help.
- Constipation may be helped by regular abdominal massage. Itching is a local contraindication to massage and should be reported to the physician. If severe, massage should be withheld. Abnormal growth of breast tissue requires caution in applying massage to the chest in both women and men. If tenderness is severe, chest massage should not be done.

ketoprofen (kee-toh-PROH-fen)

Actron caplets, Apo-Keto, Apo-Keto-E, Novo-Keto-EC, Orudis, Orudis-E, Orudis KT, Orudis SR, Oruvail, Rhodis, Rhodis-EC

Drug Class: NSAID (nonsteroidal anti-inflammatory drug) nonopioid analgesic, antipyretic, anti-inflammatory

Drug Actions

May inhibit prostaglandin synthesis. Relieves pain, fever, and inflammation.

Use

- Rheumatoid arthritis
- Osteoarthritis
- Mild-to-moderate pain
- Dysmenorrhea
- Minor aches and pain
- Fever

Side Effects

Gastrointestinal: nausea, abdominal pain, diarrhea, constipation, gas, peptic ulceration, anorexia, vomiting, stomatitis.
Nervous System: headache, dizziness, CNS excitation, or depression.
Urinary: nephrotoxicity.
Skin: rash, exfoliative dermatitis, photosensitivity.
Other: ringing in the ears, visual disturbances, laryngeal edema, prolonged bleeding time, abnormal blood profiles, shortness of breath, bronchospasm.

Onset, Peak, and Duration

Route	Onset	Peak	Duration
Oral, Rectal	1–2 hr	$^1/_2$–2 hr	3–4

 Massage Considerations

- This drug may decrease the perception of pain; therefore, deep tissue massage should be used with caution. There may be other cautions or contraindications to massage related to the client condition.
- Side effects of dizziness require care in getting the client on and off the table. Rapid effleurage or tapotement at the end of the session may help. Constipation and gas may be helped by regular abdominal massage. Rash is a local contraindication to massage and should be reported to the physician. If severe, massage should not be given.

ketorolac tromethamine (KEE-toh-roh-lak troh-METH-uh-meen)

Toradol

Drug Class: NSAID (nonsteroidal anti-inflammatory drug) analgesic

Drug Actions

May inhibit prostaglandin synthesis. Relieves pain.

Use

- Short-term management of pain

Side Effects

Cardiovascular: edema, hypertension, palpitations.
Gastrointestinal: nausea, painful digestion, GI pain, diarrhea.
Nervous System: drowsiness, insomnia, syncope, dizziness, headache.
Urinary: hematuria, increased urination.
Skin: sweating.
Other: pain at injection site, purpura, eosinophilia, anemia.

Onset, Peak, and Duration

Route	Onset	Peak	Duration
Oral	30–60 min	30–60 min	6–8 hr
I.V.	Immediate	Immediate	8 hr
I.M.	≤10 min	30–60 min	6–8 hr

Massage Considerations

- This drug may decrease the perception of pain; therefore, deep tissue massage should be used with caution. There may be other cautions and contraindications to massage related to the client condition.
- The site of I.M. injection of the drug should not be massaged for at least 1 hour after the administration of the drug.
- Side effects of drowsiness and dizziness require care in getting the client on and off the table. Using stimulation at the end of the massage with rapid effleurage or tapotement may help.

---

ketotifen fumarate (kee-toe-TYE-fen FOO-muh-rayt)

Zaditor

Drug Class: Ophthalmic antihistamine

Drug Actions

Temporary prevention of eye itching

Use

- Temporary prevention of itching of eye caused by allergic conjunctivitis

Side Effects

Nervous System: headaches.
Other: conjunctival infection, rhinitis, ocular allergic reactions, burning or stinging of eyes, conjunctivitis, eye discharge, dry eyes, eye pain, eyelid disorder, itching of eyes, keratitis, lacrimation disorder, mydriasis, photophobia, ocular rash, pharyngitis, flulike syndrome.

Onset, Peak, and Duration

Route	Onset	Peak	Duration
Ophthalmic	Within minutes	Unknown	Unknown

Massage Considerations

- There are no cautions or contraindications to massage related to this drug

L

labetalol hydrochloride (lah-BAY-tuh-lol high-droh-KLOR-ighd)

Normodyne, Presolol, Trandate

Drug Class: α-Adrenergic and beta-blocker

Drug Actions

Lowers blood pressure

Use

- Hypertension
- Severe hypertension
- Hypertensive emergency

Side Effects

Cardiovascular: orthostatic hypotension, peripheral vascular disease, bradycardia, ventricular arrhythmias.
Gastrointestinal: nausea, vomiting, diarrhea.
Nervous System: vivid dreams, dizziness, fatigue, headache, transient scalp tingling.
Urinary: sexual dysfunction, urine retention.
Skin: rash.
Other: nasal stuffiness, increased airway resistance.

Onset, Peak, and Duration

Route	Onset	Peak	Duration
Oral	≤20 min	2–4 hr	8–12 hr
I.V.	2–5 min	5 min	2–4 hr

Massage Considerations

- This drug acts to block certain receptors in the sympathetic nervous system (SNS); the action of the systemic reflex strokes such as effleurage, rocking, and friction and the relaxation effects of massage may be increased as a result. Using more stimulating and rapid application of the above strokes at the end of the session may help. If the effect is severe, using stimulating massage techniques throughout the sesssion may be needed.
- Other cautions and contraindications to massage may be related to the client condition.
- Side effects of hypotension and dizziness may be addressed as shown above.
- Rash is a local contraindication to massage and should be reported to the physician immediately. If severe, massage should be withheld.

lactulose (LAK-tyoo-lohs)

Cephulac, Cholac, Chronulac, Constilac, Constulose, Duphalac, Enulose, Generlac, Kristalose, Lac-Dol

Drug Class: Laxative

Drug Actions

Produces osmotic effect in the colon. Resulting distension promotes peristalsis. Also decreases blood ammonia. Relieves constipation, decreases symptoms of hepatic encephalopathy.

Use

- Constipation
- Prevention and treatment of hepatic encephalopathy, including hepatic precoma and coma in patients with severe hepatic disease
- To induce bowel evacuation in geriatric patients with colonic retention of barium and severe constipation after a barium meal examination
- To restore bowel movements after hemorrhoidectomy

Side Effects

Gastrointestinal: abdominal cramps, belching, diarrhea, distension, gas.

Onset, Peak, and Duration

Route	Onset	Peak	Duration
Oral	24–48 hr	Varies	Varies
Rectal	Unknown	Unknown	Unknown

 Massage Considerations

- No cautions or contraindications to massage are related to the actions of this drug. Cautions and contraindications to massage may be related to the client condition.
- Rectal administration of the drug may give quick results; therefore, it would be best to give massage before the administration of the drug.
- Side effects of gas may be helped by abdominal massage, but because this may increase the evacuation of the bowel, it should be done with caution. Quick access to the bathroom and privacy should be provided.

lamivudine (la-MI-vyoo-deen)

Epivir, Epivir-HBV

Drug Class: Antiviral

Drug Actions

Reduces the symptoms of HIV and hepatitis B virus (HBV) infection

Use

- HIV infection (with other antiretrovirals)
- Chronic hepatitis B with evidence of HBV replication and active liver inflammation

Side Effects

Gastrointestinal: nausea, diarrhea, vomiting, anorexia, abdominal pain, abdominal cramps, painful digestion, pancreatitis, hepatomegaly (children).
Nervous System: fever, headache, fatigue, neuropathy, malaise, dizziness, insomnia, sleep disorders, depressive disorders, malaise.
Skin: rash.
Other: chills; abnormal blood profiles; lymphadenopathy (in children); nasal symptoms; musculoskeletal pain; muscle pain; joint pain; cough; ear, nose, and throat infections; sore throat.

Onset, Peak, and Duration

Route	Onset	Peak	Duration
Oral	Unknown	1–3 hr	Unknown

Massage Considerations

- No cautions or contraindications to massage are related to the actions of this drug. Cautions and contraindications to massage may be related to the client condition.
- Side effects of dizziness require care in getting the client on and off the table. Using stimulation at the end of the session with friction, effleurage, or tapotement may help.
- Neuropathy is a local contraindication to deep tissue massage. If severe, no deep tissue massage should be given.
- Rash is a local contraindication to massage and should be reported to the physician immediately. If severe or widespread, no massage should be given.

lamivudine and zidovudine (la-MI-vyoo-deen and zye-DOE-vyoo-deen)

Combivir

Drug Class: Antiretroviral

Drug Actions

Reduces the symptoms of HIV infection

Use

- HIV infection

Side Effects

Gastrointestinal: nausea, diarrhea, vomiting, anorexia, abdominal pain, abdominal cramps, painful digestion.
Nervous System: fever, headache, malaise, fatigue, insomnia, dizziness, neuropathy, depression.
Skin: rash.
Other: chills, nasal signs and symptoms, neutropenia, severe anemia, musculoskeletal pain, muscle pain, joint pain, cough.

Onset, Peak, and Duration

Route	Onset	Peak	Duration
Oral	Unknown	Unknown	Unknown

Massage Considerations

- No cautions or contraindications to massage are related to the actions of this drug. Cautions and contraindications to massage may be related to the client condition.
- Side effects of dizziness require care in getting the client on and off the table. Using stimulation at the end of the session with friction, effleurage, or tapotement may help.
- Neuropathy is a local contraindication to deep tissue massage. If severe or widespread, no deep tissue massage should be given.
- Rash is a local contraindication to massage and should be reported to the physician immediately. If severe, no massage should be given.

lamotrigine (lah-MOH-trigh-jeen)

Lamictal

Drug Class: Anticonvulsant

Drug Actions

Prevents partial seizure activity

Use

- Adjunct therapy for partial seizures caused by epilepsy
- Generalized seizures of Lennox-Gastaut syndrome
- To convert patients from monotherapy with a hepatic enzyme-inducing anticonvulsant drug to lamotrigine therapy

Side Effects

Cardiovascular: palpitations.
Gastrointestinal: nausea, vomiting, diarrhea, painful digestion, abdominal pain, constipation, anorexia, dry mouth.
Nervous System: fever, dizziness, headache, ataxia, sleepiness, incoordination, insomnia, tremor, depression, anxiety, seizures, irritability, speech disorder, decreased memory, aggravated reaction, concentration disturbance, sleep disorder, emotional lability, malaise, mind racing, suicide attempts.
Skin: Stevens-Johnson syndrome, toxic epidermal necrolysis, rash, itching, hair loss, acne.
Other: hot flushes, flulike syndrome, infection, chills, tooth disorder, painful joints, muscle spasm, neck pain, double vision, blurred vision, vision abnormality, nystagmus, rhinitis, pharyngitis, dysmenorrhea, vaginitis, amenorrhea, cough, shortness of breath.

Onset, Peak, and Duration

Route	Onset	Peak	Duration
Oral	Unknown	1.5–4 .75 hr	Unknown

 Massage Considerations

- The action of this drug may decrease the transmission of nerve impulses. The local reflex strokes of compression, vibration, stretching, and friction may be less effective or may require a longer application to be effective. Also, deep tissue massage should be used with caution.
- Further cautions and contraindications to massage may be related to the client condition.
- Side effects of dizziness and sleepiness require care in getting the client on and off the table. Stimulation with rapid effleurage at the end of the session may help.
- Constipation may be helped by abdominal massage.
- Rash, itching, or acne are local contraindications to massage and should be reported to the physician immediately. If severe, massage should be withheld. If the client has to continue taking the drug and acne is a concern, massage may be given if the massage therapist wears gloves to protect against contact with blood and body fluids.
- Hair loss is a contraindication to scalp massage if the client is disturbed by hair loss during the massage or the scalp is tender.

lansoprazole (lan-soh-PRAY-zohl)

Prevacid, Prevacid SoluTab

Drug Class: Antiulcer drug

Drug Actions

Decreases gastric acid formation

Use

- Short-term therapy for active duodenal ulcer
- Maintenance of healed duodenal ulcers
- Short-term therapy for erosive esophagitis
- Short-term therapy for active benign gastric ulcer
- *Helicobacter pylori* eradication to reduce risk of duodenal ulcer recurrence
- Long-term therapy for pathologic hypersecretory conditions, including Zollinger-Ellison syndrome
- Short-term therapy for symptomatic gastroesophageal reflux disease
- Nonsteroidal anti-inflammatory drug (NSAID)-related ulcer in patients who are continuing treatment with NSAIDs
- To reduce risk of NSAID-related ulcer in patients with a history of gastric ulcer who need NSAIDs

Side Effects

Gastrointestinal: diarrhea, nausea, abdominal pain.

Onset, Peak, and Duration

Route	Onset	Peak	Duration
Oral	Unknown	2 hr	>24 hr

 **Massage Considerations**

- No cautions or contraindications to massage are indicated because a client is taking this drug.

---

leflunomide (leh-FLOO-noh-mighd)

Arava

Drug Class: Immunomodulator

Drug Actions

Reduces pain and inflammation related to rheumatoid arthritis

Use

- Active rheumatoid arthritis

Side Effects

Cardiovascular: angina pectoris, hypertension, chest pain, peripheral edema, palpitations, tachycardia, vasculitis, vasodilation, varicose veins.
Gastrointestinal: mouth ulcer, oral candidiasis, stomatitis, dry mouth, anorexia, diarrhea, painful digestion, gastroenteritis, nausea, abdominal pain, vomiting, cholelithiasis, colitis, constipation, esophagitis, gas, gastritis, melena, gingivitis, taste perversion.
Nervous System: weakness, dizziness, fever, headache, paresthesia, malaise, migraine, sleep disorder, neuritis, anxiety, depression, insomnia, neuralgia.
Urinary: urinary tract infection, albuminuria, cystitis, painful urination, hematuria, menstrual disorder, pelvic pain, vaginal candidiasis, prostate disorder, urinary frequency.
Skin: hair loss, itching, rash, dry skin, acne, eczema, contact dermatitis, fungal dermatitis, hair discoloration, hematoma, nail disorder, skin nodule, subcutaneous nodule, maculopapular rash, skin disorder, skin discoloration, skin ulcer, increased sweating, bruising.

Other: allergic reaction, flulike syndrome, injury or accident, pain, abscess, cyst, hernia, tooth disorder, herpes simplex, herpes zoster, pharyngitis, rhinitis, sinusitis, nosebleeds, enlarged salivary gland, blurred vision, cataracts, conjunctivitis, eye disorders, anemia, hyperlipidemia, weight loss, diabetes mellitus, hyperglycemia, hyperthyroidism, hypokalemia, arthrosis, back pain, bursitis, muscle cramps, muscle pain, bone necrosis, bone pain, joint pain, leg cramps, joint disorder, neck pain, synovitis, tendon rupture, tenosynovitis, bronchitis, increased cough, pneumonia, respiratory infection, asthma, shortness of breath, lung disorders.

Onset, Peak, and Duration

Route	Onset	Peak	Duration
Oral	Unknown	6–12 hr	Unknown

Massage Considerations

- No cautions or contraindications to massage are related to the actions of this drug. Cautions or contraindications to massage may be related to the client condition.
- Side effects of dizziness require care in getting the client on and off the table. Using stimulation with rapid effleurage or tapotement at the end of the session may help.
- Paresthesia, neuritis, and neuralgia are local contraindications to deep tissue massage. If severe or widespread, they may contraindicate massage completely.
- Constipation and gas may be helped by abdominal massage.
- Rash or itching are local contraindications to massage and should be reported to the physician immediately. If severe or widespread, massage should be withheld.
- Hair loss is a contraindication to scalp massage if the client is disturbed by hair loss during the massage or the scalp is tender.

leucovorin calcium (citrovorum factor, folinic acid)

(loo-kah-VOR-in KAL-see-um)

Drug Class: Vitamin, antidote

Drug Actions

Raises folic acid level

Use

- Overdose of folic acid antagonist
- Rescue after high methotrexate dose given as cancer therapy
- Megaloblastic anemia caused by congenital enzyme deficiency
- Folate-deficient megaloblastic anemia
- Hematologic toxicity caused by pyrimethamine or trimethoprim therapy
- Palliative treatment of advanced colorectal carcinoma

Side Effects

Skin: hypersensitivity reactions (rash, itching, redness).
Other: bronchospasm.

Onset, Peak, and Duration

Route	Onset	Peak	Duration
Oral	20–30 min	2–3 hr	3–6 hr
I.V.	5 min	10 min	3–6 hr
I.M.	10–20 min	<1 hr	3–6 hr

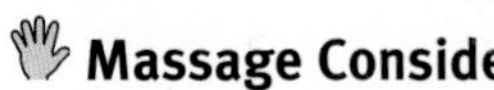

Massage Considerations

- No cautions or contraindications to massage are related to the actions of this drug. Cautions and contraindications to massage may be related to the client condition.
- The site of intramuscular (I.M.) injection of the drug should not be massaged for at least an hour to avoid increasing the rate of absorption of the drug.
- Side effects of rash, itching, or redness from hypersensitivity reactions are local contraindications to massage and should be reported to the physician immediately. In many cases, these reactions will be a complete contraindication to massage until the reactions have cleared.

---

leuprolide acetate (loo-PROH-lighd AS-ih-tayt)

Eligard, Lucrin, Lupron, Lupron Depot, Lupron Depot-Ped, Lupron Depot-3 Month, Lupron Depot-4 Month, Lupron for Pediatric Use

Drug Class: Antineoplastic, luteinizing hormone–releasing hormone analog

Drug Actions

Initially stimulates but then inhibits release of follicle-stimulating hormone and luteinizing hormone, resulting in testosterone suppression. Hinders prostatic cancer cell growth and eases signs and symptoms of endometriosis.

Use

- Advanced prostate cancer
- Endometriosis
- Central precocious puberty

Side Effects

Cardiovascular: arrhythmias, angina, heart attack, peripheral edema.
Gastrointestinal: nausea, vomiting.
Nervous System: dizziness, depression, headache.
Skin: skin reactions at injection site.
Other: hot flushes, decreased libido, abnormal growth of breast tissue, transient bone pain (during first week of treatment), impotence, pulmonary embolism.

Onset, Peak, and Duration

Route	Onset	Peak	Duration
I.M., Subcutaneous injection	Unknown	1–2 mo	1–3 mo

Massage Considerations

- No cautions or contraindications to massage are related to the actions of this drug Cautions and contraindications to massage may be related to the client condition.
- Because this is a long-acting, slowly absorbed drug, the site of I.M. or subcutaneous injection should not be massaged for at least 24 hours for daily injections and for the long-acting Depot forms for at least 1 month.
- Side effects of dizziness require care in getting the client on and off the table. Using rapid effleurage or tapotement at the end of the session may help.
- Abnormal growth of breast tissue in either men or women requires caution in chest massage. If very tender, no massage of the chest should be done.

levalbuterol hydrochloride (leev-al-BYOO-teh-rohl high-droh-KLOR-ighd)

Xopenex

Drug Class: β_2-Agonist bronchodilator

Drug Actions

Activates β_2 receptors on airway smooth muscle, which causes smooth muscle from the trachea to terminal bronchioles to relax, thereby relieving bronchospasm and reducing airway resistance. Also inhibits the release of mediators from mast cells in the airway.

Use

- To prevent or treat bronchospasm in patients with reversible obstructive airway disease

Side Effects

Cardiovascular: tachycardia.
Gastrointestinal: painful digestion.
Nervous System: dizziness, migraine, nervousness, tremor, anxiety, pain.
Other: flulike syndrome, accidental injury, viral infection, rhinitis, sinusitis, turbinate edema, leg cramps, increased cough.

Onset, Peak, and Duration

Route	Onset	Peak	Duration
Inhalation	10–17 min	90 min	5–8 hr

Massage Considerations

- This drug stimulates certain receptors of the sympathetic nervous system (SNS), and though taken by inhalation, there may be some systemic effects. This may make the systemic reflex strokes of effleurage, rocking, and friction less effective and the relaxation effects of massage a little more difficult to achieve. Applying rocking or friction at the muscle attachments for a longer period of time and using slow, rhythmic effleurage throughout the session may help to achieve the desired results.
- Cautions and contraindications to massage may be related to the client condition.
- Side effects of dizziness require care in getting the client on and off the table. Using tapotement at the end of the session may help.

levetiracetam (leev-ah-tah-RACE-ah-tam)

Keppra

Drug Class: Anticonvulsant

Drug Actions

Prevents seizure activity

Use

- Adjunctive therapy for partial seizures

Side Effects

Gastrointestinal: anorexia.
Nervous System: weakness, headache, sleepiness, dizziness, depression, paresthesia, nervousness, hostility, emotional lability, ataxia, amnesia, anxiety.

Other: infection, double vision, pharyngitis, rhinitis, sinusitis, leukopenia, neutropenia, muscukoskeletal pain, cough.

Onset, Peak, and Duration

Route	Onset	Peak	Duration
Oral	1 hr	1 hr	12 hr

 Massage Considerations

- The action of this drug decreases the transmission of nerve impulses. This may potentially decrease the effectiveness of the local reflex strokes of compression, stretching, and vibration as well as decreasing the effectiveness of deep tissue massage. Deep tissue massage should be used with caution. Applying the local reflex strokes for a longer period of time may counteract this effect, or the mechanical strokes of effleurage and pétrissage may be more effective. Tapotement, which stimulates the central nervous system (CNS), should be used with caution.
- Side effects of sleepiness and dizziness require care in getting the client on and off the table. Using rapid effleurage at the end of the session may help.
- Paresthesia is a local contraindication to deep tissue massage.

---

levodopa (lee-voh-DOH-puh)

Dopar, Larodopa

Drug Class: Precursor of dopamine antiparkinsonian

Drug Actions

Relieves signs and symptoms of parkinsonism.

Use

- Idiopathic parkinsonism
- Postencephalitic parkinsonism
- Symptomatic parkinsonism after carbon monoxide or manganese intoxication or with cerebral arteriosclerosis

Side Effects

Cardiovascular: orthostatic hypotension, cardiac irregularities, flushing, hypertension, phlebitis.
Gastrointestinal: dry mouth, excessive salivation, bitter taste, nausea, vomiting, anorexia, constipation, gas, diarrhea, epigastric pain.
Nervous System: aggressive behavior, abnormal movements (choreiform, dystonic, dyskinetic), involuntary grimacing and head movements, myoclonic body jerks, seizures, ataxia, tremor, muscle twitching, bradykinetic episodes, psychiatric disturbance, memory loss, mood changes, nervousness, anxiety, disturbing dreams, euphoria, malaise, fatigue, severe depression, suicidal tendencies, dementia, delirium, hallucinations.
Urinary: urinary frequency, urine retention, incontinence, darkened urine, priapism.
Other: dark perspiration, excessive and inappropriate sexual behavior, hemolytic anemia, leukopenia, agranulocytosis, hepatotoxicity, weight loss, hyperventilation, hiccups, blepharospasm, blurred vision, double vision, dilated pupils or abnormal constriction of the pupils, widening of palpebral fissures, activation of latent Horner syndrome, oculogyric crises, nasal discharge.

Onset, Peak, and Duration

Route	Onset	Peak	Duration
Oral	Unknown	1–3 hr	About 5 hr but varies greatly

 Massage Considerations

- No cautions or contraindications to massage are indicated because a client is taking this drug. In almost all cases, cautions and contraindications to massage will be related to the client condition.
- Side effects of hypotension require care in getting the client on and off the table. Using rapid effleurage at the end of the session may help.
- Constipation and gas may be helped by regular abdominal massage.
- Urinary frequency may require that the client get up in the middle of the session. Providing privacy and quick access to the bathroom is needed. Water fountains or water music, which could stimulate the urge to urinate, should be avoided.

levofloxacin (lee-voe-FLOX-a-sin)

Levaquin

Drug Class: Broad-spectrum antibacterial

Drug Actions

Kills susceptible bacteria

Use

- Acute maxillary sinusitis caused by susceptible bacteria
- Acute bacterial exacerbation of chronic bronchitis
- Community-acquired pneumonia
- Mild to moderate skin and skin-structure infections
- Mild to moderate uncomplicated urinary tract infections
- Mild to moderate acute pyelonephritis
- Complicated skin and skin-structure infections
- Chronic bacterial prostatitis
- Traveler's diarrhea
- Prevention of traveler's diarrhea
- Uncomplicated cervical, urethral, or rectal gonorrhea
- Disseminated gonococcal infection
- Nongonococcal urethritis
- Urogenital chlamydial infections
- Acute pelvic inflammatory disease

Side Effects

Cardiovascular: chest pain, palpitations, vasodilation, abnormal electrocardiogram (ECG).
Gastrointestinal: nausea, diarrhea, constipation, vomiting, abdominal pain, painful digestion, gas, pseudomembranous colitis.
Nervous System: headache, insomnia, dizziness, encephalopathy, paresthesia, pain, seizures.
Skin: rash, photosensitivity reactions, itching, erythema multiforme, Stevens-Johnson syndrome.
Other: hypersensitivity reactions, anaphylaxis, multisystem organ failure, eosinophilia, hemolytic anemia, lymphocytopenia, vaginitis, hypoglycemia, back pain, tendon rupture, allergic pneumonitis.

Onset, Peak, and Duration

Route	Onset	Peak	Duration
Oral, I.V.	Unknown	1–2 hr	Unknown

Massage Considerations

- No cautions or contraindications to massage are related to the actions of this drug. Cautions and contraindications to massage may be related to the client condition or the severity of the infection.
- Side effects of dizziness require care in getting the client on and off the table. Stimulating the client at the end of the session with effleurage or tapotement may help.
- Paresthesia is a local contraindication to deep tissue massage.
- Constipation and gas may be helped by abdominal massage.
- Rash is a local contraindication to massage and should be reported to the physician immediately. If severe or widespread, massage should be withheld.

---

levothyroxine sodium (T4, L-thyroxine sodium) (lee-voh-thigh-ROKS-een SOH-dee-um)

Eltroxin, Levo-T, Levothroid, Levoxine, Levoxyl, Novothyrox, Oroxine, Synthroid, ThryroTabs, Unithroid

Drug Class: Thyroid hormone replacement

Drug Actions

Raises thyroid hormone levels in body

Use

- Congenital hypothyroidism
- Myxedema coma
- Hypothyroidism
- Thyroid hormone replacement

Side Effects

Cardiovascular: tachycardia, palpitations, arrhythmias, angina pectoris, hypertension, cardiac arrest.
Gastrointestinal: appetite change, nausea, diarrhea.
Nervous System: fever, headache, nervousness, insomnia, tremor.
Skin: sweating.
Other: heat intolerance, menstrual irregularities, weight loss, leg cramps.

Onset, Peak, and Duration

Route	Onset	Peak	Duration
Oral, I.V., I.M.	24 hr	Unknown	Unknown

Massage Considerations

- No cautions or contraindications to massage are related to the actions of this drug. Cautions and contraindications to massage may be related to the client condition.
- The site of I.M. injection of the drug should not be massaged for 24 hours.

linezolid (linn-AYE-zoe-lid)

Zyvox

Drug Class: Antibiotic

Drug Actions

Hinders or kills susceptible bacteria

Use

- Vancomycin-resistant *Enterococcus faecium* infections, including those with concurrent bacteremia
- Nosocomial pneumonia
- Complicated skin and skin-structure infections, including diabetic foot infections without osteomyelitis
- Uncomplicated skin and skin-structure infections

Side Effects

Gastrointestinal: diarrhea, nausea, constipation, vomiting, altered taste, tongue discoloration, oral candidiasis, pseudomembranous colitis.
Nervous System: headache, insomnia, dizziness, fever.
Skin: rash.
Other: fungal infection, vaginal candidiasis, abnormal blood profiles.

Onset, Peak, and Duration

Route	Onset	Peak	Duration
Oral:			
Tablet	Unknown	1 hr	4.75–5.5 hr
Suspension	Unknown	1 hr	4.5 hr
I.V.	Unknown	0.5 hr	4.75 hr

 Massage Considerations

- No cautions or contraindications to massage are indicated because a client is taking this drug. Cautions and contraindications to massage may be related to the client condition and severity of infection.
- Side effects of dizziness require care in getting the client on and off the table. Stimulation with rapid effleurage or tapotement at the end of the session may help.
- Constipation may be helped by abdominal massage.
- Rash is a local contraindication to massage and should be reported to the physician immediately. If severe or widespread, massage should be withheld.

liothyronine sodium (T_3) (lee-oh-THIGH-roh-neen SOH-dee-um)

Cytomel, Tertroxin, Triostat

Drug Class: Thyroid hormone replacement

Drug Actions

Raises thyroid hormone levels in body

Use

- Congenital hypothyroidism
- Myxedema
- Myxedema coma, precoma
- Nontoxic goiter
- Thyroid hormone replacement
- T_3 suppression test to differentiate hyperthyroidism from euthyroidism

Side Effects

Cardiovascular: tachycardia, arrhythmias, angina, hypertension, cardiac arrest.
Gastrointestinal: diarrhea, abdominal cramps, vomiting.
Nervous System: irritability, nervousness, insomnia, tremor, headache.
Skin: sweating.
Other: heat intolerance, menstrual irregularities, weight loss, accelerated bone maturation in infants and children.

Onset, Peak, and Duration

Route	Onset	Peak	Duration
Oral	Unknown	2–3 days	3 days
I.V.	Unknown	Unknown	Unknown

Massage Considerations

- No cautions or contraindications to massage are indicated because a client is taking this drug. Cautions and contraindications to massage may be related to the client condition.

lisinopril (ligh-SIN-uh-pril)

Prinivil, Zestril

Drug Class: Angiotensin-converting enzyme (ACE) inhibitor antihypertensive

Drug Actions

Lowers blood pressure

Use

- Hypertension
- Adjunct therapy in heart failure (with diuretics and digoxin)
- Hemodynamically stable patients within 24 hours of acute heart attack to improve survival

Side Effects

Cardiovascular: hypotension, orthostatic hypotension, chest pain.
Gastrointestinal: diarrhea, nausea, painful digestion, painful swallowing.
Nervous System: dizziness, headache, fatigue, depression, sleepiness, paresthesia.
Skin: rash.
Other: angioedema; anaphylaxis; decreased libido; nasal congestion; impotence; hyperkalemia; muscle cramps; dry, persistent, tickling, nonproductive cough.

Onset, Peak, and Duration

Route	Onset	Peak	Duration
Oral	1 hr	7 hr	24 hr

Massage Considerations

- No cautions or contraindications to massage are indicated because a client is taking this drug. Cautions and contraindications to massage may be related to the client condition.
- Side effects of hypotension, dizziness, and sleepiness require care in getting the client on and off the table. Using stimulation with rapid effleurage and tapotement at the end of the session may help.
- Paresthesia is a local contraindication to deep tissue massage.
- Rash is a local contraindication to massage and should be reported to the physician. If severe, no massage should be given.

---

lithium carbonate (LITH-ee-um KAR-buh-nayt)

lithium carbonate

Carbolith, Duralith, Eskalith, Eskalith CR, Lithane, Lithicarb, Lithizine, Lithobid, Lithonate, Lithotabs

lithium citrate

Lithium Citrate Syrup

Drug Class: Antimanic

Drug Actions

Prevents or controls mania

Use

- Prevention or control of mania
- Major depression
- Schizoaffective disorder
- Schizophrenic disorder
- Alcohol dependence
- Apparent mixed bipolar disorder in children
- Chemotherapy-induced neutropenia in children and patients with AIDS who are receiving zidovudine

Side Effects

Cardiovascular: reversible ECG changes, arrhythmias, hypotension, ankle and wrist edema.
Gastrointestinal: dry mouth, metallic taste, nausea, vomiting, anorexia, diarrhea, thirst, abdominal pain, gas, indigestion.
Nervous System: tremor, drowsiness, headache, confusion, restlessness, dizziness, psychomotor retardation, stupor, lethargy, coma, syncope, epileptiform seizures, electroencephalogram changes, worsened organic mental syndrome, impaired speech, ataxia, weakness, incoordination.
Urinary: frequent urination, glycosuria, renal toxicity with long-term use, albuminuria.
Skin: itching, rash, diminished or absent sensation, drying and thinning of hair, psoriasis, acne, hair loss.
Other: ringing in the ears, blurred vision, leukocytosis, transient hyperglycemia, goiter, hypothyroidism, hyponatremia.

Onset, Peak, and Duration

Route	Onset	Peak	Duration
Oral	1–3 wk	30 min–3 hr	Unknown

Massage Considerations

- This drug may decrease the perception of pain; therefore, deep tissue massage should be done with great caution, if at all. Local reflex strokes such as traction, stretching, vibration, and compression as well as deep tissue massage may be less effective. They may require longer periods of application to achieve the desired results.
- This drug is extremely toxic and difficult to adjust in dosage. It is used for very serious illness. The physician should be consulted before any massage is given, and close, ongoing collaboration is essential.
- Side effects of drowsiness and dizziness require care in getting the client on and off the table. Using stimulation with effleurage and tapotement at the end of the session may help. If symptoms are severe, more stimulating massage techniques throughout the session may be used.
- Gas may be helped by regular abdominal massage.
- Frequent urination may require the client to get up in the middle of the session. Providing privacy and quick access to the bathroom is essential. Water fountains and water music, which may stimulate the urge to urinate, should be avoided.
- Itching, rash, and acne are local contraindications to massage and should be reported to the physician immediately. If severe or widespread, massage should be withheld. If the client has to continue taking the medication and acne is a problem, massage may be given if the massage therapist wears gloves.
- Diminished or absent sensation is a contraindication to deep tissue massage.
- Hair loss is a contraindication to scalp massage if the client is disturbed by hair loss during the massage or if the scalp is tender.
- The best strokes for this client will be the mechanical strokes of friction, effleurage, and pétrissage. Myofascial massage techniques may also be used.

---

lomustine (CCNU) (loh-MUH-steen)

CeeNU

Drug Class: Antineoplastic

Drug Actions

Kills selected cancer cells

Use

- Brain tumor
- Hodgkin's disease
- Lymphomas

Side Effects

Gastrointestinal: nausea, vomiting (beginning within 4 to 5 hours), stomatitis.
Urinary: nephrotoxicity, progressive azotemia, renal impairment.
Other: secondary malignant disease, anemia, abnormal blood profiles, hepatotoxicity, pulmonary fibrosis.

Onset, Peak, and Duration

Route	Onset	Peak	Duration
Oral	Unknown	Unknown	Unknown

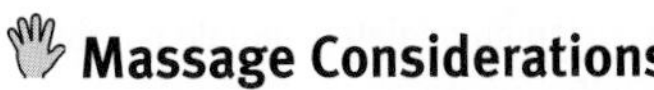

Massage Considerations

- Because of the toxic effects of this drug, deep tissue massage is contraindicated. Circulatory massage with effleurage should be used with caution and limited.
- Further cautions and contraindications to massage may be related to the client condition.
- The physician should be consulted before any massage is given, and close collaboration is essential.
- Because this drug is usually given every 4 to 6 weeks and has a half-life of 1 to 2 days, it would be best to give massage on the weeks when the drug is not being given. At a minimum, massage should not be given for at least 48 hours after administration of the drug so as not to overtax the liver and kidneys as they try to rid the body of the drug.
- The best strokes to use with this client are the systemic reflex and local reflex strokes of rocking, gentle friction, gentle compression, stretching, and vibration. Pétrissage may be used, and myofascial massage techniques may help with areas of tightness and gluteation.

---

loperamide (loh-PEH-ruh-mighd)

Imodium, Imodium A-D, Kaopectate II Caplets, Maalox Anti-Diarrheal Caplets, Neo-Diaral, Pepto Diarrhea Control

Drug Class: Antidiarrheal

Drug Actions

Inhibits peristaltic activity, prolonging transit of intestinal contents and relieving diarrhea.

Use

- Acute diarrhea
- Chronic diarrhea
- Acute diarrhea including traveler's diarrhea

Side Effects

Gastrointestinal: dry mouth; abdominal pain, distension, or discomfort; constipation; nausea; vomiting.
Nervous System: drowsiness, fatigue, dizziness.
Skin: rash.
Other: hypersensitivity reactions.

Onset, Peak, and Duration

Route	Onset	Peak	Duration
Oral	Unknown	2.5–5 hr	24 hr

Massage Considerations

- No cautions and contraindications to massage are related to the actions of this drug. Cautions and contraindications to massage may be related to the client condition. If the diarrhea is acute, it would be best to wait for it to resolve before giving massage.
- Side effects of drowsiness or dizziness require care in getting the client on and off the table. Stimulation with rapid effleurage or tapotement at the end of the session may help.
- Constipation may be helped by abdominal massage, but this should be done with caution because of the reason the drug is being taken. If no bowel movement has occurred and

pain, tenderness, or nausea is present, refer to the physician immediately and do not do massage, because this may be a sign of bowel obstruction.
- Rash is a local contraindication to massage and should be reported to the physician. If severe, massage should be withheld.

---

lopinavir and ritonavir (loe-PIN-a-veer and rih-TOH-nuh-veer)

Kaletra

Drug Class: Antiviral

Drug Actions

Inhibits the HIV protease, resulting in the production of immature, noninfectious viral particles.

Use

- HIV infection (with other antiretrovirals)

Side Effects

Cardiovascular: chest pain, deep vein thrombosis, hypertension, palpitations, peripheral edema, thrombophlebitis, vasculitis, facial edema, edema.
Gastrointestinal: abdominal pain, abnormal stools, diarrhea, nausea, vomiting, anorexia, cholecystitis, constipation, dry mouth, dyspepsia, dysphagia, enterocolitis, belching, taste perversion, esophagitis, fecal incontinence, gas, gastritis, gastroenteritis, gastrointestinal disorder, hemorrhagic colitis, increased appetite, pancreatitis, inflamed salivary glands, stomatitis, ulcerative stomatitis.
Nervous System: pain, weakness, headache, fever, insomnia, malaise, abnormal dreams, agitation, amnesia, anxiety, ataxia, confusion, depression, dizziness, dyskinesia, emotional lability, encephalopathy, hypertonia, nervousness, neuropathy, paresthesia, peripheral neuritis, sleepiness, abnormal thinking, tremor.
Urinary: abnormal ejaculation, hypogonadism, renal calculus, urine abnormality.
Skin: rash, acne, hair loss, dry skin, exfoliative dermatitis, furunculosis, nail disorder, itching, benign skin neoplasm, skin discoloration, sweating.
Other: chills, flulike syndrome, viral infection, abnormal growth of breast tissue, decreased libido, sinusitis, abnormal vision, eye disorder, otitis media, ringing in the ears, anemia, abnormal blood profiles, hyperbilirubinemia in children, Cushing syndrome, hypothyroidism, dehydration, decreased glucose tolerance, lactic acidosis, weight loss, hyperglycemia, hyperuricemia, hypercholesterolemia, hyponatremia in children, back pain, joint pain, arthrosis, muscle pain, bronchitis, shortness of breath, lung edema.

Onset, Peak, and Duration

Route	Onset	Peak	Duration
Oral	Unknown	4 hr	6 hr

 Massage Considerations

- No cautions or contraindications to massage are related to the actions of this drug. Cautions and contraindications to massage may be related to the client condition.
- Side effects of deep vein thrombosis or thrombophlebitis are a complete contraindication to massage.
- Dizziness and sleepiness require care in getting the client on and off the table. Stimulation with effleurage or tapotement at the end of the session may help.

- Paresthesia, peripheral neuritis, or neuropathy are local contraindications to deep tissue massage. If severe or widespread, no deep tissue massage should be given.
- Gas may be helped by abdominal massage.
- Rash, itching, or acne are local contraindications to massage and should be reported to the physician immediately. If severe or widespread, no massage should be given. If the client's acne is severe and the client desires massage, the therapist should wear gloves to massage the affected areas.
- Hair loss is a contraindication to scalp massage if the client is disturbed by hair loss during the massage or the scalp is tender.

---

loracarbef (loh-ruh-KAR-bef)

Lorabid

Drug Class: Antibiotic

Drug Actions

Kills susceptible bacteria

Use

- Secondary bacterial infections of acute bronchitis
- Acute bacterial exacerbations of chronic bronchitis
- Pneumonia
- Pharyngitis
- Sinusitis
- Tonsillitis
- Acute otitis media
- Uncomplicated skin and skin-structure infections
- Impetigo
- Uncomplicated cystitis
- Uncomplicated pyelonephritis

Side Effects

Cardiovascular: vasodilation.
Gastrointestinal: diarrhea, nausea, vomiting, abdominal pain, anorexia, pseudomembranous colitis.
Nervous System: headache, sleepiness, nervousness, insomnia, dizziness.
Skin: rash, hives, itching, erythema multiforme.
Other: hypersensitivity reactions, anaphylaxis, vaginal candidiasis, transient thrombocytopenia, leukopenia, eosinophilia.

Onset, Peak, and Duration

Route	Onset	Peak	Duration
Oral	Unknown	30–60 min	Unknown

 Massage Considerations

- No cautions or contraindications to massage are indicated because a client is taking this drug. Cautions or contraindications to massage may be related to the client condition and severity of infection.
- Side effects of sleepiness or dizziness require care in getting the client on and off the table. Using stimulation with effleurage or tapotement at the end of the session may help.

- Rash, itching, or hives are local contraindications to massage and should be reported to the physician immediately. If severe or widespread, massage should be withheld.

loratadine (loo-RAH-tuh-deen)

Alavert, Claratyne, Claritin, Claritin RediTabs, Claritin Syrup, Claritin-D 12-hour, Claritin-D 24 Hour, Tavist ND Allergy

Drug Class: Antihistamine

Drug Actions

Blocks effects of histamine at H_1-receptor sites. Drug's chemical structure prevents entry into CNS, preventing sedation. Relieves allergy symptoms.

Use

- Allergic rhinitis
- Chronic idiopathic hives

Side Effects

Gastrointestinal: dry mouth.
Nervous System: headache, drowsiness, fatigue, insomnia, nervousness.

Onset, Peak, and Duration

Route	Onset	Peak	Duration
Oral	1 hr	4–6 hr	24 hr

 Massage Considerations

- No cautions or contraindications to massage are indicated because a client is taking this drug. Cautions and contraindications to massage may be related to the client condition.
- Side effects of drowsiness require care in getting the client on and off the table. Using stimulation with effleurage and tapotement at the end of the session may help.

lorazepam (loo-RAZ-eh-pam)

Apo-Lorazepam, Ativan, Lorazepam Intensol, Novo-Lorazem, Nu-Loraz

Drug Class: Benzodiazepine anxiolytic, sedative-hypnotic

Drug Actions

Relieves anxiety and promotes calmness and sleep

Use

- Anxiety
- Insomnia caused by anxiety
- Premedication before operative procedure
- Nausea and vomiting caused by emetogenic cancer chemotherapy
- Status epilepticus

Side Effects

Cardiovascular: transient hypotension.
Gastrointestinal: dry mouth, abdominal discomfort.
Nervous System: drowsiness, lethargy, hangover, fainting, anterograde amnesia, restlessness, psychosis.

Urinary: incontinence, urine retention.
Other: acute withdrawal syndrome (after suddenly stopping drug in physically dependent patients), visual disturbances.

Onset, Peak, and Duration

Route	Onset	Peak	Duration
Oral	1 hr	2 hr	12–24 hr
I.V.	1–5 min	1–1.5 hr	6–8 hr
I.M.	15–30 min	1–1.5 hr	6–8 hr

 Massage Considerations

- This drug depresses the CNS; therefore, deep tissue massage should be used with great caution. The local reflex strokes of compression, stretching, vibration, and deep tissue massage may be less effective and require longer application to be effective. The systemic reflex strokes of rocking, friction, and effleurage may have increased effect and the relaxation effects of massage may be increased. Using stimulation at the end of the session with rapid effleurage, tapotement, and friction may help. If symptoms are severe, using more stimulating massage techniques throughout the session may be required.
- The site of I.M. injection of the drug should not be massaged for at least $1^1/_2$ hours to 2 hours to avoid increasing the rate of absorption of the drug.
- Side effects of drowsiness and hypotension may be addressed as noted above.

losartan potassium (loh-SAR-tan poh-TAH-see-um)

Cozaar

Drug Class: Angiotensin II receptor antagonist antihypertensive

Drug Actions

Inhibits vasoconstricting and aldosterone-secreting effects of angiotensin II and lowers blood pressure.

Use

- Nephropathy in type 2 diabetes mellitus
- Hypertension
- To reduce risk of stroke in patients with hypertension and left ventricular hypertrophy

Side Effects

Cardiovascular: edema, chest pain, hypotension, orthostatic hypotension, diabetic vascular disease.
Gastrointestinal: abdominal pain, nausea, diarrhea, painful digestion, gastritis.
Nervous System: dizziness, weakness, fatigue, headache, insomnia, fever, hypersthesia, diabetic neuropathy.
Urinary: urinary tract infections.
Skin: cellulitis.
Other: angioedema, nasal congestion, sinusitis, pharyngitis, sinus disorder, muscle cramps, muscle pain, back or leg pain, cough, upper respiratory tract infection, sinusitis, cataract, anemia, hyperkalemia, hypoglycemia, weight gain, muscle weakness, cough, bronchitis, infection, flulike syndrome, trauma.

Onset, Peak, and Duration

Route	Onset	Peak	Duration
Oral	Unknown	1–4 hr	Unknown

 **Massage Considerations**

- No cautions or contraindications to massage are related to the actions of this drug. Cautions and contraindications to massage may be related to the client condition.
- Side effects of dizziness and hypotension require care in getting the client on and off the table. Stimulation with rapid effleurage or tapotement at the end of the session may help.
- Neuropathy is a contraindication locally to deep tissue massage.

lovastatin (mevinolin) (loh-vuh-STAH-tin)

Altocor, Mevacor

Drug Class: Cholesterol-lowering drug

Drug Actions

Lowers low density lipoprotein and total cholesterol levels

Use

- Primary prevention of coronary artery disease
- Coronary artery disease
- Hyperlipidemia
- Heterozygous familial hypercholesterolemia

Side Effects

Gastrointestinal: constipation, diarrhea, painful digestion, gas, abdominal pain or cramps, heartburn, painful swallowing, nausea.
Nervous System: headache, dizziness, peripheral neuropathy.
Skin: rash, itching.
Other: blurred vision, muscle cramps, muscle pain, myositis, rhabdomyolysis.

Onset, Peak, and Duration

Route	Onset	Peak	Duration
Oral	Unknown	2–6 hr	4–6 wk
Extended-release	Unknown	14 hr	Unknown

 **Massage Considerations**

- No cautions or contraindications to massage are indicated because a client is taking this drug. Cautions and contraindications to massage may be related to the client condition.
- Side effects of dizziness require care in getting the client on and off the table. Stimulation with effleurage or tapotement at the end of the session may help.
- Neuropathy is a local contraindication to deep tissue massage.
- Constipation and gas may be helped by abdominal massage.
- Rash or itching is a local contraindication to massage and should be reported to the physician. If severe, massage should be withheld.
- Rhabdomyolysis is a serious and potentially life-threatening disorder of muscle tissue. If the client presents with worsening muscle pain with no apparent cause, notify the physician immediately and do no massage until the client condition has been evaluated and cleared.

lymphocyte immune globulin (antithymocyte globlin [equine], ATG), (LIG) (LIM-foh-sight ih-MYOON GLOH-byoo-lin)

Atgam

Drug Class: Immunoglobulin immunosuppressant

Drug Actions

Prevents or relieves signs and symptoms of renal allograft rejection; also relieves signs and symptoms of aplastic anemia.

Use

- Prevention of acute renal allograft rejection
- Acute renal allograft rejection
- Aplastic anemia
- Skin allotransplantation

Side Effects

Cardiovascular: hypotension, chest pain, thrombophlebitis, tachycardia, edema, iliac vein obstruction, renal artery stenosis.
Gastrointestinal: nausea, vomiting, diarrhea, epigastric pain, abdominal distension, stomatitis.
Nervous System: malaise, seizures, headache.
Skin: rash.
Other: febrile reactions, serum sickness, anaphylaxis, infection, night sweats, laryngospasm, abnormal blood profiles, lymphadenopathy hyperglycemia, joint pain, shortness of breath, hiccups, pulmonary edema.

Onset, Peak, and Duration

Route	Onset	Peak	Duration
I.V.	Unknown	5 days	Unknown

Massage Considerations

- No cautions or contraindications to massage are related to the actions of this drug. In most cases, cautions and contraindications to massage will be related to the client condition.
- The physician should be consulted before any massage is given.
- Care should be taken to not expose the client to any infections by scheduling the client as the first client of the day. No massage should be given if the massage therapist has any infections.
- Side effects of hypotension require care in changing position and getting the client on and off the table. Stimulation with effleurage or tapotement at the end of the session may help.
- Thrombophlebitis is a complete contraindication to massage.
- Rash is a local contraindication to massage and should be reported to the physician immediately. If severe or widespread, massage should be withheld.

M

magaldrate (aluminum-magnesium complex)

(muh-GAL-drayt)

Losopan, Riopan

Drug Class: Antacid

Drug Actions

Reduces total acid load in GI tract, elevates gastric pH to reduce pepsin activity, strengthens gastric mucosal barrier, and increases esophageal sphincter tone.

Use

- Antacid

Side Effects

Gastrointestinal: mild constipation, diarrhea.

Onset, Peak, and Duration

Route	Onset	Peak	Duration
Oral			
Fasting	≤20 min	Unknown	20–60 min
Nonfasting	≤20 min	3 hr	20–60 min

Massage Considerations

- There are no cautions or contraindications to massage related to this drug.
- Side effects of constipation may be helped by abdominal massage.

magnesium (mag-NEE-see-um KLOR-ighd)

magnesium chloride

Slow-Mag

magnesium sulfate

Drug Class: Anticonvulsant, electrolyte supplement, antiarrhythmic

Drug Actions

Raises magnesium levels, alleviates seizure activity, and restores normal sinus rhythm

Use

- Mild hypomagnesemia
- Severe hypomagnesemia
- Magnesium supplementation
- Magnesium supplementation in total parenteral nutrition (TPN)
- Hypomagnesemic seizures
- Seizures caused by hypomagnesemia in acute nephritis
- Paroxysmal atrial tachycardia in patients unresponsive to other treatments
- To reduce morbidity and mortality from acute heart attack

Side Effects

Cardiovascular: flushing; slow, weak pulse; arrhythmias; hypotension; circulatory collapse.
Nervous System: weak or absent deep tendon reflexes, flaccid paralysis, hypothermia, drowsiness, perioral paresthesia, twitching carpopedal spasm, tetany, seizures.
Skin: sweating.
Other: hypocalcemia, respiratory paralysis.

Onset, Peak, and Duration

Route	Onset	Peak	Duration
Oral	Unknown	4 hr	4–6 hr
I.V., I.M.	Unknown	Unknown	4–6 hr

 Massage Considerations

- There are no cautions or contraindications to massage related to this drug. There may be cautions or contraindications to massage related to the client condition.
- The site of I.M. injection should not be massaged for at least 4 hours to avoid increasing the rate of absorption of the drug into the body.
- Side effects of drowsiness and hypotension require care in getting the client on and off the table. Stimulation with effleurage and tapotement at the end of the session may help.

magnesium citrate (citrate of magnesia) (mag-NEE-see-um SIH-trayt)

Citro-Mag, Evac-Q-Mag

magnesium hydroxide (milk of magnesia)

Milk of Magnesia, Milk of Magnesia Concentrate, Phillips' Milk of Magnesia, Phillips' Milk of Magnesia Concentrated

magnesium sulfate (epsom salts)

Drug Class: Saline laxative

Drug Actions

Reduces total acid load in GI tract, elevates gastric pH to reduce pepsin activity, strengthens gastric mucosal barrier, and increases esophageal sphincter tone. Soothes stomach upset, relieves constipation, and raises magnesium level.

Use

- Constipation
- To evacuate bowel before surgery
- Acid indigestion
- Gastroesophageal reflux disease
- Peptic ulcer disease
- Heartburn

Side Effects

Gastrointestinal: abdominal cramping, nausea, diarrhea, laxative dependence with long-term or excessive use.
Other: fluid and electrolyte disturbances.

Onset, Peak, and Duration

Route	Onset	Peak	Duration
Oral	30 min–3 hr	Varies	Varies

 Massage Considerations

- Although there are no cautions or contraindications to massage related to this drug, if the drug is being used for evacuation or constipation, massage should be given before drug administration or after the drug has had its effect

---

magnesium oxide (mag-NEE-see-um OKS-ighd)

Mag-Ox 400, Maox, Uro-Mag

Drug Class: Antacid, laxative

Drug Actions

Reduces total acid load in GI tract, elevates gastric pH to reduce pepsin activity, strengthens gastric mucosal barrier, and increases esophageal sphincter tone. Soothes stomach upset, relieves constipation, and raises magnesium level.

Use

- Antacid use
- Constipation
- Mild hypomagnesemia

Side Effects

Gastrointestinal: diarrhea, nausea, abdominal pain.
Other: hypermagnesemia.

Onset, Peak, and Duration

Route	Onset	Peak	Duration
Oral			
Fasting	20 min	Unknown	20–60 min
Nonfasting	20 min	3 hr	20–60 min

 Massage Considerations

- There are no cautions or contraindications to massage related to this drug.

---

magnesium sulfate (mag-NEE-see-um SUL-fayt)

Drug Class: Anticonvulsant

Drug Actions

Prevents or controls seizures, raises magnesium level, stops paroxysmal atrial tachycardia, and alleviates selected symptoms of acute nephritis in children.

Use

- Control of seizures caused by epilepsy, glomerulonephritis, or hypothyroidism
- Control of seizures in preeclampsia or eclampsia
- Hypomagnesemia

- Prevention of hypomagnesia as part of Total Parenteral Nutrition (TPN)
- Seizures, hypertension, and encephalopathy linked to acute nephritis in children
- Management of paroxysmal atrial tachycardia
- Management of life-threatening ventricular arrhythmias, such as sustained ventricular tachycardia or torsades de pointes
- Management of preterm labor
- Asthma

Side Effects

Cardiovascular: hypotension, flushing, circulatory collapse, depressed cardiac function, heart block.
Nervous System: drowsiness, depressed reflexes, flaccid paralysis, hypothermia.
Skin: sweating.
Other: hypocalcemia, respiratory paralysis.

Onset, Peak, and Duration

Route	Onset	Peak	Duration
I.V.	1–2 min	Almost immediate	30 min
I.M.	1 hr	Unknown	3–4 hr

 Massage Considerations

- There are no cautions or contraindications to massage related to the action of this drug. In most cases, there will be cautions and contraindications to massage related to the client condition.
- The physician should be consulted before any massage is given.
- The action of the drug may decrease the effectiveness of the local reflex strokes of compression, stretching and vibration and of deep tissue massage. Applying for longer periods may achieve the desired results or using mechanical strokes such as effleurage and pétrissage can be used.
- Side effects of drowsiness and hypotension require care in getting the client on and off the table. Using stimulation with rapid effleurage and tapotement at the end of the session may help.

---

mannitol (MAN-ih-tol)

Osmitrol

Drug Class: Osmotic diuretic

Drug Actions

Increases water excretion, decreases intracranial or intraocular pressure, prevents or treats kidney dysfunction, and alleviates drug intoxication

Use

- Test dose for marked oliguria or suspected inadequate kidney function
- Oliguria
- Prevention of oliguria or acute renal impairment
- Edema
- Ascites caused by renal, hepatic, or cardiac failure
- Reduction of intraocular or intracranial pressure
- Diuresis in drug intoxication

Side Effects

Cardiovascular: transient expansion of plasma volume during infusion, causing circulatory overload and heart failure; tachycardia; chest pains.
Gastrointestinal: thirst, nausea, vomiting, diarrhea.
Nervous System: headache, confusion, seizures.
Urinary: urine retention.
Other: water intoxication, cellular dehydration, blurred vision, rhinitis.

Onset, Peak, and Duration

Route	Onset	Peak	Duration
I.V.	30–60 min	≤1 hr	6–8 hr

 Massage Considerations

- This drug changes the fluid balance in the body to encourage excretion of fluids.
- Circulatory massage with effleurage should be used with great caution and be very limited so as not to tax the kidneys any further. Deep tissue massage should be used with great caution, if at all.
- In most cases, there will be further cautions and contraindications to massage related to the client condition.
- The physician should be consulted before any massage is given.
- The best strokes to use with this client are rocking, gentle friction, gentle compression, stretching and traction, and gentle pétrissage.

---

mebendazole (meh-BEN-duh-zohl)

Vermox

Drug Class: Anthelmintic

Drug Actions

Kills helminth infestation

Use

- Pinworm
- Roundworm
- Whipworm
- Hookworm
- Trichinosis
- Capillariasis
- Toxocariasis
- Dracunculiasis

Side Effects

Gastrointestinal: transient abdominal pain, diarrhea.

Onset, Peak, and Duration

Route	Onset	Peak	Duration
Oral	Unknown	2–5 hr	Varies

Massage Considerations

- Because this drug treats infections with parasites that may be spread through contact, massage should be withheld until the treatment is completed and the infestation resolved.
- If massage is given, special care should be taken in handling the sheets, washing them immediately, and in disinfecting the table and hands after the massage.

---

mechlorethamine hydrochloride (nitrogen mustard)

(meh-klor-ETH-uh-meen high-droh-KLOR-ighd)

Mustargen

Drug Class: Antineoplastic

Drug Actions

Kills certain cancer cells

Use

- Hodgkin's disease
- Polycythemia vera
- Chronic lymphocytic leukemia
- Chronic myelocytic leukemia
- Bronchogenic cancer
- Lymphosarcoma
- Mycosis fungoides
- Malignant effusions

Side Effects

Cardiovascular: thrombophlebitis.
Gastrointestinal: metallic taste, nausea, vomiting, anorexia.
Nervous System: headache, weakness, drowsiness, dizziness.
Skin: hair loss, rash, sloughing, severe irritation if drug extravasates or touches skin.
Other: precipitation of herpes zoster, anaphylaxis, secondary malignant disease, ringing in the ears, hearing loss with high doses, abnormal blood profiles, myelosuppression, mild anemia.

Onset, Peak, and Duration

Route	Onset	Peak	Duration
I.V., intracavitary	Rapid	Unknown	Unknown

Massage Considerations

- Because of the toxic effects of this drug, deep tissue massage is contraindicated and circulatory massage with effleurage should be used with caution and limited.
- There may be further cautions and contraindications to massage related to the client condition.
- The physician should be consulted before any massage is given, and close collaboration is essential.
- This drug is usually given every 3–4 weeks and metabolizes quickly. Massage should be done on the weeks that the drug is not being given or before the drug is given on the week it is to be administered. This will help avoid overtaxing the already taxed liver and kidneys as they work to remove the drug from the body.

- Side effects of thrombophlebitis is a complete contraindication to massage. If the client presents with pain, redness, heat, and/or swelling, especially in the lower leg, refer to the physican immediately and withhold massage until the client is evaluated for possible blood clot. Drowsiness and dizziness require care in getting the client on and off the table. Using tapotement or friction to the legs at the end of the session may help. Rash is a local contraindication to massage and should be reported to the physician immediately. If severe or widespread, massage should be withheld. Hair loss is a contraindication to scalp massage if the client is disturbed by hair loss during the massage or if the scalp is tender.
- The best strokes to use with this client are the reflex strokes of rocking, stretching, gentle compression, gentle friction, and vibration. Myofascial massage techniques may be used for areas of tightness or gluteation.

meclizine hydrochloride (meclozine hydrochloride)

(MEK-lih-zeen high-droh-KLOR-ighd)

Ancolan, Antivert, Antivert/25, Antivert/50, Antrizine, Bonamine, Bonine, Dramamine Less Drowsy Formula, Meni-D, Vergon

Drug Class: Antiemetic, antivertigo drug

Drug Actions

Relieves vertigo and nausea

Use

- Vertigo, dizziness
- Motion sickness

Side Effects

Gastrointestinal: dry mouth.
Nervous System: drowsiness, fatigue.
Other: blurred vision.

Onset, Peak, and Duration

Route	Onset	Peak	Duration
Oral	1 hr	Unknown	8–24 hr

 Massage Considerations

- There are no cautions or contraindications to massage related to this drug.
- Side effects of drowsiness require care in getting the client on and off the table.
- Stimulation with rapid effleurage or tapotement at the end of the session may help. If symptom is severe or worsened with massage, a more stimulating massage technique should be used throughout the session.

medroxyprogesterone acetate (med-roks-ee-proh-JES-ter-ohn AS-ih-tayt)

Amen, Cycrin, Depo-Provera, Provera

Drug Class: Progestin antineoplastic

Drug Actions

Stops abnormal uterine bleeding, reverses secondary amenorrhea, prevents pregnancy, and hinders cancer cell growth

Use

- Abnormal uterine bleeding caused by hormonal imbalance
- Secondary amenorrhea
- Endometrial or renal carcinoma
- Contraception
- Paraphilia

Side Effects

Cardiovascular: hypertension, thrombophlebitis, pulmonary embolism, edema, thromboembolism, stroke.
Gastrointestinal: nausea, vomiting, abdominal cramps.
Nervous System: dizziness, migraine, lethargy, depression.
Skin: melasma, rash, pain, induration, sterile abscesses, acne, hair loss.
Other: breast tenderness, enlargement, or secretion; decreased libido, hypersensitivity reactions, intolerance to contact lenses. nervousness, weakness, breakthrough bleeding, dysmenorrhea, amenorrhea, cervical erosion, abnormal secretions, uterine fibromas, vaginal candidiasis, cholestatic jaundice, tumors, gallbladder disease, hyperglycemia, weight gain.

Onset, Peak, and Duration

Route	Onset	Peak	Duration
Oral, I.M.	Unknown	Unknown	Unknown

Massage Considerations

- There are no cautions or contraindications to massage related to the actions of this drug.
- There may be cautions or contraindications to massage related to the client condition.
- It is unclear how long it takes for the drug to absorb from the site of I.M. injection. It is best to avoid massage to the area for as long as possible depending on the frequency of the drug administration. If given daily or more than once daily, avoid the last area of injection. If it is given weekly or less often, avoid the area for a week after injection.
- Side effects of thrombophlebitis, embolism or thrombus are complete contraindications to massage. If the client exhibits pain, redness, swelling, or heat, especially in the lower leg, refer to the physician and do not massage until the client has been evaluated for possible blood clot. Dizziness requires care in gettting the client on and off the table. Friction to the legs or tapotement at the end of the session may help. Rash or acne are local contraindications to massage and should be reported to the physician. If the drug is continued and the client still wants massage, gloves may be worn for protection while working over the affected areas. Hair loss is a contraindication to scalp massasge if the client is disturbed by hair loss during the session or if the scalp is tender. Breast tenderness requires caution with depth in massage of the chest. If severe, avoid massage of the area.

mefloquine hydrochloride (MEF-loh-kwin high-droh-KLOR-ighd)

Lariam

Drug Class: Antimalarial

Drug Actions

Kills malaria-causing organisms

Use

- Acute malaria infections
- Malaria prevention

Side Effects

Cardiovascular: extrasystoles, chest pain, edema.
Gastrointestinal: loss of appetite, vomiting, nausea, loose stools, diarrhea, GI discomfort, painful digestion.
Nervous System: dizziness, fever, fatigue, syncope, headache, seizures, tremor, ataxia, mood changes, panic attacks, suicide.
Skin: rash.
Other: chills, ringing in the ears.

Onset, Peak, and Duration

Route	Onset	Peak	Duration
Oral	Unknown	7–24 hr	Unknown

Massage Considerations

- There are no cautions or contraindications to massage related to the actions of this drug.
- There may be cautions or contraindications to massage related to the client condition.
- Side effects of dizziness require care in getting the client on and off the table. Stimulation with rapid effleurage and tapotement at the end of the session may help. Rash is a local contraindication to massage and should be reported to the physician immediately. If severe, massage should be withheld.

---

megestrol acetate (meh-JES-trol AS-ih-tayt)

Megace, Megostat

Drug Class: Antineoplastic

Drug Actions

Hinders cancer cell growth and increases appetite

Use

- Breast cancer
- Endometrial cancer
- Anorexia, cachexia, or unexplained significant weight loss in patients with AIDS
- Anorexia or cachexia in patients with neoplastic disease

Side Effects

Cardiovascular: hypertension, thrombophlebitis, heart failure, thromboembolic phenomena.
Gastrointestinal: nausea, vomiting, abdominal pain.
Skin: hair loss, abnormal growth of hair on the body.
Other: breast tenderness, weight gain, increased appetite, breakthrough menstrual bleeding, carpal tunnel syndrome, back pain, pulmonary embolism.

Onset, Peak, and Duration

Route	Onset	Peak	Duration
Oral	Unknown	Unknown	Unknown

Massage Considerations

- There are no cautions or contraindications to massage related to this drug. There may be cautions or contraindications to massage related to the client condition.
- The physician should be consulted before any massage is given.

- Side effects of thromboembolism is a complete contraindication to massage. If the client presents with redness, heat, swelling, or pain, do not give massage and refer to the physician immediately for evaluation. Hair loss is a contraindication to scalp massage if the client is disturbed by hair loss during the massage or if the scalp is tender. Breast tenderness requires caution in the depth of massage of the chest. If severe, massage of the area should be avoided.

meloxicam (mell-OX-ih-kam)

Mobic

Drug Class: Enolic acid nonsteroidal anti-inflammatory drug (NSAID)

Drug Actions

Mechanism of action may be related to prostaglandin (cyclooxygenase) synthetase inhibition. Relieves of signs and symptoms of osteoarthritis.

Use

- To relieve signs and symptoms of osteoarthritis

Side Effects

Cardiovascular: arrhythmias, palpitations, tachycardia, angina, heart failure, hypertension, hypotension, heart attack, edema.
Gastrointestinal: abdominal pain, diarrhea, painful digestion, gas nausea, constipation, colitis, dry mouth, duodenal ulcer, esophagitis, gastric ulcer, gastritis, GI reflux, hemorrhage, pancreatitis, vomiting, increased appetite, taste perversion.
Nervous System: dizziness, headache, fatigue, seizures, paresthesia, fever, tremor, anxiety, confusion, depression, nervousness, sleepiness, malaise, syncope.
Urinary: albuminuria, hematuria, urinary frequency, renal impairment, urinary tract infection.
Skin: rash, itching, hives, hair loss, bullous eruption, photosensitivity reactions, sweating.
Other: accidental injury, allergic reaction, angioedema, flulike symptoms, pharyngitis, abnormal vision, conjunctivitis, ringing in the ears, abnormal blood profiles, purpura, upper respiratory tract infection, asthma, bronchospasm, shortness of breath, cough, bilirubinemia, hepatitis, dehydration, weight changes, joint pain, back pain.

Onset, Peak, and Duration

Route	Onset	Peak	Duration
Oral	Unknown	Unknown	Unknown

Massage Considerations

- This drug may decrease the perception of pain; therefore, deep tissue massage should be used with caution.
- There may be other cautions or contraindications to massage related to the client condition.
- Side effects of hypotension, dizziness, and sleepiness require care in getting the client on and off the table. Using stimulation with effleurage or tapotement at the end of the session may help. Paresthesia is a local contraindication to deep tissue massage.
- Constipation and gas may be helped by abdominal massage. Urinary frequency may require the client to get up in the middle of a session. Providing privacy and quick access to the bathroom is appropriate. Water fountains or music that may stimulate the urge to urinate should be avoided. Rash, itching, or hives are local contraindications to massage and should be reported to the physician. If severe or widespread, no massage should be given. Hair loss is a contraindication to massage if the client is disturbed by hair loss during the massage or if the scalp is tender.

melphalan (L-phenylalanine mustard) (MEL-feh-len)

Alkeran

Drug Class: Antineoplastic

Drug Actions

Kills certain cancer cells

Use

- Multiple myeloma
- Nonresectable advanced ovarian cancer

Side Effects

Skin: itching, rash, hair loss.
Other: anaphylaxis, hypersensitivity reactions, abnormal blood profiles, bone marrow suppression, hepatotoxicity, pneumonitis, pulmonary fibrosis.

Onset, Peak, and Duration

Route	Onset	Peak	Duration
Oral, I.V.	Unknown	Unknown	Unknown

Massage Considerations

- Because this drug is very toxic, deep tissue massage is contraindicated and circulatory massage with effleurage should be used with caution and limited.
- There may be other cautions or contraindications to massage related to the client condition.
- The physician should be consulted before any massage is given, and close collaboration is essential.
- The drug is most often given daily for a period of a few weeks followed by a few weeks off. So as not to overtax the liver and kidneys as they try to rid the body of the drug, massage would best be given on the weeks that the drug is not being given. If massage is desired during the time when the drug is being given, it would best be done before the administration of the drug. If this is not possible, 4–6 hours after administration would be best, as the half-life is 2 hours.
- Side effects of rash and itching are local contraindications to massage and should be reported to the physician immediately. If severe or widespread, massage should be withheld. Hair loss is a contraindication to scalp massage if the client is disturbed by hair loss during the massage or if the scalp is tender.
- The best strokes for this client are the reflex strokes of rocking, gentle compression, gentle friction, stretching, and vibration.

memantine hydrochloride (MEHM-en-tyn high-droh-KLOR-ighd)

Namenda

Drug Class: Alzheimer's disease drug

Drug Actions

Antagonizes NMDA receptors, the persistent activation of which seems to increase Alzheimer's symptoms. Decreases dementia related to Alzheimer's disease.

Use

- Moderate to severe Alzheimer's-type dementia.

Side Effects

Cardiovascular: edema, heart failure, hypertension.
Gastrointestinal: anorexia, constipation, diarrhea, nausea, vomiting.
Nervous System: abnormal gait, aggressiveness, agitation, anxiety, ataxia, confusion, stroke, depression, dizziness, fatigue, hallucinations, headache, hypokinesia, insomnia, pain, sleepinesss, syncope, TIA.
Urinary: incontinence, urinary frequency, urinary tract infection.
Skin: rash.
Other: falls, flulike symptoms, inflicted injury, cataracts, conjunctivitis, anemia, weight loss, joint pain, back pain, bronchitis, coughing, shortness of breath, pneumonia, upper respiratory tract infection.

Onset, Peak, and Duration

Route	Onset	Peak	Duration
Oral	Unknown	3–7 hr	Unknown

Massage Considerations

- There are no cautions or contraindications to massge related to the action of this drug.
- There may be cautions or contraindications to massage related to the client condition.
- Side effects of dizziness and sleepiness require care in getting the client on and off the table. Stimulation with rapid effleurage at the end of the session may help. Constipation may be helped by abdominal massage. Urinary frequency may require the client to get up during the massage. Privacy and quick access to the bathroom should be provided. Water fountains and music that may stimulate the urge to urinate should be avoided. Rash is a local contraindication to massage and should be reported to the physician. If severe, massage should be withheld.

menotropins (meh-noh-TROH-pins)

Humegon, Pergonal, Repronex

Drug Class: Gonadotropin ovulation stimulant, spermatogenesis stimulant

Drug Actions

Stimulates ovulation and fertility

Use

- Anovulation
- Infertility with ovulation
- Infertility in men

Side Effects

Cardiovascular: stroke, fever, tachycardia.
Gastrointestinal: nausea, vomiting, diarrhea.
Other: abnormal growth of breast tissue, hypersensitivity reactions, anaphylaxis., ovarian enlargement with pain and abdominal distention, multiple births, ovarian hyperstimulation syndrome (sudden ovarian enlargement, ascites, or pleural effusion), hemoconcentration with fluid loss into abdomen, atelectasis, acute respiratory distress syndrome, pulmonary embolism, pulmonary infarction, arterial occlusion.

Onset, Peak, and Duration

Route	Onset	Peak	Duration
I.M.	9–12 days	Unknown	Unknown

 Massage Considerations

- There are no cautions or contraindications to massage related to the action of this drug.
- There may be cautions and contraindication to massage related to the client condition.
- The physician approval should be obtained before any massage is given.
- The site of I.M. injection should not be massaged for 24 hours after adminstration.
- Side effects of abnormal growth of breast tissue requires caution with chest massage. If the area is too tender, no massage should be done in the area.

---

meperidine hydrochloride (meh-PER-uh-deen high-droh-KLOR-ighd)

Demerol

Drug Class: Opioid analgesic, adjunct to anesthesia

Drug Actions

Binds with opioid receptors in CNS, altering both perception of and emotional response to pain through unknown mechanism

Use

- Moderate to severe pain
- Preoperatively
- Adjunct to anesthesia
- Obstetric analgesia

Side Effects

Cardiovascular: hypotension, bradycardia, tachycardia, cardiac arrest, shock.
Gastrointestinal: nausea, vomiting, constipation, ileus.
Nervous System: sedation, sleepiness, clouded sensorium, euphoria, paradoxical excitement, tremors, dizziness, seizures.
Urinary: urine retention.
Skin: local tissue irritation and induration (after Subcutaneous injection), phlebitis (after I.V. use).
Other: pain at injection site, physical dependence, muscle twitching, respiratory depression, respiratory arrest.

Onset, Peak, and Duration

Route	Onset	Peak	Duration
Oral	15 min	60–90 min	2–4 hr
I.V.	1 min	5–7 min	2–4 hr
I.M., S.C. Injection	10–15 min	30–50 min	2–4 hr

 Massage Considerations

- This drug decreases the perception of pain; therefore, deep tissue massage is contraindicated.

- There may be further cautions and contraindications to massage related to the client condition.
- The depressant effect on the CNS may decrease the effectiveness of the local reflex strokes of stretching, compression, and vibration and may increase the effects of the systemic reflex strokes of rocking, effleurage, and friction. Using more stimulating strokes and techniques throughout the session may help. Using mechanical strokes such as pétrissage and more rapid effleurage may be the most effective.
- The site of I.M. or subcutaneous injection of the drug should not be massaged for at least 1 hour so as not to increase the absorption rate of the drug.
- Side effects of hypotension, dizziness, sleepiness may be addressed as noted above. Constipation may be helped by abdominal massage.

---

mercaptopurine (6-mercaptopurine, 6-MP) (mer-cap-toh-PYOO-reen)

Purinethol

Drug Class: Antineoplastic

Drug Actions

Inhibits growth of certain cancer cells

Use

- Acute lymphoblastic leukemia in children
- Chronic myelocytic leukemia
- Acute myeloblastic leukemia

Side Effects

Gastrointestinal: nausea, vomiting, anorexia, painful oral ulcers.
Skin: rash, hyperpigmentation.
Other: abnormal blood profiles, biliary stasis, jaundice, hepatotoxicity, hyperuricemia.

Onset, Peak, and Duration

Route	Onset	Peak	Duration
Oral	Unknown	Unknown	Unknown

Massage Considerations

- Because of the toxic effects of this drug, deep tissue massage should be used with caution. Circulatory massage with effleurage also should be used with caution.
- There may be other cautions and contraindications to massage related to the client condition.
- The physician should be consulted before any massage is given, and close collaboration is essential.
- Side effects of rash is a local contraindication to massage and should be reported to the physician immediately. If severe or widespread, massage should be withheld.

---

meropenem (mer-oh-PEN-em)

Merrem I.V.

Drug Class: Antibiotic

Drug Actions

Bactericidal

Use

- Complicated appendicitis and peritonitis

Side Effects

Cardiovascular: thrombophlebitis at injection site.
Gastrointestinal: diarrhea, nausea, vomiting, constipation, oral candidiasis, pseudomembranous colitis, glossitis.
Nervous System: seizures, headache.
Skin: rash, itching, phlebitis.
Other: hypersensitivity reactions, anaphylaxis, inflammation, anemia, eosinophilia, apnea.

Onset, Peak, and Duration

Route	Onset	Peak	Duration
I.V.	Unknown	Within 1 hr	Unknown

 Massage Considerations

- There are no cautions or contraindications to massage related to the actions of this drug. In most cases, there will be cautions and contraindications to massage related to the client condition.
- The physician should be consulted before any massage is given.
- Sid effects of thrombophlebitis is a complete contraindication to massage. Constipation may be helped by abdominal massage. Rash or itching is a local contraindication to massage and should be reported to the physician immediately. If severe or widespread, massage should be withheld.

---

mesalamine (mez-AL-uh-meen)

Asacol, Canasa, Pentasa, Rowasa

Drug Class: Salicylate anti-inflammatory

Drug Actions

Unknown; probably acts topically by inhibiting prostaglandin production in colon. Relieves inflammation in lower GI tract.

Use

- Active mild to moderate distal ulcerative colitis
- Proctitis
- Proctosigmoiditis
- Maintenance of remission of ulcerative colitis

Side Effects

Gastrointestinal: abdominal pain, cramps, or discomfort; gas; diarrhea; rectal pain; bloating; nausea; vomiting; belching; pancolitis; pancreatitis.
Nervous System: headache, dizziness, fatigue, fever, malaise.
Skin: rash, itching, hives, hair loss, acne.
Other: anaphylaxis, wheezing.

Onset, Peak, and Duration

Route	Onset	Peak	Duration
Oral, Rectal	Unknown	3–12 hr	Unknown

Massage Considerations

- There are no cautions or contraindications to massage related to this drug. There may be cautions or contraindications to massage related to the client condition.
- Side effects of dizziness require care in getting the client on and off the table. Stimulation with effleurage or tapotement at the end of the session may help. Gas may be helped by abdominal massage. Rash, itching, hives, or acne are local contraindications to massage and should be reported to the physician. If severe or widespread, no massage should be given. In the case of acne, if the client is still taking the drug, massage may be given with gloves on when working on the affected areas. Hair loss is a contraindication to scalp massage if the client is disturbed by hair loss during the massage or if the scalp is tender.

---

mesna (MEZ-nah)

MESNEX

Drug Class: Uroprotectant

Drug Actions

Prevents ifosfamide from adversely affecting bladder tissue

Use

- Prevention of hemorrhagic cystitis in patients receiving ifosfamide
- Prevention of hemorrhagic cystitis in bone marrow recipients receiving cyclophosphamide

Side Effects

Cardiovascular: chest pain, edema, hypotension, tachycardia, flushing.
Gastrointestinal: nausea, vomiting, diarrhea, constipation, anorexia, abdominal pain, painful digestion.
Nervous System: fatigue, fever, weakness, dizziness, headache, sleepiness, anxiety, confusion, insomnia, pain.
Urinary: hematuria.
Skin: hair loss, increased sweating, pallor.
Other: allergy, injection site reaction, abnormal blood profiles, hypokalemia, dehydration, back pain, shortness of breath, coughing, pneumonia.

Onset, Peak, and Duration

Route	Onset	Peak	Duration
Oral, I.V.	Unknown	Unknown	Unknown

Massage Considerations

- There are no cautions or contraindications to massage related to the actions of this drug.
- There may be cautions and contraindications to massage related to the client condition.
- Side effects of hypotension, dizziness, and drowsiness require care in getting the client on and off the table. Stimulation with rapid effleurage and tapotement at the end of the session may help. Constipation may be helped by abdominal massage. Hair loss contraindicates scalp massage if the client is disturbed by hair loss during the massage or if the scalp is tender.

mesoridazine besylate (mes-oh-RID-eh-zeen BES-eh-layt)

Serentil, Serentil Concentrate

Drug Class: Antipsychotic

Drug Actions

Relieves psychotic signs and symptoms

Use

- Management of psychotic disorders and for schizophrenic patients who do not show an acceptable response to other antipsychotics

Side Effects

Cardiovascular: orthostatic hypotension, tachycardia, ECG changes, prolonged QT interval, torsades de pointes, sudden death.
Gastrointestinal: dry mouth, constipation, increased appetite.
Nervous System: extrapyramidal reactions, drowsiness, tardive dyskinesia, sedation, EEG changes, dizziness, neuroleptic malignant syndrome.
Urinary: urine retention, dark urine, menstrual irregularities, inhibited ejaculation.
Skin: mild photosensitivity reactions, sterile abscess.
Other: allergic reactions, abnormal growth of breast tissue, pain at I.M. injection site, ocular changes, blurred vision, retinitis pigmentosa, abnormal blood profiles, cholestatic jaundice, weight gain.

Onset, Peak, and Duration

Route	Onset	Peak	Duration
Oral, I.M.	Up to several wk	Unknown	Unknown

Massage Considerations

- This drug acts in blocking neurotransmittors in the brain and may decrease perception of pain. Deep tissue massage is contraindicated.
- In most cases, there will be further cautions and contraindications to massage related to the client condition.
- The physician should be consulted before any massage is given, and close collaboration is essential.
- The site of I.M. injection of the drug should not be massaged for at least 1 hour, if possible avoid longer than 1 hour.
- Side effects of hypotension, drowsiness, and dizziness require care in getting the client on and off the table. Stimulating the client at the end of the session with rapid effleurage may be helpful. If the symptom is severe, more stimulating massage techniques should be used throughout the session. Constipation may be helped by regular abdominal massage.
- Abnormal growth of breast tissue in men and women requires caution with depth in massage of the chest. If too tender, avoid massage of the area completely.

metaproterenol sulfate (met-uh-proh-TER-eh-nul SUL-fayt)

Alupent

Drug Class: Beta-adrenergic agonist bronchodilator

Drug Actions

Relaxes bronchial smooth muscle by acting on $beta_2$-adrenergic receptors. Improves breathing.

Use

- Acute episodes of bronchial asthma
- Bronchial asthma and reversible bronchospasm

Side Effects

Cardiovascular: tachycardia, hypertension, ECG changes, palpitations, cardiac arrest.
Gastrointestinal: vomiting, nausea, bad taste.
Nervous System: nervousness, weakness, drowsiness, tremors.
Other: paradoxical bronchoconstriction.

Onset, Peak, and Duration

Route	Onset	Peak	Duration
Oral	1 min	≤1 hr	1–4 hr
Inhalation	15 min	≤1 hr	2–6 hr
Nebulization	5–30 min	≤1 hr	2–6 hr

Massage Considerations

- There are no cautions or contraindications to massage related to this drug. There may be cautions and contraindications to massage related to the client condition.
- The drug acts to stimulate certain sympathetic nervous system (SNS) receptors and may decrease the effectiveness of the systemic reflex strokes rocking, effleurage, and friction and make the relaxation effects of massage more difficult to achieve. Using these strokes for a longer period of time during the massage may help to achieve the desired effects.
- Side effects of drowsiness may be helped by stimulation with effleurage and tapotement at the end of the session.

metformin hydrochloride (met-FOR-min high-droh-KLOR-ighd)

Glucophage, Glucophage XR, Riomet

Drug Class: Antidiabetic

Drug Actions

Decreases hepatic glucose production and intestinal absorption of glucose and improves insulin sensitivity (increases peripheral glucose uptake and utilization). Lowers glucose level.

Use

- Adjunct to diet and exercise to lower glucose level in patients with type 2 (non–insulin-dependent) diabetes mellitus.

Side Effects

Gastrointestinal: diarrhea, nausea, vomiting, abdominal discomfort, gas, indigestion, unpleasant or metallic taste.
Nervous System: headache, dizziness, weakness.
Other: megaloblastic anemia, lactic acidosis.

Onset, Peak, and Duration

Route	Onset	Peak	Duration
Oral	Unknown	Unknown	Unknown
Oral Extended-Release	Unknown	4–8 hr	Unknown
Oral Solution	Unknown	2 1/2 hr	Unknown

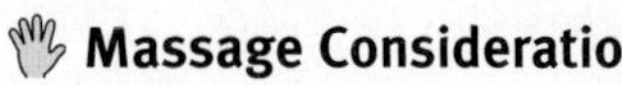

Massage Considerations

- There are no cautions or contraindications to massage related to this drug. There may be cautions or contraindications to massage related to the client condition.
- Side effects of dizziness may be helped by stimulation with effleurage or tapotement at the end of the session. Gas may be helped by abdominal massage.

---

methadone hydrochloride (METH-eh-dohn high-droh-KLOR-ighd)

Dolophine, Methadose, Physeptone

Drug Class: Opioid analgesic, opioid detoxification adjunct

Drug Actions

Binds to opioid receptors at many sites in CNS, altering both perception of and emotional response to pain through unknown mechanism

Use

- Severe pain
- Opiate withdrawal syndrome

Side Effects

Cardiovascular: hypotension, bradycardia, shock, cardiac arrest, arrhythmias.
Gastrointestinal: nausea, vomiting, constipation, ileus.
Nervous System: sedation, sleepiness, clouded sensorium, euphoria, dizziness, chorea, seizures.
Urinary: urine retention.
Skin: sweating.
Other: decreased libido, physical dependence, pain at injection site, tissue irritation, induration after subcutaneous injection, respiratory depression, respiratory arrest, visual disturbances.

Onset, Peak, and Duration

Route	Onset	Peak	Duration
Oral	30–60 min	$\frac{1}{2}$–1 hr	4–6 hr
I.M.	10–20 min	1–2 hr	4–5 hr
Subcutaneous Injection	Unknown	Unknown	Unknown

Massage Considerations

- This drug decreases the perception of pain; therefore, deep tissue massage is contraindicated.
- There may be further cautions and contraindications to massage related to the client condition.
- The physician should be consulted before any massage is given.
- The depressive effects of the drug on the CNS may decrease the effectiveness of the local reflex strokes of compression, stretching, and vibration. Applying them for longer than usual amounts of time may help. Also, the systemic reflex strokes of effleurage, rocking, and friction may have an increased effect and the relaxation effects of massage may be increased. Using more stimulating and rapid application techniques throughout the session may help.

- The site of I.M. or subcutaneous injection of the drug should not be massaged for at least 2 hours to avoid increasing the rate of absorption of the drug.
- Side effects of hypotension, drowsiness, and dizziness may be addressed as noted above.
- Constipation may be helped by abdominal massage.

---

methamphetamine hydrochloride (meth-am-FET-uh-meen high-droh-KLOR-ighd)

Desoxyn

Drug Class: Amphetamine CNS stimulant, short-term adjunct anorexigenic, sympathomimetic amine

Drug Actions

Unknown; probably promotes nerve impulse transmission by releasing stored norepinephrine from nerve terminals in brain. Main sites of activity appear to be cerebral cortex and reticular activating system. In hyperkinetic children, drug has paradoxical calming effect.

Use

- Attention deficit hyperactivity disorder
- Short-term adjunct in exogenous obesity

Side Effects

Cardiovascular: hypertension, hypotension, tachycardia, palpitations, arrhythmias.
Gastrointestinal: metallic taste, dry mouth, nausea, vomiting, abdominal cramps, diarrhea, constipation, anorexia.
Nervous System: nervousness, insomnia, irritability, talkativeness, dizziness, headache, hyperexcitability, tremors.
Skin: hives.
Other: altered libido, blurred vision, dilated pupils, impotence.

Onset, Peak, and Duration

Route	Onset	Peak	Duration
Oral	Unknown	Unknown	≤24 hr

Massage Considerations

- This drug is a CNS stimulant; tapotement should be used with caution. There may be further cautions and contraindications to massage related to the client condition.
- Side effects of dizziness and hypotension require care in getting on and off the table.
- Using friction to the legs or effleurage at the end of the session may help. Constipation may be helped by regular abdominal massage. Hives are a local contraindication to massage and should be reported to the physician immediately. If severe or widespread, massage should be withheld.
- The best approach to this client is to use systemic reflex strokes extensively throughout the massage. Rocking and slow rhythmic effleurage along with pétrissage will best achieve relaxation.

---

methimazole (meth-IH-muh-zohl)

Tapazole

Drug Class: Antithyroid drug

Drug Actions

Reduces thyroid hormone level

Use

- Hyperthyroidism

Side Effects

Gastrointestinal: diarrhea, nausea, vomiting, salivary gland enlargement, loss of taste.
Nervous System: headache, drowsiness, dizziness.
Skin: abnormal hair loss, rash, hives, skin discoloration.
Other: drug-induced fever, abnormal blood profiles, lymphadenopathy, jaundice, hypothyroidism, joint pain, muscle pain.

Onset, Peak, and Duration

Route	Onset	Peak	Duration
Oral	≤5 days	30 min-1 hr	Unknown

 Massage Considerations

- There are no cautions or contraindications to massage related to this drug. There may be caution and contraindications to massage related to the client condition.
- Side effects of drowsiness and dizziness require care in getting the client on and off the table. Stimulation with effleurage or tapotement at the end of the session may help. Rash or hives are local contraindications to massage and should be reported to the physician. If severe or widespread, massage should be withheld. Hair loss is a contraindication to scalp massage if the client is disturbed by hair loss during the session or if the scalp is tender.

---

methocarbamol (meth-oh-KAR-buh-mol)

Robaxin, Robaxin-750

Drug Class: Centrally acting skeletal muscle relaxant

Drug Actions

Unknown; probably modifies central perception of pain without modifying pain reflexes

Use

- As adjunct in acute, painful musculoskeletal conditions
- Supportive therapy in tetanus management

Side Effects

Cardiovascular: hypotension, bradycardia with I.M. or I.V. use, thrombophlebitis, flushing.
Gastrointestinal: nausea, anorexia, GI upset, metallic taste.
Nervous System: drowsiness, dizziness, headache, syncope, fever, mild muscle incoordination with I.M. or I.V. use, seizures with I.V. use.
Urinary: hematuria with I.V. use, discoloration of urine.
Skin: hives, itching, rash.
Other: extravasation with I.V. use, anaphylaxis with I.M. or I.V. use, blurred vision, hemolysis.

Onset, Peak, and Duration

Route	Onset	Peak	Duration
Oral	≤30 min	≤2 hr	Unknown
I.V.	Immediate	Immediate	Unknown
I.M.	Unknown	Unknown	Unknown

 Massage Considerations

- This drug decreases the perception of pain; therefore, deep tissue massage should be used with great caution if at all. There may be further cautions and contraindications to massage related to the client condition.
- Because of the action of this drug, the local reflex strokes of compression, stretching, and vibration may be less effective. Applying them for longer than usual periods of time may be needed.
- The site of I.M. injection should not be massaged for at least 2 hours, longer if possible.
- Side effects of hypotension, drowsiness, and dizziness may be helped by stimulating strokes such as rapid effleurage and tapotement at the end of the session.
- Thrombophlebitis is a complete contraindication to massage. Rash, hives, or itching are local contraindications to massage and should be reported to the physician. If severe or widespread, no massage should be given.

methotrexate (amethopterin, MTX) (meth-oh-TREKS-ayt)

Trexall

methotrexate sodium

Methotrexate LPF, Rheumatrex Dose Pack

Drug Class: Antineoplastic, immunosuppressant, antirheumatic

Drug Actions

Kills certain cancer cells and reduces inflammation

Use

- Trophoblastic tumors (choriocarcinoma, hydatidiform mole)
- Acute lymphoblastic and lymphatic leukemia
- Meningeal leukemia
- Burkitt's lymphoma (stage I or stage II)
- Lymphosarcoma (stage III)
- Osteosarcoma
- Mycosis fungoides
- Psoriasis
- Rheumatoid arthritis
- Head and neck carcinoma

Side Effects

Gastrointestinal: stomatitis, diarrhea, enteritis, intestinal perforation, nausea, vomiting. *Nervous System:* arachnoiditis (within hours of intrathecal use), subacute neurotoxicity (may begin few weeks later), demyelination, leukoencephalopathy.

Urinary: nephropathy, tubular necrosis, renal impairment.
Skin: hives, itching, hair loss, hyperpigmentation, psoriatic lesions, rash, photosensitivity reactions.
Other: sudden death, pharyngitis, WBC and platelet count nadirs on day 7, anemia, leukopenia, thrombocytopenia, acute toxicity, chronic toxicity, cirrhosis, hepatic fibrosis, hyperuricemia, osteoporosis in children with long-term use, pulmonary fibrosis, pulmonary interstitial infiltrates, pneumonitis.

Onset, Peak, and Duration

Route	Onset	Peak	Duration
Oral	Unknown	1–2 hr	Unknown
I.V., Intrathecal	Unknown	Immediate	Unknown
I.M.	Unknown	30 min-1 hr	Unknown

 Massage Considerations

- Because of the toxic effects of this drug, deep tissue massage and circulatory massage with effleurage should be used with caution.
- There may be further cautions or contraindications to massage related to the client condition.
- The physician should be consulted before any massage is given.
- The site of I.M. injection of the drug should not be massaged for at least 1 hour to avoid increasing the rate of absorption of the drug into the body.
- Side effects of hives, rash, and itching are local contraindications to massage and should be reported to the physician immediately. If severe or widespread, massage should not be given. Hair loss is a contraindication to scalp massage if the client is disturbed by hair loss during the session or if the scalp is tender.

methylcellulose (meth-il-SEL-yoo-lohs)

Citrucel, Citrucel Sugar Free

Drug Class: Bulk-forming laxative

Drug Actions

Absorbs water and expands to increase bulk and moisture content of stool, which encourages peristalsis and bowel movement

Use

- Chronic constipation

Side Effects

Gastrointestinal: nausea, vomiting, and diarrhea with excessive use; esophageal, gastric, small intestinal, or colonic strictures when drug is chewed or taken in dry form; abdominal cramps, especially in severe constipation; laxative dependence with long-term or excessive use.

Onset, Peak, and Duration

Route	Onset	Peak	Duration
Oral	12–24 hr	≤3 days	Varies

Massage Considerations

- There are no cautions or contraindications to massage related to this drug

---

methyldopa (meth-il-DOH-puh)

Aldomet, Apo-Methyldopa, Dopamet, Hydopa, Novomedopa, Nu-Medopa

methyldopate hydrochloride

Aldomet

Drug Class: Centrally acting antiadrenergic antihypertensive

Drug Actions

Unknown; thought to involve inhibition of central vasomotor centers, thereby decreasing sympathetic outflow to heart, kidneys, and peripheral vasculature. Lowers blood pressure.

Use

- Hypertension
- Hypertensive crisis

Side Effects

Cardiovascular: bradycardia, heart failure, orthostatic hypotension, aggravated angina, myocarditis, edema.
Gastrointestinal: nausea, vomiting, diarrhea, pancreatitis, dry mouth.
Nervous System: sedation, headache, weakness, dizziness, decreased mental acuity, involuntary choreoathetoid movements, psychic disturbances, depression, nightmares.
Skin: rash.
Other: abnormal growth of breast tissue, abnormal breast milk production, drug-induced fever, nasal congestion, impotence, hemolytic anemia, reversible agranulocytosis, thrombocytopenia, hepatic necrosis, gain.

Onset, Peak, and Duration

Route	Onset	Peak	Duration
Oral	Unknown	4–6 hr	12–48 hr
I.V.	Unknown	4–6 hr	10–16 hr

Massage Considerations

- This drug acts centrally to block sympathetic nervous system (SNS) activity. This may increase the effects of the systemic reflex strokes such as effleurage, rocking, and friction and increase the relaxation effects of massage. Using stimulating strokes such as tapotement and rapid friction, effleurage, and pétrissage at the end of the session may help. If symptoms are severe, using these more stimulating massage techniques throughout the session may be needed.
- There may be other cautions and contraindications to massage related to the client condition.
- Side effects of sedation, dizziness, and hypotension require care in getting the client on and off the table and may be addressed as noted above. Rash is a local contraindication to massage and should be reported to the physician. If severe, massage should be withheld.
- Abnormal growth of breast tissue in men or women and or breast secretions requires caution in chest massage. If too tender, no chest massage should be given.

methylphenidate hydrochloride (meth-il-FEN-ih-dayt high-droh-KLOR-ighd)

Concerta, Metadate CD, Metadate ER, Methylin, Methylin ER, Ritalin, Ritalin LA, Ritalin ER

Drug Class: CNS stimulant (analeptic)

Drug Actions

Unknown; probably promotes nerve impulse transmission by releasing stored norepinephrine from nerve terminals in brain. Main site of activity appears to be cerebral cortex and reticular activating system. In hyperkinetic children, drug has paradoxical calming effect. Promotes calmness and prevents sleep.

Use

- Attention deficit hyperactivity disorder (ADHD)
- Narcolepsy

Side Effects

Cardiovascular: palpitations, angina, tachycardia, changes in blood pressure and pulse rate.
Gastrointestinal: vomiting; nausea, abdominal pain, and anorexia.
Nervous System: nervousness, insomnia, Tourette syndrome, dizziness, headache, akathisia, dyskinesia, seizures.
Skin: rash, hives, exfoliative dermatitis, erythema multiforme.
Other: dry throat, pharyngitis and sinusitis, abnormal blood profiles, weight loss, delayed growth, upper respiratory tract infection, cough.

Onset, Peak, and Duration

Route	Onset	Peak	Duration
Oral:			
Concerta	Unknown	6–8 hr	8–12 hr
Metadate CD	Unknown	1st peak 1 1/2 hr; 2nd peak 4 1/2 hr	8–12 hr
Methylin, Ritalin	Unknown	2 hr	3–6 hr
Methylin ER, Ritalin-SR	Unknown	4 3/4 hr	3–8 hr
Ritalin LA	Unknown	1st peak 1–3 hr; 2nd peak 4–7 hr	8–12 hr

Massage Considerations

- Although there are no cautions or contraindications to massage related to the actions of this drug, the stimulant effect of the drug may decrease the effectiveness of the systemic reflex strokes of effleurage, rocking, and friction, and the overall relaxation effects of massage. Using these strokes for longer periods and using slow and rhythmic effleurage throughout the session may help achieve the desired effects.
- There may be other cautions and contraindications to massage related to the client condition.
- Side effects of dizziness require care in getting the client on and off the table. Using friction to the legs at the end of the session is recommended. Rash or hives are a local contraindication to massage and should be reported to the physician immediately. If severe or widespread, massage should be withheld.

methylprednisolone (meth-il-pred-NIS-uh-lohn)

Medrol, Meprolone

methylprednisolone acetate

depMedalone 40, depMedalone 80, Depo-Medrol, Depopred-40, Depopred-80

methylprednisolone sodium succinate

A-MethaPred, Solu-Medrol

Drug Class: Glucocorticoid anti-inflammatory, immunosuppressant

Drug Actions

Not clear; decreases inflammation, suppresses immune response, stimulates bone marrow, and influences protein, fat, and carbohydrate metabolism

Use

- Severe inflammation
- Immunosuppression
- Shock
- Acute exacerbations of multiple sclerosis
- Severe lupus nephritis
- To minimize motor and sensory defects caused by acute spinal cord injury
- Adjunct to moderate-to-severe *Pneumocystis carinii* pneumonia

Side Effects

Cardiovascular: heart failure, hypertension, edema, thromboembolism, fatal arrest or circulatory collapse after rapid administration of large I.V. doses.
Gastrointestinal: peptic ulceration, GI irritation, increased appetite, pancreatitis.
Nervous System: euphoria, insomnia, psychotic behavior, pseudotumor cerebri.
Skin: abnormal hair growth, delayed wound healing, acne, various skin eruptions.
Other: susceptibility to infections, acute adrenal insufficiency with increased stress (infection, surgery, or trauma) or abrupt withdrawal after long-term therapy, cataracts, glaucoma, hypokalemia, hyperglycemia, carbohydrate intolerance, growth suppression in children, muscle weakness, osteoporosis.

Onset, Peak, and Duration

Route	Onset	Peak	Duration
Oral	Rapid	1–2 hr	30–36 hr
I.V.	Immediate	Immediate	Unknown
I.M.	6–48 hr	Unknown	4–8 days

Massage Considerations

- The actions of this drug when taken long-term (longer than 2 weeks) change the metabolism and effect changes in both fat and connective tissues, as well as bone and muscle tissue. Because of this, deep tissue massage is contraindicated. Myofascial massage techniques should be used with great caution.
- In most cases, there will be further cautions and contraindications to massage related to the client condition.
- The physician should be consulted before any massage is given.

- The site of I.M. injection of the drug should not be massaged for at least 24 hours to avoid speeding up the absorption of the drug into the body.
- Side effects of acne and skin eruptions are local contraindications to massage and should be reported to the physician. If the client needs to continue to take the drug and still desires massage, gloves should be worn to massage the affected sites. Osteoporosis requires caution in the amount of pressure applied during massage and use of stretching and traction techniques. If severe, massage may be contraindicated completely.
- The best approach to this client is to use the systemic reflex strokes and mechanical strokes of rocking, rhythmic effleurage, gentle friction, and pétrissage.

---

metoclopramide hydrochloride (met-oh-KLOH-preh-mighd high-droh-KLOR-ighd)

Apo-Metoclop, Clopra, Maxeran, Maxolon, Octamide, Octamide PFS, Pramin, Reclomide, Reglan

Drug Class: Antiemetic, GI stimulant

Drug Actions

Stimulates motility of upper GI tract by increasing lower esophageal sphincter tone and blocks dopamine receptors at chemoreceptor trigger zone. Prevents or minimizes nausea and vomiting from chemotherapy or surgery. Also reduces gag reflex in small-bowel intubation and radiologic examinations, improves gastric emptying when diabetic gastroparesis is present, and reduces gastric reflux.

Use

- Prevention or reduction of nausea and vomiting induced by cisplatin alone or with other chemotherapeutics
- Prevention or reduction of postoperative nausea and vomiting
- To facilitate small-bowel intubation and aid in radiologic examinations
- Delayed gastric emptying caused by diabetic gastroparesis
- Gastroesophageal reflux disease

Side Effects

Cardiovascular: transient hypertension.
Gastrointestinal: nausea, bowel disturbances.
Nervous System: restlessness, anxiety, drowsiness, fatigue, fever, lassitude, insomnia, suicide ideation, seizures, headache, dizziness, extrapyramidal symptoms, tardive dyskinesia, dystonic reactions, sedation.
Skin: rash.
Other: prolactin secretion, loss of libido, agranulocytosis, neutropenia.

Onset, Peak, and Duration

Route	Onset	Peak	Duration
Oral	30–60 min	1–2 hr	1–2 hr
I.V.	1–3 min	Unknown	1–2 hr
I.M.	10–15 min	Unknown	1–2 hr

Massage Considerations

- There are no cautions or contraindications to massage related to the actions of this drug.
- There may be cautions or contraindications to massage related to the client condition.
- The site of I.M. injection of the drug should not be massaged for at least 1 hour after administration.
- Side effects of drowsiness and dizziness require care in getting the client on and off table.
- Using stimulation with effleurage and tapotement at the end of the session may help.
- Rash is a local contraindication to massage and should be reported to the physician. If severe, no massage should be given.

---

metolazone (meh-TOH-luh-zohn)

Mykrox, Zaroxolyn

Drug Class: Diuretic, antihypertensive

Drug Actions

Promotes water and sodium elimination and lowers blood pressure

Use

- Edema in heart failure or renal disease
- Mild to moderate essential hypertension

Side Effects

Cardiovascular: volume depletion, orthostatic hypotension, palpitations, chest pain.
Gastrointestinal: anorexia, nausea, pancreatitis.
Nervous System: dizziness, headache, fatigue.
Urinary: increased urination at night, frequent urination.
Skin: photosensitivity reactions, rash.
Other: hypersensitivity reactions, abnormal blood profiles, hepatic encephalopathy, hyperglycemia and glucose tolerance impairment; hyperuricemia, fluid and electrolyte imbalances, including hypokalemia, metabolic alkalosis, hypercalcemia, and dilutional hyponatremia and hypochloremia, dehydration, acute gouty attacks, muscle cramps, swelling.

Onset, Peak, and Duration

Route	Onset	Peak	Duration
Oral	1 hr	2–8 hr	12–24 hr

Massage Considerations

- There are no cautions or contraindications to massage related to this drug. There may be cautions and contraindications to massage related to the client condition.
- Side effects of dizziness and hypotension require care in getting the client on and off the table. Using rapid effleurage and tapotement at the end of the session may help. Frequent urination may require the client to get up in the middle of the session. Privacy and quick access to the bathroom should be provided. Water fountains and music that may stimulate the urge to urinate should be avoided. Rash is a local contraindication to massage and should be reported to the physician. If severe or widespread, massage should be withheld.

metoprolol succinate (meh-TOH-pruh-lol SUHK-seh-nayt)

Toprol-XL

metoprolol tartrate (meh-TOH-pruh-lol TAR-trayt)

Apo-Metoprolol, Apo-Metoprolol (Type L), Betaloc, Betaloc Durules, Lopresor, Lopressor, Minax, Novometoprol, Nu-Metop

Drug Class: $Beta_1$ selective blocker antihypertensive, adjunct treatment of acute MI

Drug Actions

Reduces blood pressure and angina and helps to prevent myocardial tissue damage

Use

- Hypertension
- Early intervention in acute heart attack
- Angina pectoris
- Stable, symptomatic heart failure (New York Heart Association class II) resulting from ischemia, hypertension, or cardiomyopathy
- Atrial tachyarrhythmias after acute heart attack
- Unstable angina or non–ST-segment elevation heart attack at high risk for ischemic events

Side Effects

Cardiovascular: bradycardia, hypotension, heart failure, AV block, peripheral vascular disease.
Gastrointestinal: nausea, vomiting, diarrhea.
Nervous System: fatigue, lethargy, dizziness, fever.
Skin: rash.
Other: joint pain, shortness of breath, bronchospasm.

Onset, Peak, and Duration

Route	Onset	Peak	Duration
Oral	≤15 min	1–12 hr	6–24 hr
I.V.	≤5 min	20 min	5–8 hr

Massage Considerations

- The action of this drug as a blocker of sympathetic nervous system (SNS) receptors is very specific; however, there may be an increase in the effects of the systemic reflex strokes and the relaxation effect of massage. Using stimulation at the end of the massage with rapid effleurage and friction may help.
- There may be other cautions and contraindications to massage related to the client condition.
- Side effects of dizziness and hypotension require care in getting the client on and off the table and may be addressed as noted above. Rash is a local contraindication to massage and should be reported to the physician. If severe, massage should be withheld.

metronidazole (met-roh-NIGH-duh-zohl)

Apo-Metronidazole, Flagyl, Flagyl ER, Flagyl 375, Metric 21, Metrogyl, Metrozine, Novonidazol, Protostat, Trikacide

metronidazole hydrochloride

Flagyl I.V. RTU, Metro I.V., Novonidazol

Drug Class: Antibacterial, antiprotozoal, amebicide

Drug Actions

Hinders growth of selected organisms, including most anaerobic bacteria and protozoa

Use

- Amebic hepatic abscess
- Intestinal amebiasis
- Trichomoniasis
- Refractory trichomoniasis
- Bacterial infections caused by anaerobic microorganisms
- Prevention of postoperative infection in contaminated or potentially contaminated colorectal surgery
- Pelvic inflammatory disease
- Bacterial vaginosis
- Active Crohn's disease
- Prevention of sexually transmitted disease in sexual assault victims
- Helicobacter pylori with peptic ulcer disease

Side Effects

Cardiovascular: flattened T wave, edema, flushing, thrombophlebitis after I.V. infusion.
Gastrointestinal: abdominal cramping, stomatitis, nausea, vomiting, anorexia, diarrhea, constipation, proctitis, dry mouth, metallic taste.
Nervous System: dizziness, headache, ataxia, fever, incoordination, confusion, irritability, depression, restlessness, weakness, fatigue, drowsiness, insomnia, sensory neuropathy, paresthesia of limbs, psychic stimulation, seizures.
Urinary: darkened urine, increased urination, painful urination, pus in the urine, incontinence, cystitis, dyspareunia, dry vagina and vulva, sense of pelvic pressure.
Skin: itching, rash.
Other: decreased libido, abnormal growth of breast tissue, overgrowth of nonsusceptible organisms, especially *Candida* (glossitis, furry tongue), abnormal blood profiles.

Onset, Peak, and Duration

Route	Onset	Peak	Duration
Oral	Unknown	1–2 hr	Unknown
I.V.	Immediate	Immediate	Unknown

 Massage Considerations

- There are no cautions or contraindications to massage related to the actions of this drug.
- There may be cautions and contraindications to massage related to the client condition and severity of infection. Side effects of dizziness and drowsiness require care in getting the client on and off the table. Using stimulation at the end of the session with rapid effleurage and tapotement may help. Paresthesia and neuropathy are local contraindications to deep tissue massage. Thrombophlebitis is a complete contraindication to massage. Constipation may be helped by abdominal massage.
- Increased urination may require the client to get up in the middle of the massage. Privacy and quick access to the bathroom should be provided. Water fountains and music that may stimulate the urge to urinate should be avoided. Rash or itching is a local contraindication

to massage and should be reported to the physician immediately. If severe or widespread, no massage should be given. Abnormal growth of breast tissue in men or women requires caution in depth and pressure of chest massage. If too tender, massage to the chest should be avoided.

---

mexiletene hydrochloride (MEKS-il-eh-teen high-droh-KLOR-ighd)

Mexitil

Drug Class: Class IB ventricular antiarrhythmic

Drug Actions

Abolishes ventricular arrhythmias

Use

- Refractory life-threatening ventricular arrhythmias, including ventricular tachycardia and PVCs
- Diabetic neuropathy

Side Effects

Cardiovascular: hypotension, bradycardia, widened QRS complex, arrhythmias, palpitations, chest pain.
Gastrointestinal: nausea, vomiting.
Nervous System: tremor, dizziness, blurred vision, ataxia, double vision, confusion, nystagmus, nervousness, headache.
Skin: rash.

Onset, Peak, and Duration

Route	Onset	Peak	Duration
Oral	$^1/_2$–2 hr	2–3 hr	Unknown

Massage Considerations

- There are no cautions or contraindications to massage related to the action of this drug.
- There will, however, be cautions and contraindications to massage related to the client condition.
- Side effects of dizziness and hypotension require care in getting the client on and off the table. Stimulation with effleurage and tapotement at the end of the session may help.
- Rash is a local contraindication to massage and should be reported to the physician. If severe, massage should be withheld.

---

miglitol (MIG-lih-tall)

Glyset

Drug Class: Antidiabetic

Drug Actions

Lowers glucose level through reversible inhibition of alpha glucosidases in the small intestine; they convert oligosaccharides and disaccharides to glucose. Inhibiting these enzymes delays glucose absorption. Drug has no effect on insulin secretion.

Use

- Monotherapy as an adjunct to diet to improve glycemic control in patients with type 2 diabetes mellitus

Side Effects

Gastrointestinal: abdominal pain, diarrhea, gas.
Skin: rash.

Onset, Peak, and Duration

Route	Onset	Peak	Duration
Oral	Unknown	2–3 hr	Unknown

 Massage Considerations

- There are no cautions or contraindications to massage related to this drug. In most cases, there will be cautions and contraindications to massage related to the client condition.
- Side effects of gas may be helped with abdominal massage. Rash is a local contraindication to massage and should be reported to the physician. If severe or widespread, massage should be withheld.

---

minocycline hydrochloride (migh-noh-SIGH-kleen high-droh-KLOR-ighd)

Akamin, Alti-Minocycline, Apo-Minocycline, Dynacin, Minocin, Minomycin, Novo-Minocycline, PMS-Minocycline

Drug Class: Antibiotic

Drug Actions

Hinders bacterial cell growth

Use

- Infections caused by sensitive gram-negative and gram-positive organisms
- Trachoma
- Amebiasis
- Gonorrhea in patients sensitive to penicillin
- Syphilis in patients sensitive to penicillin
- Meningococcal carrier state
- Uncomplicated urethral, endocervical, or rectal infection
- Uncomplicated gonococcal urethritis in men
- Multibacillary leprosy
- Nocardiosis
- Nongonococcal urethritis

Side Effects

Cardiovascular: pericarditis, thrombophlebitis.
Gastrointestinal: anorexia, epigastric distress, oral candidiasis, nausea, vomiting, diarrhea, enterocolitis, inflammatory lesions in anogenital region.
Nervous System: light-headedness or dizziness from vestibular toxicity, intracranial hypertension (pseudotumor cerebri).

Skin: rashes, photosensitivity reactions, increased pigmentation, hives.
Other: permanent discoloration of teeth, enamel defects, hypersensitivity reactions (anaphylaxis), difficulty swallowing, glossitis, abnormal blood profiles, bone growth retardation if used in children younger than age 8; superinfection.

Onset, Peak, and Duration

Route	Onset	Peak	Duration
Oral	Unknown	1–4 hr	Unknown
I.V.	Immediate	Immediate	Unknown

Massage Considerations

- There are no cautions or contraindications to massage related to this drug. There may be cautions or contraindications to massage related to the client condition and severity of infection.
- Side effects of thrombophlebitis are a complete contraindication to massage. Dizziness requires care in positioning and getting the client on and off the table. Stay with the client as they sit up after the session until certain that there are no symptoms of light-headedness.
- Rash is a local contraindication to massage and should be reported to the physician immediately. If severe or widespread, no massage should be given.

---

minoxidil (migh-NOKS-uh-dil)

Loniten

Drug Class: Antihypertensive

Drug Actions

Unknown; produces direct arteriolar vasodilation. Lowers blood pressure.

Use

- Severe hypertension

Side Effects

Cardiovascular: edema, tachycardia, pericardial effusion and tamponade, heart failure, ECG changes.
Skin: hypertrichosis (elongation, thickening, and enhanced pigmentation of fine body hair), rash, Stevens-Johnson syndrome.
Other: breast tenderness, weight gain.

Onset, Peak, and Duration

Route	Onset	Peak	Duration
Oral	About 30 min	≤1 hr	2–5 days

Massage Considerations

- There are no cautions or contraindications to massage related to this drug. There may be cautions and contraindications to massage related to the client condition.
- The vasodilating action of the drug may increase the effects of circulatory massage with effleurage. Using friction to the legs or more rapid effleurage and tapotement at the end of the session may prevent problems with dizziness.
- Side effects of breast tenderness require caution with depth and pressure of chest massage. If too tender, the area should be avoided. Rash is a local contraindication to massage and should be reported to the physician. If severe, massage should be withheld.

mirtazapine (mir-TAH-zuh-peen)

Remeron, Remeron SolTab

Drug Class: Antidepressant

Drug Actions

Relieves depression

Use

- Depression

Side Effects

Cardiovascular: edema, peripheral edema.
Gastrointestinal: nausea, increased appetite, dry mouth, constipation.
Nervous System: sleepiness, dizziness, weakness, abnormal dreams, abnormal thinking, tremor, confusion.
Urinary: urinary frequency.
Other: flulike syndrome, neutropenia, agranulocytosis, weight gain, back pain, muscle pain, shortness of breath.

Onset, Peak, and Duration

Route	Onset	Peak	Duration
Oral	Unknown	Within 2 hr	Unknown

Massage Considerations

- There are no cautions or contraindications to massage related to the action of this drug.
- There may be cautions or contraindications to massage related to the client condition.
- Side effects of sleepiness and drowsiness require care in getting the client on and off the table. Stimulation with rapid effleurage or tapotement at the end of the session may help. Constipation may be helped by abdominal massage.

misoprostol (mee-SOH-pruh-stol)

Cytotec

Drug Class: Gastric mucosal protectant

Drug Actions

Protects gastric mucosa from ulcerating

Use

- Prevention of NSAID-induced gastric ulcer in elderly or debilitated patients at high risk for complications from gastric ulcer and in patients with history of NSAID-induced ulcer
- Duodenal or gastric ulcer

Side Effects

Gastrointestinal: diarrhea, abdominal pain, nausea, gas, painful digestion, vomiting, constipation.
Nervous System: headache.
Other: hypermenorrhea, dysmenorrhea, spotting, cramps, menstrual disorders.

Onset, Peak, and Duration

Route	Onset	Peak	Duration
Oral	30 min	10–15 min	3 hr

Massage Considerations

- There are no cautions and contraindications to massage related to the actions of this drug.
- Side effects of gas and constipation may be helped by regular abdominal massage.

---

mitomycin (mitomycin-C) (might-oh-MIGH-sin)

Mitozytrex, Mutamycin

Drug Class: Antineoplastic

Drug Actions

Kills certain cancer cells

Use

- Disseminated pancreatic and stomach cancers
- Bladder cancer

Side Effects

CNS: headache, neurologic abnormalities, confusion, drowsiness, fatigue, fever.
Gastrointestinal: nausea, vomiting, anorexia, stomatitis.
Nervous System: headache, neurologic abnormalities, confusion, drowsiness, fatigue, fever.
Urinary: renal toxicity, hemolytic uremic syndrome.
Skin: pealing, induration, itching, and pain at injection site; septicemia, cellulitis, ulceration, and sloughing with extravasation; reversible hair loss; purple coloration of nail beds.
Other: abnormal blood profiles, pulmonary edema, shortness of breath, nonproductive cough, acute respiratory distress syndrome, interstitial pneumonitis.

Onset, Peak, and Duration

Route	Onset	Peak	Duration
I.V.	Unknown	Unknown	Unknown

Massage Considerations

- Because of the toxic effects of this drug, deep tissue massage is contraindicated and circulatory massage with effleurage should be used with caution and limited.
- There may be further cautions and contraindications to massage related to the client condition.
- The physician should be consulted before any massage is given, and close collaboration is essential.
- This drug is usually given every 6–8 weeks and has a very short half-life. Massage would best be given on weeks that the drug is not given and prior to administration during the week that it is given.
- Side effects of drowsiness require stimulation at the end of the session with friction to the legs or tapotement. Neurological abnormalities, if they include neuropathies or paresthesia require caution in depth and pressure of massage to the affected areas. Itching is a local contraindication to massage and should be reported to the physician immediately.

If severe, massage may be completely contraindicated. Hair loss is a contraindication to scalp massage if the client is disturbed by hair loss during the massage or if the scalp is tender.
- The best approach to massage for this client is to use the systemic reflex strokes and mechanical strokes of rocking, friction, pétrissage, and local reflex strokes of stretching, traction, and gentle compression.

---

mitoxantrone hydrochloride (migh-toh-ZAN-trohn high-droh-KLOR-ighd)

Novantrone

Drug Class: Antineoplastic

Drug Actions

Hinders susceptible cancer cell growth

Use

- Combination initial therapy for acute nonlymphocytic leukemia
- To reduce neurologic disability and frequency of relapse in chronic progressive, progressive relapsing, or worsening relapsing-remitting multiple sclerosis
- Combination initial therapy for pain from advanced hormone-refractory prostate cancer

Side Effects

Cardiovascular: heart failure, arrhythmias, tachycardia.
Gastrointestinal: bleeding, abdominal pain, diarrhea, nausea, mucositis, vomiting, stomatitis.
Nervous System: seizures, headache.
Urinary: uric acid nephropathy, renal impairment.
Skin: petechiae, bruising, hair loss.
Other: conjunctivitis, myelosuppression, jaundice, hyperuricemia, shortness of breath, cough.

Onset, Peak, and Duration

Route	Onset	Peak	Duration
I.V.	Unknown	Unknown	Unknown

Massage Considerations

- Because of the toxic effects of this drug, deep tissue massage and circulatory massage with effleurage should be used with caution and limited.
- In most cases, there will be further cautions and contraindications to massage related to the client condition.
- The physician should be consulted before any massage is given, and close collaboration is essential.
- This drug may be given daily for anywhere from 3 to 21 days, or may be given every few months. It has a long half-life of over 5 days. It is best to give massage on the weeks when the drug is not being given. If given during the weeks the drug is administered, the massage should be given before the administration, and effleurage should be severely limited so as not to overtax the liver and kidney as they try to rid the body of the drug.
- Side effects of bruising requires caution in the depth and pressure of the massage. Hair loss is a contraindication to scalp massage if the client is disturbed by hair loss during the massage or the scalp is tender.
- The best approach for this client is to use local reflex and mechanical strokes such as stretching, traction, pétrissage, and gentle friction and compression.

modafinil (moh-DAF-ih-nil)

Provigil

Drug Class: Nonamphetamine CNS stimulant

Drug Actions

Unknown. It has wake-promoting actions similar to those of sympathomimetics, including amphetamines, but it is structurally distinct from amphetamines and does not appear to alter the release of either dopamine or norepinephrine to produce CNS stimulation. Improves daytime wakefulness.

Use

- To improve wakefulness in patients with excessive daytime sleepiness caused by narcolepsy

Side Effects

Cardiovascular: hypotension, hypertension, vasodilation, arrhythmias, chest pain.
Gastrointestinal: nausea, diarrhea, dry mouth, mouth ulcer, gingivitis, thirst, anorexia, vomiting.
Nervous System: headache, nervousness, dizziness, depression, anxiety, fever, cataplexy, insomnia, paresthesia, dyskinesia, hypertonia, confusion, amnesia, emotional lability, ataxia, syncope, tremor.
Urinary: abnormal urine, urine retention, abnormal ejaculation.
Skin: herpes simplex, dry skin.
Other: chills, rhinitis, pharyngitis, nose bleed, amblyopia, abnormal vision, eosinophilia, hyperglycemia, neck pain, rigid neck, joint disorder, lung disorders, shortness of breath, asthma.

Onset, Peak, and Duration

Route	Onset	Peak	Duration
Oral	Unknown	2–4 hr	Unknown

Massage Considerations

- There are no cautions or contraindications to massage related to the actions of this drug.
- Although the drug produces stimulation of the CNS, the exact mechanism is unknown. It may potentially decrease the effectiveness of systemic reflex strokes such as rocking, effleurage and friction and may decrease the relaxing effects of massage. Applying these strokes for longer than usual periods may help, or focus on the mechanical effects of the strokes such as effleurage given slow and rhythmically, as well as pétrissage and compression.
- Side effects of hypotension and dizziness require care in getting the client on and off the table. Using tapotement and rapid effleurage at the end of the session may help.

moexipril hydrochloride (moh-EKS-eh-pril high-droh-KLOR-ighd)

Univasc

Drug Class: ACE (angiotensin converting enzyme) inhibitor antihypertensive

Drug Actions

Unknown; may suppress renin-angiotensin-aldosterone system. Inhibits ACE, thereby inhibiting production of angiotensin II (a potent vasoconstrictor and stimulator of aldosterone secretion). Lowers blood pressure.

Use

- Hypertension

Side Effects

Cardiovascular: peripheral edema, hypotension, orthostatic hypotension, chest pain, flushing.
Gastrointestinal: diarrhea, painful digestion, nausea.
Nervous System: dizziness, headache, fatigue, pain.
Urinary: urinary frequency.
Skin: rash.
Other: anaphylaxis, angioedema, flulike syndrome, pharyngitis, rhinitis, sinusitis, neutropenia, hyperkalemia, muscle pain, persistent, nonproductive cough; upper respiratory tract infection.

Onset, Peak, and Duration

Route	Onset	Peak	Duration
Oral	1 hr	3–6 hr	24 hr

Massage Considerations

- There are no cautions or contraindications to massage related to this drug. There may be cautions or contraindications to massage related to the client condition.
- Side effects of hypotension and dizziness require care in getting the client on and off the table. Using stimulation with rapid effleurage or tapotement at the end of the session may help. Urinary frequency may require the client to get up in the middle of the session.
- Privacy and quick access to the bathroom should be provided. Water fountains or music that may stimulate the need to urinate should not be used. Rash is a local contraindication to massage and should be reported to the physician immediately. If severe or widespread, massage should be withheld.

---

montelukast sodium (mon-tih-LOO-kist SOH-dee-um)

Singulair

Drug Class: Antiasthmatic

Drug Actions

Reduces early- and late-phase bronchoconstriction caused by antigen challenge. Improves breathing.

Use

- Asthma
- Seasonal allergic rhinitis
- Prevention of exercise-induced bronchoconstriction

Side Effects

Gastrointestinal: painful digestion, infectious gastroenteritis, abdominal pain.
Nervous System: headache, dizziness, fatigue, fever, weakness.
Urinary: pus in the urine.
Skin: rash.
Other: trauma, influenza, dental pain, nasal congestion.

Onset, Peak, and Duration

Route	Onset	Peak	Duration
Oral:			
Coated	Unknown	3–4 hr	Unknown
Chewable	Unknown	$2\text{–}2^1/_2$ hr	Unknown

 Massage Considerations

- There are no cautions or contraindications to massage related to the actions of this drug. There may be cautions and contraindications to massage related to the client condition.
- Side effects of dizziness may be helped by using stimulation at the end of the massage with rapid effleurage or tapotement. Rash is a local contraindication to massage and should be reported to the physician. If severe or widespread, massage should be withheld.

---

morphine hydrochloride (MOR-feen high-droh-KLOR-ighd)

M.O.S., M.O.S.-SR

morphine sulfate

Astramorph PF, Avinza, DMS Concentrate, Duramorph PF, Infumorph 200, Infumorph 500, Kadian, Morphine H.P., MS Contin, MSIR, MS/L, MS/L concentrate, OMS concentrate, Oramorph SR, RMS Uniserts, Roxanol, Roxanol 100, Roxanol T, Statex

morphine tartrate

Drug Class: Opioid analgesic

Drug Actions

Binds with opioid receptors in CNS, altering both perception of and emotional response to pain through unknown mechanism

Use

- Severe pain
- Severe pain associated with terminal cancer

Side Effects

Cardiovascular: hypotension, flushing, bradycardia, shock, cardiac arrest.
Gastrointestinal: nausea, vomiting, constipation, ileus.
Nervous System: sedation, sleepiness, clouded sensorium, euphoria, seizures (with large doses), dizziness, nightmares (with long-acting oral forms).
Urinay: urine retention.
Skin: itching and flushing with epidural administration.
Other: physical dependence, thrombocytopenia, respiratory depression, respiratory arrest.

Onset, Peak, and Duration

Route	Onset	Peak	Duration
Oral	1 hr	1–2 hr	4–12 hr
I.V.	<5 min	20 min	4–5 hr
I.M.	10–30 min	30–60 min	4–5 hr
S.C. Injection	10–30 min	50–90 min	4–5 hr
Rectal	20–60 min	20–60 min	4–5 hr
Epidural	15–60 min	15–60 min	24 hr
Intrathecal	15–60 min	Unknown	24 hr

Massage Considerations

- This drug changes the perception of pain and depresses the CNS. Deep tissue massage should be used with great caution if at all.
- There may be further cautions and contraindications to massage related to the client condition.
- The action of this drug may decrease the effectiveness of the local reflex strokes of stretching, traction, compression and vibration, as well as of deep tissue massage. These strokes may need to be applied for longer periods than usual to be effective. This drug may increase the actions of the systemic reflex strokes of effleurage, rocking, and friction as well as the relaxation effects of massage. Using the strokes such as effleurage and friction in a more rapid and stimulating manner throughout the massage may help.
- The site of I.M. or subcutaneous injection of the drug should not be massaged for at least 2 hours.
- Side effects of hypotension, sleepiness, and dizziness may be addressed as noted above. Constipation may be helped by regular abdominal massage. Itching is a local contraindication to massage and should be reported to the physician. It occurs more often with I.V. dosing than with other methods of administration. If severe, massage may be contraindicated completely until the condition has resolved.
- The best approach to this client is to use the mechanical strokes. Applying stimulating effleurage, pétrissage, and friction may be the most effective.

moxifloxacin hydrochloride (mox-ih-FLOX-uh-sin high-droh-CLOR-ighd)

Avelox, Avelox I.V.

Drug Class: Antibiotic

Drug Actions

Kills susceptible bacteria

Use

- Acute bacterial sinusitis
- Acute bacterial exacerbation of chronic bronchitis
- Community-acquired pneumonia
- Uncomplicated skin and skin-structure infections

Side Effects

Cardiovascular: prolonged QT interval, chest pain, palpitations, tachycardia, hypertension, peripheral edema.

Gastrointestinal: pseudomembranous colitis, nausea, diarrhea, abdominal pain, vomiting, painful digestion, dry mouth, constipation, oral candidiasis, anorexia, stomatitis, glossitis, gas, gastrointestinal disorder, taste perversion.
Nervous System: dizziness, headache, weakness, pain, malaise, insomnia, nervousness, anxiety, confusion, sleepiness, tremor, paresthesia.
Skin: rash itching, sweating.
Other: candidiasis, allergic reaction, injection site reaction. Abnormal blood profiles, liver dysfunction, cholestatic jaundice, vaginitis, vaginal candidiasis, leg pain, back pain, joint pain, muscle pain, tendon rupture, shortness of breath.

Onset, Peak, and Duration

Route	Onset	Peak	Duration
Oral, I.V.	Unknown	1–3 hr	Unknown

Massage Considerations

- There are no cautions or contraindications to massage related to this drug. There may be cautions and contraindications to massage related to the client condition and severity of infection.
- Side effects of dizziness and sleepiness may be helped by stimulation at the end of the session with rapid effleurage or tapotement. Paresthesia is a contraindication to deep tissue massage. Constipation and gas may be helped by abdominal massage. Rash is a local contraindication to massage and should be reported to the physician immediately. If severe or widespread, massage should be withheld.

---

moxifloxacin hydrochloride ophthalmic solution

(mocks-ih-FLOCKS-ah-sin high-droe-KLOR-ighd off-THAL-mick suh-LOO-shun)

Vigamox

Drug Class: Antibiotic

Drug Actions

Kills susceptible bacteria causing infection

Use

- Bacterial conjunctivitis

Side Effects

Skin: rash.
Other: infection, fever, conjunctivitis; dry eyes; increased lacrimation; keratitis; ocular hyperemia; ocular discomfort, pain, and pruritus; otitis media; pharyngitis; reduced visual acuity; rhinitis; subconjunctival hemorrhage, increased cough.

Onset, Peak, and Duration

Route	Onset	Peak	Duration
Ocular	Unknown	Unknown	Unknown

Massage Considerations

- There are no cautions or contraindications to massage related to the actions of this drug.
- Side effects of rash are a local contraindication to massage and should be reported to the physician immediately.

muromonab-CD3 (myoo-roh-MOH-nab see dee three)

Orthoclone OKT3

Drug Class: Monoclonal antibody immunosuppressive

Drug Actions

Halts acute allograft rejection in kidney transplantation

Use

- Acute allograft rejection in heart, liver, or kidney transplant

Side Effects

Cardiovascular: vasodilation, arrhythmia, bradycardia, hypertension, hypotension, chest pain, tachycardia, vascular occlusion, edema, cardiac arrest, shock, heart failure.
Gastrointestinal: anorexia, diarrhea, nausea, abdominal pain, GI pain, vomiting.
Nervous System: weakness, fatigue, lethargy, malaise, fever, seizures, dizziness, headache, meningitis, tremor, confusion, depression, nervousness, sleepiness.
Urinary: renal dysfunction.
Skin: diaphoresis, itching, rash.
Other: chills, pain in trunk area, cytokine release syndrome, hypersensitivity reactions, photophobia, ringing in the ears, abnormal blood profiles, joint pain, muscle pain,shortness of breath, hyperventilation, hypoxia, pneumonia, pulmonary edema, respiratory congestion, wheezing, acute respiratory distress syndrome.

Onset, Peak, and Duration

Route	Onset	Peak	Duration
I.V.	Almost immediately	Unknown	1 wk after therapy stops

Massage Considerations

- There are no cautions or contraindications to massage related to the actions of this drug.
- In most cases, there will be cautions and contraindications to massage related to the client condition.
- The physician should be consulted before any massage is given, and close collaboration is essential.
- Because this drug suppresses the immune system, it would be best to schedule the client as the first session of the day so as not to expose the client to other people. If the massage therapist has any infection, no massage should be given.
- Side effects of hypotension, dizziness, and sleepiness require care in getting the client on and off the table. Using stimulation at the end of the massage with effleurage and tapotement may help. Rash or itching is a local contraindication to massage and should be reported to the physician immediately. If severe or widespread, no massage should be given.

mycophenolate mofetil (migh-koh-FEN-oh-layt MOH-feh-til)

CellCept

mycophenolate mofetil hydrochloride

CellCept Intravenous

Drug Class: Immunosuppressant

Drug Actions

Prevents organ rejection

Use

- Prevention of organ rejection in patients receiving allogeneic renal transplants
- Prevention of organ rejection in patients receiving allogeneic cardiac transplants
- Prevention of organ rejection in patients receiving allogeneic hepatic transplants

Side Effects

Cardiovascular: chest pain, hypertension, edema, peripheral edema.
Gastrointestinal: diarrhea, constipation, nausea, painful digestion, vomiting, oral candidiasis, abdominal pain, hemorrhage.
Nervous System: tremor, insomnia, dizziness, headache, pain, fever, weakness.
Urinary: urinary tract infections, hematuria, kidney tubular necrosis.
Skin: acne, rash.
Other: infection, sepsis, pharyngitis, abnormal blood profiles, hypercholesteremia, hypophosphatemia, hypokalemia, hyperkalemia, hyperglycemia, back pain, shortness of breath, cough, infection, bronchitis, pneumonia.

Onset, Peak, and Duration

Route	Onset	Peak	Duration
Oral	Unknown	Unknown	Unknown
I.V.	Unknown	Unknown	10–17 hr

Massage Considerations

- There are no cautions or contraindications to massage related to the actions of this drug.
- In most cases, there will be cautions and contraindications to massage related to the client condition.
- The physician should be consulted before any massage is given, and close collaboration is essential.
- Because this drug suppresses the immune system, it would be best to schedule the client as the first session of the day so as not to expose the client to other people. If the massage therapist has any infection, no massage should be given.
- Side effects of hypotension, dizziness, and sleepiness require care in getting the client on and off the table. Using stimulation at the end of the massage with effleurage and tapotement may help. Constipation may be helped by abdominal massage. Rash or acne is a local contraindication to massage and should be reported to the physician immediately. If severe or widespread, no massage should be given. If acne persists and the client wishes to receive massage, gloves may be worn while working on the affected areas.

N

nabumetone (nuh-BYOO-meh-tohn)

Apo-Nabumetone, Relafen

Drug Class: NSAID (nonsteroidal anti-inflammatory drug)

Drug Actions

May inhibit prostaglandin synthesis, relieving inflammation and pain.

Use

- Rheumatoid arthritis
- Osteoarthritis

Side Effects

Cardiovascular: vasculitis, edema.
Gastrointestinal: diarrhea, painful digestion, abdominal pain, constipation, gas, nausea, dry mouth, gastritis, stomatitis, vomiting, bleeding, ulceration.
Nervous System: dizziness, headache, fatigue, insomnia, nervousness, sleepiness.
Skin: itching, rash, increased sweating.
Other: ringing in the ears, shortness of breath, pneumonitis.

Onset, Peak, and Duration

Route	Onset	Peak	Duration
Oral	Unknown	2–4 hr	Unknown

Massage Considerations

- This drug decreases the perception of pain; therefore, deep tissue massage should be done with caution.
- Further cautions and contraindications to massage may be related to the client condition.
- Side effects such as dizziness may be helped by stimulation at the end of the massage with effleurage and tapotement. Care should be taken in getting the client on and off the table.
- Constipation and gas may be helped by abdominal massage.
- Rash or itching are local contraindications to massage and should be reported to the physician. If severe or widespread, massage should be withheld.

nadolol (nay-DOH-lol)

Apo-Nadol, Corgard

Drug Class: Nonselective beta-blocker antihypertensive, antianginal

Drug Actions

Reduces cardiac oxygen demand by blocking catecholamine-induced increases in heart rate, blood pressure, and myocardial contraction. Depresses renin secretion. Lowers blood pressure and relieves angina.

Use

- Angina pectoris
- Hypertension
- Arrhythmias
- Prevention of vascular headaches

Side Effects

Cardiovascular: bradycardia, hypotension, heart failure, peripheral vascular disease.
Gastrointestinal: nausea, vomiting, diarrhea, constipation.
Nervous System: fatigue, lethargy, dizziness, fever.
Skin: rash.
Other: increased airway resistance.

Onset, Peak, and Duration

Route	Onset	Peak	Duration
Oral	Unknown	2–4 hr	Unknown

Massage Considerations

- No cautions or contraindications to massage are indicated because a client is taking this drug. Cautions and contraindications to massage may be related to the client condition.
- The action of this drug blocks certain sympathetic nervous system receptors. This blockage may potentially increase the effects of systemic reflex strokes such as effleurage, rocking, and friction and increase the relaxation effects of massage. Using stimulation with tapotement, rapid effleurage, and friction, especially at the end of the session, may help balance this effect.
- Side effects of hypotension and dizziness may be addressed as above.
- Constipation may be helped by abdominal massage.
- Rash is a local contraindication to massage and should be reported to the physician. If severe, massage should not be given.

---

nafcillin sodium (naf-SIL-in Soh-dee-um)

Drug Class: Penicillin antibiotic

Drug Actions

Kills susceptible bacteria

Use

- Systemic infections caused by susceptible organisms
- Meningitis
- Acute or chronic osteomyelitis caused by susceptible organisms
- Native valve endocarditis caused by susceptible organisms

Side Effects

Gastrointestinal: nausea, vomiting, diarrhea.
Other: hypersensitivity reactions (chills, fever, rash, itching, hives, anaphylaxis), vein irritation, thrombophlebitis, abnormal blood profiles.

Onset, Peak, and Duration

Route	Onset	Peak	Duration
I.V.	Immediate	Immediate	Unknown

Massage Considerations

- No cautions or contraindications to massage are indicated because a client is taking this drug. Cautions and contraindications to massage may be related to the client condition.
- Side effects of thrombophlebitis are a complete contraindication to massage.
- Rash, itching, and hives are local contraindications to massage and should be reported to the physician immediately. If severe or widespread, massage should be withheld.

---

nalbuphine hydrochloride (NAL-byoo-feen high-droh-KLOR-ighd)

Nubain

Drug Class: Opioid analgesic, adjunct to anesthesia

Drug Actions

Binds with opioid receptors in the central nervous system (CNS), altering pain perception and response to pain by an unknown mechanism.

Use

- Moderate to I.M. severe pain
- Adjunct in balanced anesthesia

Side Effects

Cardiovascular: hypertension, hypotension, tachycardia, bradycardia.
Gastrointestinal: cramps, painful digestion, bitter taste, dry mouth, nausea, vomiting, constipation.
Nervous System: headache, sedation, dizziness, nervousness, depression, restlessness, crying, euphoria, hostility, unusual dreams, confusion, hallucinations, speech difficulty, delusions.
Urinary: urinary urgency.
Skin: itching; burning; hives; sweaty, clammy feeling.
Other: blurred vision, respiratory depression, pulmonary edema.

Onset, Peak, and Duration

Route	Onset	Peak	Duration
I.V.	2–3 min	≤30 min	3–4 hr
I.M.	≤15 min	≤60 min	3–6 hr
Subcutaneous Injection	≤15 min	Unknown	3–6 hr

Massage Considerations

- This drug decreases the perception of pain; therefore, deep tissue massage should be used with great caution, if at all.
- Further cautions and contraindications to massage may be related to the client condition.
- This drug depresses the CNS. Local reflex strokes such as stretching, compression, vibration, and even deep tissue massage may be less effective. Using them for a longer time may help. The relaxation effects of massage and the systemic reflex strokes of effleurage, rocking, and friction may have increased effects. Using a more rapid manner in applying these strokes may help to balance this effect.
- The site of intramuscular or subcutaneous injections should not be massaged for at least 1 to 3 hours to avoid increasing the rate of absorption of the drug into the body.
- Side effects of hypotension and dizziness require care in getting the client on and off the table. Stimulation with rapid effleurage and tapotement at the end of the session may help. If the symptom is severe, using more stimulating and rapid massage techniques throughout the session may be needed.

- Constipation may be helped by abdominal massage.
- Urinary urgency may require the client to get up in the middle of the session. Privacy and quick access to the bathroom are essential. Water fountains or water music, which may stimulate the need to urinate, should be avoided.
- Itching, burning, or hives are local contraindications to massage and should be reported to the physician. If severe or widespread, no massage should be given.
- The best approach to this client is to use mechanical strokes of pétrissage, friction, and effleurage applied in a slightly more stimulating and rapid manner.

---

naltrexone hydrochloride (nal-TREKS-ohn high-droh-KLOR-ighd)

Depade, ReVia

Drug Class: Adjunct in opioid detoxification

Drug Actions

Unknown; may reversibly block subjective effects of intravenous opioids by occupying opioid receptors in brain.

Use

- Adjunct in maintaining opioid-free state in detoxified patients
- Alcohol dependence

Side Effects

Gastrointestinal: nausea, vomiting, anorexia, abdominal pain.
Nervous System: insomnia, anxiety, nervousness, headache, depression, suicidal ideation.
Other: lymphocytosis, hepatotoxicity, muscle and joint pain.

Onset, Peak, and Duration

Route	Onset	Peak	Duration
Oral	15–30 min	>12 hr	24 hr

Massage Considerations

- No cautions or contraindications to massage are indicated because a client is taking this drug. Cautions and contraindications to massage may be related to the client condition.
- The actions of this drug may make the systemic reflex strokes of rocking, effleurage, or friction less effective. Using these strokes for longer periods of time may help. Using slow, rhythmic effleurage throughout the session may balance this effect.

---

nandrolone decanoate (NAN-druh-lohn deh-kuh-NOH-ayt)

Androlone-D, Deca-Durabolin, Hybolin Decanoate, Kabolin, Neo-Durabolic

nandrolone phenpropionate

Durabolin, Hybolin Improved

Drug Class: Pharmacologic class: Anabolic steroid

Drug Actions

Promotes tissue building, reverses catabolism, and stimulates erythropoiesis; hinders growth of breast cancer cells (phenpropionate).

Use

- Severe debility or disease states
- Refractory anemias
- Metastatic breast cancer

Side Effects

Cardiovascular: edema.
Gastrointestinal: gastroenteritis, nausea, vomiting, diarrhea, change in appetite.
Urinary: bladder irritability.
Other: androgenic effects in women (acne, edema, weight gain, abnormal hair growth, hoarseness, clitoral enlargement, decreased breast size, altered libido, male pattern baldness, oily skin or hair), hypoestrogenic effects in women (flushing, sweating, vaginitis, vaginal bleeding, nervousness, emotional lability, menstrual irregularities), excessive hormonal effects in prepubertal men (premature epiphyseal closure, acne, priapism, growth of body and facial hair, phallic enlargement), excessive hormonal effects in postpubertal men (testicular atrophy, oligospermia, decreased ejaculatory volume, impotence, abnormal growth of breast tissue, epididymitis), pain, induration at injection site, thrombocytopenia, reversible jaundice, peliosis hepatis, liver cell tumors, hypercalcemia, muscle cramps or spasms.

Onset, Peak, and Duration

Route	Onset	Peak	Duration
I.M.			
Decanoate	Unknown	3–6 days	Unknown
Phenpropionate	Unknown	1–2 days	Unknown

Massage Considerations

- This drug affects the metabolism of all the tissues in the body, changing connective, muscle, and tendon tissue. Deep tissue massage is contraindicated. Stretching and traction should be used with caution. Myofascial massage techniques may be less effective and should be used with great caution, if at all.
- Further cautions and contraindications to massage may be related to the client condition.
- The physician should be consulted before any massage is given, and close collaboration is essential.
- The site of intramuscular injection of the drug should not be massaged for 1 week.
- Side effects of acne are a local contraindication to massage. If severe and the client desires massage, the massage therapist may wear gloves when working on the affected areas.
- Abnormal growth of breast tissue requires care in massage of the chest. If the chest is too tender, massage of the area should be avoided.
- The best approach to this client is to use rocking and the mechanical strokes of effleurage, pétrissage, and gentle compression and friction.

---

naproxen (nuh-PROK-sin)

Apo-Naproxen, EC-Naprosyn, Naprosyn, Naprosyn SR, Naxen, Novo-Naprox, Nu-Naprox

naproxen sodium

Aleve, Anaprox, Anaprox DS, Apo-Napro-Na, Apo-Napro-Na DS, Naprelan, Novo-Naprox Sodium, Synflex, Synflex DS

Drug Class: NSAID (nonsteroidal anti-inflammatory drug)

Drug Actions

Unknown; produces anti-inflammatory, analgesic, and antipyretic effects, possibly by inhibiting prostaglandin synthesis.

Use

- Rheumatoid arthritis
- Osteoarthritis
- Ankylosing spondylitis
- Juvenile arthritis
- Acute gout
- Mild to moderate pain
- Primary dysmenorrhea
- Acute tendinitis and bursitis

Side Effects

Cardiovascular: peripheral edema, palpitations, digital vasculitis.
Gastrointestinal: epigastric distress, occult blood loss, nausea, peptic ulceration.
Nervous System: headache, drowsiness, dizziness, ringing in the ears, cognitive dysfunction, aseptic meningitis.
Urinary: nephrotoxicity.
Skin: itching, rash, hives.
Other: visual disturbances, abnormal blood profiles, hyperkalemia, shortness of breath.

Onset, Peak, and Duration

Route	Onset	Peak	Duration
Oral	≤1 hr	1–6 hr	7–12 hr
Rectal	Unknown	Unknown	Unknown

Massage Considerations

- This drug decreases the perception of pain. Deep tissue massage should be used with caution.
- Further cautions and contraindications to massage may be related to the client condition.
- Side effects of dizziness and drowsiness require care in getting the client on and off the table. Using stimulation with rapid effleurage and tapotement at the end of the session may help.
- Itching, rash, or hives are local contraindications to massage and should be reported to the physician. If severe or widespread, massage should be withheld.

naratriptan hydrochloride (nah-rah-TRIP-tin high-droh-KLOR-ighd)

Amerge, Naramig

Drug Class: Antimigraine drug

Drug Actions

May activate receptors in intracranial blood vessels, leading to vasoconstriction and relief of migraine headache; activation of receptors on sensory nerve endings in trigeminal system may inhibit proinflammatory neuropeptide release.

Use

- Acute migraine headaches with or without aura

Side Effects

Cardiovascular: palpitations, increased blood pressure, tachyarrhythmias, abnormal electrocardiogram (ECG) changes (PR and QT interval prolongation, ST/T wave abnormalities, premature ventricular contractions, atrial flutter or fibrillation), coronary vasospasm, coronary artery vasospasm, transient myocardial ischemia, heart attack, ventricular tachycardia, ventricular fibrillation.
Gastrointestinal: nausea, hyposalivation, vomiting.
Nervous System: paresthesias, dizziness, drowsiness, malaise, fatigue, syncope.
Other: warm or cold temperature sensations; pressure, tightness, and heaviness sensations; ear, nose, and throat infections; photophobia.

Onset, Peak, and Duration

Route	Onset	Peak	Duration
Oral	Unknown	2–3 hr	Unknown

 Massage Considerations

- No cautions or contraindications to massage are indicated because a client is taking this drug. Cautions and contraindications to massage may be related to the client condition.
- Side effects of dizziness and drowsiness require care in getting the client on and off the table. Using stimulation with effleurage and taptotement at the end of the session may help.
- Paresthesia is a local contraindication to deep tissue massage.

---

nateglinide (na-TEG-li-nide)

Starlix

Drug Class: Antidiabetic

Drug Actions

Stimulates insulin secretion from the pancreas. Lowers glucose level.

Use

- Alone or with metformin or a thiazolidinedione to lower glucose levels in patients with type 2 diabetes.

Side Effects

Gastrointestinal: diarrhea.
Nervous System: dizziness.
Other: flulike symptoms, accidental trauma, hypoglycemia, back pain, arthropathy, upper respiratory tract infection, bronchitis, coughing.

Onset, Peak, and Duration

Route	Onset	Peak	Duration
Oral	20 min	1 hr	4 hr

Massage Considerations

- No cautions or contraindications to massage are related to the actions of this drug. Cautions and contraindications to massage may be related to the client condition.
- Side effects of dizziness require care in getting the client on and off the table. Stimulation with effleurage or tapotement at the end of the session may help.

nefazodone hydrochloride (nef-AZ-oh-dohn high-droh-KLOR-ighd)

Serzone

Drug Class: Antidepressant

Drug Actions

Not precisely defined. Drug inhibits neuronal uptake of serotonin ($5\text{-}HT_2$) and norepinephrine; it also occupies serotonin and α_1-adrenergic receptors in CNS. Relieves depression.

Use

- Depression

Side Effects

Cardiovascular: vasodilation, orthostatic hypotension, hypotension, peripheral edema.
Gastrointestinal: dry mouth, nausea, constipation, painful digestion, diarrhea, increased appetite, vomiting, taste perversion.
Nervous System: headache, fever, sleepiness, dizziness, weakness, insomnia, light-headedness, confusion, memory impairment, paresthesia, abnormal dreams, decreased concentration, ataxia, incoordination, psychomotor retardation, tremor, hypertonia.
Urinary: urinary frequency, urinary tract infection, urine retention, vaginitis.
Skin: itching, rash.
Other: infection, flulike syndrome, chills, thirst, breast pain, blurred vision, abnormal vision, pharyngitis, ringing in the ears, visual field defect, hyponatremia, neck rigidity, joint pain, cough.

Onset, Peak, and Duration

Route	Onset	Peak	Duration
Inhalation	10–17 min	90 min	5–8 hr

Massage Considerations

- No cautions or contraindications to massage are related to the actions of this drug. Cautions and contraindications to massage may be related to the client condition.
- Side effects of hypotension, dizziness, and sleepiness require care in getting the client on and off the table. Using stimulation with rapid effleurage and tapotement at the end of the session may help. If the symptom is severe, using more rapid and stimulating massage strokes throughout the session may be needed.
- Paresthesia is a local contraindication to deep tissue massage.
- Constipation may be helped by abdominal massage.
- Urinary frequency requires privacy and quick access to the bathroom. Water fountains or water music, which may stimulate urination, should be avoided.
- Rash and itching are local contraindications to massage and should be reported to the physician. If severe, massage should be withheld.

nelfinavir mesylate (nel-FIN-uh-veer MES-ih-layt)

Viracept

Drug Class: HIV protease inhibitor antiviral

Drug Actions

Reduces viral replication and spread

Use

- HIV infection when antiretroviral therapy is warranted
- Postexposure prophylaxis following occupational exposure to HIV

Side Effects

Gastrointestinal: nausea, diarrhea, gas, pancreatitis.
Nervous System: seizures, suicidal ideation.
Skin: rash.
Other: redistribution or accumulation of body fat, abnormal blood profiles, hepatitis, dehydration, diabetes mellitus, hyperlipidemia, hyperuricemia, hypoglycemia.

Onset, Peak, and Duration

Route	Onset	Peak	Duration
Oral	Unknown	2–4 hr	Unknown

 Massage Considerations

- No cautions or contraindications to massage are related to the actions of this drug. Cautions and contraindications to massage may be related to the client condition.
- Side effects of gas may be helped by abdominal massage.
- Rash is a local contraindication to massage and should be reported to the physician. If severe or widespread, massage should be withheld.

---

neostigmine bromide (nee-oh-STIG-meen BROH-mighd)

Prostigmin

neostigmine methylsulfate

Prostigmin

Drug Class: Cholinesterase inhibitor muscle stimulant

Drug Actions

Inhibits destruction of acetylcholine released from parasympathetic and somatic efferent nerves. Acetylcholine accumulates, promoting increased stimulation of receptor. Stimulates muscle contraction.

Use

- Myasthenia gravis
- To diagnose myasthenia gravis
- Postoperative abdominal distension and bladder atony
- Antidote for nondepolarizing neuromuscular blockers
- Supraventricular tachycardia from tricyclic antidepressant overdose
- To decrease small bowel transit time during radiography

Side Effects

Cardiovascular: bradycardia, hypotension, cardiac arrest.
Gastrointestinal: nausea, vomiting, diarrhea, abdominal cramps, excessive salivation.
Nervous System: dizziness, headache, mental confusion, jitters.
Urinary: urinary frequency.
Skin: rash (with bromide), sweating.

Other: hypersensitivity reactions (anaphylaxis), blurred vision, lacrimation, miosis, muscle cramps, muscle weakness, muscle fasciculations, depressed respiratory drive, bronchospasm, bronchoconstriction, respiratory arrest.

Onset, Peak, and Duration

Route	Onset	Peak	Duration
Oral	45–75 min	1–2 hr	2–4 hr
I.V.	4–8 min	1–2 hr	2–4 hr
I.M.	20–30 min	1–2 hr	2–4 hr
Subcutaneous Injection	Unknown	1–2 hr	2–4 hr

Massage Considerations

- No cautions or contraindications to massage are related to the actions of this drug. Cautions and contraindications to massage may be related to the client condition.
- The action of this drug may make the local reflex strokes of stretching, compression, and vibration as well as deep tissue massage less effective. Using them for longer periods than usual may produce the desired results. Using mechanical strokes of pétrissage and effleurage may be more effective.
- Side effects of hypotension or dizziness require care in getting the client on and off the table. Stimulation with rapid effleurage and tapotement at the end of the session may help.
- Urinary frequency may require the client to go to the bathroom in the middle of the session. Privacy and quick access to the bathroom are essential. Water fountains or water music, which may stimulate urination, should be avoided.
- Rash is a local contraindication to massage and should be reported to the physician. If severe, massage should be withheld.

---

nevirapine (neh-VEER-uh-peen)

Viramune

Drug Class: Nonnucleoside reverse transcriptase inhibitor antiviral

Drug Actions

May inhibit replication of HIV-1

Use

- Adjunct for patients with HIV-1 infection whose condition is deteriorating
- Adjunct therapy in children infected with HIV-1
- Prevention of maternal-fetal transmission of HIV

Side Effects

Gastrointestinal: nausea, diarrhea, abdominal pain, ulcerative stomatitis.
Nervous System: headache, paresthesia, fever.
Skin: rash, blistering, Stevens-Johnson syndrome.
Other: hepatitis, hepatotoxicity, muscle pain.

Onset, Peak, and Duration

Route	Onset	Peak	Duration
Oral	Unknown	4 hr	Unknown

Massage Considerations

- No cautions or contraindications to massage are related to the actions of this drug. Cautions and contraindications to massage may be related to the client condition.
- Side effects of paresthesia are a local contraindication to deep tissue massage.
- Rash or blistering are local contraindications to massage and should be reported to the physician immediately. If severe or widespread, massage should be withheld.

niacin (vitamin B_3, nicotinic acid) (NIGH-uh-sin)

niacin

Niacin TR Tablets, Niacor, Niaspan, Nico-400, Nocobid, Nicolar, Nocotinex, Slo-Niacin

niacinamide (nicotinamide)

Drug Class: Vitamin B_3, antilipemic, peripheral vasodilator

Drug Actions

Niacin and niacinamide stimulate lipid metabolism, tissue respiration, and glycogenolysis; niacin decreases synthesis of low density lipoproteins and inhibits lipolysis in adipose tissue. Restores normal level of vitamin B_3, lowers triglyceride and cholesterol levels, and dilates peripheral blood vessels.

Use

- Daily vitamin supplement
- Pellagra
- Hartnup disease
- Niacin deficiency
- Hyperlipidemias, especially with hypercholesterolemia

Side Effects

Cardiovascular: flushing, excessive peripheral vasodilation, arrhythmias.
Gastrointestinal: nausea, vomiting, diarrhea, possible activation of peptic ulceration, epigastric or substernal pain.
Nervous System: dizziness, transient headache.
Skin: itching, dryness, tingling.
Other: hepatic dysfunction, hyperglycemia, hyperuricemia.

Onset, Peak, and Duration

Route	Onset	Peak	Duration
Oral	Unknown	45 min	Unknown
I.V., I.M., Subcutaneous Injection	Unknown	Unknown	Unknown

Massage Considerations

- No cautions or contraindications to massage are related to the actions of this drug. Cautions and contraindications to massage may be related to the client condition.
- The site of intramuscular or subcutaneous injection should not be massaged for at least 2 to 3 hours.
- Side effects of dizziness may be helped by using stimulation at the end of the massage with effleurage and tapotement.

- Itching is a local contraindication to massage and should be reported to the physician. If severe, massage should be withheld.

nicardipine hydrochloride (nigh-KAR-dih-peen high-droh-KLOR-ighd)

Cardene, Cardene I.V., Cardene SR

Drug Class: Calcium channel blocker antianginal, antihypertensive

Drug Actions

Inhibits calcium ion influx across cardiac and smooth muscle cells, decreasing myocardial contractility and oxygen demand. Also dilates coronary arteries and arterioles. Lowers blood pressure and relieves angina.

Use

- Chronic stable angina (alone or with other antianginals)
- Hypertension

Side Effects

Cardiovascular: peripheral edema, palpitations, angina, tachycardia, flushing.
Gastrointestinal: nausea, abdominal discomfort, dry mouth.
Nervous System: dizziness, headache (intravenous form), paresthesia, drowsiness, weakness.
Skin: rash.

Onset, Peak, and Duration

Route	Onset	Peak	Duration
Oral	≤20 min	30 min–4 hr	6–12 hr
I.V.	Immediate	Within minutes	Soon after therapy stops

Massage Considerations

- No cautions or contraindications to massage are indicated because a client is taking this drug. Cautions and contraindications to massage may be related to the client condition.
- Side effects of dizziness may be helped by using stimulation with rapid effleurage and tapotement at the end of the sesssion.
- Paresthesia is a local contraindication to deep tissue massage.
- Rash is a local contraindication to massage and should be reported to the physician.

nifedipine (nigh-FEH-duh-peen)

Adalat, Adalat CC, Adalat P.A., Adalat XL, Nifedical XL, Nu-Nifed, Procardia, Procardia XL

Drug Actions: Calcium channel blocker antianginal

Drug Actions

Unknown; may inhibit calcium ion influx across cardiac and smooth muscle cells, decreasing myocardial contractility and oxygen demand. Also may dilate coronary arteries and arterioles. Reduces blood pressure and prevents angina.

Use

- Vasospastic angina (also called Prinzmetal [variant] angina)
- Classic chronic stable angina pectoris
- Hypertension

Side Effects

Cardiovascular: flushing, peripheral edema, hypotension, palpitations, heart failure, heart attack.
Gastrointestinal: nausea, heartburn, diarrhea.
Nervous System: dizziness, headache, weakness, syncope.
Skin: rash, itching.
Other: nasal congestion, hypokalemia, muscle cramps, shortness of breath, pulmonary edema.

Onset, Peak, and Duration

Route	Onset	Peak	Duration
Oral	20 min	30 min–2 hr	4–24 hr

Massage Considerations

- No cautions or contraindications to massage are related to the actions of this drug. Cautions and contraindications to massage may be related to the client condition.
- Side effects of hypotension and dizziness require care in getting the client on and off the table. Stimulation with rapid effleurage or tapotement at the end of the session may help.
- Rash and itching are local contraindications to massage and should be reported to the physician immediately. If severe or widespread, massage should be withheld.

nisoldipine (nigh-SOHL-dih-peen)

Sular

Drug Class: Calcium channel blocker antihypertensive

Drug Actions

Prevents entry of calcium ions into vascular smooth muscle cells, causing dilation of arterioles, which decreases peripheral vascular resistance. Lowers blood pressure.

Use

- Hypertension

Side Effects

Cardiovascular: vasodilation, palpitations, chest pain, peripheral edema.
Gastrointestinal: nausea.
Nervous System: headache, dizziness.
Skin: rash.
Other: sinusitis, pharyngitis.

Onset, Peak, and Duration

Route	Onset	Peak	Duration
Oral	Unknown	6–12 hr	Unknown

Massage Considerations

- No cautions or contraindications to massage are indicated because a client is taking this drug. Cautions and contraindications to massage may be related to the client condition.
- Side effects of dizziness require care in getting the client on and off the table. Stimulation with effleurage or tapotement at the end of the session may help.
- Rash is a local contraindication to massage and should be reported to the physician. If severe or widespread, massage should not be given.

---

nitrofurantoin macrocrystals (nigh-troh-fyoo-RAN-toyn MAH-kroh-kris-tuls)

Macrobid, Macrodantin

nitrofurantoin microcrystals

Apo-Nitrofurantoin, Furadantin, Furalan, Macrodantin

Drug Class: Urinary tract anti-infective

Drug Actions

Hinders growth of many common Gram-positive and Gram-negative urinary pathogens

Use

- Urinary tract infection
- Long-term suppression therapy

Side Effects

Gastrointestinal: anorexia, nausea, vomiting, abdominal pain, diarrhea.
Nervous System: peripheral neuropathy, headache, dizziness, drowsiness, ascending polyneuropathy with high doses or renal impairment.
Skin: rash, itching, hives, exfoliative dermatitis, Stevens-Johnson syndrome.
Other: hypersensitivity reactions, anaphylaxis, transient hair loss, drug fever, overgrowth of nonsusceptible organisms in urinary tract, hemolysis in patients with G6PD deficiency (reversed after stopping drug), agranulocytosis, thrombocytopenia, hepatitis, hepatic necrosis, asthmatic attacks in patients with history of asthma, pulmonary sensitivity (cough, chest pains, fever, chills, shortness of breath).

Onset, Peak, and Duration

Route	Onset	Peak	Duration
Oral	Unknown	Unknown	Unknown

Massage Considerations

- No cautions or contraindications to massage are related to the actions of this drug. Cautions and contraindications to massage may be related to the client condition and severity of infection.
- Side effects of dizziness and drowsiness require care in getting the client on and off the table. Stimulation with rapid effleurage or tapotement at the end of the session may help.
- Peripheral neuropathy is a local contraindication to deep tissue massage.
- Rash, itching, or hives are local contraindications to massage and should be reported to the physician immediately. If severe or widespread, no massage should be given.

- Hair loss is a contraindication to scalp massage if the client in disturbed by hair loss during the massage or if the scalp is tender.

nitroglycerin (glyceryl trinitrate) (nigh-troh-GLIH-suh-rin)

Anginine, Deponit, GTN-Poh, Minitran, Nitradisc, Nitro-Bid IV, Nitrodisc, Nitro-Dur, Nitrogard, Nitroglyn, Nitroject, Nitrolingual, Nitrong, NitroQuick, Nitrostat, Nitro-Time, Transderm-Nitro, Transiderm-Nitro, Tridil

Drug Class: Antianginal, vasodilator

Drug Actions

Prevents or relieves acute angina, lowers blood pressure, and helps minimize heart failure caused by heart attack.

Use

- Prevention of chronic anginal attacks
- Acute angina pectoris
- To prevent or minimize anginal attacks when taken immediately before stressful events
- Hypertension related to surgery
- Heart failure linked to heart attack
- Angina pectoris in acute situations
- To produce controlled hypotension during surgery (by intravenous infusion)
- Hypertensive crisis

Side Effects

Cardiovascular: orthostatic hypotension, tachycardia, flushing, palpitations, fainting.
Gastrointestinal: nausea, vomiting.
Nervous System: headache, sometimes with throbbing; dizziness; weakness.
Skin: cutaneous vasodilation, contact dermatitis (patch), rash.
Other: hypersensitivity reactions, sublingual burning.

Onset, Peak, and Duration

Route	Onset	Peak	Duration
Oral	20–45 min	Unknown	8–12 hr
I.V.	Immediate	Immediate	3–5 min
Topical	30 min	Unknown	4–8 hr
Transdermal	30 min	Unknown	≤24 hr
Sublingual	1–3 min	Unknown	30–60 min
Buccal	3 min	Unknown	5 hr
Translingual	2–4 min	Unknown	30–60 min

Massage Considerations

- No cautions or contraindications to massage are related to the actions of this drug. Cautions and contraindications to massage may be related to the client condition.
- The action of this drug in dilating blood vessels may increase the effects of the systemic strokes such as rocking, effleurage, and friction and increase the relaxation and vasodilation effects of massage. Using stimulation with rapid effleurage and tapotement at the end of the session may help. If the symptom is severe, using more rapid and stimulating massage techniques throughout the session may be needed.

- The site of topical application of the drug should not be massaged for up to 8 hours. The site of transdermal patches should not be massaged until the patch is removed.
- Side effects of hypotension and dizziness may be addressed as noted above.
- Rash is a local contraindication to massage and should be reported to the physician.

nizatidine (nigh-ZAT-ih-deen)

Axid, Axid AR, Tazac

Drug Class: Histamine$_2$ (H_2)-receptor antagonist antiulcer drug

Drug Actions

Competitively inhibits action of H_2 at receptor sites of parietal cells. Decreases gastric acid secretion.

Use

- Active duodenal ulcer
- Maintenance therapy for duodenal ulcer
- Benign gastric ulcer
- Gastroesophageal reflux disease

Side Effects

Cardiovascular: arrhythmias.
Nervous System: sleepiness, fever.
Skin: sweating, rash, hives, exfoliative dermatitis.
Other: thrombocytopenia, liver damage, hyperuricemia.

Onset, Peak, and Duration

Route	Onset	Peak	Duration
Oral	≤30 min	30 min–3 hr	≤12 hr

Massage Considerations

- No cautions or contraindications to massage are indicated because a client is taking this drug.
- Side effects of sleepiness may be helped by stimulation with tapotement or rapid effleurage at the end of the session.
- Rash and hives are local contraindications to massage and should be reported to the physician.

norethindrone (nor-ETH-in-drohn)

Camila, Errin, Jolivette, Micronor, Nora-BE, Nor-Q.D.

norethindrone acetate

Aygestin, Norlutate

Drug Class: Contraceptive

Drug Actions

Prevents pregnancy and relieves symptoms of endometriosis, amenorrhea, and abnormal uterine bleeding.

Use

- Amenorrhea
- Abnormal uterine bleeding
- Endometriosis
- To prevent pregnancy

Side Effects

Cardiovascular: hypertension, thrombophlebitis, pulmonary embolism, thromboembolism, stroke, edema.
Gastrointestinal: nausea, vomiting, abdominal cramps.
Nervous System: dizziness, migraine, lethargy, depression.
Skin: abnormal skin discoloration, rash.
Other: decreased libido; breast tenderness, enlargement, or secretion; breakthrough bleeding; dysmenorrhea; amenorrhea; cervical erosion; abnormal secretions; uterine fibromas; vaginal candidiasis; cholestatic jaundice; hyperglycemia.

Onset, Peak, and Duration

Route	Onset	Peak	Duration
Oral	Unknown	Unknown	Unknown

Massage Considerations

- No cautions or contraindications to massage are related to the actions of this drug.
- Side effects of thrombophlebitis or embolism are a complete contraindication to massage. If the client presents with redness, heat, swelling, or pain, especially in the lower extremities, massage should be withheld until the client is evaluated by the physician for possible blood clot.
- Dizziness requires care in getting the client on and off the table. Stimulation with tapotement at the end of the session may help.
- Rash is a local contraindication to massage and should be reported to the physician. If severe or widespread, massage should be withheld.

---

norfloxacin (nor-FLOKS-uh-sin)

Noroxin

Drug Class: Broad-spectrum antibiotic

Drug Actions

Kills certain bacteria

Use

- Urinary tract infection
- Cystitis
- Acute, uncomplicated gonorrhea
- Gastroenteritis
- Traveler's diarrhea

Side Effects

Gastrointestinal: nausea, constipation, gas, heartburn, dry mouth.
Nervous System: fatigue, sleepiness, headache, fever, dizziness, seizures.
Urinary: crystalluria.

Skin: rash, photosensitivity reaction.
Other: hypersensitivity reactions (rash, anaphylactoid reactions), eosinophilia, joint pain, arthritis, muscle pain, joint swelling.

Onset, Peak, and Duration

Route	Onset	Peak	Duration
Oral	Unknown	1–2 hr	Unknown

Massage Considerations

- No cautions or contraindications to massage are related to the actions of this drug. Cautions and contraindications to massage may be related to the client condition and severity of infection.
- Side effects of sleepiness and dizziness require care in getting the client on and off the table. Using rapid effleurage and tapotement at the end of the session may help.
- Constipation and gas may be helped by abdominal massage.
- Rash is a local contraindication to massage and should be reported to the physician immediately. If severe or widespread, massage should be withheld.

---

nortriptyline hydrochloride (nor-TRIP-teh-leen high-droh-KLOR-ighd)

Allegron, Aventyl, Pamelor

Drug Class: Tricyclic antidepressant

Drug Actions

Unknown; increases amount of norepinephrine, serotonin, or both in CNS by blocking their reuptake by presynaptic neurons. Relieves depression.

Use

- Depression
- Panic disorder

Side Effects

Cardiovascular: tachycardia, ECG changes, hypertension, heart block, stroke, heart attack.
Gastrointestinal: dry mouth, constipation, nausea, vomiting, anorexia, paralytic ileus.
Nervous System: drowsiness, dizziness, excitation, seizures, tremor, weakness, confusion, headache, nervousness,electroencephalogram changes, extrapyramidal reactions.
Urinary: urine retention.
Skin: sweating, rash, hives, photosensitivity.
Other: hypersensitivity reaction, blurred vision, ringing in the ears, abnormal pupil dilation, bone marrow depression, abnormal blood profiles.

Onset, Peak, and Duration

Route	Onset	Peak	Duration
Oral	Unknown	7–8.5 hr	Unknown

Massage Considerations

- No cautions or contraindications to massage are related to the actions of this drug. Cautions and contraindications to massage may be related to the client condition.

- Side effects of dizziness and drowsiness require care in getting the client on and off the table. Stimulation with rapid effleurage or tapotement at the end of the session may help. If the symptom is severe, using more rapid and stimulating massage techniques throughout the session may be needed.
- Constipation may be helped by abdominal massage.
- Rash or hives are local contraindications to massage and should be reported to the physician immediately. If severe or widespread, massage should be withheld.

nystatin (nigh-STAT-in)

Mycostatin, Nilstat, Nystex

Drug Class: Antifungal

Drug Actions

Kills susceptible yeasts and fungi

Use

- Gastrointestinal tract infections
- Oral, vaginal, and intestinal infections caused by *Candida*
- Vaginal infections

Side Effects

Gastrointestinal: transient nausea, vomiting, diarrhea (with large oral dosage).

Onset, Peak, and Duration

Route	Onset	Peak	Duration
Oral, topical, vaginal	Unknown	Unknown	Unknown

Massage Considerations

- No cautions or contraindications to massage are indicated because a client is taking this drug. Cautions and contraindications to massage may be related to the client condition.

O

octreotide acetate (ok-TREE-oh-tighd AS-ih-tayt)

Sandostatin, Sandostatin LAR Depot

Drug Class: Somatotropic hormone

Drug Actions

Relieves flushing and diarrhea caused by certain tumors and treats acromegaly

Use

- Flushing and diarrhea caused by carcinoid tumors
- Watery diarrhea caused by vasoactive intestinal polypeptide secreting tumors (vipomas).

- Acromegaly
- GI fistula
- Variceal bleeding
- AIDS-related diarrhea
- Short bowel (ileostomy) syndrome
- Chemotherapy- and radiation-induced diarrhea
- Pancreatic fistula
- Irritable bowel syndrome
- Dumping syndrome

Side Effects

Cardiovascular: flushing, arrhythmias, bradycardia.
Gastrointestinal: nausea, diarrhea, abdominal pain or discomfort, loose stools, vomiting, fat malabsorption, gallbladder abnormalities.
Nervous System: pain, dizziness, headache, fatigue.
Skin: edema, wheal, erythema and pain at injection site.
Other: burning at S.C. injection site, hyperglycemia, hypoglycemia, hypothyroidism.

Onset, Peak, and Duration

Route	Onset	Peak	Duration
I.M., Subcutaneous Injection	≤30 min	30–60 min	12 hr–6 wk

 Massage Considerations

- Although there are no cautions or contraindications to massage related to the actions of this drug, there will, in almost all cases, be contraindications to massage related to the client condition.
- The physician should be consulted before any massage is given.
- The site of I.M. or subcutaneous injection of the drug should not be massaged for at least 1 hour.
- Side effects of dizziness require care in getting the client on and off the table. Stimulation with rapid effleurage or tapotement at the end of the session may help.

ofloxacin (oh-FLOKS-eh-sin)

Apo-Oflox, Floxin

Drug Class: Antibiotic

Drug Actions

Kills susceptible aerobic gram-positive and gram-negative organisms

Use

- Lower respiratory tract infections
- Cervicitis or urethritis
- Acute, uncomplicated gonorrhea
- Mild to moderate skin and skin-structure infections
- Cystitis
- Urinary tract infections
- Prostatitis
- Adjunct to brucella infections

- Typhoid fever
- Antituberculosis drug (adjunct)
- Postoperative sternotomy or soft tissue wounds
- Acute Q fever pneumonia
- Mediterranean spotted fever
- Traveler's diarrhea

Side Effects

Cardiovascular: chest pain.
Gastrointestinal: nausea, anorexia, abdominal pain or discomfort, diarrhea, vomiting, dry mouth, gas, painful digestion.
Nervous System: headache, dizziness, fever, fatigue, lethargy, malaise, drowsiness, sleep disorders, nervousness, insomnia, seizures.
Skin: rash, itching, photosensitivity reaction.
Other: hypersensitivity reactions, anaphylaxis, abnormal blood profiles, vaginitis, vaginal discharge, genital itching, hypoglycemia, hyperglycemia, trunk pain, transient joint pain, muscle pain, visual disturbances.

Onset, Peak, and Duration

Route	Onset	Peak	Duration
Oral	Unknown	1–2 hr	Unknown

Massage Considerations

- There are no cautions or contraindications to massage related to the actions of this drug. There may be cautions or contraindications to massage related to the client condition and severity of infection.
- Side effects of dizziness and drowsiness may be helped by stimulation with effleurage or tapotement at the end of the session. Gas may be helped by abdominal massage. Rash or itching is a local contraindication to massage and should be reported to the physician immediately. If severe or widespread, massage should be withheld.

---

olanzapine (oh-LAN-za-peen)

Zyprexa, Zyprexa Zydis

Drug Class: Antipsychotic

Drug Actions

Relieves signs and symptoms of psychosis

Use

- Short-term therapy for acute manic episodes related to bipolar I disorder
- Long-term therapy for schizophrenia
- Short-term therapy for acute manic episodes of bipolar I disorder, given with lithium or valproate
- Long-term therapy for bipolar I disorder

Side Effects

Cardiovascular: orthostatic hypotension, chest pain, tachycardia, hypertension, peripheral edema.
Gastrointestinal: constipation, dry mouth, painful digestion, increased appetite, vomiting, increased salivation and thirst.

Nervous System: dizziness, sleepiness, weakness, insomnia, personality disorder, akathisia, tremor, fever, abnormal gait, speech impairment, tardive dyskinesia, parkinsonism, neuroleptic malignant syndrome, suicide attempt.
Urinary: urinary incontinence, urinary tract infection, hematuria.
Skin: bruising, sweating.
Other: dental pain, flu syndrome, injury, leukopenia, weight gain, hyperglycemia, joint pain, joint stiffness and twitching, extremity pain, back pain, hypertonia. metrorrhagia, vaginitis, amenorhea, increased cough, shortness of breath, rhinitis, pharyngitis, amblyopia, conjunctivitis.

Onset, Peak, and Duration

Route	Onset	Peak	Duration
Oral	Unknown	6 hr	Unknown

 Massage Considerations

- There are no cautions or contraindications to massage related to this drug. There will be, in most cases, cautions and contraindications to massage related to the client condition.
- The physician should be consulted before any massage is given.
- Side effects of dizziness and sleepiness, as well as hypotension require care in getting the client on and off the table. Using stimulating strokes such as rapid effleurage and friction to the legs at the end of the session may help. If the symptoms are severe, applying more rapid and stimulating massage techniques throughout the session may be needed.
- Constipation may be helped by abdominal massage. Bruising is a contraindication to deep tissue massage.

---

olmesartan medoxomil (ol-meh-SAHR-tan me-DOKS-oh-mil)

Benicar

Drug Class: Angiotensin II receptor antagonist antihypertensive

Drug Actions

Blocks the vasoconstrictor and aldosterone-secreting effects of angiotensin II lowering blood pressure

Use

- Hypertension

Side Effects

Gastrointestinal: diarrhea.
Nervous System: headache.
Urinary: hematuria.
Other: flulike symptoms, accidental injury, hyperglycemia, hypertriglyceridemia, back pain, pharyngitis, rhinitis, sinusitis, bronchitis, upper respiratory tract infection.

Onset, Peak, and Duration

Route	Onset	Peak	Duration
Oral	Rapid	1–2 hr	24 hr

 Massage Considerations

- There are no cautions or contraindications to massage related to this drug. There may be cautions or contraindications to massage related to the client condition.

- This drug may potentially increase the vasodilating effects of massage. Using stimulation with rapid effleurage and friction to the legs at the end of the session may help prevent problems.

---

olsalazine sodium (olh-SAL-uh-zeen SOH-dee-um)

Dipentum

Drug Class: Salicylate anti-inflammatory

Drug Actions

Unknown; converts to 5-aminosalicylic acid (5-ASA or mesalamine) in colon, where it has local anti-inflammatory effect

Use

- Maintenance of remission of ulcerative colitis in patients intolerant of sulfasalazine

Side Effects

Gastrointestinal: diarrhea, nausea, abdominal pain, heartburn.
Nervous System: headache, depression, dizziness.
Skin: rash, itching.
Other: joint pain.

Onset, Peak, and Duration

Route	Onset	Peak	Duration
Oral	Unknown	1 hr	Unknown

Massage Considerations

- This drug may decrease the perception of pain; therefore, deep tissue massage should be used with caution.
- There may be further cautions and contraindications to massage related to the client condition.
- Side effects of dizziness require care in getting the client on and off the table. Using stimulation with rapid effleurage or tapotement at the end of the session may help. Rash or itching is a local contraindication to massage and should be reported to the physician. If severe or widespread, massage should be withheld.

---

omalizumab (oh-mah-LIZZ-uh-mahb)

Xolair

Drug Class: Monoclonal antibody antiasthmatic

Drug Actions

Reduces the release of mediators of the allergic response and treats asthma symptoms

Use

- Moderate to severe persistent asthma

Side Effects

Nervous System: headache, pain, fatigue, dizziness.
Skin: itching, rash.
Other: sinusitis, pharyngitis, earache, joint pain, fracture, leg pain, arm pain, upper respiratory tract infection, injection site reaction, viral infections.

Onset, Peak, and Duration

Route	Onset	Peak	Duration
Subcutaneous Injection	Unknown	7–8 days	Unknown

Massage Considerations

- There are no cautions or contraindications to massage related to the actions of this drug. There may be cautions or contraindications to massage related to the client condition.
- The site of subcutaneous injection of the drug should not be massaged for up to 1 week.
- Side effects of dizziness may be helped by stimulation at the end of the session with rapid effleurage and tapotement. Itching and rash are local contraindications to massage and should be reported to the physician immediately. If severe or widespread, massage should be withheld.

---

omeprazole (oh-MEH-pruh-zohl)

Losec, Prilosec, Prilosec OTC

Drug Class: Gastric acid suppressant

Drug Actions

Inhibits activity of acid (proton) pump block formation of gastric acid

Use

- Erosive esophagitis
- Symptomatic, poorly responsive gastroesophageal reflux disease (GERD)
- Pathologic hypersecretory conditions (such as Zollinger-Ellison syndrome)
- Duodenal ulcer (short-term therapy)
- Gastric ulcer
- *Helicobacter pylori* eradication to reduce risk of duodenal ulcer recurrence as part of triple therapy with clarithromycin and amoxicillin
- Posterior laryngitis
- Heartburn on 2 or more days per week

Side Effects

Gastrointestinal: diarrhea, abdominal pain, nausea, vomiting, constipation, gas.
Nervous System: headache, dizziness.
Skin: rash.
Other: back pain, cough.

Onset, Peak, and Duration

Route	Onset	Peak	Duration
Oral	≤1 hr	2 hr	<3 days

Massage Considerations

- There are no cautions or contraindications to massage related to this drug.
- Side effects of dizziness require care in getting the client on and off the table. Using stimulation with rapid effleurage or tapotement at the end of the session may help.
- Constipation and gas may be helped by abdominal massage. Rash is a local contraindication to massage and should be reported to the physician.

ondansetron hydrochloride (on-DAN-seh-tron high-droh-KLOR-ighd)

Zofran, Zofran ODT

Drug Class: Antiemetic

Drug Actions

Prevents nausea and vomiting from emetogenic chemotherapy or surgery

Use

- Prevention of nausea and vomiting caused by moderately emetogenic chemotherapy
- Prevention of nausea and vomiting caused by highly emetogenic chemotherapy
- Prevention of postoperative nausea and vomiting
- Prevention of nausea and vomiting related to radiotherapy, either total body irradiation or single high-dose fraction or daily fractions to the abdomen

Side Effects

Gastrointestinal: diarrhea, constipation.
Nervous System: headache.
Skin: rash.

Onset, Peak, and Duration

Route	Onset	Peak	Duration
Oral, I.V.	Unknown	Unknown	Unknown

Massage Considerations

- There are no cautions or contraindications to massage related to this drug. There may be cautions or contraindications to massage related to the client condition.
- Side effects of constipation may be helped by abdominal massage. Rash is a local contraindication to massage and should be reported to the physician immediately. If severe or widespread, massage should be withheld.

opium tincture (OH-pee-um TINK-shur)

opium tincture

opium tincture, camphorated (paregoric)

Drug Class: Opiate antidiarrheal

Drug Actions

Increases smooth-muscle tone in GI tract, inhibits motility and propulsion, and diminishes secretions thus relieving diarrhea

Use

- Acute, nonspecific diarrhea
- Severe opiate withdrawal symptoms in neonates born to women addicted to opiates

Side Effects

Gastrointestinal: nausea, vomiting.
Nervous System: dizziness.
Other: physical dependence after long-term use.

Onset, Peak, and Duration

Route	Onset	Peak	Duration
Oral	Unknown	Unknown	Unknown

Massage Considerations

- This drug is an opiate and suppresses the CNS. Deep tissue massage should be done with great caution if at all.
- There may be further cautions and contraindications to massage related to the client condition.
- The actions of this drug may potentially decrease the effectiveness of the local reflex strokes of compression, stretching and vibration, as well as deep tissue massage. Using these strokes for longer periods of time than usual may achieve the desired results, or using the mechanical strokes of effleurage and pétrissage may be more effective. It may increase the effect of the systemic reflex strokes such as rocking, rythmic effleurage and friction, as well as increase the relaxation effects of massage in general. Using a more rapid application of these strokes to stimulate either at the end of the session or throughout the session may be needed.
- Side effects of dizziness may be addressed as noted earlier.

orlistat (OR-lih-stat)

Xenical

Drug Class: Antiobesity drug

Drug Actions

Bonds with the active site of gastric and pancreatic lipases. These inactivated enzymes are thus unavailable to hydrolyze dietary fat, in the form of triglycerides, into absorbable free fatty acids and monoglycerides. Because the undigested triglycerides are not absorbed, the resulting caloric deficit may help with weight control.

Use

- Management of obesity, including weight loss and weight maintenance, given with a reduced-calorie diet
- Reduction of risk of weight regain after weight loss

Side Effects

Cardiovascular: pedal edema.
Gastrointestinal: oily spotting, gas with discharge, fecal urgency, fatty or oily stool, oily evacuation, increased defecation, abdominal pain, fecal incontinence, nausea, infectious diarrhea, rectal pain, vomiting.
Nervous System: headache, dizziness, fatigue, sleep disorder, anxiety, depression.
Urinary: Urinary tract infections.
Skin: rash, dry skin.
Other: tooth and gingival disorders, back pain, leg pain, arthritis, muscle pain, joint disorder, tendinitis, otitis, menstrual irregularities, vaginitis, influenza, upper respiratory tract infection, lower respiratory tract infection.

Onset, Peak, and Duration

Route	Onset	Peak	Duration
Oral	Unknown	Unknown	Unknown

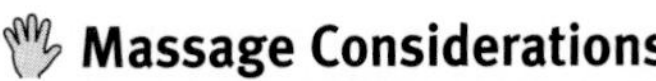

Massage Considerations

- There are no cautions or contraindications to massage related to the actions of this drug. There may be cautions or contraindications to massage related to the client condition.
- Side effects of dizziness require care in getting the client on and off the table. Using stimulation with rapid effleurage or tapotement at the end of the session may help. Gas and fecal urgency may require the client to get up in the middle of the session. Privacy and quick access to the bathroom is essential. Using candles or incense may help if the odor of gas is a problem, as massage may increase this side effect. Abdominal massage may help with cramping and gas, but should be done with caution as it may increase these effects in some clients. Rash is a local contraindication to massage and should be reported to the physician.

---

oxaliplatin (ox-ah-leh-PLA-tin)

Eloxatin

Drug Class: Antineoplastic

Drug Actions

Inhibits cancer cell formation

Use

- Metastatic colon or rectal cancer

Side Effects

Cardiovascular: chest pain, thromboembolism, edema, flushing, peripheral edema.
Gastrointestinal: GI: nausea, vomiting, diarrhea, stomatitis, abdominal pain, anorexia, constipation, painful digestion, taste perversion, gastroesophageal reflux, gas, mucositis.
Nervous System: pain, peripheral neuropathy, fatigue, headache, dizziness, insomnia, fever.
Urinary: painful urination, hematuria.
Skin: rash, hair loss.
Other: injection site reaction, anaphylaxis, hand-foot syndrome, allergic reaction, rigors, rhinitis, pharyngitis, epistaxis, abnormal lacrimation, abnormal blood profiles, hypokalemia, dehydration, back pain, joint pain, shortness of breath, cough, upper respiratory tract infection, hiccups, pulmonary toxicity.

Onset, Peak, and Duration

Route	Onset	Peak	Duration
I.V.	Unknown	Unknown	Unknown

Massage Considerations

- Because of the toxic effects of this drug, deep tissue massage is contraindicated and circulatory massage with effleurage should be used with caution and limited.
- There may be further cautions and contraindications to massage related to the client condition.
- The physician should be consulted before any massage is given and close collaboration is essential.
- This drug is usually given in every other week cycles. The Onset, Peak, and Duration of action, as well as the half-life of the drug are unknown. Therefore, it would be best to give massage on the weeks that the drug is not being given. If given during the week that the drug is given, massage should be given before the drug is received or at least 48 hours after the drug has been administered.

- Side effects of thromboembolism are a complete contraindication to massage. If the client presents with redness, heat, swelling, or pain, massage should be withheld and the client evaluated by the physician for possible blood clots immediately. Dizziness requires care in getting the client on and off the table. Friction to the legs at the end of the session may help. Peripheral neuropathy is a contraindication to deep tissue massage and caution to the depth and pressure of massage. Constipation and gas may be helped by abdominal massage if the client condition allows it. Rash is a local contraindication to massage and should be reported to the physician immediately. If severe or widespread, massage should be withheld. Hair loss is a contraindication to scalp massage if the client is disturbed by hair loss during the massage or the scalp is tender.
- The best approaches to this client are to use the systemic and local reflex strokes of rocking, gentle friction, gentle compression, vibration, and stretching. Pétrissage and myofascial massage techniques also may be used.

---

oxaprozin potassium (oks-uh-PROH-zin)

Apo-Oxaprozin, Daypro, Daypro ALTA, Rhoxal-Oxaprozin

Drug Class: NSAID (nonsteroidal anti-inflammatory drug)

Drug Actions

May inhibit prostaglandin synthesis relieving pain, fever, and inflammation

Use

- Osteoarthritis
- Rheumatoid arthritis

Side Effects

Gastrointestinal: nausea, painful digestion, diarrhea, constipation, abdominal pain or distress, anorexia, gas, vomiting, GI hemorrhage.
Nervous System: depression, sedation, sleepiness, confusion, sleep disturbances.
Urinary: painful urination, renal insufficiency, urinary frequency.
Skin: rash, photosensitivity.
Other: ringing in the ears, visual disturbances.

Onset, Peak, and Duration

Route	Onset	Peak	Duration
Oral	Unknown	2 hr	Unknown

Massage Considerations

- This drug decreases the perception of pain; therefore, deep tissue massage should be used with caution. There may be further cautions and contraindications to massage related to the client condition.
- Side effects of sleepiness may be helped by stimulation at the end of the massage with effleurage and tapotement. Constipation and gas may be helped by abdominal massage. Urinary frequency may require the client to get up in the middle of the massage. Privacy and quick access to the bathroom are essential. Water fountains and music that may stimulate the need to urinate should be avoided. Rash is a local contraindication to massage and should be reported to the physician.

oxazepam (oks-AZ-ih-pam)

Alepam, Apo-Oxazepam, Murelax, Novoxapam, Serax, Serepax

Drug Class: Benzodiazepine antianxiety, sedative-hypnotic

Drug Actions

Believed to stimulate gamma-aminobutyric receptors in ascending reticular activating system relieving anxiety and promoting calmness

Use

- Alcohol withdrawal
- Severe anxiety
- Mild-to-moderate anxiety
- Older patients with anxiety, tension, irritability, and agitation

Side Effects

Cardiovascular: transient hypotension.
Gastrointestinal: nausea, vomiting, abdominal discomfort.
Nervous System: drowsiness, lethargy, hangover, fainting, mental status changes.
Other: increased risk for falls, hepatic dysfunction.

Onset, Peak, and Duration

Route	Onset	Peak	Duration
Oral	Unknown	3 hr	Unknown

 Massage Considerations

- This drug has a sedating effect on the CNS. Deep tissue massage should be used with caution.
- There may be further cautions and contraindications to massage related to the client condition.
- The action of the drug may increase the relaxing effects of massage and may potentially increase the effects of the systemic reflex strokes of rocking, effleurage, and friction.
- Using these less, or applying them in a more rapid and stimulating manner throughout the session, may be needed. The effects of the local reflex strokes of compression, stretching, and vibration, as well as the effects of deep tissue massage may be decreased. It may be necessary to apply these strokes for longer periods of time than usual to achieve the desired effects.
- Side effects of hypotension and drowsiness may be addressed as noted earlier.

oxcarbazepine (ox-car-bay-zah-peen)

Trileptal

Drug Class: Antiepileptic

Drug Actions

Controls partial seizures

Use

- Adjunctive therapy for partial seizures in patients with epilepsy
- Conversion to monotherapy for partial seizures in patients with epilepsy
- Initial monotherapy for partial seizures in patients with epilepsy

Side Effects

Cardiovascular: hypotension, edema, chest pain.
Gastrointestinal: nausea, vomiting, abdominal pain, diarrhea, painful digestion, constipation, gastritis, anorexia, dry mouth, rectal hemorrhage, taste perversion, thirst.
Nervous System: fatigue, fever, weakness, feeling abnormal, headache, dizziness, sleepiness, ataxia, abnormal gait, insomnia, tremor, nervousness, agitation, abnormal coordination, speech disorder, confusion, anxiety, amnesia, aggravated seizures, hypoesthesia, emotional lability, impaired concentration.
Urinary: urinary tract infection, urinary frequency.
Skin: acne, rash, bruising, increased sweating.
Other: allergic reaction, hot flushes, toothache nystagmus, double vision, abnormal vision, abnormal accommodation, rhinitis, sinusitis, pharyngitis, epistaxis, vaginitis, hyponatremia, weight gain, muscle weakness, back pain, upper respiratory tract infection, coughing, bronchitis, chest infection.

Onset, Peak, and Duration

Route	Onset	Peak	Duration
Oral	Unknown	Variable	Unknown

 Massage Considerations

- This drug slows the transmission of nerve impulses in the CNS. Deep tissue massage should be used with great caution if at all.
- There may be further cautions and contraindications to massage related to the client condition.
- The action of this drug may potentially decrease the effectiveness of deep tissue massage and of the local reflex strokes of stretching, compression, and vibration. Applying these strokes for longer than usual periods of time may achieve the desired effects. Using mechanical strokes of pétrissage, friction, and effleurage may be the best approach.
- Side effects of hypotension, dizziness, and sleepiness require care in getting the client on and off the table. Stimulation with rapid effleurage and friction to the legs at the end of the session may help. Constipation may be helped by regular abdominal massage. Urinary frequency may require the client to get up during the session. Privacy and quick access to the bathroom should be provided. Water fountains and music that may stimulate the urge to urinate should be avoided. Acne or rash is a local contraindication to massage and should be reported to the physician. In the case of acne, if widespread and the client still wishes massage, gloves may be worn when working on the affected areas. Bruising is a contraindication to deep tissue massage.

---

oxybutynin chloride (oks-ee-BYOO-tih-nin KLOR-ighd)

Apo-Oxybutynin, Ditropan, Ditropan XL, Oxytrol

Drug Class: Antispasmodic

Drug Actions

Produces direct spasmolytic effect and antimuscarinic (atropine-like) effect on smooth muscles of urinary tract, increasing bladder capacity and providing some local anesthesia and mild analgesia

Use

- Antispasmodic for uninhibited or reflex neurogenic bladder
- Overactive bladder

Side Effects

Cardiovascular: flushing, palpitations, tachycardia.
Gastrointestinal: nausea, vomiting, constipation, bloated feeling, dry mouth, diarrhea, abdominal pain, gas.
Nervous System: drowsiness, fever, dizziness, insomnia, restlessness, impaired alertness, fatigue, headache.
Urinary: impotence, urinary hesitancy, urine retention, painful urination.
Skin: decreased sweating, rash, hives, itching, redness, burns.
Other: suppressed lactation, allergic reactions, transient blurred vision, abnormal dilation of pupils, cycloplegia, abnormal vision, back pain.

Onset, Peak, and Duration

Route	Onset	Peak	Duration
Oral	30–60 min	3–4 hr	6–10 hr
Transdermal	24–48 hr	Varies	96 hr

Massage Considerations

- There are no cautions or contraindications to massage related to this drug.
- The site of transdermal patch should not be massaged until the patch is removed.
- Side effects of drowsiness and dizziness require care in getting the client on and off the table. Using stimulation with effleurage and tapotement at the end of the session may help. Constipation and gas may be helped by abdominal massage. Rash, hives, or itching are local contraindications to massage and should be reported to the physician.

---

oxycodone hydrochloride (oks-ee-KOH-dohn high-droh-KLOR-ighd)

Endocodone, Endone, M-Oxy, OxyContin, Oxydose, OxyFAST, OxyIR, OxyNorm, Percolone, Roxicodone, Roxicodone Intensol, Supeudol

oxycodone pectinate

Proladone

Drug Class: Opioid analgesic

Drug Actions

Binds with opioid receptors in CNS, altering response to pain via unknown mechanism

Use

- Moderate to severe pain

Side Effects

Cardiovascular: hypotension, bradycardia.
Gastrointestinal: nausea, vomiting, constipation, ileus.
Nervous System: sedation, sleepiness clouded sensorium, euphoria, dizziness.
Urinary: urine retention.
Other: physical dependence, respiratory depression.

Onset, Peak, and Duration

Route	Onset	Peak	Duration
Oral	10–15 min	$\leq$1 hr	3–6 hr
Rectal	Unknown	Unknown	Unknown

Massage Considerations

- This drug depresses the CNS and decreases the perception of pain and sensation. Deep tissue massage is contraindicated.
- There may be further cautions and contraindications to massage related to the client condition.
- This drug may increase the relaxation effects of massage in general and may also increase the effects of the systemic reflex strokes of rocking, effleurage and friction. Using these strokes in a more rapid and stimulating manner throughout the session may be needed.
- The effectiveness of local reflex strokes such as stretching, compression, and vibration may be decreased. Applying them for longer than usual periods of time may produce the desired effects. Using the mechanical strokes of pétrissage, effleurage, and friction in a more stimulating manner throughout the session may be the best approach.
- Side effects of hypotension, dizziness, and sleepiness may be approached as noted earlier. Constipation may be helped by regular abdominal massage.

---

oxymorphone hydrochloride (oks-ee-MOR-fohn high-droh-KLOR-ighd)

Numorphan

Drug Class: Opioid analgesic

Drug Actions

Binds with opioid receptors in CNS, altering response to pain via unknown mechanism

Use

- Moderate to severe pain

Side Effects

Cardiovascular: hypotension, bradycardia.
Gastrointestinal: nausea, vomiting, constipation, ileus.
Nervous System: sedation, sleepiness, clouded sensorium, euphoria, dizziness, seizures with large doses.
Urinary: urine retention.
Other: physical dependence, respiratory depression.

Onset, Peak, and Duration

Route	Onset	Peak	Duration
I.V.	5–10 min	15–30 min	3–4 hr
I.M.	10–15 min	30–90 min	3–6 hr
Subcutaneous Injection	10–20 min	60–90 min	3–6 hr
Rectal	15–30 min	2 hr	3–6 hr

Massage Considerations

- This drug depresses the CNS and decreases the perception of pain and sensation. Deep tissue massage is contraindicated.
- There may be further cautions and contraindications to massage related to the client condition.

- This drug may increase the relaxation effects of massage in general and may also increase the effects of the systemic reflex strokes of rocking, effleurage, and friction. Using these strokes in a more rapid and stimulating manner throughout the session may be needed.
- The effectiveness of local reflex strokes such as stretching, compression, and vibration may be decreased. Applying them for longer than usual periods of time may produce the desired effects. Using the mechanical strokes of pétrissage, effleurage, and friction in a more stimulating manner throughout the session may be the best approach.
- Side effects of hypotension, dizziness, and sleepiness may be approached as noted earlier. Constipation may be helped by regular abdominal massage.

P

paclitaxel (pak-lih-TAK-sil)

Onxol, Taxol

Drug Class: Antineoplastic

Drug Actions

Stops ovarian and breast cancer cell activity

Use

- First-line and subsequent treatment of advanced ovarian cancer
- Breast cancer
- Initial treatment of advanced non–small cell lung cancer
- AIDS-related Kaposi sarcoma

Side Effects

Cardiovascular: bradycardia, hypotension, abnormal electrocardiogram (ECG).
Gastrointestinal: nausea, vomiting, diarrhea, mucositis.
Nervous System: peripheral neuropathy.
Skin: hair loss, phlebitis, cellulitis at injection site.
Other: hypersensitivity reactions (anaphylaxis), abnormal blood profiles, bleeding, joint pain, muscle pain.

Onset, Peak, and Duration

Route	Onset	Peak	Duration
I.V.	Unknown	Unknown	Unknown

Massage Considerations

- Because of the toxic effects of this drug, deep tissue massage is contraindicated and circulatory massage with effleurage should be used with caution and limited.
- Further cautions and contraindications to massage may be related to the client condition.
- The physician should be consulted before any massage is given, and close collaboration is essential.

- This drug is usually given every 2 to 3 weeks and has a short half-life (about 5 hours). Massage would best be given on the weeks that the drug is not administered. If massage is given the week the drug is administered, it should be done before the drug is given or at least 24 hours after the drug has been administered.
- Side effects of hypotension may be helped by stimulation at the end of the session with friction to the legs.
- Peripheral neuropathy is a contraindication to deep tissue massage and a caution for depth and pressure of massage in general.
- Hair loss is a contraindication to scalp massage if the client is disturbed by hair loss during the massage or if the scalp is tender.
- The best approach to this client is to use the systemic and local reflex strokes of rocking, stretching, gentle compression, gentle friction, and vibration. Pétrissage and myofascial massage techniques may also be used.

---

palivizumab (pal-ih-VYE-zoo-mab)

Synagis

Drug Class: Recombinant monoclonal antibody immunoglobulin (Ig)$G1_k$

Drug Actions

Inhibits respiratory syncytial virus (RSV) replication.

Use

- Prevention of serious lower respiratory tract disease caused by RSV in children at high risk

Side Effects

Gastrointestinal: diarrhea, vomiting, gastroenteritis, oral candidiasis.
Nervous System: nervousness, pain.
Skin: rash, fungal dermatitis, eczema, seborrhea.
Other: hernia, failure to thrive, injection site reaction, viral infection, flulike syndrome, anemia, upper respiratory tract infection, cough, wheeze, bronchiolitis, apnea, pneumonia, bronchitis, asthma, croup, shortness of breath, otitis media, rhinitis, pharyngitis, sinusitis, conjunctivitis.

Onset, Peak, and Duration

Route	Onset	Peak	Duration
I.M.	Unknown	Unknown	Unknown

Massage Considerations

- No cautions or contraindications to massage are indicated because a client is taking this drug. Cautions and contraindications to massage may be related to the client condition.
- The site of intramuscular injection of the drug is difficult to determine but should be avoided for at least a week.
- Side effects of rash or other skin eruptions are local contraindications to massage and should be reported to the physician immediately.

---

palonosetron hydrochloride (pa-LOW-no-suh-tron high-droh-KLOHR-ighd)

Aloxi

Drug Class: Antiemetic

Drug Actions

Prevents vomiting because of chemotherapy

Use

- Prevention of acute and delayed nausea and vomiting

Side Effects

Cardiovascular: bradycardia, hypotension, nonsustained ventricular tachycardia.
Gastrointestinal: constipation, diarrhea.
Nervous System: anxiety, dizziness, headache, weakness.
Other: hyperkalemia.

Onset, Peak, and Duration

Route	Onset	Peak	Duration
I.V.	30 min	Unknown	5 days

 Massage Considerations

- No cautions or contraindications to massage are indicated because a client is taking this drug. Cautions and contraindications to massage may be related to the client condition.
- Side effects of dizziness and hypotension require care in getting the client on and off the table. Using stimulation at the end of the session with friction to the legs or tapotement may help.
- Constipation may be helped by abdominal massage.

---

pamidronate disodium (pam-ih-DROH-nayt digh-SOH-dee-um)

Aredia

Drug Class: Antihypercalcemic

Drug Actions

Inhibits bone resorption. Lowers calcium levels.

Use

- Moderate to severe hypercalcemia related to malignancy (with or without metastases)
- Osteolytic bone lesions of multiple myeloma
- Osteolytic bone lesions of breast cancer
- Moderate to severe Paget disease

Side Effects

Cardiovascular: hypertension, atrial fibrillation.
Gastrointestinal: abdominal pain, anorexia, constipation, nausea, vomiting, diarrhea, painful digestion, gastrointestinal (GI) hemorrhage.
Nervous System: pain, fever, fatigue, headache, insomnia, anxiety, seizures.
Urinary: urinary tract infection, renal failure.
Other: abnormal blood profiles, hypophosphatemia, hypokalemia, hypomagnesemia, hypocalcemia, bone pain, joint pain, muscle pain.

Onset, Peak, and Duration

Route	Onset	Peak	Duration
I.V.	Unknown	Unknown	Unknown

 Massage Considerations

- Because this drug acts on calcium levels in blood and tissue, deep tissue massage should be used with caution.
- Further cautions and contraindications to massage may be related to the client condition.
- This drug may potentially decrease the effectiveness of local reflex strokes such as traction, stretching, compression, and vibration and decrease the effectiveness of deep tissue massage. The systemic reflex strokes of rocking, effleurage, and friction and the mechanical strokes of pétrissage are recommended.

---

pantoprazole sodium (pan-TOE-pra-zole SOH-dee-um)

Protonix, Protonix I.V.

Drug Class: Proton pump inhibitor

Drug Actions

Suppresses gastric acid secretion

Use

- Short-term treatment of erosive esophagitis related to gastroesophageal reflux disease (GERD)
- Short-term treatment of GERD related to history of erosive esophagitis
- Long-term maintenance of healing erosive esophagitis and reduction in relapse rates of daytime and nighttime heartburn symptoms in patients with GERD
- Short-term treatment of pathologic hypersecretion conditions related to Zollinger-Ellison syndrome or other neoplastic conditions
- Long-term treatment of pathologic hypersecretory conditions, including Zollinger-Ellison syndrome

Side Effects

Cardiovascular: chest pain.
Gastrointestinal: diarrhea, gas, abdominal pain, eructation, constipation, painful digestion, gastroenteritis, gastrointestinal disorder, nausea, vomiting.
Nervous System: headache, insomnia, weakness, migraine, anxiety, dizziness, pain.
Urinary: rectal disorder, urinary frequency, urinary tract infection.
Skin: rash.
Other: flulike syndrome, infection, pharyngitis, rhinitis, sinusitis, hyperglycemia, hyperlipidemia, back pain, neck pain, joint pain, hypertonia, bronchitis, increased cough, shortness of breath, upper respiratory tract infection.

Onset, Peak, and Duration

Route	Onset	Peak	Duration
Oral	Unknown	2.5 hr	Unknown
I.V.	15–30 min	Unknown	24 hr

 Massage Considerations

- No cautions or contraindications to massage are indicated because a client is taking this drug.
- Side effects of dizziness require care in getting the client on and off the table. Using stimulation at the end of the sesssion with effleurage and tapotement may help.
- Gas and constipation may be helped by abdominal massage.
- Rash is a local contraindication to massage and should be reported to the physician.

papaverine hydrochloride (puh-PAV-eh-reen high-droh-KLOR-ighd)

Pavabid Plateau Caps, Pavagen TD

Drug Class: Peripheral vasodilator

Drug Actions

Has direct, nonspecific relaxant effect on vascular, cardiac, and other smooth muscle and relieves vascular spasms.

Use

- Relief of cerebral and peripheral ischemia from arterial spasm and myocardial ischemia
- Coronary occlusion
- Cerebral angiospastic states
- Impotence

Side Effects

Cardiovascular: flushing, increased heart rate, increased blood pressure (parenteral use), depressed atrioventricular and intraventricular conduction, hypotension, arrhythmias.
Gastrointestinal: constipation, dry mouth, nausea.
Nervous System: headache, depression, malaise.
Skin: sweating.
Other: hepatitis, cirrhosis, increased depth of respiration, apnea.

Onset, Peak, and Duration

Route	Onset	Peak	Duration
Oral	Rapid	1–2 hr	12 hr
I.V., I.M.	Unknown	Unknown	Unknown

 Massage Considerations

- No cautions or contraindications to massage are indicated because a client is taking this drug. In many cases, cautions or contraindications to massage will be related to the client condition.
- The site of intramuscular injection of the drug should not be massaged for at least 2 to 3 hours.
- Side effects of constipation may be helped by abdominal massage.
- Hypotension may be helped by using stimulation with rapid effleurage or tapotement at the end of the session.

paroxetine hydrochloride (par-OKS-eh-teen high-droh-KLOR-ighd)

Paxil, Paxil CR

Drug Class: Selective serotonin reuptake inhibitor antidepressant

Drug Actions

Unknown; presumed to be linked to inhibition of central nervous system (CNS) neuronal uptake of serotonin.

Use

- Major depressive disorder
- Obsessive-compulsive disorder

- Panic disorder
- Social anxiety disorder
- Generalized anxiety disorder
- Posttraumatic stress disorder
- Premenstrual dysphoric disorder
- Diabetic neuropathy
- Headache
- Premature ejaculation

Side Effects

Cardiovascular: palpitations, vasodilation, orthostatic hypotension.
Gastrointestinal: dry mouth, nausea, constipation, diarrhea, taste perversion, increased or decreased appetite, gas, vomiting, painful digestion.
Nervous System: weakness, blurred vision, sleepiness, dizziness, insomnia, tremor, headache, nervousness, anxiety, paresthesia, confusion.
Urinary: abnormal ejaculation, male genital disorders (including anorgasmy, erectile difficulties, delayed ejaculation or orgasm, impotence, and sexual dysfunction), urinary frequency, other urinary disorder, female genital disorder (including anorgasmy, difficulty with orgasm).
Skin: excessive sweating, rash.
Other: decreased libido, yawning, lump or tightness in throat, painful swallowing, hyponatremia, myopathy, muscle pain, myasthenia.

Onset, Peak, and Duration

Route	Onset	Peak	Duration
Oral:			
Immediate-release	1–4 wk	2–8 hr	Unknown
Controlled-release	Unknown	6–10 hr	Unknown

 Massage Considerations

- No cautions or contraindications to massage are related to the actions of this drug. Cautions and contraindications to massage may be related to the client condition.
- Side effects of hypotension, sleepiness, and dizziness require care in getting the client on and off the table. Using stimulation with rapid effleurage and tapotement at the end of the session may help.
- Paresthesia is a local contraindication to deep tissue massage.
- Constipation and gas may be helped by abdominal massage.
- For urinary frequency, provide privacy for the client and quick access to the bathroom. Water fountains and water music, which may stimulate urination, should be avoided.
- Rash is a local contraindication to massage and should be reported to the physician.

---

pegaspargase (peg-AHS-per-jays)

Oncaspar

Drug Class: Antineoplastic

Drug Actions

Destroys cancer cells

Use

- Acute lymphoblastic leukemia

Side Effects

Cardiovascular: hypotension, tachycardia, chest pain, subacute bacterial endocarditis, hypertension, edema.
Gastrointestinal: nausea, vomiting, abdominal pain, anorexia, diarrhea, constipation, indigestion, gas, GI pain, mucositis, pancreatitis (sometimes fulminant and fatal), colitis, mouth tenderness.
Nervous System: seizures, headache, paresthesia, status epilepticus, sleepiness, coma, mental status changes, dizziness, emotional lability, mood changes, parkinsonism, confusion, disorientation, fatigue, malaise.
Urinary: increased urinary frequency, hematuria, severe hemorrhagic cystitis, renal dysfunction, renal failure.
Skin: bruising, itching, hair loss, fever blister, purpura, white hands, hives, fungal changes, nail whiteness and ridging, erythema simplex, rash, nighttime sweating.
Other: hypersensitivity reactions (including anaphylaxis, pain, fever, chills, peripheral edema, infection); sepsis; septic shock; injection pain or reaction; localized edema; thrombosis; abnormal blood profiles; disseminated intravascular coagulation; hemolytic anemia; hemorrhage; jaundice; bilirubinemia; ascites; hypoalbuminemia; fatty changes in liver; liver failure; hyperuricemia; hyponatremia; uric acid nephropathy; hypoproteinemia; proteinuria; weight loss; metabolic acidosis; hyperglycemia; hypoglycemia; joint pain; muscle pain; musculoskeletal pain; joint stiffness; cramps; cough; severe bronchospasm; upper respiratory tract infection; nosebleed.

Onset, Peak, and Duration

Route	Onset	Peak	Duration
I.V., I.M.	Unknown	Unknown	Unknown

 Massage Considerations

- Because of the toxic effects of this drug, deep tissue massage is contraindicated, and circulatory massage with effleurage should be used with caution and limited.
- Further cautions or contraindications to massage may be related to the client condition.
- The physician should be consulted before any massage is given, and close collaboration is essential.
- This drug is usually given every 2 weeks and has a long half-life (up to 6 days). It would be best to massage on the weeks the drug is not given. Give massage before the drug is administered on the week the drug is being given.
- Side effects of hypotension, dizziness, and sleepiness require care in getting the client on and off the table. Using stimulation at the end of the session with friction to the legs and tapotement may help.
- Paresthesia is a contraindication to deep tissue massage and requires care with depth and pressure.
- Constipation and gas may be helped by regular abdominal massage.
- Increased urinary frequency requires quick access to the bathroom and privacy. Water fountains or water music, which may stimulate urination, should be avoided.
- Thrombosis is a complete contraindication to massage.
- Bruising requires care with depth and pressure.
- Rash and itching are local contraindications to massage and should be reported to the physician. If severe or widespread, massage should be withheld.
- Hair loss is a contraindication to scalp massage if the client is disturbed by hair loss during the session or the scalp is tender.
- The best approach to this client is to use reflex strokes of rocking, stretching, traction, gentle compression, gentle friction, and vibration. Myofascial massage techniques should be used with caution because of easy bruising and petechiae.

pegfilgrastim (peg-FILL-grass-tihm)

Neulasta

Drug Class: Colony-stimulating factor, neutrophil-growth stimulator

Drug Actions

Increases white blood cell count

Use

- To reduce frequency of infection in patients with nonmyeloid malignancies who are receiving myelosuppressive anticancer drugs that may cause febrile neutropenia.

Side Effects

Cardiovascular: peripheral edema.
Gastrointestinal: nausea, diarrhea, vomiting, constipation, anorexia, taste perversion, painful digestion, abdominal pain, stomatitis, mucositis.
Nervous System: dizziness, headache, fatigue, insomnia, fever.
Skin: hair loss.
Other: granulocytopenia, neutropenia, skeletal pain, generalized weakness, joint pain, muscle pain, bone pain, acute respiratory distress syndrome.

Onset, Peak, and Duration

Route	Onset	Peak	Duration
Subcutaneous Injection	Unknown	Unknown	Unknown

Massage Considerations

- No cautions or contraindications to massage are related to the actions of this drug. In most cases, cautions and contraindications to massage will be related to the client condition.
- The physician should be consulted before any massage is given.
- The site of subcutaneous injection should not be massaged for at least 24 hours or longer.
- Side effects of dizziness require care in getting the client on and off the table. Stimulation with effleurage and tapotement at the end of the session may help.
- Constipation may be helped by abdominal massage.
- Hair loss is a contraindication to scalp massage if the client is disturbed by hair loss during the session or if the scalp is tender.

peginterferon alfa-2a (peg-inter-FEAR-on AL-fah TOO AY)

Pegasys

Drug Class: Antiviral

Drug Actions

Inhibits viral replication in infected cells

Use

- Chronic hepatitis C in patients not previously treated with interferon alfa

Side Effects

Cardiovascular: pulmonary embolism.
Gastrointestinal: nausea, diarrhea, abdominal pain, vomiting, dry mouth, anorexia, pancreatitis.

Nervous System: fever, pain, fatigue, weakness, headache, insomnia, dizziness, concentration and memory impairment, depression, irritability, anxiety, suicide, cerebral hemorrhage, coma.
Skin: hair loss, itching, increased sweating, rash.
Other: rigors, injection site reaction, neutropenia, thrombocytopenia, muscle pain, joint pain, back pain.

Onset, Peak, and Duration

Route	Onset	Peak	Duration
Subcutaneous Injection	Unknown	72–96 hr	Up to 1 wk

Massage Considerations

- No cautions or contraindications to massage are indicated because a client is taking this drug. Cautions and contraindications to massage may be related to the client condition.
- The site of subcutaneous injection of the drug should not be massaged for up to 1 week.
- Side effects of dizziness require care in getting the client on and off the table. Stimulation at the end of the session with effleurage or tapotement may help.
- Rash and itching are local contraindications to massage and should be reported to the physician.
- Hair loss is a contraindication to scalp massage if the client is disturbed by hair loss during the session or if the scalp is tender.

peginteferon alfa-2b (pehg-in-ter-FEAR-ahn AL-fah TOO BEE)

PEG-Intron

Drug Class: Antiviral

Drug Actions

Inhibits virus replication in infected cells

Use

- Chronic hepatitis C

Side Effects

Cardiovascular: flushing.
Gastrointestinal: nausea, anorexia, diarrhea, abdominal pain, vomiting, painful digestion, right upper quadrant pain.
Nervous System: dizziness, hypertonia, fever, depression, insomnia, anxiety, emotional lability, irritability, headache, fatigue, malaise, suicidal behavior.
Skin: hair loss, itching, dry skin, rash, increased sweating.
Other: injection site reaction (inflammation), injection site pain, viral infection, flulike symptoms, rigors, pharyngitis, sinusitis, neutropenia, thrombocytopenia, hepatomegaly, hypothyroidism, hyperthyroidism, weight decrease, musculoskeletal pain, cough.

Onset, Peak, and Duration

Route	Onset	Peak	Duration
Subcutaneous Injection	Unknown	15–44 hr	Unknown

Massage Considerations

- No cautions or contraindications to massage are indicated because a client is taking this drug. Cautions and contraindications to massage may be related to the client condition.

- The site of subcutaneous injection of the drug should not be massaged for at least 48 hours.
- Side effects of dizziness require care in getting the client on and off the table. Stimulation with effleurage and tapotement at the end of the session may help.
- Rash and itching are local contraindications to massage and should be reported to the physician.
- Hair loss is a contraindication to scalp massage if the client is disturbed by hair loss during the session or the scalp is tender.

---

pemoline (PEH-moh-leen)

Cylert, Cylert Chewable, PemADD, PemADD CT

Drug Class: CNS stimulant

Drug Actions

Releases stored norepinephrine from nerve terminals in brain (mainly in the cerebral cortex and reticular activating system), which may promote transmission of nerve impulses. Promotes calmness in children with attention deficit hyperactivity disorder (ADHD).

Use

- ADHD
- Narcolepsy

Side Effects

Gastrointestinal: anorexia, abdominal pain, nausea, diarrhea.
Nervous System: insomnia, malaise, dyskinetic movements, irritability, fatigue, mild depression, dizziness, headache, drowsiness, hallucinations, nervousness, seizures, Tourette syndrome, psychosis.
Skin: rash.
Other: aplastic anemia, hepatitis, jaundice, hepatic failure, growth suppression.

Onset, Peak, and Duration

Route	Onset	Peak	Duration
Oral	Unknown	2–4 hr	Unknown

Massage Considerations

- This drug is a CNS stimulant; therefore, tapotement should be used with great caution and limited.
- Further cautions and contraindications to massage may be related to the client condition.
- The stimulating action of this drug may decrease the relaxation effects of massage and may potentially decrease the effectiveness of the systemic reflex strokes of rocking and the systemic reflex effects of friction and slow, rhythmic effleurage. Using these strokes for longer periods of time may be more effective. The local reflex strokes (such as compression, stretching, traction, and vibration) may also be less effective. Deep tissue massage may also be less effective. Using these strokes for longer periods of time than usual may make them more effective. The best strokes may be the mechanical strokes of pétrissage and the mechanical effects of effleurage and friction.
- Side effects of dizziness and drowsiness require care in getting the client on and off the table. Use stimulation at the very end of the massage with friction to the legs.
- Rash is a local contraindication to massage and should be reported to the physician.

penicillamine (pen-ih-SIL-uh-meen)

Cuprimine, Depen

Drug Class: Heavy metal antagonist, antirheumatic

Drug Actions

Chelates heavy metals and may inhibit collagen formation; unknown for rheumatoid arthritis.

Use

- Wilson disease
- Cystinuria
- Rheumatoid arthritis
- Adjunct in heavy metal poisoning
- Primary biliary cirrhosis

Side Effects

Gastrointestinal: anorexia, epigastric pain, nausea, vomiting, diarrhea, loss of taste or altered taste perception, stomatitis, oral ulcerations.
Urinary: nephrotic syndrome, glomerulonephritis, proteinuria, hematuria.
Skin: hair loss; friability, especially at pressure spots; wrinkling; redness; hives; bruising.
Other: lupuslike syndrome, myasthenia gravis syndrome with long-term use, allergic reactions, ringing in the ears, optic neuritis, abnormal blood profiles, lymphadenopathy, hepatotoxicity, joint pain, pneumonitis.

Onset, Peak, and Duration

Route	Onset	Peak	Duration
Oral	Unknown	1 hr	Unknown

Massage Considerations

- The actions of this drug on collagen tissue contraindicate myofascial massage techniques. Circulatory massage with effleurage should be used with great caution and limited. Deep tissue massage should be used with caution.
- Further cautions and contraindications to massage may be related to the client condition.
- The physician should be consulted before any massage is given.
- The side effect of hair loss is a contraindication to scalp massage if the client is disturbed by hair loss during the session or if the scalp is tender.
- Friability is easy tearing of the outer layer of the skin. This requires great caution with all massage strokes. Friction should not be used. If severe, this side effect may contraindicate massage completely.
- Hives and itching are local contraindications to massage and should be reported to the physician immediately. If severe or widespread, massage should be withheld.
- Bruising is a contraindication to deep tissue massage and a caution to depth and pressure of massage in general.

penicillin G benzathine (pen-ih-SIL-in gee BENZ-uh-theen)

Bicillin L-A, Permapen

Drug Class: Antibiotic

Drug Actions

Kills susceptible bacteria

Use

- Congenital syphilis
- Group A streptococcal upper respiratory tract infections
- Prophylaxis of poststreptococcal rheumatic fever
- Syphilis

Side Effects

Nervous System: pain, neuropathy, seizures.
Other: hypersensitivity reactions (maculopapular and exfoliative dermatitis, chills, fever, edema, anaphylaxis), sterile abscess at injection site, eosinophilia, hemolytic anemia, thrombocytopenia, leukopenia.

Onset, Peak, and Duration

Route	Onset	Peak	Duration
I.M.	Unknown	13–24 hr	1–4 wk

 Massage Considerations

- No cautions or contraindications to massage are indicated because a client is taking this drug. Cautions or contraindications to massage may be related to the client condition and severity of infection.
- The site of intramuscular injection of the drug should not be massaged for 24 hours.
- Side effects of neuropathy are a local contraindication to deep tissue massage.

---

penicillin G potassium (pen-ih-SIL-in gee poh-TAH-see-um)

Pfizerpen

Drug Class: Antibiotic

Drug Actions

Kills susceptible bacteria

Use

- Moderate to severe systemic infections
- Anthrax

Side Effects

Cardiovascular: thrombophlebitis.
Nervous System: neuropathy, seizures.
Other: hypersensitivity reactions (rash, hives, maculopapular eruptions, exfoliative dermatitis, chills, fever, edema, anaphylaxis), overgrowth of nonsusceptible organisms, pain at injection site, hemolytic anemia, thrombocytopenia, leukopenia, severe potassium poisoning with high doses (hyperreflexia, seizures, coma).

Onset, Peak, and Duration

Route	Onset	Peak	Duration
I.V.	Immediate	Immediate	Unknown
I.M.	Unknown	15–30 min	Unknown

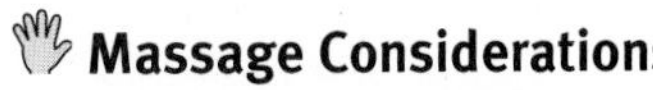

Massage Considerations

- No cautions or contraindications to massage are indicated because a client is taking this drug. Cautions or contraindications to massage may be related to the client condition and severity of infection.
- The site of intramuscular injection of the drug should not be massaged for 30 minutes.
- Side effects of thrombophlebitis are a complete contraindication to massage.
- Neuropathy is a local contraindication to deep tissue massage.

---

penicillin G procaine (benzylpenicillin procaine) (pen-ih-SIL-in gee PROH-kayn)

Drug Class: Antibiotic

Drug Actions

Kills susceptible bacteria

Use

- Moderate to severe systemic infections
- Uncomplicated gonorrhea
- Pneumococcal pneumonia
- Anthrax
- Cutaneous anthrax

Side Effects

Nervous System: seizures.
Other: hypersensitivity reactions (rash, urticaria, chills, fever, edema, prostration, anaphylaxis), overgrowth of nonsusceptible organisms, thrombocytopenia, hemolytic anemia, leukopenia, joint pain.

Onset, Peak, and Duration

Route	Onset	Peak	Duration
I.M.	Unknown	1–4 hr	1–2 days

Massage Considerations

- No cautions or contraindications to massage are indicated because a client is taking this drug. Cautions or contraindications to massage may be related to the client condition and severity of infection.
- The site of intramuscular injection of the drug should not be massaged for 4 hours.

---

penicillin G sodium (pen-ih-SIL-in gee SOH-dee-um)

Crystapen

Drug Class: Antibiotic

Drug Actions

Kills susceptible bacteria

Use

- Moderate to severe systemic infections
- Endocarditis prophylaxis for dental surgery

Side Effects

Cardiovascular: thrombophlebitis.
Nervous System: neuropathy, seizures.
Other: hypersensitivity reactions (exfoliative dermatitis, urticaria, anaphylaxis), overgrowth of nonsusceptible organisms, vein irritation, pain at injection site, hemolytic anemia, leukopenia, thrombocytopenia, joint pain.

Onset, Peak, and Duration

Route	Onset	Peak	Duration
I.V.	Immediate	Immediate	Unknown
I.M.	Unknown	15–30 min	Unknown

 Massage Considerations

- No cautions or contraindications to massage are indicated because a client is taking this drug. Cautions or contraindications to massage may be related to the client condition and severity of infection.
- The site of intramuscular injection of the drug should not be massaged for 30 minutes.
- Side effects of thrombophlebitis are a complete contraindication to massage.
- Neuropathy is a local contraindication to deep tissue massage.

---

penicillin V (phenoxymethylpenicillin) (pen-ih-SIL-in VEE)

penicillin V potassium (phenoxymethylpenicillin potassium)

Abbocillin VK, Apo-Pen-VK, Beepen-VK, Cilicaine VK, Nadopen-V, Nadopen-V-200, Nadopen-V 400, Novo-Pen-VK, Nu-Pen-VK, Pen-Vee K, PVF K, PVK, V-Cillin K, Veetids

Drug Class: Antibiotic

Drug Actions

Kills susceptible bacteria

Use

- Mild to moderate systemic infections
- Endocarditis prophylaxis for dental surgery
- Necrotizing ulcerative gingivitis
- Prophylaxis for rheumatic fever
- Prophylaxis for pneumococcal infections
- Lyme disease

Side Effects

Gastrointestinal: epigastric distress, vomiting, diarrhea, nausea.
Nervous System: neuropathy, seizures.
Other: hypersensitivity reactions (rash, hives, chills, fever, edema, anaphylaxis), overgrowth of nonsusceptible organisms, abnormal blood profiles.

Onset, Peak, and Duration

Route	Onset	Peak	Duration
Oral	Unknown	30–60 min	Unknown

 Massage Considerations

- No cautions or contraindications to massage are indicated because a client is taking this drug. Cautions or contraindications to massage may be related to the client condition and severity of infection.
- Side effects of neuropathy are a local contraindication to deep tissue massage.

---

pentamidine isethionate (pen-TAM-eh-deen ighs-eh-THIGH-oh-nayt)

NebuPent, Pentacarinat, Pentam 300

Drug Class: Antiprotozoal

Drug Actions

Hinders growth of susceptible organisms

Use

- *Pneumocystis carinii* pneumonia
- Prevention of *P. carinii* pneumonia in high-risk patients

Side Effects

Cardiovascular: chest pain, severe hypotension, hypotension, facial flushing, tachycardia.
Gastrointestinal: pancreatitis, nausea, pharyngitis, vomiting, metallic taste.
Nervous System: confusion, fever, hallucinations, fatigue, dizziness.
Urinary: renal toxicity, acute renal failure.
Skin: itching, Stevens-Johnson syndrome, rash.
Other: sterile abscess, pain and induration at injection site, night sweats, chills, decreased appetite, shortness of breath, chest congestion, cough, broncospasm, leukopenia, thrombocytopenia, anemia, hepatic dysfunction, hepatitis, hepatomegaly, hypoglycemia, hyperglycemia, hypocalcemia.

Onset, Peak, and Duration

Route	Onset	Peak	Duration
I.V.	Unknown	Immediate	Unknown
I.M.	Unknown	30 min–1 hr	Unknown
Aerosol	Unknown	Unknown	Unknown

 Massage Considerations

- No cautions or contraindications to massage are indicated because a client is taking this drug. Cautions or contraindications to massage may be related to the client condition and severity of infection.
- The site of intramuscular injection of the drug should not be massaged for at least 1 hour after administration of the drug.
- Side effects of hypotension and dizziness require care in getting the client on and off the table. Using stimulation with effleurage and tapotement at the end of the session may help. Itching and rash are local contraindications to massage and should be reported to the physician immediately. If severe or widespread, massage should be withheld.

pentazocine hydrochloride (pen-TAZ-oh-seen high-droh-KLOR-ighd)

Fortral

pentazocine hydrochloride and acetaminophen

Talacen

pentazocine hydrochloride and aspirin

Talwin Compound

pentazocine hydrochloride and naloxone hydrochloride

Talwin NX

pentazocine lactate

Fortral, Talwin

Drug Class: Opioid analgesic

Drug Actions

Binds with opioid receptors at many sites in CNS, altering pain response by unknown mechanism and relieves pain.

Use

- Moderate to severe pain
- Labor

Side Effects

Cardiovascular: hypotension, shock.
Gastrointestinal: nausea, vomiting, constipation.
Nervous System: sedation, visual disturbances, hallucinations, drowsiness, dizziness, confusion, euphoria, headache, psychotomimetic effects.
Urinary: urine retention.
Skin: induration, nodules, sloughing, and sclerosis of injection site.
Other: hypersensitivity reactions (anaphylaxis), physical and psychological dependence, dry mouth, painful swallowing, respiratory depression.

Onset, Peak, and Duration

Route	Onset	Peak	Duration
Oral	15–30 min	60–90 min	2–3 hr
I.V.	2–3 min	15–30 min	2–3 hr
I.M. Subcutaneous Injection	15–20 min	15–60 min	4–6 hr

Massage Considerations

- This drug alters the perception of pain and sensation; therefore, deep tissue massage is contraindicated.
- Further cautions and contraindications to massage may be related to the client condition.
- The action of the drug depresses the CNS. The relaxation effects of massage and the effects of the systemic reflex strokes such as rhythmic effleurage, rocking, and friction

may be increased. Using stimulation with rapid strokes at the end of the session may help. If the effect is severe, stimulation with rapid strokes of effleurage and pétrissage may be needed throughout the session. The effects of the local reflex strokes of stretching, traction, compression, and vibration may be less effective. Using these strokes for a longer than usual time may help.

- The site of intramuscular or subcutaneous injection of the drug should not be massaged for at least 1 hour.
- Side effects of hypotension, dizziness, and drowsiness may be addressed as noted above.
- Constipation may be helped by abdominal massage.

pentostatin (2'–deoxycoformycin) (pen-toh-STAH-tin)

Nipent

Drug Class: Antineoplastic

Drug Actions

Kills certain leukemic cells

Use

- Hairy cell leukemia refractory to interferon-α

Side Effects

Cardiovascular: chest pain, arrhythmias, abnormal ECG, thrombophlebitis, peripheral edema, hemorrhage.
Gastrointestinal: abdominal pain, nausea, vomiting, anorexia, diarrhea, constipation, gas, stomatitis.
Nervous System: pain, weakness, malaise, fever, headache, neurologic symptoms, anxiety, confusion, depression, dizziness, insomnia, nervousness, paresthesia, sleepiness, abnormal thinking, fatigue.
Urinary: hematuria, painful urination.
Skin: sweating, photosensitivity reaction, contact dermatitis, bruising, rash, eczema, dry skin, herpes simplex or zoster, itching, seborrhea, discoloration.
Other: infections, hypersensitivity reactions, neoplasm, chills, sepsis, flulike syndrome, abnormal vision, conjunctivitis, ear pain, eye pain, nosebleeds, pharyngitis, rhinitis, sinusitis, myelosuppression, abnormal blood profiles, lymphadenopathy, weight loss, back pain, muscle pain, joint pain, cough, bronchitis, shortness of breath, pulmonary edema, pneumonia.

Onset, Peak, and Duration

Route	Onset	Peak	Duration
I.V.	Unknown	Unknown	Unknown

 Massage Considerations

- Because of the toxic effects of this drug, deep tissue massage is contraindicated and circulatory massage with effleurage should be used with caution and limited.
- Other cautions and contraindications to massage will be related to the client condition.
- The physician should be consulted before any massage is given, and close collaboration is essential.
- This drug is usually given every other week and has a half-life of about 6 hours. Massage would best be given either before the drug is administered or at least 24 hours after the drug has been administered.
- Side effects of thrombophlebitis are a complete contraindication to massage.

- Dizziness and sleepiness require care in getting the client on and off the table. Stimulation with friction to the legs or tapotement at the end of the session may help.
- Paresthesia requires local care with depth and pressure. No deep tissue massage should be done.
- Constipation and gas may be helped by abdominal massage.
- Bruising requires care in depth and pressure and contraindicates deep tissue massage.
- Rash and itching are local contraindications to massage and should be reported to the physician. If severe or widespread, massage should be withheld.

---

pentoxifylline (pen-tok-SIH-fi-lin)

Trental

Drug Class: Hemorrheologic

Drug Actions

Unknown; thought to increase red blood cell flexibility and lower blood viscosity, thus improving capillary blood flow.

Use

- Intermittent claudication caused by chronic occlusive vascular disease

Side Effects

Gastrointestinal: painful digestion, nausea, vomiting.
Nervous System: headache, dizziness.

Onset, Peak, and Duration

Route	Onset	Peak	Duration
Oral	Unknown	2–4 hr	Unknown

 Massage Considerations

- Because this drug acts on blood viscosity, deep tissue massage should be used with great caution and no deep tissue massage should be used on the lower extremities.
- The physician should be consulted before any massage is given.
- Side effects of dizziness require care in getting the client on and off the table. Stimulation with tapotement or effleurage at the end of the session may help.

---

pergolide mesylate (PER-goh-lighd MES-ih-layt)

Permax

Drug Class: Antiparkinsonian

Drug Actions

Directly stimulates dopamine receptors and helps to relieve signs and symptoms of Parkinson's disease.

Use

- Adjunct treatment with levodopa-carbidopa in management of symptoms caused by Parkinson's disease

Side Effects

Cardiovascular: chest pain; orthostatic hypotension; vasodilation; palpitations; hypotension; hypertension; arrhythmias; heart attack; facial, peripheral, or generalized edema.

Gastrointestinal: dry mouth, painful digestion, abdominal pain, nausea, constipation, diarrhea, painful swallowing, anorexia, vomiting.
Nervous System: headache, weakness, dyskinesia, dizziness, hallucinations, dystonia, confusion, sleepiness, syncope, insomnia, anxiety, depression, tremor, abnormal dreams, personality disorder, psychosis, abnormal gait, akathisia, extrapyramidal syndrome, incoordination, akinesia, hypertonia, neuralgia, speech disorder, twitching, paresthesia.
Urinary: urinary frequency, urinary tract infection, hematuria.
Skin: sweating, rash.
Other: flulike syndrome, chills, infection, rhinitis, nosebleed, abnormal vision, double vision, eye disorder, weight gain, neck and back pain, bursitis, joint pain, muscle pain.

Onset, Peak, and Duration

Route	Onset	Peak	Duration
Oral	Unknown	Unknown	Unknown

Massage Considerations

- No cautions or contraindications to massage are related to the actions of this drug. Cautions and contraindications to massage may be related to the client condition.
- Side effects of hypotension, dizziness, and sleepiness require care in getting the client on and off the table. Using stimulation with rapid effleurage at the end of the session and staying with the client until he or she is sitting up and steady will help.
- Neuralgia and paresthesia are local contraindications to deep tissue massage. If severe, massage may be completely contraindicated.
- Constipation may be helped by abdominal massage.
- Urinary frequency requires privacy and quick access to the bathroom for the client. Water fountains or water music, which stimulate urination, should be avoided.
- Rash is a local contraindication to massage and should be reported to the physician.

---

perindopril erbumine (PER-in-doh-pril ER-buh-mighn)

Aceon

Drug Class: Angiotensin-converting enzyme (ACE) inhibitor antihypertensive

Drug Actions

Probably inhibits ACE activity, resulting in decreased vasoconstriction and decreased aldosterone, reduced sodium and water retention, and lowered blood pressure.

Use

- Essential hypertension

Side Effects

Cardiovascular: palpitations, edema, chest pain, abnormal ECG.
Gastrointestinal: painful digestion, diarrhea, abdominal pain, nausea, vomiting, gas.
Nervous System: dizziness, weakness, fever, sleep disorder, paresthesia, depression, sleepiness, nervousness, headache.
Urinary: proteinuria, urinary tract infection, sexual dysfunction in men, menstrual disorder.
Skin: rash.
Other: viral infection, injury, seasonal allergy, rhinitis, sinusitis, ear infection, pharyngitis, ringing in the ears, hyperkalemia, back pain, hypertonia, neck pain, joint pain, muscle pain, arthritis, leg or arm pain, cough, upper respiratory tract infection.

Onset, Peak, and Duration

Route	Onset	Peak	Duration
Oral	Unknown	1 hr	Unknown

 Massage Considerations

- No cautions or contraindications to massage are related to the actions of this drug. Cautions and contraindications to massage may be related to the client condition.
- Side effects of dizziness and sleepiness require care in getting the client on and off the table. Using stimulation with rapid effleurage and tapotement at the end of the session may help.
- Paresthesia is a local contraindication to deep tissue massage.
- Gas may be helped by abdominal massage.
- Rash is a local contraindication to massage and should be reported to the physician.

---

perphenazine (per-FEN-uh-zeen)

Apo-Perphenazine, Trilafon, Trilafon Concentrate

Drug Class: Antipsychotic, antiemetic

Drug Actions

Relieves signs and symptoms of psychosis; also relieves nausea and vomiting.

Use

- Psychosis in nonhospitalized patients
- Psychosis in hospitalized patients
- Severe nausea and vomiting

Side Effects

Cardiovascular: orthostatic hypotension, tachycardia, ECG changes, cardiac arrest.
Gastrointestinal: dry mouth, constipation.
Nervous System: extrapyramidal reaction, tardive dyskinesia, sedation, pseudoparkinsonism, electroencephalogram (EEG) changes, dizziness, seizures, neuroleptic malignant syndrome.
Urinary: urine retention, dark urine, menstrual irregularities, inhibited ejaculation.
Skin: mild photosensitivity reaction, sterile abscess.
Other: allergic reactions, pain at intramuscular injection site, abnormal growth of breast tissue, ocular changes, blurred vision, abnormal blood profiles, cholestatic jaundice, weight gain, increased appetite.

Onset, Peak, and Duration

Route	Onset	Peak	Duration
Oral, I.M.	Varies	Unknown	Unknown

 Massage Considerations

- Although the action of this drug is not clearly understood, there is a strong depressant action on the CNS. Deep tissue massage should be used with great caution, if at all.
- In most, if not all, cases, further cautions and contraindications to massage will be related to the client condition.
- The physician should be consulted before any massage is given, and close collaboration is essential.
- The onset and peak action of the drug are unknown. The site of intramuscular injection of the drug should not be massaged for at least 6 hours or until the next dose is in a different site.

- The depressive action of this drug may increase the relaxation effects of massage in general and increase the effect of the systemic reflex strokes of rocking, effleurage, and friction. Using these strokes in a more rapid and stimulating manner throughout the session may help. The action of the drug may also decrease the effectiveness of the local reflex strokes of compression, stretching, traction, and vibration as well as the effectiveness of deep tissue massage. Using these strokes for a longer time than usual may achieve the desired effects.
- Side effects of hypotension and dizziness may be addressed as noted above.
- Constipation may be helped by regular abdominal massage.
- The best approach to this client will be using the primarily mechanical strokes of pétrissage, effleurage, and friction. Some myofascial massage techniques may also be effective.

---

phenazopyridine hydrochloride (phenylazo diamino pyridine hydrochloride) (fen-eh-soh-PEER-eh-deen high-droh-KLOR-ighd)

Azo-Dine, Azo-Gesic, Azo-Standard, Baridium, Geridium, Phenazol, Prodium, Pyridiate, Pyridium, Pyridium Plus, Re-Azo, Urodine, Urogesic, UTI Relief

Drug Class: Urinary analgesic

Drug Actions

Has local anesthetic effect on urinary mucosa, thus relieving urinary tract pain.

Use

- Urinary tract irritation or infection

Side Effects

Gastrointestinal: nausea, mild GI disturbance.
Nervous System: headache, dizziness.
Skin: rash, itching.
Other: staining of contact lenses.

Onset, Peak, and Duration

Route	Onset	Peak	Duration
Oral	Unknown	Unknown	Unknown

Massage Considerations

- No cautions or contraindications to massage are related to the actions of this drug. The anesthetic effect is specific to the urinary tract.
- Side effects of dizziness requires care in getting the client on and off the table. Stimulation with effleurage and tapotement at the end of the session may help.
- Rash and itching are local contraindications to massage and should be reported to the physician. If severe or widespread, massage should be withheld.

---

phenobarbital (phenobarbitone) (feen-oh-BAR-bih-tol)

Solfoton

phenobarbital sodium (phenobarbitone sodium)

Luminal Sodium

Drug Class: Barbiturate anticonvulsant/sedative-hypnotic

Drug Actions

May depress CNS synaptic transmission and interfere with transmission of impulses from thalamus to brain cortex, stopping seizure activity and promoting calmness and sleep.

Use

- All forms of epilepsy except absence seizures
- Febrile seizures in children
- Status epilepticus
- Sedation
- Insomnia
- Preoperative sedation

Side Effects

Cardiovascular: bradycardia, hypotension.
Gastrointestinal: GI: nausea, vomiting.
Nervous System: drowsiness, lethargy, hangover.
Skin: rash, erythema multiforme, Stevens-Johnson syndrome, hives.
Other: angioedema, pain, swelling, thrombophlebitis, necrosis, nerve injury at injection site, exacerbation of porphyria, respiratory depression, apnea.

Onset, Peak, and Duration

Route	Onset	Peak	Duration
Oral	20–60 min	Unknown	10–12 hr
I.V.	5 min	≥15 min	10–12 hr
I.M.	>60 min	Unknown	10–12 hr

 Massage Considerations

- This drug has a depressant effect on the CNS. Deep tissue massage is contraindicated.
- In most cases, further cautions and contraindications to massage will be related to the client condition.
- The physician should be consulted before any massage is given.
- The action of the drug may increase the relaxation effects of massage in general and increase the effects of the systemic reflex strokes of rocking, effleurage, and friction. Using these strokes in a more rapid and stimulating manner throughout the session will help. The local reflex strokes of stretching, traction, vibration, and compression may be less effective. Using these strokes for a longer time than usual may achieve the desired effects.
- The site of intramuscular injection of the drug should not be massaged for at least 1 hour (the time of onset of the drug action) but probably should not be massaged for up to 10 hours.
- Side effects of hypotension and drowsiness may be addressed as noted above.
- Rash is a local contraindication to massage and should be reported to the physician immediately. If severe or widespread, massage should be withheld.
- Thrombophlebitis is a complete contraindication to massage.
- The best approach to this client is to use the mechanical strokes of effleurage, pétrissage, and friction. Myofascial massage techniques may also be helpful.

---

phentermine hydrochloride (FEN-ter-meen high-droh-KLOR-ighd)

Adipex-P, Duromine, Ionamin, Pro-Fast HS, Pro-Fast SA, Pro-Fast SR

Drug Class: Indirect-acting sympathomimetic amine

Drug Actions

Probably works by releasing stored norepinephrine from nerve terminals in the brain (primarily in the cerebral cortex and reticular activating system), thus promoting nerve impulse transmission and depressing appetite.

Use

- Short-term adjunct in exogenous obesity

Side Effects

Cardiovascular: palpitations, tachycardia, increased blood pressure.
Gastrointestinal: dry mouth, painful swallowing, constipation, diarrhea, other GI disturbances.
Nervous System: overstimulation, headache, euphoria, dysphoria, dizziness, insomnia.
Skin: hives.
Other: altered libido, abnormal dilation of the pupil, eye irritation, blurred vision, impotence.

Onset, Peak, and Duration

Route	Onset	Peak	Duration
Oral	Unknown	Unknown	12–14 hr

 Massage Considerations

- Because this drug stimulates the CNS, tapotement should be used with caution.
- Cautions and contraindications to massage may be related to the client condition.
- The action of this drug is to stimulate the CNS. This may potentially decrease the relaxation effects of massage and the effects of the systemic reflex strokes of effleurage, rocking, and friction. Using these strokes for a longer time than usual and using slow, rhythmic effleurage throughout the session may help achieve the desired effects.
- Side effects of dizziness require care in getting the client on and off the table. Stimulation with effleurage at the end of the session may be needed.
- Constipation may be helped by abdominal massage.
- Hives are a local contraindication to massage and should be reported to the physician immediately. If severe or widespread, massage should be withheld.

---

phenylephrine hydrochloride (intranasal) (fen-il-EF-rin high-droh-KLOR-ighd)

Afrin Children's Pump Mist, Alconefrin 12, Alconefrin 25, Alconefrin 50, Duration, Little Colds for Infants and Children, Little Noses Gentle Formula, Neo-Synephrine 4 Hour, Nostril, Rhinall, Vicks Sinex

Drug Class: Adrenergic vasoconstrictor

Drug Actions

Causes local vasoconstriction of dilated arterioles, reducing blood flow and relieving nasal congestion.

Use

- Nasal congestion

Side Effects

Cardiovascular: palpitations, tachycardia, premature ventricular contractions (PVCs), hypertension, pallor.

Gastrointestinal: nausea.
Nervous System: headache, tremor, dizziness, nervousness.
Other: transient burning or stinging, dry nasal mucosa, rebound nasal congestion with chronic use.

Onset, Peak, and Duration

Route	Onset	Peak	Duration
Intranasal	Rapid	Unknown	30 min–4 hr

 Massage Considerations

- No cautions or contraindications to massage are indicated because a client is taking this drug. Cautions and contraindications to massage may be related to the client condition.
- Side effects of dizziness require care in getting the client on and off the table. Stimulation with friction to the legs at the end of the session may help.

---

phenytoin (diphenylhydantoin) (FEN-uh-toyn)

Dilantin-125, Dilantin Infatabs

phenytoin sodium (extended)

Dilantin Kapseals, Phenytek

phenytoin sodium (prompt)

Dilantin

Drug Class: Anticonvulsant

Drug Actions

Probably limits seizure activity by either increasing efflux or decreasing influx of sodium ions across cell membranes in motor cortex.

Use

- Control of tonic-clonic (grand mal) and complex partial (temporal lobe) seizures
- Prevention and treatment of seizures occurring during neurosurgery
- Status epilepticus

Side Effects

Cardiovascular: hypotension.
Gastrointestinal: nausea, vomiting.
Nervous System: ataxia, slurred speech, confusion, dizziness, insomnia, nervousness, twitching, headache.
Skin: rash; Stevens-Johnson syndrome; abnormal hair growth; toxic epidermal necrolysis; photosensitivity reaction; hypertrichosis.
Other: periarteritis nodosa; lupus erythematosus; pain, necrosis, or inflammation at injection site; discoloration (purple glove syndrome) if given by intravenous infusion push in back of hand, nystagmus, diplopia, blurred vision, gingival hyperplasia, abnormal blood profiles, lymphadenopathy, toxic hepatitis, hyperglycemia, osteomalacia.

Onset, Peak, and Duration

Route	Onset	Peak	Duration
Oral	Unknown	30 min–2 hr	Unknown
Oral:			
Extended	Unknown	4–12 hr	Unknown
I.V.	Immediate	1–2 hr	Unknown
I.M.	Unknown	Unknown	Unknown

Massage Considerations

- Because this drug affects nerve impulse transmission in the CNS, deep tissue massage should be used with caution.
- Further cautions and contraindications to massage may be related to the client condition.
- The action of the drug may potentially decrease the effectiveness of the local reflex strokes of stretching, traction, compression, and vibration and of deep tissue massage. Using these strokes for a longer time than usual may achieve the desired effects.
- The site of intramuscular injection of the drug should not be massaged for 2 to 4 hours or until the next dose is given at another site.
- Side effects of hypotension and dizziness require care in getting the client on and off the table. Using stimulation with rapid effleurage at the end of the session may help.
- Rash is a local contraindication to massage and should be reported to the physician immediatlely. If severe or widespread, massage should be withheld.
- Osteomalacia, or softening of the bone, contraindicates deep tissue massage, and traction or stretching should be used with great caution. If severe, massage may be completely contraindicated.

---

pimecrolimus (py-meck-roh-LY-muhs)

Elidel

Drug Class: Topical immunomodulator

Drug Actions

Improves skin integrity

Use

- Short-term and intermittent long-term therapy for mild to moderate atopic dermatitis in nonimmunocompromised patients, in whom the use of alternative, conventional therapies is deemed inadvisable or for patients who are not adequately responding to or are intolerant of conventional therapies

Side Effects

Gastrointestinal: gastroenteritis, abdominal pain, sore throat, tonsillitis, vomiting, diarrhea, nausea, toothache, constipation, loose stools.
Nervous System: headache.
Skin: skin infections, impetigo, folliculitis, molluscum contagiosum, varicella, skin papilloma, hives, acne.
Other: herpes simplex, application site reaction (burning, irritation, erythema, pruritus), influenza, pyrexia, influenzalike illness, hypersensitivity reaction, bacterial infection, dysmenorrhea, staphylococcal infection, viral infection, nasopharyngitis, otitis media, sinusitis,

pharyngitis, eye infection, nasal congestion, rhinorrhea, sinus congestion, rhinitis, back pain, joint pain, upper respiratory tract infections, pneumonia, bronchitis, cough, asthma, wheezing, shortness of breath, nosebleeds, conjunctivitis, earache.

Onset, Peak, and Duration

Route	Onset	Peak	Duration
Topical	Unknown	Unknown	Unknown

Massage Considerations

- No cautions or contraindications to massage are related to the actions of this drug. Cautions and contraindications to massage may be related to the client condition.
- The site of topical application of the drug should not be massaged.
- If the skin condition is widespread and the client still desires massage, the physician should be consulted, gloves should be worn when working the affected areas, and massage should be given as long as possible after application of the drug or just before application.
- Side effects of hives, acne, or other skin eruptions should be reported to the physician immediately and, depending on severity, may contraindicate massage completely. At a minimum, the site of the outbreak should not be massaged.

---

pimozide (PIH-mih-zighd)

Orap

Drug Class: Antipsychotic

Drug Actions

May block dopamine nonselectively at presynaptic and postsynaptic receptors on neurons in CNS. Stops tics linked to Tourette syndrome.

Use

- Suppression of motor and phonic tics in patients with Tourette syndrome refractory to first-line therapy

Side Effects

Cardiovascular: ECG changes (prolonged QT interval), hypotension.
Gastrointestinal: dry mouth, constipation.
Nervous System: parkinsonianlike symptoms, other extrapyramidal symptoms (dystonia, akathisia, hyperreflexia, opisthotonos, oculogyric crisis), tardive dyskinesia, sedation, neuroleptic malignant syndrome.
Urinary: impotence.
Other: muscle rigidity, visual disturbances.

Onset, Peak, and Duration

Route	Onset	Peak	Duration
Oral	Unknown	4–12 hr	Unknown

Massage Considerations

- The action of this drug slows nerve impulse transmission; therefore, deep tissue massage should be used with caution.
- Other cautions and contraindications to massage may be related to the client condition.
- The actions of this drug may potentially decrease the effectiveness of the local reflex strokes of stretching, traction, compression, and vibration and of deep tissue massage.

Applying these strokes for a longer time than usual may achieve the desired effects. Using more mechanical strokes such as effleurage and pétrissage may also be effective.
- Side effects of hypotension require care in getting the client on and off the table. Stimulation with effleurage or friction to the lower legs may help.
- Constipation may be helped by abdominal massage.

pindolol (PIN-duh-lol)

Novo-Pindol, Visken

Drug Class: Beta-blocker antihypertensive

Drug Actions

Lowers blood pressure

Use

- Hypertension
- Angina

Side Effects

Cardiovascular: edema, bradycardia, heart failure, peripheral vascular disease, hypotension.
Gastrointestinal: nausea, vomiting, diarrhea.
Nervous System: insomnia, fatigue, dizziness, nervousness, vivid dreams, hallucinations, lethargy.
Skin: rash.
Other: visual disturbances, hypoglycemia without tachycardia, muscle pain, joint pain, increased airway resistance.

Onset, Peak, and Duration

Route	Onset	Peak	Duration
Oral	Unknown	1–2 hr	24 hr

 Massage Considerations

- The action of this drug is unknown. No clear cautions or contraindications to massage are related to this drug. Cautions and contraindications to massage may be related to the client condition.
- Side effects of hypotension and dizziness require care in getting the client on and off table. Stimulation with rapid effleurage and tapotement at the end of the session may help.
- Rash is a local contraindication to massage and should be reported to the physician.

pioglitazone hydrochloride (pigh-oh-GLIH-tah-zohn high-droh-KLOR-ighd)

Actos

Drug Class: Antidiabetic

Drug Actions

Decreases insulin resistance in the periphery and in the liver, resulting in lower glucose levels.

Use

- Monotherapy adjunct to diet and exercise to improve glycemic control in patients with type 2 diabetes mellitus

- Combination therapy with a sulfonylurea, metformin, or insulin when diet and exercise plus the single drug does not yield adequate glycemic control

Side Effects

Cardiovascular: edema, heart failure.
Nervous System: headache.
Other: tooth disorder, sinusitis, pharyngitis, anemia, hypoglycemia with combination therapy, aggravated diabetes mellitus, weight gain, muscle pain, upper respiratory tract infection.

Onset, Peak, and Duration

Route	Onset	Peak	Duration
Oral	Unknown	Within 2 hr	Unknown

 Massage Considerations

- No cautions or contraindications to massage are related to the actions of this drug. Cautions and contraindications to massage may be related to the client condition.

---

piperacillin sodium and tazobactam sodium (pigh-PER-uh-sil-in SOH-dee-um and taz-oh-BAK-tem SOH-dee-um)

Zosyn

Drug Class: Antibiotic

Drug Actions

Kills susceptible bacteria

Use

- Moderate to severe infections
- Appendicitis (complicated by rupture or abscess)
- Peritonitis
- Skin and skin-structure infections
- Moderately severe community-acquired pneumonia
- Moderate to severe nosocomial pneumonia

Side Effects

Cardiovascular: hypertension, tachycardia, chest pain, edema.
Gastrointestinal: diarrhea, nausea, constipation, vomiting, painful digestion, stool changes, abdominal pain.
Nervous System: pain, headache, insomnia, agitation, fever, dizziness, anxiety.
Skin: rash, itching.
Other: anaphylaxis, candidiasis, inflammation and phlebitis at intravenous site, rhinitis, thrombocytopenia, shortness of breath.

Onset, Peak, and Duration

Route	Onset	Peak	Duration
I.V.	Immediate	Immediate	Unknown

 Massage Considerations

- No cautions or contraindications to massage are related to the actions of this drug. Cautions and contraindications to massage may be related to the client condition and severity of infection.

- Side effects of dizziness require care in getting the client on and off the table. Using stimulation at the end of the session with effleurage and tapotement may help.
- Constipation may be helped by abdominal massage.
- Rash and itching are local contraindications to massage and should be reported to the physician immediately. If severe or widespread, massage should be withheld.

---

pirbuterol acetate (pir-BYOO-teh-rol AS-ih-tayt)

Maxair

Drug Class: β-Adrenergic agonist bronchodilator

Drug Actions

Relaxes bronchial smooth muscle by acting on β_2-adrenergic receptors and improves breathing ability.

Use

- Prevention and reversal of bronchospasm
- Asthma

Side Effects

Cardiovascular: tachycardia, palpitations, increased blood pressure.
Nervous System: tremor, nervousness, dizziness, insomnia, headache.
Other: dry or irritated throat.

Onset, Peak, and Duration

Route	Onset	Peak	Duration
Inhalation	≤5 min	30–60 min	5–8 hr

Massage Considerations

- No cautions or contraindications to massage are related to the actions of this drug. Cautions and contraindications to massage may be related to the client condition.
- The action of this drug in stimulating certain sympathetic nervous system (SNS) receptors is fairly specific to the lungs; however, some systemic effects may be felt. This could potentially decrease the effectiveness of the systemic reflex strokes of effleurage, rocking, and friction and the general relaxation effects of massage. Using the above strokes for a longer time than usual and using slow, rhythmic effleurage throughout the session may help to achieve the desired results.
- Side effects of dizziness require care in getting the client on and off the table. Stimulation with a little friction to the legs at the end of the session may help.

---

piroxicam (peer-OK-sih-cam)

Apo-Piroxicam, Feldene, Novo-Pirocam

Drug Class: Nonsteroidal anti-inflammatory drug , nonopioid analgesic, antipyretic, anti-inflammatory

Drug Actions

Relieves pain, fever, and inflammation, possibly by inhibiting prostaglandin synthesis.

Use

- Osteoarthritis
- Rheumatoid arthritis
- Juvenile rheumatoid arthritis

Side Effects

Cardiovascular: peripheral edema.
Gastrointestinal: epigastric distress, nausea, occult blood loss, peptic ulceration, severe GI bleeding.
Nervous System: headache, drowsiness, dizziness, paresthesia, sleepiness.
Urinary: nephrotoxicity.
Skin: itching, rash, hives, photosensitivity reaction.
Other: auditory disturbances, abnormal blood profiles, hyperkalemia, acidosis, dilutional hypernatremia, bronchospasm.

Onset, Peak, and Duration

Route	Onset	Peak	Duration
Oral	15–30 min	3–5 hr	24 hr

 Massage Considerations

- This drug decreases the perception of pain; therefore, deep tissue massage should be used with caution.
- Further cautions and contraindications to massage may be related to the client condition.
- Side effects of drowsiness, dizziness, and sleepiness require care in getting the client on and off the table. Stimulation with rapid effleurage and tapotement at the end of the session may help.
- Paresthesia is a local contraindication to deep tissue massage.
- Itching, rash, or hives are local contraindications to massage and should be reported to the physician. If severe or widespread, massage should be withheld.

---

polysaccharide iron complex (pol-ee-SAK-uh-righd IGH-ern KOM-pleks)

Hytinic, Ferrex 150, Niferex, Niferex-150, Nu-Iron, Nu-Iron 150

Drug Class: Oral iron supplement

Drug Actions

Restores normal iron levels in body

Use

- Uncomplicated iron deficiency anemia

Side Effects

Gastrointestinal: nausea, constipation, black stools, epigastric pain.

Onset, Peak, and Duration

Route	Onset	Peak	Duration
Oral	≤3 days	5–30 days	2 mo

Massage Considerations

- No cautions or contraindications to massage are related to the actions of this drug. Cautions and contraindications to massage may be related to the client condition.
- Side effects of constipation may be helped by abdominal massage.

---

potassium bicarbonate (puh-TAS-ee-um bigh-KAR-buh-nayt)

K+ Care ET

Drug Class: Potassium supplement

Drug Actions

Replaces and maintains potassium level

Use

- Hypokalemia

Side Effects

Cardiovascular: arrhythmias, cardiac arrest, heart block, ECG changes (prolonged PR interval, widened QRS complex, ST-segment depression, and tall, tented T waves).
Gastrointestinal: nausea, vomiting, abdominal pain, diarrhea, ulcerations, hemorrhage, obstruction, perforation.
Nervous System: paresthesia of limbs, listlessness, mental confusion, weakness or heaviness of legs, flaccid paralysis.

Onset, Peak, and Duration

Route	Onset	Peak	Duration
Oral	Unknown	$\leq$4 hr	Unknown

Massage Considerations

- No cautions or contraindications to massage are indicated because a client is taking this drug. Cautions and contraindications to massage may be related to the client condition.
- Side effects of paresthesias are a local contraindication to deep tissue massage.

---

potassium chloride (puh-TAS-ee-um KLOR-ighd)

Apo-K, Cena-K, Gen-K, K-8, K-10, K+ 10, Kaochlor, Kaochlor S-F, Kaon-CL, Kaon-Cl-10, Kaon-Cl 20%, Kay Ciel, K+ Care, K- Dur 10, K-Dur 20, K-Lease, K-Lor, Klor-Con, Klor-Con 8, Klor-Con 10, Klor-Con/25, Klorvess, Klotrix, K-Lyte/Cl, K-Norm, K-Tab, K-vescent Potassium Chloride, Micro-K Extencaps, Micro-K 10 Extencaps, Micro-K LS, Potasalan, Slow-K, Ten-K

Drug Class: Potassium supplement

Drug Actions

Replaces and maintains potassium level

Use

- Prevention of hypokalemia
- Hypokalemia
- Severe hypokalemia
- Acute heart attack

Side Effects

Cardiovascular: arrhythmias, heart block, cardiac arrest, ECG changes (prolonged PR interval, widened QRS complex, ST-segment depression, and tall, tented T waves).
Gastrointestinal: nausea, vomiting, abdominal pain, diarrhea, GI ulcerations (stenosis, hemorrhage, obstruction, perforation).
Nervous System: paresthesia of limbs, listlessness, mental confusion, weakness or heaviness of limbs, flaccid paralysis.
Urinary: oliguria.
Skin: cold skin, gray pallor, phlebitis.
Other: respiratory paralysis.

Onset, Peak, and Duration

Route	Onset	Peak	Duration
Oral	Unknown	≤4 hr	Unknown
I.V.	Immediate	Immediate	Unknown

Massage Considerations

- No cautions or contraindications to massage are indicated because a client is taking this drug. Cautions and contraindications to massage may be related to the client condition.
- Side effects of paresthesias are a local contraindication to deep tissue massage.

---

potassium gluconate (puh-TAS-ee-um GLOO-kuh-nayt)

Kaon, Kaylixir, K-G Elixir

Drug Class: Potassium supplement

Drug Actions

Replaces and maintains potassium level

Use

- Hypokalemia

Side Effects

Cardiovascular: arrhythmias, ECG changes (prolonged PR interval, widened QRS complex, ST-segment depression, and tall, tented T waves).
Gastrointestinal: nausea and vomiting; abdominal pain; diarrhea; GI ulcerations that may be accompanied by stenosis, hemorrhage, obstruction or perforation (with oral products, especially enteric-coated tablets).
Nervous System: paresthesia of limbs, listlessness, mental confusion, weakness or heaviness of legs, flaccid paralysis.

Onset, Peak, and Duration

Route	Onset	Peak	Duration
Oral	Unknown	≤4 hr	Unknown

Massage Considerations

- No cautions or contraindications to massage are indicated because a client is taking this drug. Cautions and contraindications to massage may be related to the client condition.
- Side effects of paresthesias are a local contraindication to deep tissue massage.

potassium iodide (puh-TAS-ee-um IGH-uh-dighd)

Iosat, Pima, Thyro-Block

potassium iodide, saturated solution (SSKI)

strong iodine solution (Lugal's Solution)

Drug Class: Antithyroid

Drug Actions

Lowers thyroid hormone levels

Use

- Preparation for thyroidectomy
- Thyrotoxic crisis
- Radiation protectant for thyroid gland
- Hyperthyroidism

Side Effects

Gastrointestinal: burning, irritation, nausea, vomiting, diarrhea (sometimes bloody), metallic taste.
Nervous System: fever, frontal headache.
Skin: acneform rash, mucous membrane ulceration.
Other: hypersensitivity reactions, tooth discoloration, acute rhinitis, inflammation of salivary glands, periorbital edema, conjunctivitis, hyperemia, potassium toxicity (confusion, irregular heartbeat, numbness, tingling, pain or weakness in hands and feet, tiredness).

Onset, Peak, and Duration

Route	Onset	Peak	Duration
Oral	≤24 hr	10–15 days	Unknown

Massage Considerations

- No cautions or contraindication to massage are related to the actions of this drug.
- In most cases, cautions and contraindications to massage will be related to the client condition.
- Side effects of rash are a local contraindication to massage and should be reported to the physician. If severe or widespread, massage should be withheld.
- Because numbness or tingling and pain in the extremities may be related to serious potassium toxicity, massage is contraindicated until the client has been evaluated by the physician for this side effect.

pramipexole dihydrochloride (pram-ih-PEKS-ohl digh-high-droh-KLOR-ighd)

Mirapex

Drug Class: Antiparkinsonian

Drug Actions

Probably stimulates dopamine receptors and relieves symptoms of idiopathic Parkinson's disease.

Use

- Signs and symptoms of idiopathic Parkinson's disease

Side Effects

Cardiovascular: chest pain, peripheral edema, general edema, orthostatic hypotension.
Gastrointestinal: dry mouth, anorexia, constipation, difficulty swallowing, nausea.
Nervous System: malaise, akathisia, amnesia, weakness, confusion, delusions, dizziness, dream abnormalities, dyskinesia, dystonia, extrapyramidal syndrome, gait abnormalities, hallucinations, hypesthesia, hypertonia, insomnia, myoclonus, paranoid reaction, sleepiness, sleep disorders, thought abnormalities, fever.
Urinary: impotence, urinary frequency, urinary tract infections, urinary incontinence.
Skin: skin disorders.
Other: decreased libido, accidental injury, accommodation abnormalities, double vision, rhinitis, vision abnormalities, weight loss, arthritis, bursitis, twitching, myasthenia, shortness of breath, pneumonia.

Onset, Peak, and Duration

Route	Onset	Peak	Duration
Oral	Rapid	2 hr	8–12 hr

Massage Considerations

- No cautions or contraindications to massage are indicated because a client is taking this drug. Cautions and contraindications to massage may be related to the client condition.
- Side effects of hypotension, dizziness, and sleepiness require care in getting the client on and off the table. Stimulation with effleurage and tapotement at the end of the session may help. Hypesthesia, or decreased sensation, is a contraindication to deep tissue massage.
- Constipation may be helped by abdominal massage.
- Urinary frequency requires providing privacy and quick access to the bathroom when the client needs it. Water fountains and water music, which stimulate urination, should be avoided.
- Skin disorders should be evaluated by the physician and are a local contraindication to massage.

---

pravastatin sodium (PRAH-vuh-stat-in SOH-dee-um)

Pravachol

Drug Class: Antilipemic

Drug Actions

Inhibits the synthesis of cholesterol, lowering low density lipoproteins and total cholesterol levels in some patients.

Use

- Primary hypercholesterolemia
- Mixed dyslipidemia
- Primary and secondary prevention of coronary events
- Hyperlipidemia
- Homozygous familial hypercholesterolemia
- Heterozygous familial hypercholesterolemia

Side Effects

Cardiovascular: chest pain.
Gastrointestinal: vomiting, diarrhea, heartburn, nausea.
Nervous System: headache, fatigue, dizziness.
Urinary: renal failure secondary to myoglobinuria.
Skin: rash.
Other: flulike symptoms, rhinitis, myositis, myopathy, localized muscle pain, myalgia, rhabdomyolysis, cough.

Onset, Peak, and Duration

Route	Onset	Peak	Duration
Oral	Unknown	1 hr	Unknown

 Massage Considerations

- No cautions or contraindications to massage are indicated because a client is taking this drug.
- Cautions and contraindications to massage may be related to the client condition.
- Side effects of dizziness require care in getting the client on and off the table. Stimulation with effleurage or tapotement at the end of the sesssion may help.
- Rash is a local contraindication to massage and should be reported to the physician.
- Rhabdomyolysis is an extremely serious muscular degenerative condition that may present as increasing pain and tenderness of the muscles with no clear cause. Massage should not be given and the client should be referred to the physician for immediate evaluation to rule out this condition.

prazosin hydrochloride (PRAH-zoh-sin high-droh-KLOR-ighd)

Minipress

Drug Class: α-Adrenergic blocker antihypertensive

Drug Actions

α-Adrenergic blocking activity lowers blood pressure

Use

- Mild to moderate hypertension, alone or with diuretic or other antihypertensive
- Benign prostatic hypertrophy

Side Effects

Cardiovascular: orthostatic hypotension, palpitations.
Gastrointestinal: vomiting, diarrhea, abdominal cramps, constipation, nausea, dry mouth.
Nervous System: dizziness, headache, drowsiness, weakness, first-dose syncope, depression.
Other: priapism, impotence, blurred vision.

Onset, Peak, and Duration

Route	Onset	Peak	Duration
Oral	30–90 min	2–4 hr	7–10 hr

 Massage Considerations

- No cautions or contraindications to massage are indicated because a client is taking this drug. Cautions and contraindications to massage may be related to the client condition.

- Side effects of hypotension, dizziness, and drowsiness require care in getting the client on and off the table. Stimulation with effleurage and tapotement at the end of the session may help.
- Constipation may be helped by abdominal massage.

---

prednisolone (systemic) (pred-NIS-uh-lohn)

Delta-Cortef, Prelone

prednisolone acetate

Cotolone, Key-Pred-25, Predalone 50, Predcor-50

prednisolone sodium phosphate

Hydeltrasol, Key-Pred SP, Orapred, Pediapred

prednisolone tebutate

Nor-Pred TBA, Predate TBA, Predcor-TBA, Prednisol TBA

Drug Class: Glucocorticoid, mineralocorticoid, anti-inflammatory, immunosuppressant

Drug Actions

Decreases inflammation; suppresses immune response; stimulates bone marrow; and influences protein, fat, and carbohydrate metabolism.

Use

- Severe inflammation
- Modification of body's immune response to disease
- Acute exacerbations of multiple sclerosis
- Nephrotic syndrome
- Uncontrolled asthma in patients taking inhaled corticosteroids and long-acting bronchodilators

Side Effects

Cardiovascular: heart failure, thromboembolism, hypertension, edema.
Gastrointestinal: peptic ulceration, GI irritation, increased appetite, pancreatitis.
Nervous System: euphoria, insomnia, psychotic behavior, pseudotumor cerebri, seizures.
Skin: abnormal hair growth, delayed wound healing, acne, various skin eruptions.
Other: susceptibility to infections, acute adrenal insufficiency with increased stress (infection, surgery, or trauma) or abrupt withdrawal after long-term therapy, cataracts, glaucoma, hypokalemia, hyperglycemia, carbohydrate intolerance, growth suppression in children, muscle weakness, osteoporosis.

Onset, Peak, and Duration

Route	Onset	Peak	Duration
Oral	Rapid	1–2 hr	30–36 hr
I.V.	Rapid	<1hr	Unknown
I.M.	Rapid	<1hr	<4 wk
Rectal	Unknown	Unknown	Unknown
Intra-articular, intralesional	1–2 days	Unknown	3 days–4 wk

Massage Considerations

- When this drug is taken long term, longer than 2 weeks, the metabolism of the body is changed and muscle, connective, and fatty tissues of the body are also changed. Because of this, deep tissue massage is contraindicated. Stretching and traction should be used with caution. Myofascial massage techniques should be used with great caution and may not be as effective.
- Further cautions and contraindications to massage may be related to the client condition.
- The site of intramuscular injection of the drug should not be massaged for at least 1 hour. The site of intra-articular (into the joint) or intralesional injection should not be massaged for at least 3 days.
- Side effects of thromboembolism are a complete contraindication to massage.
- Symptoms of pain, redness, swelling, and heat, especially in the lower extremities, should be referred to the physician for evaluation immediately and massage withheld.
- Acne and skin eruptions are local contraindications to massage and should be reported to the physician. If the client must continue to take the drug and acne is severe, massage may be given with the massage therapist wearing gloves when working the affected areas.
- Susceptibility to infections requires extra attention to cleanliness. Scheduling the client as the first client of the day to avoid exposure to others may help. If the massage therapist has any symptoms of infection, massage should not be given that day.
- Osteoporosis is a caution to depth and pressure of massage and, if severe, may contraindicate massage completely.
- The best approach to this client is to use the systemic reflex strokes and mechanical strokes of rocking, effleurage, gentle friction, and pétrissage.

---

prednisone (PRED-nih-sohn)

Apo-Prednisone, Deltasone, Liquid Pred, Meticorten, Novo-Prednisone, Orasone, Panafcort, Panasol-S, Prednicen-M, Prednisone Intensol, Sone, Sterapred, Winpred

Drug Class: Adrenocorticoid steroid, anti-inflammatory, immunosuppressant

Drug Actions

Decreases inflammation; suppresses immune response; stimulates bone marrow; and influences protein, fat, and carbohydrate metabolism.

Use

- Severe inflammation
- Immunosuppression
- Acute exacerbations of multiple sclerosis

Side Effects

Cardiovascular: heart failure, thromboembolism, hypertension, edema.
Gastrointestinal: peptic ulceration, GI irritation, increased appetite, pancreatitis.
Nervous System: euphoria, insomnia, psychotic behavior, pseudotumor cerebri, seizures.
Skin: abnormal hair growth, delayed wound healing, acne, various skin eruptions.
Other: susceptibility to infections, cataracts, glaucoma, hypokalemia, hyperglycemia, carbohydrate intolerance, growth suppression in children, muscle weakness, osteoporosis.

Onset, Peak, and Duration

Route	Onset	Peak	Duration
Oral	Varies	Varies	Varies

 Massage Considerations

- When this drug is taken long term, longer than 2 weeks, the metabolism of the body is changed and muscle, connective, and fatty tissues of the body are also changed. Because of this, deep tissue massage is contraindicated. Stretching and traction should be used with caution. Myofascial massage techniques should be used with great caution and may not be as effective.
- Further cautions and contraindications to massage may be related to the client condition.
- The site of intramuscular injection of the drug should not be massaged for at least 1 hour. The site of intra-articular (into the joint) or intralesional injection should not be massaged for at least 3 days.
- Side effects of thromboembolism are a complete contraindication to massage.
- Symptoms of pain, redness, swelling, and heat, especially in the lower extremities, should be referred to the physician for evaluation immediately and massage withheld.
- Acne and skin eruptions are local contraindications to massage and should be reported to the physician. If the client must continue to take the drug and acne is severe, massage may be given with the massge therapist wearing gloves when working the affected areas.
- Susceptibility to infections requires extra attention to cleanliness. Scheduling the client as the first client of the day to avoid exposure to others may help. If the massage therapist has any symptoms of infection, massage should not be given that day.
- Osteoporosis is a caution to depth and pressure of massage and, if severe, may contraindicate massage completely.
- The best approach to this client is to use the systemic reflex strokes and mechanical strokes of rocking, effleurage, gentle friction, and pétrissage.

---

primidone (PRIH-mih-dohn)

Apo-Primidone, Mysoline, PMS Primidone, Sertan

Drug Class: Anticonvulsant

Drug Actions

Prevents seizures.

Use

- Generalized tonic-clonic, focal, and complex-partial (psychomotor) seizures
- Benign familial tremor (essential tremor)

Side Effects

Cardiovascular: edema.
Gastrointestinal: anorexia, nausea, vomiting, thirst.
Nervous System: drowsiness, ataxia, emotional disturbances, hyperirritability, fatigue.
Urinary: impotence, polyuria.
Skin: rash, hair loss.
Other: double vision, nystagmus, edema of eyelids, abnormal blood profiles.

Onset, Peak, and Duration

Route	Onset	Peak	Duration
Oral	Unknown	3–4 hr	Unknown

 Massage Considerations

- Although the action of this drug is unknown, it has a CNS depressant effect. Deep tissue massage should be done with caution.

- Other cautions and contraindications to massage may be related to the client condition.
- The depressant effect of this drug may increase the effects of the systemic reflex strokes of effleurage, rocking, and friction and the relaxation effects of massage in general. Using these strokes in a more rapid and stimulating manner throughout the session may help. A decrease in the effectiveness of the local reflex strokes of stretching, traction, compression, and vibration, and even of deep tissue massage, may occur. Using these strokes for a longer than usual time may help achieve the desired effects.
- Side effects of drowsiness require care in getting the client on and off table and may be addressed as noted above.
- Rash is a local contraindication to massage and should be reported to the physician.
- Hair loss is a contraindication to scalp massage if the client is disturbed by hair loss during the massage or if the scalp is tender.

---

probenecid (proh-BEN-uh-sid)

Benemid, Benuryl, Probalan

Drug Class: Uricosuric

Drug Actions

Blocks renal tubular reabsorption of uric acid, increasing excretion, and inhibits active renal tubular secretion of many weak organic acids, such as penicillins and cephalosporins, thus lowering uric acid and prolonging penicillin action.

Use

- Adjunct to penicillin therapy
- Gonorrhea
- Hyperuricemia of gout
- Gouty arthritis
- To diagnose parkinsonian syndrome or mental depression

Side Effects

Cardiovascular: flushing, hypotension.
Gastrointestinal: anorexia, nausea, vomiting, sore gums, gastric distress.
Nervous System: headache, fever, dizziness.
Urinary: urinary frequency, renal colic.
Skin: hair loss, rash, itching.
Other: hypersensitivity reaction, anaphylaxis, hemolytic anemia, aplastic anemia, hepatic necrosis.

Onset, Peak, and Duration

Route	Onset	Peak	Duration
Oral	Unknown	2–4 hr	8 hr

Massage Considerations

- No cautions or contraindications to massage are related to the actions of this drug. Cautions and contraindications to massage may be related to the client condition.
- Side effects of hypotension and dizziness require using stimulation with effleurage and tapotement at the end of the sesssion.
- Urinary frequency may require the client to get up in the middle of the session. Privacy and quick access to the bathroom is needed. Water fountains and water music, which may stimulate urination, should be avoided.

- Hair loss is a contraindication to scalp massage if the client is disturbed by hair loss during the massage or if the scalp is tender.
- Rash and itching are local contraindications to massage and should be reported to the physician.

---

procainamide hydrochloride (proh-KAYN-uh-mighd high-droh-KLOR-ighd)

Procainamide Durules, Procan SR, Procanbid, Promine, Pronestyl, Pronestyl SR

Drug Class: Ventricular antiarrhythmic, supraventricular antiarrhythmic

Drug Actions

Restores normal sinus rhythm.

Use

- Symptomatic PVCs
- Life-threatening ventricular tachycardia
- Maintenance of normal sinus rhythm after conversion of atrial flutter
- Loading dose to prevent atrial fibrillation or paroxysmal atrial tachycardia
- Malignant hyperthermia

Side Effects

Cardiovascular: hypotension, ventricular asystole, bradycardia, atrioventricular block, ventricular fibrillation after parenteral use, heart failure.
Gastrointestinal: nausea, vomiting, anorexia, diarrhea, bitter taste with large doses.
Nervous System: hallucinations, fever, confusion, depression, dizziness.
Skin: rash.
Other: lupus-like syndrome (especially after prolonged use), abnormal blood profiles, joint pain.

Onset, Peak, and Duration

Route	Onset	Peak	Duration
Oral	2 hr	1–1.5 hr	Unknown
I.V.	Immediate	Immediate	Unknown
I.M.	10–30 min	15–60 min	Unknown

Massage Considerations

- No cautions or contraindications to massage are related to the actions of this drug. Cautions and contraindications to massage will be related to the client condition.
- The physician should be consulted before any massage is given.
- The site of intramuscular injection should not be massaged for at least 1 hour.
- Side effects of hypotension and dizziness require care in getting the client on and off the table. Using gentle stimulation with tapotement at the end of the session may help.
- Rash is a local contraindication to massage and should be reported to the physician.

---

procarbazine hydrochloride (proh-KAR-buh-zeen high-droh-KLOR-ighd)

Matulane, Natulan

Drug Class: Antibiotic antineoplastic

Drug Actions

Kills selected cancer cells

Use

- Hodgkin's disease
- Lymphoma
- Brain and lung cancer

Side Effects

Gastrointestinal: nausea, vomiting, anorexia, stomatitis, dry mouth, difficulty swallowing, diarrhea, constipation.
Nervous System: nervousness, depression, insomnia, nightmares, paresthesia, neuropathy, hallucinations, confusion, seizures, coma.
Skin: rash, hair loss, retinal hemorrhage, nystagmus, photophobia, bleeding tendency, abnormal blood profiles, hepatotoxicity, pleural effusion, pneumonitis.

Onset, Peak, and Duration

Route	Onset	Peak	Duration
Oral	Unknown	Unknown	Unknown

 Massage Considerations

- Because of the toxic effects of this drug, deep tissue massage is contraindicated, and circulatory massage with effleurage should be used with caution and limited.
- Further cautions and contraindications to massage may be related to the client condition.
- The physician should be consulted before any massage is given, and close collaboration is essential.
- This drug is usually taken daily and has a very short half-life. Massage should be given before the drug is administered if possible; if not, massage may be given a few hours after the drug is administered.
- Side effects of paresthesia and neuropathy are local contraindications to deep tissue massage, and care should be taken with depth and pressure at all times.
- Constipation may be helped by abdominal massage.
- Rash is a local contraindication to massage and should be reported to the physician immediately. If severe or widespread, massage should be withheld.
- Hair loss is a contraindication to scalp massage if the client is disturbed by hair loss during the massage or if the scalp is tender.
- The best approach to this client is to use systemic and local reflex strokes of rocking, friction, gentle compression, stretching, traction, and vibration.

---

prochlorperazine (proh-klor-PER-ah-zeen)

Compazine, PMS Prochlorperazine, Prorazin, Stemetil

prochlorperazine edisylate

Compa-Z, Compazine Syrup, Cotranzine, Ultrazine-10

prochlorperazine maleate

Anti-Naus, Compazine Spansule, PMS Prochlorperazine, Prorazin, Stemetil

Drug Class: Antipsychotic, antiemetic, anxiolytic

Drug Actions

Relieves nausea and vomiting, signs and symptoms of psychosis, and anxiety.

Use

- Preoperative nausea control
- Severe nausea and vomiting
- To manage symptoms of psychotic disorders
- To manage symptoms of severe psychoses
- Nonpsychotic anxiety

Side Effects

Cardiovascular: orthostatic hypotension, tachycardia, ECG changes.
Gastrointestinal: dry mouth, constipation.
Nervous System: extrapyramidal reactions, sedation, pseudoparkinsonism, EEG changes, dizziness.
Urinary: urine retention, dark urine, menstrual irregularities, inhibited ejaculation.
Skin: mild photosensitivity, exfoliative dermatitis.
Other: allergic reactions, abnormal growth of breast tissue, ocular changes, blurred vision, abnormal blood profiles, cholestatic jaundice, weight gain, increased appetite.

Onset, Peak, and Duration

Route	Onset	Peak	Duration
Oral	30–40 min	Unknown	3–12 hr
I.V.	Immediate	Immediate	Unknown
I.M.	10–20 min	Unknown	3–4 hr
Rectal	60 min	Unknown	3–4 hr

 Massage Considerations

- No cautions or contraindications to massage are related to the actions of this drug.
- In most cases, cautions and contraindications to massage will be related to the client condition.
- The physician should be consulted before any massage is given.
- The site of intramuscular injection should not be massaged for 1 to 3 hours.
- Side effects of hypotension and dizziness require care in getting the client on and off the table. Stimulation with effleurage or tapotement at the end of the session may help.
- Constipation may be helped by abdominal massage.
- Dermatitis is a local contraindication to massage and should be reported to the physician. If severe or widespread, massage should be withheld.
- Abnormal growth of breast tissue in men or women requires care in depth and pressure when doing chest massage, and no deep tissue massage should be done in the area. If too tender, the area should be avoided completely.

progesterone (proh-JES-teh-rohn)

Crinone 4%, Crinone 8%, Gesterol 50, PMS-Progesterone, Progestasert, Prometrium

Drug Class: Hormone

Drug Actions

Suppresses ovulation and forms thick cervical mucus, alleviating amenorrhea and dysfunctional uterine bleeding.

Use

- Amenorrhea
- Secondary amenorrhea
- Prevention of endometrial hyperplasia
- Dysfunctional uterine bleeding
- Contraception (with an intrauterine device)
- Infertility

Side Effects

Cardiovascular: hypertension, thrombophlebitis, thromboembolism, pulmonary embolism, cerebrovascular accident, edema.
Gastrointestinal: nausea, vomiting, abdominal cramps.
Nervous System: dizziness, migraine, lethargy, depression.
Skin: discoloration of the skin, rash.
Other: breast tenderness, enlargement, or secretion; decreased libido; pain at injection site; cholestatic jaundice; hyperglycemia; breakthrough bleeding; dysmenorrhea; amenorrhea; cervical erosion; abnormal secretions; uterine fibromas; vaginal candidiasis.

Onset, Peak, and Duration

Route	Onset	Peak	Duration
Oral	Unknown	1–2 hr	Unknown
I.M.	Unknown	24 hr	Unknown
Intravaginal	Unknown	3–6 hr	Unknown

 Massage Considerations

- No cautions or contraindications to massage are related to the actions of this drug. Cautions and contraindications to massage may be related to the client condition.
- The site of intramuscular injection should not be massaged for at least 24 hours.
- Side effects of thrombophlebitis or embolism are complete contraindications to massage. If the client presents with symptoms of heat, redness, swelling, or pain, especially in the legs, do not massage and refer to the physician for evaluation immediately.
- Dizziness requires care in getting the client on and off the table. Stimulation with effleurage at the end of the session may help.
- Rash is a local contraindication to massage and should be reported to the physician.
- Breast tenderness or enlargement requires caution in depth and pressure of chest massage. No deep tissue massage should be done in the area. If the area is too tender, massage there is completely contraindicated.

---

promethazine hydrochloride (proh-METH-uh-zeen high-droh-KLOR-ighd)

Anergan 50, Phenergan

promethazine theoclate

Avomine

Drug Class: Antiemetic, antivertigo drug, antihistamine (H_1-receptor antagonist), sedative

Drug Actions

Competes with histamine for H_1-receptor sites on effector cells, which prevents motion sickness and relieves nausea, nasal congestion, and allergy symptoms. Also promotes calmness.

Use

- Motion sickness
- Nausea and vomiting
- Rhinitis, allergy symptoms
- Sedation
- Routine preoperative or postoperative sedation or adjunct to analgesics

Side Effects

Cardiovascular: hypotension, ECG changes.
Gastrointestinal: anorexia, nausea, vomiting, constipation, dry mouth.
Nervous System: sedation, confusion, restlessness, tremors, drowsiness (especially geriatric patients).
Urinary: urine retention.
Skin: photosensitivity, venous thrombosis at injection site.
Other: transient myopia, nasal congestion, abnormal blood profiles.

Onset, Peak, and Duration

Route	Onset	Peak	Duration
Oral	15–60 min	Unknown	≤12 hr
I.V.	3–5 min	Unknown	≤12 hr
I.M., rectal	20 min	Unknown	≤12 hr

Massage Considerations

- No contraindications to massage are related to this drug. Because of the sedative effects of the drug, deep tissue massage should be used with caution.
- Further cautions or contraindications to massage may be related to the client condition.
- The site of intramuscular injection of the drug should not be massaged for at least 1 hour.
- Side effects of hypotension, dizziness, and drowsiness require care in getting the client on and off the table. Stimulation with effleurage and tapotement at the end of the session may help.
- Constipation may be helped by abdominal massage.
- Thrombosis of any kind is a complete contraindication to massage.

---

propoxyphene hydrochloride (dextropropoxyphene hydrochloride) (proh-POK-sih-feen high-droh-KLOR-ighd)

Darvon, 642

propoxyphene napsylate (dextropropoxyphene napsylate)

Darvon-N

Drug Class: Opioid analgesic

Drug Actions

Binds with opioid receptors in CNS, altering both perception of and emotional response to pain through unknown mechanism.

Use

- Mild to moderate pain

Side Effects

Gastrointestinal: nausea, vomiting, constipation.
Nervous System: dizziness, headache, sedation, euphoria, paradoxical excitement, insomnia.
Other: psychological and physical dependence, respiratory depression.

Onset, Peak, and Duration

Route	Onset	Peak	Duration
Oral	15–60 min	2–2.5 hr	4–6 hr

 Massage Considerations

- This drug decreases the perception of pain and sensation. Deep tissue massage is contraindicated.
- Further cautions and contraindications to massage may be related to the client condition.
- The depressant effect on the CNS may potentially increase the relaxation effects of massage in general and increase the effects of the systemic reflex strokes of effleurage, rocking, and friction. Using these strokes in a more rapid and stimulating manner throughout the session may help. The drug may decrease the effects of the local reflex strokes of stretching, traction, compression, and vibration. Using these strokes for longer than usual may achieve the desired results.
- Side effects of dizziness require care in getting the client on and off the table and may be addressed as noted above.
- Constipation may be helped by abdominal massage.

---

propranolol hydrochloride (proh-PRAH-nuh-lohl high-droh-KLOR-ighd)

Apo-Propranolol, Detensol, Inderal, Inderal LA, InnoPran XL, Novopranol, PMS Propranolol

Drug Class: Beta-blocker antihypertensive, antianginal, antiarrhythmic, adjunct therapy for migraine, adjunct

Drug Actions

Relieves anginal and migraine pain, lowers blood pressure, restores normal sinus rhythm, and helps limit heart attack damage; therapy for heart attack.

Use

- Angina pectoris
- Mortality reduction after heart attack
- Supraventricular, ventricular, and atrial arrhythmias
- Tachyarrhythmias caused by excessive catecholamine action during anesthesia
- Hypertension
- Prevention of frequent, severe, uncontrollable, or disabling migraine or vascular headache
- Essential tremor
- Hypertrophic subaortic stenosis
- Adjunct therapy in pheochromocytoma
- Adjunctive treatment to anxiety

Side Effects

Cardiovascular: bradycardia, hypotension, heart failure, intermittent claudication.
Gastrointestinal: nausea, vomiting, diarrhea, constipation (InnoPran XL).
Nervous System: fatigue, lethargy, vivid dreams, fever, hallucinations, mental depression, dizziness (InnoPran XL).
Skin: rash.
Other: agranulocytosis, joint pain, increased airway resistance.

Onset, Peak, and Duration

Route	Onset	Peak	Duration
Oral	30 min	60–90 min	12 hr
Oral:			
InnoPran XL	Unknown	12–14 hr	24 hr
I.V.	≤1 min	≤1 min	<5 min

Massage Considerations

- No cautions or contraindications to massage are related to the actions of this drug. Cautions and contraindications to massage may be related to the client condition.
- The action of this drug blocks certain sympathetic nervous system (SNS) effects in the body. This may potentially increase the relaxation effects of massage in general. Using a slightly more stimulating application of massage techniques throughout the session may be helpful.
- Side effects of hypotension and dizziness may be addressed as noted above.
- Constipation may be helped by abdominal massage.
- Rash is a local contraindication to massage and should be reported to the physician.

propylthiouracil (PTU) (proh-pil-thigh-oh-YOOR-uh-sil)

Propyl-Thyracil

Drug Class: Antihyperthyroid drug

Drug Actions

Lowers thyroid hormone level

Use

- Hyperthyroidism
- Thyrotoxic crisis

Side Effects

Cardiovascular: vasculitis.
Gastrointestinal: diarrhea, nausea, vomiting (may be dose related), salivary gland enlargement, loss of taste.
Nervous System: headache, drowsiness, dizziness.
Skin: rash, hives, skin discoloration, itching.
Other: drug-induced fever, visual disturbances, abnormal blood profiles, lymphadenopathy, jaundice, hepatotoxicity, dose-related hypothyroidism (mental depression; cold intolerance; hard, nonpitting edema), joint pain, muscle pain.

Onset, Peak, and Duration

Route	Onset	Peak	Duration
Oral	Unknown	1–1.5 hr	Unknown

Massage Considerations

- No cautions or contraindications to massage are related to the actions of this drug. Cautions and contraindications to massage may be related to the client condition.
- Side effects of drowsiness and dizziness require care in getting the client on and off the table. Stimulation with effleurage or tapotement at the end of the session may help.
- Rash, itching, and hives are local contraindications to massage and should be reported to the physician immediately. If severe or widespread, massage should be withheld.

---

pseudoephedrine hydrochloride (soo-doh-eh-FED-rin high-droh-KLOR-ighd)

Cenafed, Children's Sudafed Liquid, Decofed, DeFed-60, Dimetapp, Dorcol Children's Decongestant, Drixoral Non-Drowsy Formula, Eltor 120, Genaphed, Halofed, Halofed Adult Strength, Maxenal, Myfedrine, Novafed, PediaCare Infants' Oral Decongestant Drops, Pseudo, Pseudofrin, Pseudogest, Robidrine, Sudafed, Sudafed 12 Hour, Sudafed 60, Sufedrin, Triaminic

pseudoephedrine sulfate

Afrin, Drixoral, Drixoral 12 Hour Non-Drowsy Formula

Drug Class: Adrenergic decongestant

Drug Actions

Stimulates (-adrenergic receptors in respiratory tract, resulting in vasoconstriction. Acts to relieve congestion of nasal and eustachian tube.

Use

- Nasal and eustachian tube decongestion

Side Effects

Cardiovascular: arrhythmias, palpitations, tachycardia, hypertension.
Gastrointestinal: anorexia, nausea, vomiting, dry mouth.
Nervous System: anxiety, transient stimulation, tremor, dizziness, headache, insomnia, nervousness.
Urinary: difficulty urinating.
Skin: pallor.
Other: respiratory difficulty.

Onset, Peak, and Duration

Route	Onset	Peak	Duration
Oral	15–30 min	30–60 min	3–12 hr

Massage Considerations

- No cautions or contraindications to massage are related to the actions of this drug.
- Side effects of dizziness require care in positioning the client, and using stimulation at the end of the session with effleurage may help.

psyllium (SIL-ee-um)

Fiberall, Genfiber, Hydrocil Instant, Konsyl, Konsyl-D, Metamucil, Modane Bulk, Perdiem Fiber Therapy, Reguloid, Serutan, Syllact

Drug Class: Bulk laxative

Drug Actions

Absorbs water and expands to increase bulk and moisture content of stool, thus encouraging peristalsis and bowel movement.

Use

- Constipation
- Bowel management
- Irritable bowel syndrome

Side Effects

Gastrointestinal: nausea, vomiting, and diarrhea with excessive use; esophageal, gastric, small intestinal, or colonic strictures with dry form; abdominal cramps in severe constipation.

Onset, Peak, and Duration

Route	Onset	Peak	Duration
Oral	12–24 hr	≤3 days	Varies

Massage Considerations

- No cautions or contraindications to massage are indicated because a client is taking this drug.
- For abdominal cramps and severe constipation, refer for evaluation to rule out obstruction before doing any massage.

pyrantel embonate (peer-AN-tul EM-boh-nayt)

Anthel, Combantrin, Early Bird

pyrantel pamoate

Antiminth, Combantrin, Pin-Rid, Pin-X, Reese's Pinworm Medicine

Drug Class: Anthelmintic

Drug Actions

Relieves roundworm and pinworm infestation

Use

- Roundworm
- Pinworm

Side Effects

Gastrointestinal: anorexia, nausea, vomiting, gastralgia, cramps, diarrhea, tenesmus.
Nervous System: headache, dizziness, fever, drowsiness, insomnia, weakness.
Skin: rash.

Onset, Peak, and Duration

Route	Onset	Peak	Duration
Oral	Varies	1–3 hr	Varies

Massage Considerations

- No cautions or contraindications to massage are related to the actions of this drug. However, because pinworms and roundworm can be found on sheets, it would be best to not give massage until the treatment is complete and the infection resolved.

---

pyrazinamide (peer-uh-ZIN-uh-mighd)

PMS-Pyrazinamide, Tebrazid, Zinamide

Drug Class: Antituberculotic

Drug Actions

Helps eradicate tuberculosis. Only active against *Mycobacterium tuberculosis.*

Use

- Adjunct for tuberculosis when primary and secondary antituberculotics cannot be used or have failed

Side Effects

Gastrointestinal: anorexia, nausea, vomiting, diarrhea.
Nervous System: malaise, fever.
Urinary: painful urination.
Other: sideroblastic anemia, thrombocytopenia, hepatitis, hepatotoxicity, hyperuricemia, joint pain.

Onset, Peak, and Duration

Route	Onset	Peak	Duration
Oral	Unknown	1–2 hr	Unknown

Massage Considerations

- No cautions or contraindications to massage are related to the actions of this drug. Cautions and contraindications to massage may be related to the client condition.
- The physician should be consulted before any massage is given.

---

pyridostigmine bromide (peer-ih-doh-STIG-meen BROH-mighd)

Mestinon, Mestinon SRI, Mestinon Timespans, Regonol

Drug Class: Cholinesterase inhibitor muscle stimulant

Drug Actions

Inhibits destruction of acetylcholine released from parasympathetic and somatic efferent nerves. This allows acetylcholine to accumulate and strengthen muscle contraction.

Use

- Antidote for nondepolarizing neuromuscular blockers
- Myasthenia gravis
- To increase survival after exposure to the nerve agent Soman

Side Effects

Cardiovascular: bradycardia, hypotension, thrombophlebitis.
Gastrointestinal: abdominal cramps, nausea, vomiting, diarrhea, excessive salivation.
Nervous System: headache with large doses, weakness, sweating, seizures.
Skin: rash.
Other: abnormal constriction of the pupil, muscle cramps, muscle fasciculations, bronchospasm, bronchoconstriction, increased bronchial secretions.

Onset, Peak, and Duration

Route	Onset	Peak	Duration
Oral	20–60 min	1–2 hr	3–12 hr
I.V.	2–5 min	Unknown	2–3 hr
I.M.	15 min	Unknown	2–3 hr

 **Massage Considerations**

- When used for myasthenia gravis, no cautions or contraindications to massage are related to this drug.
- The site of intramuscular injection should not be massaged for up to 2 hours.
- Side effects of thrombophlebitis are a complete contraindication to massage.
- Hypotension requires stimulation at the end of the session with effleurage and tapotement.
- Rash is a local contraindication to massage and should be reported to the physician immediately.

---

pyridoxine hydrochloride (peer-ih-DOKS-een high-droh-KLOR-ighd)

Aminoxin, Beesix, Nestrex, Rodex

Drug Class: Water-soluble vitamin

Drug Actions

Vitamin B_6 stimulates various metabolic functions, including amino acid metabolism. Raises pyridoxine levels, prevents and relieves seizure activity related to pyridoxine deficiency or dependency, and blocks effects of isoniazid poisoning.

Use

- Daily vitamin supplement
- Dietary vitamin B_6 deficiency
- Seizures related to vitamin B_6 deficiency or dependency
- Vitamin B_6-responsive anemias or dependency syndrome (inborn errors of metabolism). Prevention of vitamin B_6 deficiency during drug therapy
- Drug-induced vitamin B_6 deficiency
- Antidote for isoniazid poisoning
- Premenstrual syndrome
- Carpal tunnel syndrome
- Hyperoxaluria type I

Side Effects

Nervous System: drowsiness, paresthesia, unstable gait.

Onset, Peak, and Duration

Route	Onset	Peak	Duration
Oral, I.V., I.M.	Unknown	Unknown	Unknown

Massage Considerations

- No cautions or contraindications to massage are indicated because a client is taking this drug. Cautions and contraindications to massage may be related to the client condition.
- Side effects of drowsiness require stimulation with effleurage at the end of the session.
- Paresthesia is a local contraindication to deep tissue massage.

---

pyrimethamine (peer-ih-METH-uh-meen)

Daraprim

pyrimethamine with sulfadoxine

Fansidar

Drug Class: Antimalarial

Drug Actions

Prevents malaria and treats malaria and toxoplasmosis infections.

Use

- Malaria prophylaxis and transmission control
- Acute attacks of malaria
- Acute attacks of malaria
- Malaria prophylaxis
- Toxoplasmosis
- Isosporiasis

Side Effects

Gastrointestinal: anorexia, vomiting, diarrhea, atrophic glossitis.
Nervous System: stimulation, seizures.
Skin: rash, erythema multiforme, Stevens-Johnson syndrome, toxic epidermal necrolysis.
Other: abnormal blood profiles.

Onset, Peak, and Duration

Route	Onset	Peak	Duration
Oral	Unknown	1.5–8 hr	Unknown

Massage Considerations

- No cautions or contraindications to massage are related to the actions of this drug. Cautions and contraindications to massage may be related to the client condition.
- Side effects of rash or other skin eruptions are local contraindications to massage and should be reported to the physician immediately. If severe or widespread, massage should be withheld.

Q

quetiapine fumarate (KWET-ee-uh-peen FYOO-muh-rayt)

Seroquel

Drug Class: Antipsychotic

Drug Actions

Affects dopamine and serotonin in the CNS and reduces symptoms of psychotic disorders

Use

- Schizophrenia

Side Effects

Cardiovascular: orthostatic hypotension, tachycardia, palpitations, peripheral edema.
Gastrointestinal: dry mouth, painful digestion, abdominal pain, constipation, anorexia.
Nervous System: fever, weakness, dizziness, headache, seizures, sleepiness, hypertonia, dysarthria, neuroleptic malignant syndrome, tardive dyskinesia.
Urinary: urine retention.
Skin: rash, sweating.
Other: flulike syndrome, pharyngitis, rhinitis, ear pain, cataracts, sinusitis, nasal congestion, leukopenia, weight gain, hypothyroidism, hyperglycemia, back pain, increased cough, shortness of breath.

Onset, Peak, and Duration

Route	Onset	Peak	Duration
Oral	Unknown	$1\frac{1}{2}$ hr	Unknown

Massage Considerations

- This drug has a sedative effect on the CNS; therefore. deep tissue massage should be used with caution.
- There may be further cautions and contraindications to massage related to the client condition.
- The physician should be consulted before any massage is given.
- Side effects of hypotension, dizziness, and sleepiness require care in getting the client on and off the table. Stimulation with effleurage and tapotement at the end of the session may help. Constipation may be helped by regular abdominal massage. Rash is a local contraindication to massage and should be reported to the physician

quinapril hydrochloride (KWIN-eh-pril high-droh-KLOR-ighd)

Accupril, Asig

Drug Class: Antihypertensive

Drug Actions

May inhibit conversion of angiotensin I to angiotensin II, which lowers peripheral arterial resistance and decreases aldosterone secretion and lowers blood pressure

Use

- Hypertension
- Heart failure

Side Effects

Cardiovascular: palpitations, vasodilation, tachycardia, hypertensive crisis, angina, orthostatic hypotension, arrhythmias.
Gastrointestinal: dry mouth, abdominal pain, constipation, GI hemorrhage.
Nervous System: sleepiness, dizziness syncope, malaise, nervousness, depression.
Skin: itching, exfoliative dermatitis, photosensitivity reaction, sweating.
Other: angioedema, dry throat, hyperkalemia, back pain, dry, persistent, tickling, nonproductive cough.

Onset, Peak, and Duration

Route	Onset	Peak	Duration
Oral	≤1 hr	1–2 hr	2 hr

 Massage Considerations

- There are no cautions or contraindications to massage related to the actions of this drug.
- There may be cautions or contraindications to massage related to the client condition.
- Side effects of hypotension, dizziness, and sleepinesss may be addressed by stimulation at the end of the session with effleurage and tapotement. Constipation may be helped by abdominal massage. Itching or other skin eruptions are a local contraindication to massage and should be reported to the physician.

---

quinidine bisulfate (KWIN-eh-deen bigh-SUL-fayt)

quinidine bisulfate (66.4% quinidine base)

Biquin Durules, Kinidin Durules

quinidine gluconate (62% quinidine base)

Quinaglute Dura-Tabs, Quinalan, Quinate

quinidine sulfate (83% quinidine base)

Apo-Quinidine, Cin-Quin, Quinidex Extentabs, Quinora

Drug Class: Antiarrhythmic

Drug Actions

Has direct and indirect (anticholinergic) effects on cardiac tissue that restores normal sinus rhythm. Also relieves signs and symptoms of malaria infection.

Use

- Atrial flutter or fibrillation
- Paroxysmal supraventricular tachycardia
- Premature atrial and ventricular contractions
- Paroxysmal AV junctional rhythm
- Paroxysmal atrial tachycardia
- Paroxysmal ventricular tachycardia
- Maintenance after cardioversion of atrial fibrillation or flutter
- Severe plasmodium falciparum malaria

Side Effects

Cardiovascular: PVCs, ventricular tachycardia, atypical ventricular tachycardia (torsades de pointes), severe hypotension, SA and AV block, ventricular fibrillation, cardiotoxicity, tachycardia, aggravated heart failure, ECG changes (widening of QRS complex, notched P waves, widened QT interval, ST-segment depression).
Gastrointestinal: diarrhea, nausea, vomiting, excessive salivation, anorexia, petechial hemorrhage of buccal mucosa, abdominal pain.
Nervous System: dizziness, headache, light-headedness, confusion, restlessness, cold sweats, pallor, fainting, fever, dementia.
Skin: rash, itching.
Other: angioedema, cinchonism, hypersensitivity reaction, lupus erythematosus, ringing in the ears, blurred vision, abnormal blood profiles, hepatotoxicity, acute asthma attack, respiratory arrest.

Onset, Peak, and Duration

Route	Onset	Peak	Duration
Oral	1–3 hr	1–2 hr	6–8 hr
I.V.	Immediate	Immediate	Unknown
I.M.	Unknown	Unknown	Unknown

 Massage Considerations

- There are no cautions or contraindications to massage related to this drug. There will be, in most cases, cautions and contraindications to massage related to the client condition.
- The physician should be consulted before any massage is given.
- The action of this drug in blocking cholinergic effects is fairly specific to the cardiac system. Because its anticholinergic effects may block the PNS, is possible the relaxation effects of massage in general and the effects of the systemic reflex strokes of rocking, effleurage, and friction may be lessened. Simply applying these strokes for a longer period of time will help achieve the desired results.
- Side effects of dizziness require care in getting the client on and off the table. Using rapid effleurage at the end of the session may help. Rash or itching is a local contraindication to massage and should be reported to the physician. If severe or widespread, massage should be withheld.

quinupristin and dalfopristin (QUIN-uh-pris-tin and DALF-oh-pris-tin)

Synercid

Drug Class: Antibiotic

Drug Actions

Inhibits or destroys susceptible bacteria

Use

- Serious or life-threatening infections linked to vancomycin-resistant Enterococcus faecium bacteremia
- Complicated skin and skin-structure infections caused by Staphylococcus aureus (methicillin susceptible) or Streptococcus pyogenes

Side Effects

Cardiovascular: thrombophlebitis.
Gastrointestinal: nausea, diarrhea, vomiting.
Nervous System: headache, pain.
Skin: inflammation, pain, and edema at infusion site; rash; itching.
Other: muscle pain, joint pain.

Onset, Peak, and Duration

Route	Onset	Peak	Duration
I.V.	Unknown	Unknown	Unknown

 Massage Considerations

- There are no cautions or contraindications to massage related to the actions of this drug. There will be cautions and contraindications to massage related to the client condition.
- The physician should be consulted before any massage is given.
- Side effects of thrombophlebitis are a complete contraindication to massage. Rash or itching are local contraindications to massage and should be reported to the physician immediately. If severe or widespread, massage should be withheld.

R

rabeprazole sodium (rah-BEH-pruh-zohl SOH-dee-um)

Aciphex

Drug Class: Proton pump inhibitor

Drug Actions

Blocks activity of the acid (proton) pump blocking gastric acid secretion

Use

- Healing of erosive or ulcerative gastroesophageal reflux disease (GERD)
- Maintenance of healing of erosive or ulcerative GERD
- Healing of duodenal ulcers
- Pathologic hypersecretory conditions including Zollinger-Ellison syndrome
- Symptomatic GERD, including daytime and nighttime heartburn
- *Helicobacter pylori* eradication to reduce the risk of duodenal ulcer recurrence

Side Effects

Nervous System: headache.

Onset, Peak, and Duration

Route	Onset	Peak	Duration
Oral	<1 hr	2–5 hr	>24 hr

Massage Considerations

- No cautions or contraindications to massage are indicated because a client is taking this drug.

---

raloxifene hydrochloride (rah-LOKS-ih-feen high-droh-KLOR-ighd)

Evista

Drug Class: Antiosteoporotic

Drug Actions

Prevents bone breakdown in postmenopausal women.

Use

- Prevention and treatment of osteoporosis

Side Effects

Cardiovascular: chest pain, peripheral edema.
Gastrointestinal: nausea, painful digestion, vomiting, gas, gastrointestinal disorder, gastroenteritis, abdominal pain.
Nervous System: depression, insomnia, migraine, fever.
Urinary: urinary tract infections.
Skin: rash, sweating.
Other: hot flushes, infection, flulike syndrome, breast pain, sinusitis, pharyngitis, laryngitis, weight gain, vaginitis, cystitis, leukorrhea, endometrial disorder, vaginal bleeding, joint pain, muscle pain, arthritis, leg cramps, increased cough, pneumonia.

Onset, Peak, and Duration

Route	Onset	Peak	Duration
Oral	Unknown	Unknown	24 hr

Massage Considerations

- No cautions or contraindications to massage are related to the actions of this drug. Cautions or contraindications to massage may be related to the client condition.
- Side effects of breast pain require caution in depth and pressure when doing chest massage. If the area is too tender, chest massage is contraindicated.

---

ramipril (reh-MIH-pril)

Altace, Ramace, Tritace

Drug Class: Angiotensin-converting enzyme inhibitor

Drug Actions

Decreases peripheral arterial resistance, lowers blood pressure.

Use

- Hypertension (either alone or with thiazide diuretics)
- Heart failure after heart attack
- Reduction in risk of heart attack, stroke, and death from cardiovascular causes

Side Effects

Cardiovascular: orthostatic hypotension, angina, arrhythmias, chest pain, palpitations, heart attack, edema.
Gastrointestinal: nausea, vomiting, abdominal pain, anorexia, constipation, diarrhea, painful digestion, dry mouth, gastroenteritis.
Nervous System: headache, dizziness, fatigue, syncope, weakness, malaise, light-headedness, anxiety, amnesia, seizures, depression, insomnia, nervousness, neuralgia, neuropathy, paresthesia, sleepiness, tremors.
Urinary: impotence.
Skin: rash, itching, photosensitivity reaction, increased sweating.
Other: hypersensitivity reactions; angioedema; nosebleeds; ringing in the ears; hyperkalemia; weight gain; joint pain; arthritis; muscle pain; dry, persistent, tickling, nonproductive cough; shortness of breath.

Onset, Peak, and Duration

Route	Onset	Peak	Duration
Oral	1–2 hr	<1 hr	About 24 hr

 Massage Considerations

- No cautions or contraindications to massage are related to the actions of this drug. Cautions and contraindications to massage may be related to the client condition.
- Side effects of hypotension, dizziness, and sleepiness require care in getting the client on and off the table. Stimulation with effleurage at the end of the session may help.
- Neuralgia, neuropathy, and paresthesia are local contraindications to deep tissue massage. If the symptom is severe, massage may be completely contraindicated.
- Constipation may be helped by abdominal massage.
- Rash and itching are local contraindications to massage and should be reported to the physician.

---

ranitidine hydrochloride (ruh-NIH-tuh-deen high-droh-KLOR-ighd)

Zantac, Zantac-C, Zantac EFFERdose, Zantac GELdose, Zantac 75

Drug Class: H_2-receptor antagonist

Drug Actions

Competitively inhibits action of H_2 at receptor sites of parietal cells, decreasing gastric acid secretion.

Use

- Intractable duodenal ulcer
- Pathologic hypersecretory conditions, such as Zollinger-Ellison syndrome
- Duodenal and gastric ulcer
- Maintenance therapy for healing duodenal ulcer
- GERD
- Erosive esophagitis
- Relief of occasional heartburn, acid indigestion, and sour stomach

Side Effects

Nervous System: dizziness, malaise.
Other: burning and itching at injection site, anaphylaxis, angioedema, blurred vision, abnormal blood profiles, jaundice.

Onset, Peak, and Duration

Route	Onset	Peak	Duration
Oral	≤1 hr	1–3 hr	≤13 hr
I.V., I.M.	Unknown	Unknown	≤13 hr

Massage Considerations

- No cautions or contraindications to massage are related to the actions of this drug. Cautions and contraindications to massage may be related to the client condition.
- The site of intramuscular injection of the drug should not be massaged for at least 1 to 3 hours.
- Side effects of dizziness require care in getting the client on and off the table. Stimulation with effleurage or tapotement at the end of the session should help.

---

repaglinide (reh-PAG-lih-nighd)

Prandin

Drug Class: Antidiabetic

Drug Actions

Stimulates the release of insulin from beta cells in the pancreas. Lowers glucose level.

Use

- Adjunct to diet and exercise to lower glucose levels in patients with type 2 diabetes mellitus (non–insulin-dependent diabetes mellitus) whose hyperglycemia cannot be controlled satisfactorily by diet and exercise alone
- Adjunct to diet, exercise, and metformin, rosiglitazone, or pioglitazone

Side Effects

Cardiovascular: angina, chest pain.
Gastrointestinal: constipation, diarrhea, painful digestion, nausea, vomiting.
Nervous System: headache, paresthesia.
Urinary: urinary tract infection.
Other: tooth disorder, rhinitis, sinusitis, hypoglycemia, hyperglycemia, joint pain, back pain, bronchitis, upper respiratory infection.

Onset, Peak, and Duration

Route	Onset	Peak	Duration
Oral	Unknown	1 hr	Unknown

Massage Considerations

- No cautions or contraindications to massage are related to the actions of this drug. Cautions and contraindications to massage may be related to the client condition.
- Side effects of paresthesia are a local contraindication to deep tissue massage.
- Constipation may be helped by abdominal massage.
- Hypoglycemia may appear as sweating, shakiness, confusion, and lethargy. If the client is prone to episodes, it would be best if the client takes a snack before the massage. If a hypoglycemic episode occurs, a form of sugar such as candy, juice, or sugar should be given. If no relief of symptoms occurs, emergency help should be called.
- For hyperglycemic episodes, the symptoms are similar to those of hypoglycemia, although often no sweating occurs. Emergency help should be called as soon as possible.

ribavirin (righ-beh-VIGH-rin)

Copegus, Rebetol, Virazole

Drug Class: Antiviral

Drug Actions

Inhibits viral activity

Use

- Hospitalized infants and young children infected by respiratory syncytial virus
- Chronic hepatitis C

Side Effects

Cardiovascular: cardiac arrest, hypotension, chest pains.
Gastrointestinal: nausea.
Nervous System: headache, dizziness, seizures, weakness.
Skin: rash.
Other: conjunctivitis, rhinitis, pharyngitis, lacrimation, rash or erythema of eyelids, reticulocytosis, severe anemia, hemolytic anemia, worsening of respiratory state, bronchospasms, apnea, bacterial pneumonia, pneumothorax.

Onset, Peak, and Duration

Route	Onset	Peak	Duration
Inhalation	Immediate	Immediate	Unknown

 Massage Considerations

- No cautions or contraindications to massage are related to the actions of this drug. Cautions and contraindications to massage may be related to the client condition.
- Side effects of hypotension and dizziness require care in getting the client on and off the table. Stimulation with effleurage at the end of the session may help.
- Rash is a local contraindication to massage and should be reported to the physician immediately. If severe or widespread, massage should be withheld.

rifabutin (rif-uh-BYOO-tin)

Mycobutin

Drug Class: Antibiotic

Drug Actions

Blocks bacterial protein synthesis

Use

- Prevention of disseminated *Mycobacterium avium* complex in patients with advanced HIV infection

Side Effects

Cardiovascular: electrocardiogram changes.
Gastrointestinal: painful digestion, belching, flatulence, diarrhea, nausea, vomiting, abdominal pain.
Nervous System: fever, headache.

Urinary: discolored urine.
Skin: rash.
Other: abnormal blood profiles, muscle pain.

Onset, Peak, and Duration

Route	Onset	Peak	Duration
Oral	Unknown	1.5–4 hr	Unknown

Massage Considerations

- No cautions or contraindications to massage are related to the actions of this drug. Cautions and contraindications to massage may be related to the client condition and severity of infection.
- Side effects of gas may be helped by abdominal massage.
- Rash is a local contraindication to massage and should be reported to the physician. If severe or widespread, massage should be withheld.

---

rifampin (rifampicin) (rih-FAM-pin)

Rifadin, Rifadin IV, Rimactane, Rimycin, Rofact

Drug Class: Antituberculotic

Drug Actions

Kills susceptible bacteria

Use

- Pulmonary tuberculosis
- Meningococcal carriers
- Prophylaxis of *Haemophilus influenzae* type B
- Leprosy

Side Effects

Cardiovascular: shock.
Gastrointestinal: epigastric distress, anorexia, nausea, vomiting, abdominal pain, diarrhea, gas, sore mouth and tongue, pseudomembranous colitis, pancreatitis.
Nervous System: ataxia, behavioral changes, confusion, dizziness, fatigue, headache, drowsiness, generalized numbness.
Urinary: hemoglobinuria, hematuria, acute renal failure, menstrual disturbances.
Skin: itching, hives, rash.
Other: flulike syndrome, discoloration of body fluids, visual disturbances, exudative conjunctivitis, abnormal blood profiles, hepatotoxicity, worsening of porphyria, hyperuricemia, osteomalacia, shortness of breath, wheezing.

Onset, Peak, and Duration

Route	Onset	Peak	Duration
Oral	Unknown	2–4 hr	Unknown
I.V.	Unknown	Unknown	Unknown

Massage Considerations

- No cautions or contraindications to massage are related to the actions of this drug. Cautions and contraindications to massage may be related to the client condition.

- Side effects of drowsiness and dizziness require care in getting the client on and off the table. Stimulation with effleurage or tapotement at the end of the session may help.
- Numbness that is generalized is a complete contraindication to deep tissue massage and requires caution in depth and pressure of any massage given.
- Gas may be helped by abdominal massage.
- Itching, hives, and rash are local contraindications to massage. If severe or widespread, massage should be withheld.

rifapentine (rif-ah-PEN-tin)

Priftin

Drug Class: Antituberculotic

Drug Actions

Kills susceptible bacteria

Use

- Pulmonary tuberculosis, with at least one other antituberculotic to which the isolate is susceptible

Side Effects

Cardiovascular: hypertension.
Gastrointestinal: anorexia, nausea, vomiting, painful digestion, diarrhea, pseudomembranous colitis.
Nervous System: pain, headache, dizziness.
Urinary: pus in the urine, proteinuria, hematuria, urinary casts.
Skin: rash, itching, acne.
Other: abnormal blood profiles, hyperuricemia, joint pain, hemoptysis.

Onset, Peak, and Duration

Route	Onset	Peak	Duration
Oral	Unknown	5–6 hr	Unknown

Massage Considerations

- No cautions or contraindications to massage are related to the actions of this drug. Cautions and contraindications to massage may be related to the client condition.
- Side effects of dizziness require care in getting the client on and off the table. Stimulation with effleurage or tapotement at the end of the session may help.
- Itching, acne, and rash are local contraindications to massage. If severe or widespread, massage should be withheld. If the client needs to continue the drug and has widespread acne, massage may be given with the massage therapist wearing gloves when working on the affected areas.

riluzole (RIGH-loo-zohl)

Rilutek

Drug Class: Neuroprotector

Drug Actions

Improves signs and symptoms of amyotrophic lateral sclerosis (ALS).

Use

- ALS

Side Effects

Cardiovascular: hypertension, tachycardia, palpitations, orthostatic hypotension, peripheral edema.
Gastrointestinal: abdominal pain, nausea, vomiting, painful digestion, anorexia, diarrhea, gas, stomatitis, dry mouth, oral candidiasis.
Nervous System: headache, aggravation reaction, weakness, hypertonia, depression, dizziness, insomnia, malaise, sleepiness, circumoral paresthesia.
Urinary: urinary tract infection, painful urination.
Skin: itching, eczema, hair loss, exfoliative dermatitis.
Other: tooth disorder, phlebitis, rhinitis, sinusitis, neutropenia, weight loss, back pain, joint pain, decreased lung function, increased cough.

Onset, Peak, and Duration

Route	Onset	Peak	Duration
Oral	Unknown	Unknown	Unknown

 Massage Considerations

- No cautions or contraindications to massage are related to the actions of this drug. Cautions and contraindications to massage may be related to the client condition.
- The physician should be consulted before any massage is given.
- Side effects of hypotension, dizziness, and sleepiness require care in getting the client on and off the table. Stimulation with effleurage and tapotement at the end of the session may help.
- Gas may be helped by abdominal massage.
- Itching and dermatitis are local contraindications to massage and should be reported to the physician. If severe or widespread, massage should be withheld.
- Hair loss is a contraindication to scalp massage if the client is disturbed by hair loss during the session or if the scalp is tender.

rimantadine hydrochloride (righ-MAN-tuh-deen high-droh-KLOR-ighd)

Flumadine

Drug Class: Antiviral

Drug Actions

Inhibits viral reproduction of influenza A virus

Use

- Prevention of influenza A virus
- Influenza A virus infection

Side Effects

Gastrointestinal: nausea, vomiting, anorexia, dry mouth, abdominal pain.
Nervous System: insomnia, headache, dizziness, nervousness, fatigue, weakness.

Onset, Peak, and Duration

Route	Onset	Peak	Duration
Oral	Unknown	1–4 hr	Unknown

Massage Considerations

- No cautions or contraindications to massage are related to the actions of this drug. Cautions and contraindications to massage may be related to the client condition.
- Side effects of dizziness may be helped by stimulation with effleurage at the end of the session.

---

risedronate sodium (ri-SEH-droe-nate SOE-dee-um)

Actonel

Drug Class: Osteoporotic drug

Drug Actions

Reverses the loss of bone mineral density

Use

- Prevention and treatment of postmenopausal osteoporosis
- Glucocorticoid-induced osteoporosis
- Paget disease

Side Effects

Cardiovascular: hypertension, cardiovascular disorder, chest pain, peripheral edema.
Gastrointestinal: nausea, diarrhea, abdominal pain, gas, gastritis, rectal disorder, constipation.
Nervous System: weakness, headache, depression, dizziness, insomnia, anxiety, neuralgia, hypertonia, paresthesia, pain.
Urinary: urinary tract infections, cystitis.
Skin: bruising, rash, itching, skin carcinoma.
Other: tooth disorder, infection, pharyngitis, rhinitis, sinusitis, cataract, conjunctivitis, otitis media, amblyopia, ringing in the ears, anemia, joint pain, neck pain, back pain, muscle pain, bone pain, leg cramps, bursitis, tendon disorder, shortness of breath, pneumonia, bronchitis.

Onset, Peak, and Duration

Route	Onset	Peak	Duration
Oral	1 hr	Unknown	Unknown

Massage Considerations

- No cautions or contraindications to massage are indicated because a client is taking this drug. Cautions and contraindications to massage may be related to the client condition.
- Side effects of dizziness may be helped by stimulation with effleurage at the end of the session.
- Paresthesia and neuralgia are contraindications to deep tissue massage. If severe, they may contraindicate massage completely.
- Bruising is a contraindication to deep tissue massage.
- Rash and itching are local contraindications to massage and should be reported to the physician.

risperidone (ris-PER-ih-dohn)

Risperdal, Risperdal M-Tab

Drug Class: Antipsychotic

Drug Actions

Blocks dopamine and serotonin receptors as well as α_1, α_2, and H_1 receptors in the central nervous system (CNS). Relieves signs and symptoms of psychosis.

Use

- Short-term therapy for schizophrenia
- Delaying relapse in long-term therapy for schizophrenia

Side Effects

Cardiovascular: tachycardia, chest pain, orthostatic hypotension, prolonged QT interval.
Gastrointestinal: constipation, nausea, vomiting, painful digestion.
Nervous System: sleepiness, extrapyramidal symptoms, headache, suicide attempt, insomnia, agitation, anxiety, tardive dyskinesia, aggressiveness, fever, sedation, neuroleptic malignant syndrome, stroke or transient ischemic attacks in older adult patients with dementia.
Skin: rash, dry skin, photosensitivity reaction.
Other: priapism, rhinitis, sinusitis, pharyngitis, abnormal vision, weight gain, joint pain, back pain, coughing, upper respiratory tract infection.

Onset, Peak, and Duration

Route	Onset	Peak	Duration
Oral	Unknown	1 hr	Unknown

 Massage Considerations

- This drug has sedative effects on the CNS. Deep tissue massage is contraindicated.
- Further cautions and contraindications to massage may be related to the client condition.
- The physician should be consulted before any massage is given.
- Side effects of hypotension and sleepiness require care in getting the client on and off the table. Stimulation with rapid effleurage at the end of the session may help.
- Constipation may be helped by abdominal massage.
- Rash is a local contraindication to massage and should be reported to the physician.

ritonavir (rih-TOH-nuh-veer)

Norvir

Drug Class: Antiviral

Drug Actions

Inhibits HIV activity

Use

- HIV infection

Side Effects

Cardiovascular: vasodilation.
Gastrointestinal: abdominal pain, anorexia, constipation, diarrhea, nausea, vomiting, taste perversion, painful digestion, gas pancreatitis, pseudomembranous colitis.

Nervous System: weakness, headache, circumoral paresthesia, dizziness, insomnia, paresthesia, peripheral paresthesia, sleepiness, thinking abnormality, generalized tonic-clonic seizure, depression, anxiety, pain, malaise, confusion, fever, syncope.
Skin: sweating, rash.
Other: fat redistribution/accumulation, hypersensitivity reactions, pharyngitis, thrombocytopenia, leukopenia, hepatitis, diabetes mellitus, weight loss, joint pain, muscle pain.

Onset, Peak, and Duration

Route	Onset	Peak	Duration
Oral	Unknown	2–4 hr	Unknown

 Massage Considerations

- No cautions or contraindications to massage are indicated because a client is taking this drug. Cautions and contraindications to massage may be related to the client condition.
- Side effects of dizziness and sleepiness may respond well to stimulation with effleurage at the end of the session.
- Paresthesia is a local contraindication to deep tissue massage.
- Constipation and gas may be helped by abdominal massage.
- Rash is a local contraindication to massage and should be reported to the physician immediately. If severe or widespread, massage should be withheld.

rivastigmine tartrate (ri-va-STIG-meen TAR-trayt)

Exelon

Drug Class: Alzheimer disease drug

Drug Actions

Thought to increase acetylcholine levels by reversibly inhibiting its hydrolysis by cholinesterase. Improves cognitive function.

Use

- Symptoms of mild to moderate Alzheimer disease

Side Effects

Cardiovascular: hypertension, chest pain, peripheral edema.
Gastrointestinal: nausea, vomiting, diarrhea, anorexia, abdominal pain, painful digestion, constipation, gas, belching.
Nervous System: syncope, fatigue, weakness, malaise, dizziness, headache, sleepiness, tremor, insomnia, confusion, depression, anxiety, hallucination, aggressive reaction, agitation, nervousness, delusion, paranoid reaction, pain.
Urinary: urinary tract infections, urinary incontinence.
Skin: increased sweating, rash.
Other: accidental trauma, flulike symptoms, rhinitis, pharyngitis, weight loss, back pain, joint pain, bone fracture, upper respiratory tract infection, cough, bronchitis.

Onset, Peak, and Duration

Route	Onset	Peak	Duration
Oral	Unknown	1 hr	12 hr

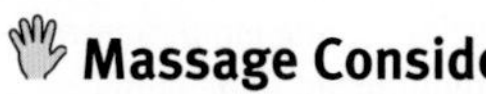

Massage Considerations

- No cautions or contraindications to massage are related to the actions of this drug. Cautions and contraindications to massage may be related to the client condition.
- Side effects of dizziness and sleepiness require care in getting the client on and off the table. Stimulation with effleurage at the end of the session may help.
- Rash is a local contraindication to massage and should be reported to the physician.

---

rizatriptan benzoate (rih-zah-TRIP-tin BEN-zoh-ayt)

Maxalt, Maxalt-MLT

Drug Class: Antimigraine drug

Drug Actions

Vasoconstricts the affected vessels, inhibits neuropeptide release, and reduces migraine pain.

Use

- Acute migraine headaches with or without aura

Side Effects

Cardiovascular: flushing, chest pain, pressure or heaviness, palpitations, coronary artery vasospasm, transient myocardial ischemia, heart attack, ventricular tachycardia, ventricular fibrillation.
Gastrointestinal: dry mouth, nausea, diarrhea, vomiting.
Nervous System: dizziness, headache, sleepiness, paresthesia, weakness, fatigue, hypesthesia, decreased mental acuity, euphoria, tremor.
Other: pain; warm or cold sensations; hot flushes; neck, throat, and jaw pain, pressure, or heaviness; shortness of breath.

Onset, Peak, and Duration

Route	Onset	Peak	Duration
Oral	Unknown	1–1.5 hr	Unknown

Massage Considerations

- Although the action of this drug is in decreasing pain in the head and face, it is appropriate to use deep tissue massage with caution throughout the body.
- Side effects of dizziness and sleepiness require care in getting the client on and off the table. Stimulation with rapid effleurage at the end of the session may help.
- Paresthesia and hypesthesia are contraindications to deep tissue massage. If severe, they may contraindicate massage completely.

---

ropinirole hydrochloride (roh-PIN-er-ohl high-droh-KLOR-ighd)

Requip

Drug Class: Antiparkinsonian

Drug Actions

Improves physical mobility in patients with parkinsonism

Use

- Idiopathic Parkinson's disease

Side Effects

Cardiovascular: hypotension, orthostatic symptoms, flushing, hypertension, edema, chest pain, extrasystoles, atrial fibrillation, palpitations, tachycardia, peripheral ischemia.
Gastrointestinal: dry mouth, nausea, vomiting, painful digestion, gas, abdominal pain, anorexia, constipation, abdominal pain,vomiting, diarrhea.
Nervous System: pain, weakness, fatigue, malaise, hallucinations, dizziness, aggravated Parkinson disease, syncope, sleepiness, headache, confusion, hyperkinesia, hypesthesia, amnesia, impaired concentration, insomnia, abnormal dreaming, tremor, anxiety, nervousness, paresthesia.
Urinary: urinary tract infection, impotence (male), pus in the urine, urinary incontinence.
Skin: increased sweating.
Other: viral infection, yawning, pharyngitis, abnormal vision, eye abnormality, xerophthalmia, rhinitis, sinusitis, bronchitis, dyspnea, double vision, increased saliva, anemia, weight loss, dyskinesia, hypokinesia, paresis, joint pain, arthritis, upper respiratory infection, falls.

Onset, Peak, and Duration

Route	Onset	Peak	Duration
Oral	Unknown	1–2 hr	6 hr

 Massage Considerations

- No cautions or contraindications to massage are related to the actions of this drug. Cautions and contraindications to massage may be related to the client condition.
- Side effects of hypotension, dizziness, and sleepiness may be helped by using stimulation with rapid effleurage and friction at the end of the session. If symptoms are severe, stimulating massage techniques throughout the session may be required.
- Hypesthesia and paresthesia are contraindications to deep tissue massage and, if severe, may contraindicate massage completely.
- Constipation and gas may be helped by abdominal massage.

---

rosiglitazone maleate (roh-sih-GLIH-tah-zohn MAL-ee-ayt)

Avandia

Drug Class: Antidiabetic

Drug Actions

Lowers glucose level by improving insulin sensitivity

Use

- Adjunct to diet and exercise (as monotherapy) to improve glycemic control in patients with type 2 diabetes mellitus
- As combination therapy with sulfonylurea, metformin, or insulin when diet, exercise, and a single drug do not result in adequate glycemic control

Side Effects

Cardiovascular: edema, heart failure, peripheral edema.
Gastrointestinal: diarrhea.
Nervous System: headache, fatigue.
Other: injury, sinusitis, anemia, hyperglycemia, back pain, upper respiratory tract infection.

Onset, Peak, and Duration

Route	Onset	Peak	Duration
Oral	Unknown	1 hr	Unknown

 Massage Considerations

- No cautions or contraindications to massage are indicated because a client is taking this drug. Cautions and contraindications to massage may be related to the client condition.

---

rosiglitazone maleate and metformin hydrochloride

(roh-si-GLI-ta-zone and met-FOR-min)

Avandamet

Drug Class: Antidiabetic

Drug Actions

Improves insulin sensitivity. Lowers glucose level.

Use

- Adjunct to diet and exercise to improve glycemic control in patients with type 2 diabetes mellitus

Side Effects

Cardiovascular: edema.
Gastrointestinal: diarrhea.
Nervous System: headache, fatigue.
Other: injury, viral infection, sinusitis, anemia, hyperglycemia, hypoglycemia, back pain, joint pain, upper respiratory tract infection.

Onset, Peak, and Duration

Route	Onset	Peak	Duration
Oral:			
Rosiglitazone	Unknown	1 hr	Unknown
Metformin	Unknown	2.5–3 hr	Unknown

 Massage Considerations

- No cautions or contraindications to massage are indicated because a client is taking this drug. Cautions and contraindications to massage may be related to the client condition.
- Side effects of hypoglycemia may present as sweating, nervousness, tremor, confusion, and dizziness. It is appropriate to give the client a form of rapidly absorbed sugar such as candy, juice, soft drinks, or similar sources of sugar. If this does not resolve symptoms quickly, emergency help should be called. Encouraging the client to take a snack before the massage may help prevent problems if the client is prone to this side effect.

rosuvastatin calcium (ro-SOO-va-stat-in KAL-see-uhm)

Crestor

Drug Class: Antihyperlipidemic

Drug Actions

Lowers total cholesterol, low density lipoprotein (LDL), apolipoprotein B (ApoB), non–high density lipoprotein (HDL), and triglyceride levels.

Use

- Adjunct to diet to reduce total cholesterol, LDL, ApoB, non-HDL, and triglyceride levels
- To increase HDL level in primary hypercholesterolemia (heterozygous familial and nonfamilial)
- Mixed dyslipidemia (Fredrickson Type IIa and IIb)
- Adjunct to diet to treat elevated triglyceride levels (Fredrickson Type IV)
- Adjunct to other lipid-lowering therapies to reduce LDL, ApoB, and total cholesterol levels in homozygous familial hypercholesterolemia

Side Effects

Cardiovascular: chest pain, hypertension, palpitation, vasodilation.
Gastrointestinal: diarrhea, painful digestion, nausea, abdominal pain, vomiting, gastritis, constipation, gastroenteritis, gas, periodontal abscess.
Nervous System: headache, weakness, dizziness, insomnia, paresthesia, depression, anxiety, pain, neuralgia, hypertonia.
Urinary: urinary tract infection.
Skin: rash, itching, bruising.
Other: flulike syndrome, accidental injury, pharyngitis, rhinitis, sinusitis, anemia, diabetes mellitus, muscle pain, back pain, pelvic pain, neck pain, pathologic fracture, arthritis, asthma, pneumonia, bronchitis, increased cough, shortness of breath.

Onset, Peak, and Duration

Route	Onset	Peak	Duration
Oral	2 wk	Unknown	Unknown

 Massage Considerations

- No cautions or contraindications to massage are indicated because a client is taking this drug. Cautions and contraindications to massage may be related to the client condition.
- Side effects of dizziness may be helped by stimulation with rapid effleurage or tapotement at the end of the session.
- Paresthesia and neuralgia are local contraindications to deep tissue massage and, if severe, may contraindicate massage completely.
- Constipation and gas may be helped by abdominal massage.
- Rash and itching are local contraindications to massage and should be reported to the physician.
- Bruising is a contraindication to deep tissue massage.

S

salmeterol xinafoate (sal-MEE-ter-ohl zee-neh-FOH-ayt)

Serevent Diskus

Drug Class: Bronchodilator

Drug Actions

Selectively activates $beta_2$-adrenergic receptors, which results in bronchodilation. Also blocks release of allergic mediators from mast cells in respiratory tract improving breathing ability.

Use

- Long-term maintenance treatment of asthma
- Prevention of bronchospasm in patients with nocturnal asthma or reversible obstructive airway disease
- Prevention of exercise-induced bronchospasm
- Maintenance treatment of bronchospasm with COPD (including emphysema and chronic bronchitis)

Side Effects

Cardiovascular: tachycardia, palpitations, ventricular arrhythmias.
Gastrointestinal: nausea, vomiting, diarrhea, heartburn.
Nervous System: headache, sinus headache, tremor, nervousness, dizziness.
Other: hypersensitivity reactions, anaphylaxis, nasopharyngitis, nasal cavity or sinus disorder, joint and back pain, muscle pain, upper respiratory tract infection, cough, lower respiratory tract infection, bronchospasm.

Onset, Peak, and Duration

Route	Onset	Peak	Duration
Inhalation	10–20 min	3 hr	12 hr

Massage Considerations

- There are no cautions or contraindications to massage related to the action of this drug.
- There may be cautions or contraindications to massage related to the client condition.
- The action of this drug is to stimulate certain receptors of the sympathetic nervous system (SNS) and is fairly specific to the lungs; however, there may be some systemic effects. This may potentially decrease the relaxation effects of massage in general and also may decrease the effectiveness of the systemic reflex strokes of rocking, effleurage, and friction. Using these strokes for a longer period of time than usual may help to achieve the desired effects.
- Side effects of dizziness require care in getting the client on and off the table. Stimulation with rapid effleurage at the end of the session may help.

saquinavir (sah-KWIN-ah-veer)

Fortovase

saquinavir mesylate

Invirase

Drug Class: Antiviral

Drug Actions

Hinders HIV activity

Use

- Adjunct treatment for advanced HIV infection in selected patients

Side Effects

Cardiovascular: chest pain.
Gastrointestinal: diarrhea, ulcerated buccal mucosa, abdominal pain, nausea, pancreatitis.
Nervous System: weakness, paresthesia, headache, dizziness.
Skin: rash.
Other: pancytopenia, thrombocytopenia, musculoskeletal pain, bronchitis, cough.

Onset, Peak, and Duration

Route	Onset	Peak	Duration
Oral	Unknown	Unknown	Unknown

Massage Considerations

- There are no cautions or contraindications to massage related to this drug.
- There may be cautions or contraindications to massage related to the client condition.
- Side effects of dizziness require care in getting the client on and off the table. Stimulation with rapid effleurage at the end of the session may help. Paresthesia is a contraindication to deep tissue massage. Rash is a local contraindication to massage and should be reported to the physician. If severe or widespread, massage should be withheld.

sargramostim (granulocyte macrophage colony-stimulating factor, GM-CSF) (sar-GRAH-moh-stim)

Leukine

Drug Class: Hematopoietic growth factor

Drug Actions

Stimulates formation of granulocytes (neutrophils, eosinophils) and macrophages

Use

- Acceleration of hematopoietic reconstitution after autologous bone marrow transplantation in patients with malignant lymphoma or acute lymphoblastic leukemia, or during autologous bone marrow transplantation in patients with Hodgkin's disease
- Bone marrow transplantation failure or engraftment delay
- Neutrophil recovery following chemotherapy in acute myelogenous leukemia

Side Effects

Cardiovascular: edema, supraventricular arrhythmia, pericardial effusion.
Gastrointestinal: nausea, vomiting, diarrhea, anorexia, hemorrhage, GI disorder, stomatitis.
Nervous System: malaise, CNS disorders, weakness, fever.
Urinary: urinary tract disorder, abnormal kidney function.

Skin: hair loss, rash.
Other: sepsis, mucous membrane disorder, blood dyscrasias, hemorrhage, liver damage, shortness of breath, lung disorders, pleural effusion.

Onset, Peak, and Duration

Route	Onset	Peak	Duration
I.V.	≤30 min	2 hr	Unknown

Massage Considerations

- Because this drug is related to blood and blood formation, deep tissue massage is contraindicated.
- There will be further cautions and contraindications to massage related to the client condition. In many cases, massage will be contraindicated completely.
- The physician should be consulted before any massage is given and close collaboration throughout is required.
- Side effects of rash is a contraindication to massage until the physician has evaluated the client. Hair loss is a contraindication to scalp massage if the client is disturbed by hair loss during the session or if the scalp is tender. Extra care needs to be taken with infection control.

---

scopolamine (hyoscine) (skoh-POL-uh-meen)

scopolamine

Scop, Transderm Scōp, Scopace

scopolamine butylbromide (hyoscine butylbromide)

Buscopan

scopolamine hydrobromide (hyoscine hydrobromide)

Drug Class: Anticholinergic

Drug Actions

Relieves spasticity, nausea, and vomiting; reduces secretions; and blocks cardiac vagal reflexes

Use

- Spastic states
- Preoperatively to reduce secretions
- Prevention of nausea and vomiting from motion sickness

Side Effects

Cardiovascular: palpitations, tachycardia, flushing, paradoxical bradycardia.
Gastrointestinal: constipation, dry mouth, nausea, vomiting, epigastric distress.
Nervous System: disorientation, restlessness, irritability, dizziness, drowsiness, headache, confusion, hallucinations, delirium, fever.
Urinary: urinary hesitancy, urine retention.
Skin: rash, dryness, contact dermatitis with transdermal patch.
Other: dilated pupils, blurred vision, photophobia, increased intraocular pressure, difficulty swallowing, bronchial plugging, depressed respirations.

Onset, Peak, and Duration

Route	Onset	Peak	Duration
Oral	30–60 min	Unknown	4–6 hr
I.V., I.M., Subcutaneous Injection	30 min	Unknown	4 hr
Rectal	Unknown	Unknown	Unknown
Transdermal	Unknown	Unknown	≤72 hr

Massage Considerations

- This drug blocks certain receptors of the PNS, especially in the G.I. tract. It also has some sedating effects. Deep tissue massage should be used with caution.
- There may be further cautions or contraindications to massage related to the client condition.
- The site of I.M. or subcutaneous injection of the drug should not be massaged for up to 4 hours. The site of transdermal application of the drug should not be massaged as long as the patch is in place, up to 72 hours.
- Side effects of dizziness and drowsiness may be helped by using stimulation with rapid effleurage either at the end of the session or throughout the session if the symptom is severe. Constipation may be helped by abdominal massage. Rash is a local contraindication to massage and should be reported to the physician.

secobarbital sodium (sek-oh-BAR-bih-tohl SOH-dee-um)

Novosecobarb, Seconal Sodium

Drug Class: Barbituate

Drug Actions

Interferes with transmission of impulses in the brain, promoting sedation and relief from seizures

Use

- Preoperative sedation
- Insomnia

Side Effects

Gastrointestinal: Nausea, vomiting.
Nervous System: drowsiness, lethargy, hangover, paradoxical excitement in geriatric patients, somnolence.
Skin: rash, hives, Stevens-Johnson syndrome.
Other: exacerbation of porphyria, respiratory depression, angioedema, physical or psychological dependence.

Onset, Peak, and Duration

Route	Onset	Peak	Duration
Oral	15 minutes	5–30 minutes	1–4 hours

Massage Considerations

- Because of the sedating effect, deep tissue should be used with caution or not at all.
- Side effects of drowsiness and lethargy may be increased by massage. Using stimulating strokes throughout the session may be needed. Rash or hives are a local contraindication and should be reported to the physician.

---

selegiline hydrochloride (L-deprenyl hydrochloride)

(see-LEJ-eh-leen high-droh-KLOR-ighd)

Atapryl, Carbex, Eldepryl, Selpak

Drug Class: MAO inhibitor antiparkinsonian

Drug Actions

May directly increase dopaminergic activity by decreasing reuptake of dopamine into nerve cells
Improves physical mobility

Use

- Adjunct treatment with levodopa-carbidopa in managing symptoms of Parkinson's disease

Side Effects

Cardiovascular: orthostatic hypotension, hypertension, hypotension, arrhythmias, palpitations, angina, tachycardia, peripheral edema.
Gastrointestinal: dry mouth, nausea, vomiting, constipation, abdominal pain, anorexia or poor appetite, painful digestion, diarrhea, heartburn.
Nervous System: dizziness, increased tremors, chorea, loss of balance, restlessness, increased bradykinesia, facial grimacing, stiff neck, dyskinesia, involuntary movements, twitching, increased apraxia, behavioral changes, fatigue, headache, confusion, hallucinations, vivid dreams, malaise, syncope.
Urinary: slow urination, transient nocturia, prostatic hyperplasia, urinary hesitancy, urinary frequency, urine retention, sexual dysfunction.
Skin: rash, hair loss, sweating.
Other: weight loss, blepharospasm.

Onset, Peak, and Duration

Route	Onset	Peak	Duration
Oral	Unknown	30 min–2 hr	Unknown

Massage Considerations

- There are no cautions or contraindications to massage related to the actions of this drug.
- There may be cautions and contraindications to massage related to the client condition.
- Side effects of hypotension and dizziness require care in getting the client on and off the table. Stimulation with rapid effleurage and tapotement at the end of the session may help. Constipation may be helped by abdominal massage. Frequent urination may require the client to get up during the session. Privacy and quick access to the bathroom should be provided. Water fountains and music that may stimulate the urge to urinate should be avoided. Rash is a local contraindication to massage and should be reported to the physician. Hair loss is a contraindication to scalp massage if the client is disturbed by hair loss during the session or the scalp is tender.

senna (SEN-uh)

Black-Draught, Fletcher's Castoria, Senexon, Senokot, Senolax, X-Prep

Drug Class: timulant laxative

Drug Actions

Increases peristalsis, probably by direct effect on smooth muscle of intestine. It also promotes fluid accumulation in colon and small intestine. Relieves constipation and cleanses bowel.

Use

- Acute constipation
- Preparation for bowel examination

Side Effects

Gastrointestinal: nausea; vomiting; diarrhea; malabsorption of nutrients; yellow or yellow-green cast to feces; abdominal cramps, especially in severe constipation; "cathartic colon" (syndrome resembling ulcerative colitis radiologically) with long-term misuse; constipation after catharsis; diarrhea in breast-feeding infants of mothers receiving senna; darkened pigmentation of rectal mucosa with long-term use (usually reversible within 4 to 12 months after stopping drug); laxative dependence; loss of normal bowel function with excessive use.
Urinary: red-pink discoloration in alkaline urine; yellow-brown color to acidic urine.
Other: protein-losing enteropathy, electrolyte imbalance.

Onset, Peak, and Duration

Route	Onset	Peak	Duration
Oral	6–10 hr	Varies	Varies
Rectal	30 min–2 hr	Varies	Varies

Massage Considerations

- There are no cautions or contraindications to massage related to this drug

sertraline hydrochloride (SER-truh-leen high-droh-KLOR-ighd)

Zoloft

Drug Class: Selective serotonin uptake inhibitor (SSRI) antidepressant

Drug Actions

Unknown; may be linked to inhibited neuronal uptake of serotonin in CNS
Relieves depression

Use

- Depression
- Posttraumatic stress disorder
- Social anxiety disorder
- Premenstrual dysphoric disorder
- Premature ejaculation

Side Effects

Cardiovascular: palpitations, chest pain, hot flushes, flushing.
Gastrointestinal: dry mouth, nausea, diarrhea, loose stools, painful digestion, vomiting, constipation, thirst, gas, anorexia, abdominal pain, increased appetite.

Nervous System: headache, tremor, dizziness, insomnia, sleepiness, paresthesia, hypesthesia, hyperesthesia, fatigue, twitching, hypertonia, nervousness, anxiety, confusion.
Urinary: male sexual dysfunction.
Skin: sweating, rash, itching.
Other: decreased libido, muscle pain.

Onset, Peak, and Duration

Route	Onset	Peak	Duration
Oral	2–4 wk	4 $^{1}/_{2}$–8 $^{1}/_{2}$ hr	Unknown

Massage Considerations

- There are no cautions or contraindications to massage related to the actions of this drug.
- There may be cautions and contraindications to massage related to the client condition.
- Side effects of dizziness and sleepiness may be helped by stimulation at the end of the session with rapid effleurage or tapotement. Paresthesia, hyperesthesia, and hypesthesia are all contraindications to deep tissue massage. Constipation and gas may be helped by abdominal massage. Rash or itching is a local contraindication to massage and should be reported to the physician.

---

sevelamer hydrochloride (seh-VEL-ah-mer high-droh-KLOR-ighd)

Renagel

Drug Class: Hyperphosphatemia drug

Drug Actions

Decreases phosphorus level

Use

- Reduction of phosphorus in patients with end-stage renal disease

Side Effects

Cardiovascular: hypertension, hypotension, thrombosis.
Gastrointestinal: vomiting, nausea, constipation, diarrhea, gas, painful digestion.
Nervous System: headache, pain.
Other: infection, cough.

Onset, Peak, and Duration

Route	Onset	Peak	Duration
Oral	Unknown	Unknown	Unknown

Massage Considerations

- This drug increases excretion of excess phosphorus in the body. Circulatory massage with effleurage should be used with great caution and limited.
- There will be other cautions and contraindications to massage related to the client condition.
- The physician should be consulted before any massage is given and close collaboration is essential.
- Side effects of thrombosis are a complete contraindication to massage. Hypotension may be helped by stimulation at the end of the session with gentle friction to the legs.
- Constipation may be helped by abdominal massage.

sibutramine hydrochloride monohydrate (sigh-BYOO-truh-meen high-droh-KLOR-ighd mah-noh-HIGH-drayt)

Meridia

Drug Class: Antiobesity drug

Drug Actions

Inhibits reuptake of norepinephrine, serotonin, and dopamine and facilitates weight loss

Use

- Management of obesity

Side Effects

Cardiovascular: tachycardia, vasodilation, hypertension, palpitations, chest pain, generalized edema.
Gastrointestinal: dry mouth, taste perversion, anorexia, constipation, increased appetite, nausea, painful digestion, gastritis, vomiting, abdominal pain, rectal disorder.
Nervous System: weakness, headache, insomnia, dizziness, nervousness, anxiety, depression, paresthesia, sleepiness, CNS stimulation, emotional lability, migraine.
Urinary: dysmenorrhea, urinary tract infection, vaginal candidiasis, metrorrhagia.
Skin: rash, acne sweating.
Other: flulike syndrome, injury, herpes simplex, accident, allergic reaction, thirst, rhinitis, pharyngitis, sinusitis, ear disorder, ear pain, laryngitis, joint pain, muscle pain tenosynovitis, joint disorder, neck or back pain, cough.

Onset, Peak, and Duration

Route	Onset	Peak	Duration
Oral	Unknown	3–4 hr	Unknown

Massage Considerations

- There are no cautions or contraindications to massage related to the actions of this drug.
- There may be cautions and contraindications to massage related to the client condition.
- The stimulant effect of the drug may make the relaxation effects of massage more difficult to achieve and decrease the effectiveness of systemic reflex strokes such as rocking, effleurage, and friction. Applying these strokes for longer periods may help achieve the desired effects, as well as using slow and rhythmic effleurage throughout the session.
- Side effects of dizziness and sleepiness may be helped by stimulation at the end of the massage session with friction to the legs. Paresthesia is a contraindication to deep tissue massage. Constipation may be helped by abdominal massage. Rash and acne are local contraindications to massage and should be reported to the physician. If acne is severe or widespread, massage may be given with the massage therapist wearing gloves when working the affected areas.

sildenafil citrate (sil-DEN-ah-fil SIGH-trayt)

Viagra

Drug Class: Therapy for erectile dysfunction

Drug Actions

Increases smooth muscle relaxation and inflow of blood to the corpus cavernosum so patient achieves an erection

Use

- Erectile dysfunction

Side Effects

Cardiovascular: heart attack, sudden cardiac death, ventricular arrhythmia, cerebrovascular hemorrhage, transient ischemic attack, hypotension, flushing.
Gastrointestinal: painful digestion, diarrhea.
Nervous System: anxiety, headache, dizziness, seizures, sleepiness.
Urinary: hematuria, prolonged erection, priapism, urinary tract infections.
Skin: rash.
Other: flulike syndrome, double vision, temporary vision loss, decreased vision, ocular redness or bloodshot appearance, increased intraocular pressure, retinal vascular disease, retinal bleeding, vitreous detachment or traction, perimacular edema, abnormal vision (photophobia, color tinged vision, blurred vision), ocular burning, ocular swelling or pressure, joint pain, back pain, respiratory tract infection.

Onset, Peak, and Duration

Route	Onset	Peak	Duration
Oral	Unknown	30 min–2 hr	4 hr

Massage Considerations

- This drug has strong effects on the circulatory system. No therapeutic massage should be given when the drug has been taken until the effects of the drug have worn off which will be at least 4 hours.

---

simethicone (sigh-METH-ih-kohn)

Extra Strength Gas-X, Gas Relief, Gas-X, Maximum Strength Gas Relief, Maximum Strength Phazyme, Mylanta Gas, Mylanta Gas Maximum Strength, Mylanta Gas Regular Strength, Mylicon-80, Mylicon-125, Ovol, Ovol-40, Oval-80, Phazyme, Phazyme 95, Phazyme 125

Drug Class: Antiflatulent

Drug Actions

Disperses or prevents formation of mucus-surrounded gas pockets in GI tract

Use

- Gas
- Functional gastric bloating

Side Effects

Gastrointestinal: excessive belching or flatus.

Onset, Peak, and Duration

Route	Onset	Peak	Duration
Oral	Immediate	Immediate	Unknown

 Massage Considerations

- There are no cautions or contraindications to massage related to this drug.

simvastatin (synvinolin) (sim-vuh-STAT-in)

Lipex, Zocor

Drug Class: Cholesterol-lowering drug

Drug Actions

Lowers LDL and total cholesterol levels

Use

- Reductions in risk of coronary artery disease mortality and cardiovascular events in patients at high risk of coronary events
- To reduce total and LDL cholesterol in patients with homozygous familial hypercholesterolemia
- Heterozygous familial hypercholesterolemia

Side Effects

Gastrointestinal: abdominal pain, constipation, diarrhea, painful digestion, gas, nausea.
Nervous System: headache, weakness.
Other: upper respiratory tract infection.

Onset, Peak, and Duration

Route	Onset	Peak	Duration
Oral	Unknown	$1\,^1/_2$–$2\,^1/_2$ hr	Unknown

 Massage Considerations

- There are no cautions or contraindications to massage related to the actions of this drug.
- There may be cautions and contraindications to massage related to the client condition.
- Side effects of constipation and gas may be helped by abdominal massage.

sirolimus (sir-AH-lih-mus)

Rapamune

Drug Class: Immunosuppressant

Drug Actions

Immunosuppression in patients receiving renal transplants

Use

- Prophylaxis of organ rejection in patients receiving renal transplants

Side Effects

Cardiovascular: facial edema, hypertension, heart failure, atrial fibrillation, tachycardia, hypotension, peripheral edema, chest pain, edema, hemorrhage, palpitations, peripheral vascular disorder, thrombophlebitis, thrombosis, vasodilation.
Gastrointestinal: diarrhea, nausea, vomiting, constipation, abdominal pain, painful digestion, enlarged abdomen, hernia, ascites, peritonitis, anorexia, difficulty swallowing, belching, esophagitis, gas, gastritis, gastroenteritis, gingivitis, gum hyperplasia, ileus, mouth ulcerations, oral candidiasis, stomatitis.

Nervous System: headache, insomnia, tremor, anxiety, depression, weakness, malaise, syncope, confusion, dizziness, emotional lability, hypertonia, hypesthesia, hypotonia, neuropathy, paresthesia, sleepiness, fever, pain.
Urinary: painful urination, hematuria, albuminuria, kidney tubular necrosis, urinary tract infections, pelvic pain, glycosuria, bladder pain, hydronephrosis, impotence, kidney pain, nocturia, oliguria, pyuria, scrotal edema, testis disorder, toxic nephropathy, urinary frequency, urinary incontinence, urine retention.
Skin: rash, acne, abnormal hair growth, fungal dermatitis, itching, skin hypertrophy, skin ulcer, bruising, sweating.
Other: abscess; cellulitis; chills; flulike syndrome; infection; sepsis; abnormal healing, pharyngitis, epistaxis, rhinitis, sinusitis, abnormal vision, cataracts, conjunctivitis, deafness, ear pain, otitis media, ringing in the ears, abnormal blood profiles, lymphadenopathy, hepatic artery thrombosis, hypercholesteremia, hyperlipidemia, hypokalemia, weight gain, hypophosphatemia, hyperkalemia, hypervolemia, Cushing syndrome, diabetes mellitus, acidosis, dehydration, hypercalcemia, hyperglycemia, hyperphosphatemia, hypocalcemia, hypoglycemia, hypomagnesemia, hyponatremia, weight loss, back pain, joint pain, muscle pain, arthrosis, bone necrosis, leg cramps, osteoporosis, tetany, shortness of breath, cough, atelectasis, upper respiratory tract infection, asthma, bronchitis, hypoxia, lung edema, pleural effusion, pneumonia.

Onset, Peak, and Duration

Route	Onset	Peak	Duration
Oral	Unknown	1–3 hr	Unknown

Massage Considerations

- There are no cautions or contraindications to massage related to the actions of this drug.
- There will be cautions and contraindications to massage related to the client condition.
- The physician should be consulted before any massage is given.
- Side effects of hypotension, dizziness and sleepiness may be helped by stimulation with tapotement or gentle friction to the legs at the end of the session. Thrombophlebitis or thrombosis are complete contraindications to massage. Neuropathy, paresthesia, or hypesthesia are contraindications to deep tissue massage. Constipation and gas may be helped by abdominal massage. Frequent urination requires privacy and quick access to the bathroom for the client. Water fountains or music that may stimulate the need to urinate should be avoided. Cushing syndrome causes changes in metabolism and in connective, fatty, and muscle tissues. Deep tissue massage is contraindicated. Stretching and traction and myofascial massage techniques should be used with great caution.
- Osteoporosis is a contraindication to deep tissue massage and if severe, may contraindicate massage completely. Rash, acne, and itching are local contraindications to massage and should be reported to the physician. If severe or widespread, massage should be withheld. Bruising is a contraindication to deep tissue massage. Extra care should be taken with infection control. Schedule the client as the first session of the day to limit exposure to others and no massage should be given if the massage therapist has any symptoms of infection.
- The best approach to this client is to use systemic reflex strokes of rocking and slow, rhythmic effleurage. Gentle compression and pétrissage may also be used.

---

somatrem (SOH-muh-trem)

Protropin

Drug Class: Anterior pituitary hormone (human growth hormone GH)

Drug Actions

Stimulates linear, skeletal muscle, and organ growth in children

Use

- Long-term treatment of children who have growth failure because of lack of adequate endogenous growth hormone secretion

Side Effects

Other: antibodies to growth hormone, leukemia, hypothyroidism, hyperglycemia.

Onset, Peak, and Duration

Route	Onset	Peak	Duration
I.M., Subcutaneous Injection	Unknown	Unknown	12–48 hr

Massage Considerations

- There are no cautions or contraindications to massage related to the actions of this drug.
- There may be cautions or contraindications to massage related to the client condition.
- The physician should be consulted before any massage is given.
- The site of I.M. or subcutaneous injection of the drug should not be massage for up to 12 hours after administration.

---

somatropin (soh-muh-TROH-pin)

Genotropin, Genotropin Miniquick, Humatrope, Norditropin, Nutropin, Nutropin AQ, Nutropin Depot, Saizen, Serostim

Drug Class: Anterior pituitary hormone (human growth hormone)

Drug Actions

Simulates linear, skeletal muscle, and organ growth

Use

- Long-term treatment of growth failure in children with inadequate secretion of endogenous growth hormone.
- Growth failure from chronic renal insufficiency up to time of kidney transplant.
- Long-term treatment of short stature related to Turner syndrome.
- Long-term treatment of growth failure in children with Prader-Willi syndrome (PWS) diagnosed by genetic testing.
- Replacement of endogenous growth hormone in adult patients with growth hormone deficiency.
- AIDS wasting or cachexia.
- Long-term treatment of growth failure in children born small for gestational age who don't achieve catch-up growth by 2 years of age.

Side Effects

Cardiovascular: mild, transient edema.
Nervous System: headache, weakness.
Other: injection site pain, antibodies to growth hormone, leukemia, mild hyperglycemia, hypothyroidism, localized muscle pain.

Onset, Peak, and Duration

Route	Onset	Peak	Duration
I.M., Subcutaneous Injection	Unknown	7 1/2 hr	12–48 hr

Massage Considerations

- There are no cautions or contraindications to massage related to the actions of this drug.
- There may be cautions or contraindications to massage related to the client condition.
- The physician should be consulted before any massage is given.
- The site of I.M. or subcutaneous injection of the drug should not be massage for up to 12 hours after administration.

sotalol hydrochloride (SOH-tuh-lol high-droh-KLOR-ighd)

Betapace, Betapace AF, Sotacor

Drug Class: Nonselective beta blocker

Drug Actions

Restores normal sinus rhythm, lowers blood pressure, and relieves angina

Use

- Documented, life-threatening ventricular arrhythmias
- Maintenance of normal sinus rhythm (delay in time to recurrence of atrial fibrillation/atrial flutter) in patients with symptomatic atrial fibrillation/atrial flutter who are currently in sinus rhythm

Side Effects

Cardiovascular: bradycardia, arrhythmias, heart failure, AV block, proarrhythmic events (ventricular tachycardia, PVCs, ventricular fibrillation), edema, palpitations, chest pain, ECG abnormalities, hypotension.
Gastrointestinal: nausea, vomiting, diarrhea, painful digestion.
Nervous System: weakness, headache, dizziness, weakness, fatigue.
Other: shortness of breath, bronchospasm.

Onset, Peak, and Duration

Route	Onset	Peak	Duration
Oral	Unknown	2 1/2–4 hr	Unknown

Massage Considerations

- There are no cautions or contraindications to massage related to the actions of this drug.
- There may be cautions and contraindications to massage related to the client condition.
- Side effects of hypotension or dizziness require care in getting the client on and off the table. Stimulation with rapid effleurage or tapotement at the end of the session may help.

spironolactone (spih-ron-uh-LAK-tohn)

Aldactone, Novospiroton, Spiractin,

Drug Class: Potassium-sparing diuretic

Drug Actions

Promotes water and sodium excretion and hinders potassium excretion, lowers blood pressure, and helps to diagnose primary hyperaldosteronism

Use

- Edema
- Essential hypertension
- Diuretic-induced hypokalemia
- Diagnosis of primary hyperaldosteronism
- Management of primary hyperaldosteronism
- Hirsutism
- Premenstrual syndrome
- Heart failure in patients receiving an ACE inhibitor and a loop diuretic with or without digoxin
- Decrease risk of metrorrhagia
- Acne vulgaris

Side Effects

Gastrointestinal: diarrhea, gastric bleeding, ulceration, cramping, gastritis, vomiting.
Nervous System: headache, drowsiness, lethargy, confusion, ataxia.
Urinary: impotence, menstrual disturbances.
Skin: hives, rash, abnormal hair growth.
Other: drug fever, abnormal growth of breast tissue, breast soreness, anaphylaxis, angioedema, agranulocytosis, hyperkalemia, hyponatremia, mild acidosis, dehydration.

Onset, Peak, and Duration

Route	Onset	Peak	Duration
Oral	Unknown	1–2 hours	Unknown

Massage Considerations

- There are no cautions or contraindications to massage related to the actions of this drug.
- There may be cautions or contraindications to massage related to the client condition.
- Because the action of this drug promotes urination, frequency may require the client to go to the bathroom in the middle of the session. Privacy and quick access to the bathroom should be provided. Water fountains and music that may stimulate the urge to urinate should be avoided.
- Side effects of drowsiness may be helped by stimulation at the end of the session with tapotement. Hives or rash are a local contraindication to massage and should be reported to the physician. Breast growth and tenderness in men and women requires caution in depth and pressure of chest massage. No deep tissue massage of the chest should be done. If too tender, avoid the area completely.

stavudine (2,3-didehydro-3-deoxythymidine, d4T)

(stay-VYOO-deen)

Zerit, Zerit XR

Drug Class: Antiviral

Drug Actions

Inhibits HIV replication

Use

- Patients with advanced HIV infection who are intolerant of or unresponsive to other antivirals

Side Effects

Cardiovascular: chest pain.
Gastrointestinal: abdominal pain, diarrhea, nausea, vomiting, anorexia, painful digestion, constipation, weight loss, pancreatitis.
Nervous System: weakness, peripheral neuropathy, headache, malaise, insomnia, anxiety, depression, nervousness, dizziness, fever.
Skin: rash, itching, sweating.
Other: chills, breast enlargement, redistribution or accumulation of body fat, conjunctivitis, abnormal blood profiles, hepatotoxicity, severe hepatomegaly with steatosis, lactic acidosis, back pain, muscle pain, joint pain, shortness of breath.

Onset, Peak, and Duration

Route	Onset	Peak	Duration
Oral	Unknown	$\leq$1 hr	Unknown

 Massage Considerations

- There are no cautions or contraindications to massage related to the actions of this drug.
- There may be cautions or contraindications to massage related to the client condition.
- Side effects of dizziness require care in getting the client on and off the table. Stimulation with effleurage at the end of the session may help. Neuropathy is a contraindication to deep tissue massage. Constipation may be helped by abdominal massage. Rash or itching is a local contraindication to massage and should be reported to the physician immediately. If severe or widespread, massage should be withheld.

---

streptomycin sulfate (strep-toh-MIGH-sin SUL-fayt)

Drug Class: Antibiotic

Drug Actions

Kills bacteria

Use

- *Streptococcal endocarditis*
- Primary and adjunct treatment in tuberculosis
- *Enterococcal endocarditis*
- Tularemia

Side Effects

Gastrointestinal: vomiting, nausea.
Nervous System: neuromuscular blockade.
Urinary: some nephrotoxicity (not as much as other aminoglycosides).
Skin: exfoliative dermatitis.
Other: hypersensitivity reactions, angioedema, anaphylaxis, ototoxicity (tinnitus, vertigo, hearing loss), abnormal blood profiles, apnea.

Onset, Peak, and Duration

Route	Onset	Peak	Duration
I.M.	Unknown	1–2 hr	Unknown

Massage Considerations

- There are no cautions or contraindications to massge related to the actions of this drug.
- There may be cautions and contraindications to massage related to the client condition and severity of infection.
- The site of I.M. injection of the drug should not be massaged for at least 2 hours.

---

sucralfate (SOO-krahl-fayt)

Carafate, SCF

Drug Class: Antiulcer drug

Drug Actions

May adhere to and protect ulcer's surface by forming barrier
Aids in duodenal ulcer healing

Use

- Maintenance therapy for duodenal ulcer
- Short-term (up to 8 weeks) treatment of duodenal ulcer
- Gastric ulcer

Side Effects

Gastrointestinal: constipation, nausea, gastric discomfort, diarrhea, bezoar formation, vomiting, gas, dry mouth, indigestion.
Nervous System: dizziness, sleepiness, headache.
Skin: rash, itching.
Other: back pain.

Onset, Peak, and Duration

Route	Onset	Peak	Duration
Oral	Unknown	≤6 hr	Unknown

Massage Considerations

- There are no cautions or contraindications to massage related to the actions of this drug.
- There may be cautions or contraindications to massage related to the client condition.
- Side effects of dizziness and sleepiness may be helped by stimulation with effleurage and tapotement at the end of the session. Constipation and gas may be helped by abdominal massage. Rash and itching are local contraindications to massage and should be reported to the physician.

---

sulfasalazine (salazosulfapyridine, sulphasalazine)
(sul-fuh-SAL-uh-zeen)

Azulfidine, Azulfidine EN-Tabs, PMS-Sulfasalazine E.C., Salazopyrin, Salazopyrin EN-Tabs, S.A.S.-500, S.A.S. Enteric-500

Drug Class: Anti-inflammatory

Drug Actions

Relieves inflammation in GI tract

Use

- Mild to moderate ulcerative colitis
- Adjunct therapy in severe ulcerative colitis
- Crohn's disease
- Rheumatoid arthritis
- Patients with polyarticular-course juvenile rheumatoid arthritis

Side Effects

Gastrointestinal: nausea, vomiting, diarrhea, abdominal pain, anorexia, stomatitis.
Nervous System: headache, depression, seizures, hallucinations.
Urinary: toxic nephrosis with oliguria and anuria, crystalluria, hematuria, oligospermia, infertility.
Skin: Stevens-Johnson syndrome, generalized skin eruption, epidermal necrolysis, exfoliative dermatitis, photosensitivity reactions, hives, itching.
Other: hypersensitivity reactions (serum sickness, drug fever, anaphylaxis), abnormal blood profiles, jaundice, hepatotoxicity.

Onset, Peak, and Duration

Route	Onset	Peak	Duration
Oral:			
Parent Drug	Unknown	$1\frac{1}{2}$–6 hr	Unknown
Metabolites	Unknown	12–24 hr	Unknown

Massage Considerations

- The reason for this drug's anti-inflammatory effects is unknown; however, deep tissue massage should be used with caution.
- There may be further cautions and contraindications to massage related to the client condition.
- Side effects of hives, itching, or skin euptions are local contraindications to massage and should be reported to the physician immediately. If severe or widespread, massage should be withheld.

---

sulfinpyrazone (sul-fin-PEER-uh-zohn)

Anturan, Anturane

Drug Class: Uricosuric, renal tubular blocker, platelet aggregation inhibitor

Drug Actions

Blocks renal tubular reabsorption of uric acid, increasing excretion, and inhibits platelet aggregation
Relieves signs and symptoms of gouty arthritis

Use

- Intermittent or chronic gouty arthritis
- Prophylaxis of thromboembolic disorders, including angina, heart attack, transient (cerebral) ischemic attacks, and presence of prosthetic heart valves

Side Effects

Gastrointestinal: nausea, painful digestion, epigastric pain, reactivation of peptic ulcerations.
Skin: rash.
Other: blood dyscrasias, bronchoconstriction in patients with aspirin-induced asthma.

Onset, Peak, and Duration

Route	Onset	Peak	Duration
Oral	Unknown	1–2 hr	4–6 hr

 Massage Considerations

- Because of this drug's action on platelets and blood clotting mechanisms, deep tissue massage should be used with caution.
- There may be further cautions and contraindications to massage related to the client condition.
- Side effects of rash are a local contraindication to massage and should be reported to the physician.

---

sulindac (SUL-in-dak)

Aclin, Apo-Sulin, Clinoril, Novo-Sundac

Drug Class: NSAID (nonsteroidal anti-inflammatory drug)

Drug Actions

Inhibits prostaglandin synthesis relieving pain, fever, and inflammation

Use

- Osteoarthritis
- Rheumatoid arthritis
- Ankylosing spondylitis
- Acute subacromial bursitis or supraspinatus tendinitis
- Acute gouty arthritis

Side Effects

Cardiovascular: hypertension, heart failure, palpitations, edema.
Gastrointestinal: epigastric distress, peptic ulceration, pancreatitis, GI bleeding, occult blood loss, nausea, constipation, gas, painful digestion, anorexia.
Nervous System: dizziness, headache, nervousness, psychosis.
Urinary: interstitial nephritis, nephrotic syndrome, renal failure.
Skin: rash, itching.
Other: drug fever, anaphylaxis, hypersensitivity syndrome, angioedema, ringing in the ears, transient visual disturbances, abnormal blood profiles.

Onset, Peak, and Duration

Route	Onset	Peak	Duration
Oral	Unknown	2–4 hr	Unknown

Massage Considerations

- This drug decreases the perception of pain; therefore, deep tissue massage should be used with caution.

- There may be further cautions or contraindications to massage related to the client condition.
- Side effects of dizziness require care in getting the client on and off the table. Using stimulation with rapid effleurage or tapotement at the end of the session may help.
- Constipation and gas may be helped by abdominal massage. Rash or itching is a local contraindication to massage and should be reported to the physician. If severe or widespread, massage should be withheld.

---

sumatriptan succinate (soo-muh-TRIP-ten SEK-seh-nayt)

Imitrex

Drug Class: Antimigraine drug

Drug Actions

Causes vasoconstriction of cerebral vessels and relieves acute migraine pain

Use

- Acute migraine attacks (with or without aura)
- Acute treatment of cluster headache episodes

Side Effects

Cardiovascular: atrial fibrillation, ventricular fibrillation, ventricular tachycardia, coronary artery vasospasm, transient myocardial ischemia, heart attack, pressure or tightness in chest.
Gastrointestinal: abdominal discomfort, difficulty swallowing, diarrhea; nausea, vomiting, unusual or bad taste (nasal spray).
Nervous System: dizziness, drowsiness, headache, anxiety, malaise, fatigue.
Skin: sweating.
Other: warm or hot sensation; burning sensation; heaviness, pressure or tightness; tight feeling in head; cold sensation; numbness; flushing, tingling, injection site reaction, muscle pain, muscle cramps, neck pain, upper respiratory inflammation and shortness of breath (oral), discomfort of throat, nasal cavity or sinus, mouth, jaw, or tongue; altered vision.

Onset, Peak, and Duration

Route	Onset	Peak	Duration
Oral	30 min	2–4 hr	Unknown
Subcutaneous Injection	10–20 min	1–2 hr	Unknown
Intranasal	Rapid	1–2 hr	Unknown

Massage Considerations

- There are no cautions or contraindications to massage related to this drug.
- There may be cautions or contraindications to massage related to the client condition.
- The site of subcutaneous injection of the drug should not be massaged for at least 2 hours after administration of the drug to avoid speeding up the absorption of the drug into the body.
- Side effects of dizziness and drowsiness require care in getting the client on and off the table. Stimulation with rapid effleurage or tapotement at the end of the session may help.

T

tacrine hydrochloride (TAK-reen high-droh-KLOR-ighd)

Cognex

Drug Class: Psychotherapeutic for Alzheimer disease

Drug Actions

Reversibly inhibits enzyme cholinesterase in central nervous system (CNS), allowing buildup of acetylcholine, and improving thinking in patients with Alzheimer disease.

Use

- Mild to moderate dementia of Alzheimer type

Side Effects

Cardiovascular: chest pain, facial flushing.
Gastrointestinal: nausea, vomiting, anorexia, diarrhea, painful digestion, loose stools, changes in stool color, constipation.
Nervous System: agitation, ataxia, insomnia, abnormal thinking, sleepiness, depression, anxiety, headache, fatigue, dizziness, confusion.
Skin: rash.
Other: rhinitis, jaundice, weight loss, muscle pain, upper respiratory tract infection, cough.

Onset, Peak, and Duration

Route	Onset	Peak	Duration
Oral	Unknown	30 min–3 hr	Unknown

 Massage Considerations

- No cautions or contraindications to massage are related to the actions of this drug. Cautions or contraindications to massage may be related to the client condition.
- Side effects of sleepiness or dizziness require care in getting the client on and off the table. Stimulation with effleurage or friction to the legs at the end of the session may help. If symptoms are severe, using a more stimulating massage technique throughout the sesssion may be needed.
- Constipation may be helped by abdominal massage.
- Rash is a local contraindication to massage and should be reported to the physician.

tacrolimus (tek-roh-LYE-mus)

Prograf

Drug Class: Immunosuppressant

Drug Actions

Suppresses the immune system and prevents organ rejection.

Use

- Prophylaxis of organ rejection in allogenic liver transplantation
- Prophylaxis of organ rejection in allogenic kidney transplantation

Side Effects

Cardiovascular: hypertension, peripheral edema.
Gastrointestinal: ascites, diarrhea, nausea, constipation, anorexia, vomiting, abdominal pain.
Nervous System: weakness, headache, tremor, insomnia, paresthesia, delirium, coma, pain, fever, neurotoxicity.
Urinary: abnormal kidney function, urinary tract infection, oliguria, nephrotoxicity.
Skin: photosensitivity reactions.
Other: anaphylaxis, anemia, leukocytosis, thrombocytopenia, hyperkalemia, hypokalemia, hyperglycemia, hypomagnesemia, back pain, pleural effusion, atelectasis, shortness of breath.

Onset, Peak, and Duration

Route	Onset	Peak	Duration
Oral, I.V.	Unknown	1.5–3.5 hr	Unknown

Massage Considerations

- No cautions or contraindications to massage are related to the actions of this drug. Cautions and contraindications to massage will be related to the client condition.
- The physician should be consulted before any massage is given.
- Side effects of paresthesia are a contraindication to deep tissue massage.
- Constipation may be helped by abdominal massage.

tacrolimus (topical) (tack-row-LYE-mus)

Protopic

Drug Class: Immunosuppressant

Drug Actions

Causes immunosuppression and inhibits the release of mediators from mast cells and basophils in skin, which improves skin condition.

Use

- Moderate to severe atopic dermatitis

Side Effects

Cardiovascular: face edema, peripheral edema.
Gastrointestinal: diarrhea, vomiting, nausea, abdominal pain, gastroenteritis, painful digestion.
Nervous System: headache, fever, hyperesthesia, weakness, insomnia, pain.
Skin: skin burning, itching, skin erythema, skin infection, eczema herpeticum, pustular rash, folliculitis, hives, maculopapular rash, rash, fungal dermatitis, acne, sunburn, tingling, benign skin neoplasm, skin disorder, vesiculobullous rash, dry skin, herpes zoster, eczema, exfoliative dermatitis, contact dermatitis.
Other: flulike symptoms, accidental injury, infection, lack of drug effect, alcohol intolerance, periodontal abscess, cyst, herpes simplex, allergic reaction, otitis media, pharyngitis, rhinitis, sinusitis, conjunctivitis, lymphadenopathy, back pain, muscle pain, increased cough, asthma, pneumonia, bronchitis.

Onset, Peak, and Duration

Route	Onset	Peak	Duration
Topical	Unknown	Unknown	Unknown

Massage Considerations

- No cautions or contraindications to massage are related to the actions of this drug.
- Cautions or contraindications to massage may be related to the client condition.

---

tadalafil (tah-DAH-lah-phil)

Cialis

Drug Class: Erectile dysfunction drug

Drug Actions

Prolongs smooth muscle relaxation and promotes blood flow into the corpus cavernosum

Use

- Erectile dysfunction

Side Effects

Cardiovascular: flushing.
Gastrointestinal: painful digestion.
Nervous System: headache.
Other: back pain, limb pain, muscle pain, nasal congestion.

Onset, Peak, and Duration

Route	Onset	Peak	Duration
Oral	Immediate	30 min–6 hr	Unknown

Massage Considerations

- Because of the effect on the cardiovascular system and the unknown duration of action of this drug, no therapeutic massage should be given until the next day after the drug has been taken.

---

tamoxifen citrate (teh-MOKS-uh-fen SIGH-trayt)

Apo-Tamox, Nolvadex, Nolvadex-D, Novo-Tamoxifen, Tamofen, Tamone

Drug Class: Antineoplastic

Drug Actions

Acts as estrogen antagonist and hinders function of breast cancer cells

Use

- Advanced postmenopausal breast cancer
- Adjunct treatment for breast cancer
- Reduction of breast cancer risk in high-risk women
- Ductal carcinoma in situ
- Stimulation of ovulation
- McCune-Albright syndrome and precocious puberty
- Mastalgia

Side Effects

Cardiovascular: hot flushes.

Gastrointestinal: nausea, vomiting, diarrhea.
Nervous System: confusion, weakness, headache, sleepiness, stroke.
Skin: skin changes, rash.
Other: temporary bone or tumor pain, corneal changes, cataracts, retinopathy, leukopenia, thrombocytopenia, vaginal discharge and bleeding, irregular menses, amenorrhea, endometrial cancer, uterine sarcoma, fatty liver, cholestasis, hepatic necrosis, hypercalcemia, weight changes, fluid retention, brief exacerbation of pain from osseous metastases, pulmonary embolism.

Onset, Peak, and Duration

Route	Onset	Peak	Duration
Oral	4–10 wk	Unknown	Several wk

 Massage Considerations

- No cautions or contraindications to massage are related to the actions of this drug. Cautions and contraindications to massage may be related to the client condition.
- Side effects of sleepiness may be helped by stimulation with tapotement at the end of the session.
- Pulmonary embolism is a complete contraindication to massage.
- Rash is a local contraindication to massage and should be reported to the physician.

tamsulosin hydrochloride (tam-soo-LOH-sin high-droh-KLOR-ighd)

Flomax

Drug Class: Benign prostatic hypertrophy (BPH) drug

Drug Actions

Selectively blocks α receptors in the prostate, leading to relaxation of smooth muscles in the bladder neck and prostate, which improves urine flow and reduces symptoms of BPH.

Use

- BPH

Side Effects

Cardiovascular: chest pain, orthostatic hypotension.
Gastrointestinal: diarrhea, nausea.
Nervous System: weakness, dizziness, headache, insomnia, sleepiness, syncope.
Other: decreased libido, infection, tooth disorder, amblyopia, pharyngitis, rhinitis, sinusitis, abnormal ejaculation, back pain, cough.

Onset, Peak, and Duration

Route	Onset	Peak	Duration
Oral	Unknown	4–5 hr	9–15 hr

 Massage Considerations

- No cautions or contraindications to massage are related to this drug. Cautions and contraindications to massage may be related to the client condition.
- Side effects of dizziness and hypotension require care in getting the client on and off the table. Stimulation with rapid effleurage or tapotement at the end of the session may help.

tegaserod maleate (teh-GAS-uh-rahd MALL-ee-ayt)

Zelnorm

Drug Class: Irritable bowel syndrome drug

Drug Actions

In the gastrointestinal (GI) tract, stimulates the peristaltic reflex and intestinal secretion, inhibits visceral sensitivity, and relieves constipation.

Use

- Short-term treatment for irritable bowel syndrome, when the primary bowel symptom is constipation

Side Effects

Gastrointestinal: abdominal pain, diarrhea, nausea, gas.
Nervous System: headache, dizziness, migraine.
Other: accidental injury, back pain, arthropathy, leg pain.

Onset, Peak, and Duration

Route	Onset	Peak	Duration
Oral	Unknown	1 hr	Unknown

 Massage Considerations

- No cautions or contraindications to massage are related to the actions of this drug. Cautions and contraindications to massage may be related to the client condition.
- Side effects of dizziness may be helped by stimulation at the end of the session with effleurage or tapotement.
- Gas may be helped by abdominal massage.

telmisartan (tel-mih-SAR-tan)

Micardis

Drug Class: Antihypertensive

Drug Actions

Chemical effect: Blocks the vasoconstrictive and aldosterone-secreting effects of angiotensin II and lowers blood pressure.

Use

- Hypertension (used alone or with other antihypertensives)

Side Effects

Cardiovascular: chest pain, hypertension, peripheral edema.
Gastrointestinal: abdominal pain, diarrhea, painful digestion, nausea.
Nervous System: dizziness, pain, fatigue, headache.
Urinary: urinary tract infection.
Other: flulike symptoms, pharyngitis, sinusitis, back pain, muscle pain, cough, upper respiratory tract infection.

Onset, Peak, and Duration

Route	Onset	Peak	Duration
Oral	Unknown	30 min–1 hr	24 hr

 Massage Considerations

- No cautions or contraindications to massage are indicated because a client is taking this drug. Cautions and contraindications to massage may be related to the client condition.
- Side effects of dizziness may be helped by stimulation at the end of the session with tapotement or effleurage.

---

temazepam (teh-MAZ-ih-pam)

Euhypnos, Normison, Restoril, Temaze

Drug Class: Benzodiazepine sedative-hypnotic

Drug Actions

May act on limbic system, thalamus, and hypothalamus of CNS to produce hypnotic effects and promote sleep.

Use

- Short-term treatment of insomnia

Side Effects

Gastrointestinal: diarrhea, nausea, dry mouth.
Nervous System: drowsiness, dizziness, lethargy, disturbed coordination, daytime sedation, confusion, nightmares, euphoria, weakness, headache, fatigue, nervousness, anxiety, depression.
Other: physical or psychological dependence, blurred vision.

Onset, Peak, and Duration

Route	Onset	Peak	Duration
Oral	Unknown	1–2 hr	Unknown

 Massage Considerations

- This drug has a depressant effect on the CNS; therefore, deep tissue massage should be used with caution.
- Side effects of drowsiness and dizziness require care in getting the client on and off the table. Stimulation with effleurage and tapotement at the end of the session may help.

---

teniposide (VM-26) (teh-NIP-uh-sighd)

Vumon

Drug Class: Antineoplastic

Drug Actions

Prevents reproduction of leukemic cells.

Use

- Refractory childhood acute lymphoblastic leukemia

Side Effects

Cardiovascular: hypotension from rapid infusion.
Gastrointestinal: nausea, vomiting, mucositis, diarrhea.
Skin: hair loss.
Other: hypersensitivity reactions (chills, fever, hives, tachycardia, bronchospasm, shortness of breath, hypotension, flushing), phlebitis at injection site with extravasation, abnormal blood profiles, myelosuppression.

Onset, Peak, and Duration

Route	Onset	Peak	Duration
I.V.	Unknown	Unknown	Unknown

 Massage Considerations

- Because of the toxic effects of this drug, deep tissue massage is contraindicated, and circulatory massage with effleurage should be used with caution and limited.
- Further cautions and contraindications to massage may be related to the client condition.
- The physician should be consulted before any massage is given, and close collaboration is essential.
- The drug is often given twice a week and has a short half-life (5 hours). Massage is best given on the days the drug is not being administered.
- Side effects of hair loss are a contraindication to scalp massage if the client is disturbed by hair loss during the massage or if the scalp is tender.
- The best approach to this client is to use the systemic and local reflex strokes of rocking, friction, stretching, traction, and vibration. Pétrissage and myofascial massage techniques may also be used.

---

tenofovir disoproxil fumarate (teh-NAH-fuh-veer diso-PRAHK-sul FOO-mah-rate)

Viread

Drug Class: Antiviral, antiretroviral

Drug Actions

Inhibits HIV replication

Use

- HIV-1 infection, with other antiretrovirals

Side Effects

Gastrointestinal: abdominal pain, anorexia, diarrhea, gas, nausea, vomiting.
Nervous System: weakness, headache.
Urinary: glycosuria.
Other: neutropenia, hyperglycemia.

Onset, Peak, and Duration

Route	Onset	Peak	Duration
Oral	Unknown	1–2 hr	Unknown

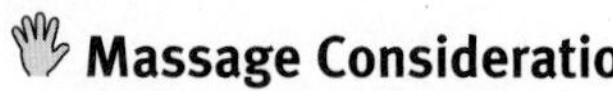

Massage Considerations

- No cautions or contraindications to massage are indicated because a client is taking this drug. No cautions or contraindications to massage are related to the client condition.
- Side effects of gas may be helped by abdominal massage.

---

terazosin hydrochloride (ter-uh-ZOH-sin high-droh-KLOR-ighd)

Hytrin

Drug Class: Selective α_1-adrenergic blocker and antihypertensive

Drug Actions

Decreases blood pressure by vasodilation produced in response to blockade of α_1-adrenergic receptors. Improves urine flow by blocking α_1-adrenergic receptors in smooth muscle of bladder, neck, and prostate, thus relieving urethral pressure and reestablishing urine flow.

Use

- Hypertension
- Symptomatic BPH

Side Effects

Cardiovascular: palpitations, orthostatic hypotension, tachycardia, peripheral edema, atrial firillation.
Gastrointestinal: nausea.
Nervous System: weakness, dizziness, headache, nervousness, paresthesia, sleepiness.
Urinary: impotence, priapism.
Other: decreased libido, nasal congestion, sinusitis, blurred vision, thrombocytopenia, back pain, muscle pain, shortness of breath.

Onset, Peak, and Duration

Route	Onset	Peak	Duration
Oral	≤15 min	2–3 hr	24 hr

Massage Considerations

- No cautions or contraindications to massage are related to the actions of this drug. Cautions and contraindications to massage may be related to the client condition.
- Side effects of hypotension, dizziness, and sleepiness require care in getting the client on and off the table. Stimulation with effleurage and tapotement at the end of the session may help.
- Paresthesia is a contraindication to deep tissue massage.

---

terbutaline sulfate (ter-BYOO-tuh-leen SUL-fayt)

Brethine, Bricanyl

Drug Class: Bronchodilator

Drug Actions

Relaxes bronchial smooth muscle by acting on β_2-adrenergic receptors and improves breathing ability.

Use

- Bronchospasm in patients with reversible obstructive airway disease
- Premature labor

Side Effects

Cardiovascular: palpitations, tachycardia, arrhythmias, flushing.
Gastrointestinal: vomiting, nausea, heartburn.
Nervous System: nervousness, tremor, headache, drowsiness, dizziness, weakness.
Skin: sweating.
Other: hypokalemia, paradoxical bronchospasm, shortness of breath.

Onset, Peak, and Duration

Route	Onset	Peak	Duration
Oral	30 min	2–3 hr	4–8 hr
Subcutaneous Injection	≤15 min	30–60 min	1.5–4 hr

 Massage Considerations

- No cautions or contraindications to massage are related to the actions of this drug. No cautions or contraindications to massage are related to the client condition.
- The site of subcutaneous injections should not be massaged for at least 1 hour to avoid increasing the rate of absorption of the drug into the body.
- This drug acts to stimulate certain receptors of the sympathetic nervous system (SNS). It is fairly specific to the lungs but may potentially decrease the relaxation effects of massage and decrease the effectiveness of systemic reflex strokes such as rocking, effleurage, and friction. Using these strokes for a longer than usual time and using slow, rhythmic effleurage throughout the session may help achieve the desired results.
- Side effects of drowsiness or dizziness may be helped by stimulation with friction to the legs at the end of the session.

---

terconazole (ter-KON-uh-zohl)

Terazol 3, Terazol 7

Drug Class: Antifungal

Drug Actions

Impairs function of *Candida* fungus

Use

- Vulvovaginal candidiasis

Side Effects

Gastrointestinal: abdominal pain.
Nervous System: headache, fever.
Skin: irritation, photosensitivity reactions, itching.
Other: chills, body aches, dysmenorrhea, vulvovaginal pain or burning.

Onset, Peak, and Duration

Route	Onset	Peak	Duration
Intravaginal	Unknown	Unknown	Unknown

Massage Considerations

- No cautions or contraindications to massage are indicated because a client is taking this drug.

---

teriparatide (rDNA origin) (tehr-ih-PAHR-uh-tyd)

Forteo

Drug Class: Osteoporosis drug

Drug Actions

A synthetic parathyroid hormone that regulates calcium and phosphorus metabolism and decreases risk of fractures in patients with osteoporosis.

Use

- Osteoporosis in postmenopausal women at high risk for fracture
- To increase bone mass in men with primary or hypogonadal osteoporosis who are at high risk for fracture

Side Effects

Cardiovascular: angina pectoris, hypertension, orthostatic hypotension.
Gastrointestinal: constipation, diarrhea, painful digestion, nausea, tooth disorder, vomiting.
Nervous System: weakness, depression, dizziness, headache, insomnia, syncope, pain.
Skin: rash, sweating.
Other: pharyngitis, rhinitis, hypercalcemia, joint pain, leg cramps, neck pain, shortness of breath, cough, pneumonia.

Onset, Peak, and Duration

Route	Onset	Peak	Duration
Subcutaneous Injection	Rapid	30 min	3 hr

Massage Considerations

- No cautions or contraindications to massage are related to the actions of this drug. Cautions and contraindications to massage will be related to the client condition.
- The physician should be consulted before massage is given.
- The site of subcutaneous injection of the drug should not be massaged for at least 30 minutes after the drug is administered.
- Side effects of hypotension and dizziness require care in getting the client on and off the table. Stimulation with rapid effleurage at the end of the session may help.
- Constipation may be helped by abdominal massage.
- Rash is a local contraindication to massage and should be reported to the physician.

---

testolactone (tes-tuh-LAK-tohn)

Teslac

Drug Class: Antineoplastic

Drug Actions

Hinders breast cancer cell activity

Use

- Advanced postmenopausal breast cancer

Side Effects

Cardiovascular: increased blood pressure, edema.
Gastrointestinal: nausea, vomiting, diarrhea, anorexia, glossitis.
Nervous System: paresthesia, peripheral neuropathy.
Skin: erythema, nail changes, hair loss.

Onset, Peak, and Duration

Route	Onset	Peak	Duration
Oral	6–12 wk	Unknown	Unknown

Massage Considerations

- Because of the toxic effects of this drug, deep tissue massage and circulatory massage with effleurage should be done with caution.
- Further cautions or contraindications to massage may be related to the client condition.
- Side effects of paresthesia and neuropathy are contraindications to deep tissue massage.
- Hair loss is a contraindication to scalp massage if the client is disturbed by hair loss during the massage or if the scalp is tender.

The massage therapist always has the responsibility to work safely. This book is a guide only and does not replace the massage therapist's own assessment of each client's safety.

---

testosterone (tes-TOS-teh-rohn)

Andronaq-50, Histerone-50, Histerone 100, Testamone 100, Testaqua, Testoject-50

testosterone cypionate

Andronate 100, Andronate 200, depAndro 100, depAndro 200, Depotest, Depo-Testosterone, Duratest-100, Duratest-200, T-Cypionate, Testred Cypionate 200, Virilon IM

testosterone enanthate

Andro L.A. 200, Andropository 200, Andryl 200, Delatest, Delatestryl, Durathate-200, Everone 200, Testrin-P.A.

testosterone propionate

Malogen in Oil, Testex

Drug Class: Androgen hormone replacement, antineoplastic

Drug Actions

Stimulates target tissues to develop normally in androgen-deficient men. Drug may have some antiestrogen properties, making it useful to treat certain estrogen-dependent breast cancers.

Use

- Hypogonadism
- Delayed puberty
- Metastatic breast cancer 1 to 5 years postmenopausal
- Postpartum breast pain and engorgement

Side Effects

Cardiovascular: edema.
Gastrointestinal: nausea.
Nervous System: headache, anxiety, depression, paresthesia, sleep apnea syndrome.
Skin: local edema, hypersensitivity skin signs and symptoms.
Other: androgenic effects in women, pain and induration at injection site, hypoestrogenic effects in women (acne; edema; oily skin; hirsutism; hoarseness; weight gain; clitoral enlargement; decreased or increased libido; flushing; diaphoresis; vaginitis, including itching, drying, and burning; vaginal bleeding; menstrual irregularities), excessive hormonal effects in boys and men (prepubertal: premature epiphyseal closure, acne, priapism, growth of body and facial hair, phallic enlargement; postpubertal: testicular atrophy, oligospermia, decreased ejaculatory volume, impotence, abnormal growth of breast tissue, epididymitis), bladder irritability, polycythemia, suppression of clotting factors, reversible jaundice, cholestatic hepatitis, hypercalcemia.

Onset, Peak, and Duration

Route	Onset	Peak	Duration
I.M.	Unknown	Unknown	Unknown

 Massage Considerations

- No cautions or contraindications to massage are related to the actions of this drug. Cautions and contraindications to massage may be related to the client condition.
- The physician should be consulted before any massage is given.
- The site of intramuscular injection should not be massaged for up to 2 hours.
- Side effects of paresthesia are a contraindication to deep tissue massage.
- Acne is a local contraindication to massage. If severe and widespread, massage may be given if the massage therapist wears gloves when working the affected areas.
- Abnormal growth of breast tissue in men and women requires care in depth and pressure of chest massage. Deep tissue massage of the chest is contraindicated. If the breast is too tender, it is best to avoid the area completely.

---

testosterone transdermal system (tes-TOS-teh-rohn tranz-DER-mal SIHS-tum)

Androderm, Testoderm, Testoderm TTS

Drug Class: Androgen hormone

Drug Actions

Stimulates target tissues to develop normally in androgen-deficient men.

Use

- Primary or hypogonadotropic hypogonadism

Side Effects

Cardiovascular: stroke, headache, depression.
Gastrointestinal: GI bleeding.
Urinary: prostatitis, prostate abnormalities, urinary tract infection.
Skin: acne, itching, irritation, blister under system, allergic contact dermatitis; burning, induration (at application site).
Other: abnormal growth of breast tissue, breast tenderness.

Onset, Peak, and Duration

Route	Onset	Peak	Duration
Transdermal	Unknown	2–4 hr	2 hr after removal

Massage Considerations

- No cautions or contraindications to massage are related to the actions of this drug. Cautions and contraindications to massage may be related to the client condition.
- The physician should be consulted before any massage is given.
- The site of the transdermal patch should not be massaged for the time it is in place and 2 hours after removal.
- Side effects of acne are local contraindications to massage. If severe and widespread, massage may be given if the massage therapist wears gloves when working the affected areas.
- Itching is a local contraindication to massage.
- Abnormal growth of breast tissue in men and women and breast tenderness require care in depth and pressure of chest massage. Deep tissue massage of the chest is contraindicated. If the breast is too tender, it is best to avoid the area completely.

tetracycline hydrochloride (tet-ruh-SIGH-kleen high-droh-KLOR-ighd)

Achromycin, Apo-Tetra, Mysteclin, Novo-Tetra, Nu-Tetra, Sumycin, Tetrex, Topicycline

Drug Class: Antibiotic

Drug Actions

Inhibiting protein synthesis, thus hindering bacterial activity

Use

- Infections caused by sensitive Gram-negative and Gram-positive organisms
- Uncomplicated urethral, endocervical, or rectal infection
- Brucellosis
- Gonorrhea in patients sensitive to penicillin
- Syphilis in nonpregnant patients sensitive to penicillin
- Acne
- Lyme disease
- Adjunct therapy for acute transmitted epididymitis (children older than age 8)
- Pelvic inflammatory disease
- Infection with *Helicobacter pylori*

Side Effects

Cardiovascular: pericarditis.
Gastrointestinal: anorexia, epigastric distress, nausea, vomiting, diarrhea, esophagitis, oral candidiasis, stomatitis, enterocolitis, inflammatory lesions in anogenital region.
Nervous System: dizziness, headache, intracranial hypertension (pseudotumor cerebri).
Skin: candidal superinfection, rash, hives, photosensitivity reactions, increased pigmentation.
Other: permanent discoloration of teeth, enamel defects, hypersensitivity reactions, sore throat, glossitis, difficulty swallowing, neutropenia, thrombocytopenia, eosinophilia, retardation of bone growth if used in children younger than age 9.

Onset, Peak, and Duration

Route	Onset	Peak	Duration
Oral	Unknown	2–4 hr	Unknown

Massage Considerations

- No cautions or contraindications to massage are related to the actions of this drug. Cautions and contraindications to massage may be related to the client condition and severity of infection.
- Side effects of dizziness require care in getting the client on and off the table.
- Stimulation with effleurage or tapotement at the end of the session may help.
- Rash and hives are local contraindications to massage and should be reported to the physician immediately. If severe or widespread, massage should be withheld.

theophylline (thee-OF-ih-lin)

Immediate-release liquids

Accurbron, Aquaphyllin, Asmalix, Bronkodyl, Elixomin, Elixophyllin, Lanophyllin, Slo-Phyllin, Theolair

Immediate-release tablets and capsules

Bronkodyl, Elixophyllin, Nuelin, Slo-Phyllin

Timed-release capsules

Elixophyllin SR, Nuelin-SR, Slo-bid Gyrocaps, Slo-Phyllin, Theo-24, Theobid Duracaps, Theochron, Theospan-SR, Theovent Long-Acting

Timed-release tablets

Quibron-T/SR Dividose, Respbid, Sustaire, T-Phyl, Theochron, Theolair-SR, Theo-Sav, Theo-Time, Theo-X, Uniphyl

theophylline sodium glycinate

Drug Class: Bronchodilator

Drug Actions

Relaxes smooth muscle of bronchial airways and pulmonary blood vessels, improving breathing ability.

Use

- Oral theophylline for acute bronchospasm in patients not already receiving theophylline
- Parenteral theophylline for patients not receiving theophylline
- Oral and parenteral theophylline for acute bronchospasm in patients receiving theophylline
- Chronic bronchospasm
- Cystic fibrosis
- Promotion of diuresis
- Cheyne-Stokes respirations
- Paroxysmal nocturnal dyspnea

Side Effects

Cardiovascular: palpitations, sinus tachycardia, extrasystoles, flushing, marked hypotension, arrhythmias.

Gastrointestinal: nausea, vomiting, diarrhea, epigastric pain.
Nervous System: restlessness, dizziness, headache, insomnia, irritability, seizures, muscle twitching.
Other: increased respiratory rate, respiratory arrest.

Onset, Peak, and Duration

Route	Onset	Peak	Duration
Oral			
Regular	15–60 min	1–2 hr	Unknown
Enteric-coated	15–60 min	1–2 hr	5 hr
Extended-release	15–60 min	1–2 hr	4–7 hr
I.V.	15 min	15–30 min	Unknown

Massage Considerations

- No cautions or contraindications to massage are related to the actions of this drug. Cautions and contraindications to massage may be related to the client condition.
- The stimulant side effects of this drug may decrease the relaxation effects of massage in general and may make the systemic reflex strokes of rocking, effleurage, and friction less effective. Using these strokes for longer than usual and using slow, rhythmic effleurage throughout the session may help achieve the desired effects.
- Side effects of dizziness or hypotension require care in getting the client on and off the table. Stimulation with gentle friction to the legs at the end of the session may help.

thioguanine (6-thioguanine, 6-TG) (thigh-oh-GWAH-neen)

Lanvis, Tabloid

Drug Class: Antineoplastic

Drug Actions

Inhibits selected leukemic cell reproduction

Use

- Acute nonlymphocytic leukemia
- Chronic myelogenous leukemia

Side Effects

Gastrointestinal: nausea, vomiting, stomatitis, diarrhea, anorexia.
Other: abnormal blood profiles, hepatotoxicity, jaundice, hepatic fibrosis, toxic hepatitis, hyperuricemia.

Onset, Peak, and Duration

Route	Onset	Peak	Duration
Oral	Unknown	Unknown	Unknown

Massage Considerations

- Because of the toxic effects of this drug, deep tissue massage should be used with caution.
- Further cautions and contraindications to massage may be related to the client condition.
- The physician should be consulted before any massage is given, and close collaboration is essential.

thioridazine hydrochloride (thigh-oh-RIGH-duh-zeen high-droh-KLOR-ighd)

Aldazine, Apo-Thioridazine, Mellaril, Mellaril Concentrate, Novo-Ridazine, PMS Thioridazine

Drug Class: Antipsychotic

Drug Actions

Unknown; probably blocks postsynaptic dopamine receptors in brain and relieves signs of psychosis, depression, anxiety, stress, fears, and sleep disturbances.

Use

- Schizophrenia in patients who have failed at least two trials with different antipsychotics
- Short-term treatment of moderate to marked depression with varying degrees of anxiety
- Dementia in geriatric patients
- Behavioral problems in children

Side Effects

Cardiovascular: orthostatic hypotension, tachycardia, electrocardiogram (ECG) changes.
Gastrointestinal: dry mouth, constipation.
Nervous System: extrapyramidal reactions, tardive dyskinesia, sedation, electroencephalogram (EEG) changes, dizziness, neuroleptic malignant syndrome.
Urinary: urine retention, dark urine, menstrual irregularities, inhibited ejaculation.
Skin: mild photosensitivity reactions.
Other: abnormal growth of breast tissue, allergic reaction, ocular changes, blurred vision, retinitis pigmentosa, abnormal blood profiles, cholestatic jaundice, weight gain, increased appetite.

Onset, Peak, and Duration

Route	Onset	Peak	Duration
Oral	Varies	Unknown	Unknown

Massage Considerations

- This drug has sedating effect on the CNS; therefore, deep tissue massage should be used with great caution.
- Further cautions or contraindications to massage may be related to the client condition.
- The physician should be consulted before any massage is given.
- Side effects of hypotension and dizziness require care in getting the client on and off the table. Stimulation with effleurage or tapotement at the end of the session may help. If the symptom is severe, using more stimulating massage techniques throughout the session may be needed.
- Constipation may be helped by abdominal massage.
- Abnormal growth of breast tissue in men or women requires care in depth and pressure of chest massage. No deep tissue massage should be done in the area. If too tender, the chest should not be massaged.

thiotepa (thigh-oh-TEE-puh)

Thioplex

Drug Class: Antineoplastic

Drug Actions

Kills certain cancer cells

Use

- Breast and ovarian cancers
- Lymphoma
- Hodgkin's disease
- Bladder tumor
- Neoplastic effusions
- Malignant meningeal neoplasm

Side Effects

Gastrointestinal: nausea, vomiting, abdominal pain, anorexia, stomatitis.
Nervous System: headache, dizziness, fatigue, weakness, fever.
Urinary: amenorrhea, decreased spermatogenesis, painful urination, urine retention, hemorrhagic cystitis.
Skin: hives, rash, dermatitis, hair loss.
Other: hypersensitivity reactions, pain at injection site, anaphylaxis, blurred vision, laryngeal edema, conjunctivitis, abnormal blood profiles, asthma.

Onset, Peak, and Duration

Route	Onset	Peak	Duration
I.V., bladder instillation, intracavitary	Unknown	Unknown	Unknown

Massage Considerations

- Because of the toxic effects of this drug, deep tissue massage is contraindicated, and circulatory massage with effleurage should be used with caution and limited in systemic administration. Deep tissue massage should be used with caution in instillation and intercavitary use.
- Further cautions and contraindications to massage may be related to the client condition.
- The physician should be consulted before any massage is given, and close collaboration is essential.
- The drug is usually given every 1 to 4 weeks and has a short half-life. It is best to give massage on days when the drug is not being administered.
- Side effects of dizziness require care in getting the client on and off the table. Stimulation with tapotement and gentle friction to the legs at the end of the session may help.
- Rash, hives, or dermatitis are local contraindications to massage and should be reported to the physician. If severe or widespread, massage should be withheld.
- Hair loss is a contraindication to scalp massage if the client is disturbed by hair loss during the session or if the scalp is tender.
- The best approach to massage for this client is to use systemic and local reflex strokes of rocking, gentle friction, stretching, traction, gentle compression, and vibration. Pétrissage and myofascial massage techniques may also be used.

thiothixene (thigh-oh-THIKS-een)

Navane

thiothixene hydrochloride

Navane

Drug Class: Antipsychotic

Drug Actions

Unknown; probably blocks postsynaptic dopamine receptors in brain, relieves signs and symptoms of psychosis.

Use

- Mild to moderate psychosis
- Severe psychosis

Side Effects

Cardiovascular: orthostatic hypotension, tachycardia, ECG changes.
Gastrointestinal: dry mouth, constipation.
Nervous System: extrapyramidal reactions, tardive dyskinesia, sedation, pseudoparkinsonism, EEG changes, dizziness, restlessness, agitation, insomnia, neuroleptic malignant syndrome.
Urinary: urine retention, menstrual irregularities, inhibited ejaculation.
Skin: mild photosensitivity reactions.
Other: pain and sterile abscesses at intramuscular injection site, abnormal growth of breast tissue, allergic reaction, abnormal blood profiles, ocular changes, blurred vision, nasal congestion, jaundice, weight gain.

Onset, Peak, and Duration

Route	Onset	Peak	Duration
Oral, I.M.	Several wk	Unknown	Unknown

 Massage Considerations

- This drug has sedating effects on the CNS; therefore, deep tissue massage should be used with great caution.
- In many cases, further cautions and contraindications to massage will be related to the client condition.
- The physician should be consulted before any massage is given.
- The site of intramuscular injection should not be massaged for at least 2 hours.
- Side effects of hypotension and dizziness require care in getting the client on and off the table. Stimulation with effleurage at the end of the session may help. If the symptom is severe, more stimulating massage techniques throughout the session may be needed.
- Constipation may be helped by abdominal massage.

---

thyroid (THIGH-royd)

Armour Thyroid, Thyroid USP

Drug Class: Thyroid hormone

Drug Actions

Not clearly defined; stimulates metabolism of body tissues by accelerating cellular oxidation, and raises thyroid hormone level in body.

Use

- Hypothyroidism
- Congenital hypothyroidism

Side Effects

Cardiovascular: tachycardia, arrhythmias, angina pectoris, increased blood pressure, cardiac decompensation and collapse.
Gastrointestinal: diarrhea, vomiting.
Nervous System: nervousness, insomnia, tremor, headache.
Skin: sweating.
Other: allergic reactions, menstrual irregularities, weight loss, heat intolerance, accelerated rate of bone maturation in infants and children.

Onset, Peak, and Duration

Route	Onset	Peak	Duration
Oral	Unknown	Unknown	Unknown

 Massage Considerations

- No cautions or contraindications to massage are related to the actions of this drug.
- Cautions and contraindications to massage may be related to the client condition.

tiagabine hydrochloride (tigh-AG-ah-been high-droh-KLOR-ighd)

Gabitril

Drug Class: Anticonvulsant

Drug Actions

May enhance activity of GABA. Prevents partial seizures

Use

- Adjunctive therapy in partial seizures

Side Effects

Cardiovascular: vasodilation.
Gastrointestinal: abdominal pain, nausea, diarrhea, vomiting, increased appetite, mouth ulcerations.
Nervous System: generalized weakness, dizziness, sleepiness, weakness, nervousness, tremor, difficulty with concentration and attention, insomnia, ataxia, confusion, speech disorder, difficulty with memory, paresthesia, depression, emotional lability, abnormal gait, hostility, language problems, agitation, pain.
Skin: rash, itching.
Other: nystagmus, pharyngitis, myasthenia, increased cough.

Onset, Peak, and Duration

Route	Onset	Peak	Duration
Oral	Rapid	45 min	7–9 hr

Side Effects

Chemical effect: Unknown; may enhance the activity of γ-aminobutyric acid (GABA), the major inhibitory neurotransmitter in the CNS. It binds to recognition sites related to the GABA uptake carrier and may thus permit more GABA to be available for binding to receptors on postsynaptic cells.
Therapeutic effect: Prevents partial seizures.

Massage Considerations

- This drug has a sedating effect on the CNS; therefore, deep tissue massage should be used with caution.
- Further cautions and contraindications to massage may be related to the client condition.
- The action of this drug may potentially increase the relaxation effects of massage and increase the effect of the systemic reflex strokes of rocking, effleurage, and friction. Using these strokes in a more rapid and stimulating manner may help. The effects of the local reflex strokes of stretching, traction, compression, vibration, and of deep tissue massage may be decreased. Using these strokes for a longer time than usual may achieve the desired effects. Using more of the mechanical strokes of effleurage and pétrissage may also be effective.
- Side effects of dizziness and sleepiness may be addressed as noted above.
- Paresthesia is a local contraindication to deep tissue massage.
- Rash and itching are local contraindications to massage and should be reported to the physician.

---

ticarcillin disodium (tigh-kar-SIL-in digh-SOH-dee-um)

Ticar, Ticillin

Drug Class: Antibiotic

Drug Actions

Inhibits cell wall synthesis, killing bacteria.

Use

- Severe systemic infections caused by susceptible strains of Gram-positive and especially Gram-negative organisms
- Uncomplicated urinary tract infection

Side Effects

Cardiovascular: vein irritation, phlebitis.
Gastrointestinal: nausea, diarrhea, vomiting.
Nervous System: seizures, neuromuscular excitability.
Other: hypersensitivity reactions (rash, itching, hives, chills, fever, edema, anaphylaxis), overgrowth of nonsusceptible organisms, pain at injection site, abnormal blood profiles, hypokalemia.

Onset, Peak, and Duration

Route	Onset	Peak	Duration
I.V.	Immediate	Immediate	Unknown
I.M.	Unknown	30–75 min	Unknown

Massage Considerations

- No cautions or contraindications to massage are related to the actions of this drug. Cautions and contraindications to massage may be related to the client condition and severity of infection.
- The site of intramuscular injection of the drug should not be massaged for at least 1.5 hours.

ticarcillin disodium and clavulanate potassium (tigh-kar-SIL-in digh-SOH-dee-um and KLAV-yoo-lan-nayt poh-TAH-see-um)

Timentin

Drug Class: Antibiotic

Drug Actions

Inhibits cell wall synthesis during microorganism replication, killing susceptible bacteria.

Use

- Systemic and urinary tract infections
- Moderate gynecologic infections
- Severe gynecologic infections

Side Effects

Cardiovascular: vein irritation, phlebitis.
Gastrointestinal: nausea, diarrhea, stomatitis, vomiting, epigastric pain, gas, pseudomembranous colitis, taste and smell disturbances.
Nervous System: seizures, neuromuscular excitability, headache, giddiness.
Other: hypersensitivity reactions (rash, itching, hives, chills, fever, edema, anaphylaxis), overgrowth of nonsusceptible organisms, pain at injection site, abnormal blood profiles, hypokalemia.

Onset, Peak, and Duration

Route	Onset	Peak	Duration
I.V.	Immediate	Immediate	Unknown

Massage Considerations

- No cautions or contraindications to massage are related to the actions of this drug. Cautions and contraindications to massage may be related to the client condition and severity of infection.
- Side effects of gas may be helped by abdominal massage.

ticlopidine hydrochloride (tigh-KLOH-peh-deen high-droh-KLOR-ighd)

Ticlid

Drug Class: Antithrombotic/anticoagulation drug

Drug Actions

Unknown; may block adenosine diphosphate–induced platelet-fibrinogen and platelet-platelet binding, prevents blood clots from forming.

Use

- To reduce risk of thrombotic stroke in patients with history of stroke or who have experienced stroke precursors

Side Effects

Cardiovascular: vasculitis.

Gastrointestinal: diarrhea, nausea, painful digestion, vomiting, gas, anorexia, abdominal pain, bleeding.
Nervous System: dizziness, intracerebral bleeding.
Urinary: hematuria, nephrotic syndrome, dark-colored urine.
Skin: rash, itching, hives, bruising.
Other: hypersensitivity reactions, postoperative bleeding, systemic lupus erythematosus, serum sickness, nosebleeds, conjunctival hemorrhage, abnormal blood profiles, hepatitis, cholestatic jaundice, hyponatremia, arthropathy, myositis, allergic pneumonitis.

Onset, Peak, and Duration

Route	Onset	Peak	Duration
Oral	Unknown	2 hr	Unknown

 Massage Considerations

- Because of the effects of this drug on blood clotting, deep tissue massage is contraindicated, and circulatory massage with effleurage should be used with caution and limited.
- Further cautions and contraindications to massage may be related to the client condition.
- The physician should be consulted before any massage is given.
- Side effects of dizziness may be helped by stimulation with friction to the legs at the end of the session.
- Gas may be helped by abdominal massage.
- Rash, hives, and itching are local contraindications to massage and should be reported to the physician.
- Bruising requires care in depth and pressure of massage.

---

timolol maleate (TIH-moh-lol MAL-ee-ayt)

Apo-Timol, Blocadren

Drug Class: Beta-blocker

Drug Actions

In heart attack, drug may decrease myocardial oxygen requirements. It also prevents arterial dilation through beta blockade for migraine headache prevention and lower blood pressure.

Use

- Hypertension
- Heart attack (long-term prophylaxis in patients who have survived acute phase)
- Prevention of migraine headache
- Angina

Side Effects

Cardiovascular: bradycardia, hypotension, peripheral vascular disease, arrhythmias, heart failure.
Gastrointestinal: nausea, vomiting, diarrhea.
Nervous System: fatigue, lethargy, dizziness.
Skin: itching.
Other: shortness of breath, bronchospasm, increased airway resistance.

Onset, Peak, and Duration

Route	Onset	Peak	Duration
Oral	15–30 min	1–2 hr	6–12 hr

 Massage Considerations

- No cautions or contraindications to massage are related to the actions of this drug. Cautions and contraindications to massage may be related to the client condition.
- Side effects of dizziness and hypotension may be helped by stimulation with effleurage and tapotement at the end of the session.
- Itching is a local contraindication to massage and should be reported to the physician. If severe or widespread, massage should be withheld.

---

tinzaparin sodium (TIN-zuh-pear-in SOE-dee-um)

Innohep

Drug Class: Anticoagulant

Drug Actions

Reduces the ability of the blood to clot

Use

- Adjunct treatment (with warfarin sodium) of symptomatic deep vein thrombosis with or without pulmonary embolism

Side Effects

Cardiovascular: arrhythmias, chest pain, hypotension, hypertension, heart attack, thromboembolism, tachycardia, dependent edema, angina pectoris.
Gastrointestinal: anorectal bleeding, constipation, gas, hematemesis, hemarthrosis, GI hemorrhage, melena, nausea, vomiting, painful digestion, retroperitoneal or intra-abdominal bleeding.
Nervous System: headache, fever, dizziness, insomnia, confusion, cerebral or intracranial bleeding, pain.
Urinary: painful urination, hematuria, urinary tract infection, urine retention, vaginal hemorrhage.
Skin: bullous eruption, cellulitis, injection site hematoma, itching, purpura, rash, skin necrosis, wound hematoma.
Other: hypersensitivity reactions, spinal or epidural hematoma, infection, impaired healing, allergic reaction, congenital anomaly, fetal death, fetal distress, nosebleed, ocular hemorrhage, abnormal blood profiles, hemorrhage, back pain, pneumonia, respiratory disorder, pulmonary embolism, shortness of breath.

Onset, Peak, and Duration

Route	Onset	Peak	Duration
Subcutaneous Injection	2–3 hr	4–5 hr	Unknown

 Massage Considerations

- This drug is given in the presence of blood clots and embolism in the body. Massage is completely contraindicated.

---

tirofiban hydrochloride (ty-roh-FYE-ban high-droh-KLOR-ighd)

Aggrastat

Drug Class: Platelet aggregation inhibitor

Drug Actions

Inhibits platelet aggregation and prevents blood clot formation

Use

- Acute coronary syndrome, with heparin, aspirin, or both, including patients who are to be managed medically and those undergoing percutaneous transluminal coronary angioplasty or atherectomy

Side Effects

Cardiovascular: bradycardia, coronary artery dissection, edema, vasovagal reaction.
Gastrointestinal: nausea, occult bleeding.
Nervous System: fever, dizziness, headache.
Skin: sweating.
Other: major bleeding at arterial access site, minor bleeding, thrombocytopenia, pelvic pain, leg pain.

Onset, Peak, and Duration

Route	Onset	Peak	Duration
I.V.	Immediate	Immediate	4–8 hr after end of infusion

 **Massage Considerations**

- Massage is completely contraindicated for the client taking this drug.

---

tobramycin sulfate (toh-breh-MIGH-sin SUL-fayt)

Nebcin

Drug Class: Antibiotic

Drug Actions

Kills susceptible bacteria

Use

- Serious infections caused by sensitive strains of bacteria

Side Effects

Gastrointestinal: nausea, vomiting, diarrhea.
Nervous System: headache, lethargy, confusion, disorientation.
Urinary: nephrotoxicity.
Other: hypersensitivity reactions (anaphylaxis), ototoxicity, abnormal blood profiles.

Onset, Peak, and Duration

Route	Onset	Peak	Duration
I.V.	Immediate	Immediate	8 hr
I.M.	Unknown	30–90 min	8 hr

 **Massage Considerations**

- No cautions or contraindications to massage are related to the actions of this drug. Cautions and contraindications to massage may be related to the client condition or severity of infection.

- The site of intramuscular injection of the drug should not be massaged for at least 1.5 hours after the drug is administered.

tolcapone (TOHL-cah-pohn)

Tasmar

Drug Class: Antiparkinson drug

Drug Actions

Increases availability of levodopa and improves physical mobility in patients with parkinsonism.

Use

- Adjunct to levodopa and carbidopa for signs and symptoms of idiopathic Parkinson's disease

Side Effects

Cardiovascular: orthostatic complaints, chest pain, chest discomfort, palpitations, hypotension.
Gastrointestinal: nausea, anorexia, diarrhea, gas, vomiting, constipation, abdominal pain, painful digestion, dry mouth.
Nervous System: dyskinesia, sleep disorder, dystonia, excessive dreaming, sleepiness, dizziness, confusion, headache, hallucinations, hyperkinesia, hypertonia, fatigue, falling, syncope, balance loss, depression, tremor, speech disorder, paresthesia, agitation, irritability, mental deficiency, hyperactivity, hypokinesia, fever.
Urinary: urinary tract infections, urine discoloration, hematuria, micturition disorder, urinary incontinence, impotence.
Skin: increased sweating, rash.
Other: burning, influenza, pharyngitis, ringing in the ears, sinus congestion, bleeding, muscle cramps, stiffness, arthritis, neck pain, bronchitis, shortness of breath, upper respiratory tract infection.

Onset, Peak, and Duration

Route	Onset	Peak	Duration
Oral	Unknown	2 hr	Unknown

Massage Considerations

- No cautions or contraindications to massage are related to the actions of this drug. Cautions and contraindications to massage may be related to the client condition.
- Side effects of hypotension, sleepiness, and dizziness require care in getting the client on and off the table. Stimulation with effleurage or tapotement at the end of the session may help.
- Paresthesia is a contraindication to deep tissue massage.
- Constipation and gas may be helped by abdominal massage.
- Rash is a local contraindication to massage and should be reported to the physician.

tolterodine tartrate (tohl-TER-oh-deen TAR-trate)

Detrol, Detrol LA

Drug Class: Anticholinergic

Drug Actions

Both urinary bladder contraction and salivation are blocked, relieving symptoms of overactive bladder.

Use

- Overactive bladder in patients with symptoms of urinary frequency, urgency, or urge incontinence

Side Effects

Cardiovascular: hypertension, chest pain.
Gastrointestinal: dry mouth, abdominal pain, constipation, diarrhea, painful digestion, gas, nausea, vomiting.
Nervous System: fatigue, paresthesia, dizziness, headache, nervousness, sleepiness.
Urinary: painful urination, urinary frequency, urine retention, urinary tract infection.
Skin: itching, rash, erythema, dry skin.
Other: flulike syndrome, falls, fungal infection, infection, abnormal vision, xerophthalmia, pharyngitis, rhinitis, sinusitis, weight gain, joint pain, back pain, bronchitis, cough, upper respiratory tract infection.

Onset, Peak, and Duration

Route	Onset	Peak	Duration
Oral	Unknown	1–2 hr	Unknown

 Massage Considerations

- No cautions or contraindications to massage are indicated because a client is taking this drug.
- Side effects of dizziness and sleepiness require care in getting the client on and off the table. Stimulation with effleurage and tapotement at the end of the session may help.
- Constipation and gas may be helped by abdominal massage.
- Urinary frequency may require that the client get up in the middle of the session. Privacy and quick access to the bathroom should be provided. Water fountains and water music, which may stimulate urination, should be avoided.
- Itching and rash are local contraindications to massage and should be reported to the physician.

---

topiramate (toh-PEER-uh-mayt)

Topamax

Drug Class: Antiepileptic

Drug Actions

Blocks CNS activity and prevents partial-onset seizures

Use

- Partial-onset seizures
- Primary generalized tonic-clonic seizures
- Adjunctive therapy for partial seizures
- Primary generalized tonic-clonic seizures
- Lennox-Gastaut syndrome

Side Effects

Cardiovascular: chest pain, palpitations, edema, hot flushes.

Gastrointestinal: taste perversion, abdominal pain, anorexia, constipation, diarrhea, dry mouth, painful digestion, gas, gastroenteritis, gingivitis, nausea, vomiting.
Nervous System: fever; fatigue; abnormal coordination; aggression; agitation; apathy; asthenia; ataxia; confusion; depression; depersonalization; dizziness; emotional lability; euphoria; generalized tonic-clonic seizures; hallucinations; hyperkinesia; hypertonia; hypesthesia; hypokinesia; insomnia; nervousness; nystagmus; paresthesia; personality disorder; psychomotor slowing; psychosis; sleepiness; speech disorders; stupor; suicide attempts; tremor; malaise; mood problems; difficulty with concentration, attention, language, or memory.
Urinary: amenorrhea, dysuria, dysmenorrhea, hematuria, impotence, intermenstrual bleeding, menstrual disorder, menorrhagia, urinary frequency, renal calculi, urinary incontinence, urinary tract infections, vaginitis, leukorrhea.
Skin: acne, hair loss, increased sweating, itching, rash.
Other: body odor, flulike syndrome, breast pain, decreased libido, abnormal vision, conjunctivitis, double vision, eye pain, hearing problems, pharyngitis, sinusitis, ringing in the ears, anemia, nosebleeds, leukopenia, weight changes, joint pain, back or leg pain, muscular weakness, myalgia, rigors, bronchitis, cough, shortness of breath, upper respiratory tract infection.

Onset, Peak, and Duration

Route	Onset	Peak	Duration
Oral	Unknown	2 hr	Unknown

Massage Considerations

- This drug has sedating effects on the CNS; therefore, deep tissue massage should be used with caution.
- Further cautions and contraindications to massage may be related to the client condition.
- Side effects of dizziness and sleepiness require care in getting the client on and off the table. Stimulation with effleurage and tapotement at the end of the session may help.
- Hypesthesia and paresthesia are local contraindications to deep tissue massage and, if severe, may contraindicate massage completely.
- Constipation and gas may be helped by abdominal massage.
- Urinary frequency requires that privacy and quick access to the bathroom be provided when needed. Water fountains and water music, which may stimulate urination, should be avoided.
- Itching, rash, and acne are local contraindications to massage and should be reported to the physician.
- Hair loss is a contraindication to scalp massage if the client is disturbed by hair loss during the session or if the scalp is tender.

---

topotecan hydrochloride (toh-poh-TEE-ken high-droh-KLOR-ighd)

Hycamtin

Drug Class: Antineoplastic

Drug Actions

Kills certain cancer cells

Use

- Metastatic carcinoma of ovary after failure of initial or subsequent chemotherapy
- Small cell lung cancer after failure of first-line chemotherapy

Side Effects

Gastrointestinal: nausea, vomiting, diarrhea, constipation, abdominal pain, stomatitis, anorexia.
Nervous System: fever, fatigue, weakness, headache, paresthesia.
Skin: hair loss.
Other: sepsis, shortness of breath.

Onset, Peak, and Duration

Route	Onset	Peak	Duration
I.V.	Unknown	Unknown	Unknown

Massage Considerations

- Because of the toxic effects of this drug, deep tissue massage is contraindicated, and circulatory massage with effleurage should be used with caution and limited.
- Further cautions and contraindications to massage may be related to the client condition.
- The physician should be consulted before any massage is given, and close collaboration is essential.
- The drug is usually given for 5 consecutive days every few weeks. It would be best to give massage on the days when the drug is not being given.
- Side effects of paresthesia require care in depth and pressure of massage and contraindicate deep tissue massage.
- Constipation may be helped by abdominal massage.
- Hair loss is a contraindication to scalp massage if the client is disturbed by hair loss during the session or if the scalp is tender.

---

torsemide (TOR-seh-mighd)

Demadex

Drug Class: Diuretic, antihypertensive

Drug Actions

Enhances excretion of sodium, chloride, and water and thus lowers blood pressure.

Use

- Diuresis in patients with heart failure
- Diuresis in patients with chronic renal impairment
- Diuresis in patients with hepatic cirrhosis
- Hypertension

Side Effects

Cardiovascular: ECG abnormalities, chest pain, edema, orthostatic hypotension.
Gastrointestinal: diarrhea, constipation, nausea, painful digestion, hemorrhage.
Nervous System: weakness, dizziness, headache, nervousness, insomnia, syncope.
Urinary: excessive urination, impotence.
Other: excessive thirst; gout; rhinitis; sore throat; dehydration; electrolyte imbalances, including hypokalemia, hypomagnesemia, hypocalcemia, hyperuricemia, hyperglycemia; hypochloremic alkalosis, joint pain, muscle pain, cough.

Onset, Peak, and Duration

Route	Onset	Peak	Duration
Oral	1 hr	1–2 hr	6–8 hr
I.V.	≤10 min	≤1 hr	6–8 hr

 Massage Considerations

- No cautions or contraindications to massage are related to the actions of this drug. Cautions and contraindications to massage may be related to the client condition.
- Side effects of dizziness and hypotension require care in getting the client on and off the table. Stimulation with effleurage and tapotement at the end of the session may help.
- Constipation may be helped by abdominal massage.

tramadol hydrochloride (TRAM-uh-dohl high-droh-KLOR-ighd)

Ultram

Drug Class: Synthetic analgesic

Drug Actions

Binds to opioid receptors and relieves pain

Use

- Moderate to moderately severe pain

Side Effects

Cardiovascular: vasodilation.
Gastrointestinal: nausea, constipation, vomiting, painful digestion, dry mouth, diarrhea, abdominal pain, anorexia, gas.
Nervous System: dizziness, headache, sleepiness, CNS stimulation, weakness, anxiety, confusion, coordination disturbance, malaise, euphoria, nervousness, sleep disorder, seizures.
Urinary: urine retention, urinary frequency, menopausal symptoms.
Skin: sweating, rash, itching.
Other: visual disturbances, hypertonia.
Respiratory: respiratory depression.

Onset, Peak, and Duration

Route	Onset	Peak	Duration
Oral	Unknown	2 hr	Unknown

 Massage Considerations

- This drug decreases the perception of pain; therefore, deep tissue massage is contraindicated.
- Further cautions and contraindications to massage may be related to the client condition.
- The sedating effects of this drug on the CNS may potentially decrease the effectiveness of the local reflex strokes of compression, vibration, stretching, and traction. Using these strokes for a longer than usual time may help achieve the desired effect, or using the mechanical strokes of effleurage and pétrissage more may be effective. The drug may also increase the relaxation effects of massage and the effects of the systemic reflex strokes of effleurage, friction, and rocking. Using these strokes in a more rapid and stimulating manner may balance this effect.

- Side effects of dizziness and sleepiness may be addressed as noted above.
- Constipation and gas may be helped by abdominal massage.
- Urinary frequency requires privacy and quick access to the bathroom for the client when needed. Water fountains and water music, which may stimulate urination, should be avoided.
- Rash and itching are local contraindications to massage and should be reported to the physician.

---

trandolapril (tran-DOH-luh-pril)

Mavik

Drug Class: Angiotensin-converting enzyme (ACE) inhibitor

Drug Actions

Inhibits circulating and tissue ACE activity, which decreases vasoconstriction and lowers blood pressure.

Use

- Hypertension
- Heart failure or left ventricular dysfunction after acute heart attack

Side Effects

Cardiovascular: chest pain, first-degree atrioventricular block, bradycardia, edema, flushing, hypotension, palpitations.
Gastrointestinal: diarrhea, painful digestion, abdominal distension, abdominal pain or cramps, constipation, vomiting, pancreatitis.
Nervous System: dizziness, headache, fatigue, drowsiness, insomnia, paresthesia, anxiety.
Urinary: urinary frequency, impotence.
Skin: rash, itching, pemphigus.
Other: anaphylaxis; angioedema; decreased libido; nosebleeds; throat irritation; neutropenia; leukopenia; hyperkalemia; hyponatremia; dry, persistent, tickling, nonproductive cough; shortness of breath; upper respiratory tract infection.

Onset, Peak, and Duration

Route	Onset	Peak	Duration
Oral			
Drug	Unknown	1 hr	Unknown
Metabolite	4–10 hr	1 hr	Unknown

Massage Considerations

- No cautions or contraindications to massage are related to the actions of this drug. Cautions and contraindications to massage may be related to the client condition.
- Side effects of hypotension, dizziness, and drowsiness require care in getting the client on and off the table. Stimulation with effleurage and tapotement at the end of the session may help.
- Paresthesia is a contraindication to deep tissue massage in the area affected.
- Constipation may be helped by abdominal massage.
- Urinary frequency may require the client to go to the bathroom in the middle of the session. Privacy and quick access to the bathroom are needed. Water fountains and water music, which may stimulate urination, should be avoided.
- Rash and itching are local contraindications to massage and should be reported to the physician.

tranylcypromine sulfate (tran-il-SIGH-proh-meen SUL-fayt)

Parnate

Drug Class: Monoamine oxidase (MAO) inhibitor antidepressant

Drug Actions

Promotes accumulation of neurotransmitters by inhibiting MAO and relieves depression.

Use

- Depression

Side Effects

Cardiovascular: orthostatic hypotension, tachycardia, paradoxical hypertension, palpitations, edema.
Gastrointestinal: dry mouth, anorexia, nausea, diarrhea, constipation, abdominal pain.
Nervous System: dizziness, headache, anxiety, agitation, drowsiness, weakness, numbness, paresthesia, tremor, jitters, confusion.
Urinary: impotence, urine retention, impaired ejaculation.
Skin: rash.
Other: SIADH (syndrome of inappropriate antidiuretic hormone), chills, abnormal blood profiles, blurred vision, ringing in the ears, hepatitis, muscle spasm, myoclonic jerks.

Onset, Peak, and Duration

Route	Onset	Peak	Duration
Oral	Unknown	1–3.5 hr	10 days after therapy stops

 Massage Considerations

- This drug may cause sedating effects on the CNS. Deep tissue massage should be used with caution.
- Further cautions and contraindications to massage may be related to the client condition.
- Side effects of hypotension, dizziness, and drowsiness require care in getting the client on and off the table. Stimulation with effleurage and tapotement at the end of the session may help. If the symptoms are severe, using a more stimulating and rapid application of massage throughout the session may be needed.
- Paresthesia is a local contraindication to deep tissue massage.
- Constipation may be helped by abdominal massage.
- Rash is a local contraindication to massage and should be reported to the physician.

trastuzumab (trahs-TOO-zuh-mab)

Herceptin

Drug Class: Monoclonal antibody antineoplastic

Drug Actions

Inhibits the proliferation of human tumor cells

Use

- Metastatic breast cancer

Side Effects

Cardiovascular: tachycardia, heart failure, peripheral edema, edema, left ventricular dysfunction.
Gastrointestinal: nausea, diarrhea, vomiting, anorexia, abdominal pain.
Nervous System: pain, fever, headache, weakness, insomnia, dizziness, paresthesia, depression, peripheral neuritis, neuropathy.
Urinary: urinary tract infections.
Skin: rash, acne.
Other: chills, infection, flulike syndrome, allergic reaction, herpes simplex, hypersensitivity reactions (including anaphylaxis), rhinitis, pharyngitis, sinusitis, anemia, leukopenia, bone pain, joint pain, back pain, cough, shortness of breath.

Onset, Peak, and Duration

Route	Onset	Peak	Duration
I.V.	Unknown	Unknown	Unknown

Massage Considerations

- Because of the toxic effects of this drug, deep tissue massage should be used with caution.
- Further cautions and contraindications to massage may be related to the client condition.
- This drug is usually given weekly and has a long half-life (up to 32 days). Massage is best given on the days that the drug is not being administered.
- Side effects of dizziness may be helped by stimulation with effleurage and tapotement at the end of the session.
- Paresthesia, neuritis, or neuropathy are local contraindications to deep tissue massage. If severe, they may contraindicate massage completely.
- Rash and acne are local contraindications to massage and should be reported to the physician immediately. If severe or widespread, massage should be withheld.

---

travoprost (TRA-voe-prost)

Travatan

Drug Class: Antiglaucoma drug, ocular antihypertensive

Drug Actions

Reduces introcular pressure

Use

- Reduction of elevated intraocular pressure in patients with open-angle glaucoma or ocular hypertension

Side Effects

Cardiovascular: angina pectoris, bradycardia, chest pain, hypertension, hypotension.
Gastrointestinal: painful digestion, GI disorder.
Nervous System: anxiety, depression, headache, pain.
Urinary: prostate disorder, urinary incontinence, urinary tract infections.
Other: accidental injury, cold syndrome, infection, ocular hyperemia, decreased visual acuity, eye discomfort, foreign body sensation, eye pain, eye itching, conjunctival hyperemia, abnormal vision, blepharitis, blurred vision, cataracts, conjunctivitis, dry eyes, eye disorders, iris discoloration, keratitis, lid margin crusting, photophobia, subconjunctival hemorrhage, tearing, sinusitis, hypercholesterolemia, arthritis, back pain, bronchitis.

Onset, Peak, and Duration

Route	Onset	Peak	Duration
Ophthalmic	Unknown	30 min	Unknown

Massage Considerations

- No cautions or contraindications to massage are indicated because a client is taking this drug.
- Side effects of hypotension require care in getting the client on and off the table. Stimulation with tapotement or friction to the legs at the end of the session may help.

trazodone hydrochloride (TRAYZ-oh-dohn high-droh-KLOR-ighd)

Desyrel, Desyrel Dividose

Drug Class: Antidepressant

Drug Actions

Inhibits serotonin uptake in brain and relieves depression

Use

- Depression
- Aggressive behavior
- Panic disorder

Side Effects

Cardiovascular: orthostatic hypotension, tachycardia, hypertension, shortness of breath.
Gastrointestinal: dry mouth, painful swallowing, constipation, nausea, vomiting, anorexia.
Nervous System: drowsiness, dizziness, nervousness, fatigue, confusion, tremor, weakness, hostility, syncope, anger, nightmares, vivid dreams, headache, insomnia.
Urinary: urine retention; priapism, possibly leading to impotence; hematuria.
Skin: rash, hives, sweating.
Other: decreased libido, blurred vision, ringing in the ears, nasal congestion, anemia.

Onset, Peak, and Duration

Route	Onset	Peak	Duration
Oral	Unknown	1–2 hr	Unknown

Massage Considerations

- Because of the sedating effects of this drug on the CNS, deep tissue massage should be used with caution.
- Further cautions and contraindications to massage may be related to the client condition.
- Side effects of hypotension, dizziness, and drowsiness require care in getting the client on and off the table. Stimulation with effleurage and tapotement at the end of the session may help. If the symptoms are severe, using more stimulating and rapid application of massage throughout the session may be needed.
- Constipation may be helped by abdominal massage.
- Rash and hives are local contraindications to massage and should be reported to the physician immediately. If severe or widespread, massage should be withheld.

triamcinolone (trigh-am-SIN-oh-lohn)

Aristocort, Atolone, Kenacort

triamcinolone acetonide

Kenaject-40, Kenalog-10, Kenalog-40, Tac-3, Tac-40, Triam-A, Triamonide 40, Tri-Kort, Trilog

triamcinolone diacetate

Amcort, Aristocort Forte, Aristocort Intralesional, Clinacort, Triam-Forte, Trilone, Tristoject

triamcinolone hexacetonide

Aristospan Intra-Articular, Aristospan Intralesional

Drug Class: Glucocorticoid anti-inflammatory, immunosuppressant

Drug Actions

Decreases inflammation, suppresses immune response; stimulates bone marrow; and influences protein, fat, and carbohydrate metabolism.

Use

- Severe inflammation or immunosuppression

Side Effects

Cardiovascular: heart failure, hypertension, edema, arrhythmias, thrombophlebitis, thromboembolism.
Gastrointestinal: peptic ulceration, GI irritation, increased appetite, pancreatitis, nausea, vomiting.
Nervous System: euphoria, insomnia, psychotic behavior, pseudotumor cerebri, dizziness, headache, paresthesia, seizures.
Urinary: menstrual irregularities.
Skin: delayed wound healing, acne, various skin eruptions.
Other: acute adrenal insufficiency during times of increased stress such as infection, surgery, trauma, abrupt withdrawal; susceptibility to infections; abnormal hair growth; cushingoid state (moonface, buffalo hump, central obesity); cataracts; glaucoma; hypokalemia; hyperglycemia; carbohydrate intolerance; muscular weakness; osteoporosis; growth suppression in children.

Onset, Peak, and Duration

Route	Onset	Peak	Duration
Oral, I.M., intralesional, intra-articular, intrasynovial	Varies	Varies	Varies

Massage Considerations

- When this drug is used long term, longer than 14 days, changes take place in the metabolism and in the connective, muscle, and fatty tissues of the body. Deep tissue massage is contraindicated. Myofascial massage should be used with caution and may be less effective.
- Further cautions and contraindications to massage may be related to the client condition.
- The site of intramuscular injection of the drug should not be massaged for 24 hours.

- Side effects of dizziness require care in getting the client on and off the table. Using stimulation with effleurage at the end of the session may help.
- Paresthesia requires care in depth and pressure of massage and contraindicates deep tissue massage.
- Thrombophlebitis or embolism is a complete contraindication to massage.
- Osteoporosis requires care in depth and pressure of massage and contraindicates deep tissue massage.
- Acne and skin eruptions are local contraindications to massage and should be reported to the physician. If the drug needs to be continued and the client still desires massage, gloves may be worn when working on the affected areas.
- The best approach for this client is to use systemic reflex strokes and mechanical strokes of rocking, effleurage, gentle friction, and pétrissage.

triamcinolone acetonide (trigh-am-SIN-oh-lohn as-EE-tuh-nighd)

Azmacort

Drug Class: Glucocorticoid anti-inflammatory, immunosuppressant

Drug Actions

Decreases inflammation, improving breathing ability.

Use

- Corticosteroid-dependent asthma

Side Effects

Cardiovascular: facial edema.
Gastrointestinal: oral candidiasis, dry or irritated tongue or mouth.
Other: hypothalamic-pituitary-adrenal function suppression, adrenal insufficiency, dry or irritated nose or throat, hoarseness, cough, wheezing.

Onset, Peak, and Duration

Route	Onset	Peak	Duration
Inhalation	1–4 wk	Unknown	Unknown

 Massage Considerations

- Even though this drug is taken by inhalation, some systemic effects can occur. When this drug is used long term, longer than 14 days, changes take place in the metabolism and in the connective, muscle, and fatty tissues of the body. Deep tissue massage should be used with caution. Myofascial massage should be used with caution and may be less effective.
- Further cautions and contraindications to massage may be related to the client condition.
- The best approach for this client is to use systemic reflex strokes and mechanical strokes of rocking, effleurage, gentle friction, and pétrissage.

triamterene (trigh-AM-tuh-reen)

Dyrenium

Drug Class: Potassium-sparing diuretic

Drug Actions

Inhibits sodium reabsorption and potassium and hydrogen excretion by direct action on distal tubule, promoting water and sodium excretion.

Use

- Edema

Side Effects

Cardiovascular: hypotension.
Gastrointestinal: dry mouth, nausea, vomiting, diarrhea.
Nervous System: dizziness, weakness, fatigue, headache.
Urinary: azotemia, interstitial nephritis, nephrolithiasis.
Skin: photosensitivity reactions, rash.
Other: anaphylaxis, megaloblastic anemia related to low folic acid levels, thrombocytopenia, agranulocytosis, jaundice, hyperkalemia, acidosis, hypokalemia, hyponatremia, hyperglycemia, muscle cramps.

Onset, Peak, and Duration

Route	Onset	Peak	Duration
Oral	2–4 hr	6–8 hr	7–9 hr

 Massage Considerations

- No cautions or contraindications to massage are related to the actions of this drug. Cautions and contraindications to massage may be related to the client condition.
- Side effects of hypotension and dizziness require care in getting the client on and off the table. Stimulation with effleurage and tapotement at the end of the session may help.
- Rash is a local contraindication to massage and should be reported to the physician immediately. If severe or widespread, massage should be withheld.

triazolam (trigh-AH-zoh-lam)

Alti-Triazolam, Apo-Triazo, Halcion, Novo-Triolam

Drug Class: Sedative-hypnotic

Drug Actions

May act on limbic system, thalamus, and hypothalamus of CNS to produce sleep.

Use

- Insomnia

Side Effects

Gastrointestinal: nausea, vomiting.
Nervous System: drowsiness, dizziness, headache, rebound insomnia, amnesia, lightheadedness, lack of coordination, confusion, depression, nervousness, ataxia.
Other: physical or psychological abuse.

Onset, Peak, and Duration

Route	Onset	Peak	Duration
Oral	Unknown	1–2 hr	Unknown

Massage Considerations

- Because of the sedating effect of this drug on the CNS, deep tissue massage should be used with caution.
- Side effects of drowsiness and dizziness require care in getting the client on and off the table. Stimulation with effleurage and tapotement at the end of the session may help. If the symptom is severe, using a more stimulating and rapid application of massage strokes throughout the session may be needed.

---

trifluoperazine hydrochloride (trigh-floo-oh-PER-eh-zeen high-droh-KLOR-ighd)

Apo-Trifluoperazine, Novo-Flurazine, PMS Trifluoperazine

Drug Class: Antipsychotic

Drug Actions

Probably blocks postsynaptic dopamine receptors in brain, relieving anxiety and signs and symptoms of psychotic disorders.

Use

- Anxiety
- Schizophrenia and other psychotic disorders

Side Effects

Cardiovascular: orthostatic hypotension, tachycardia, ECG changes.
Gastrointestinal: dry mouth, constipation, nausea.
Nervous System: extrapyramidal reactions, tardive dyskinesia, pseudoparkinsonism, dizziness, drowsiness, insomnia, fatigue, headache, neuroleptic malignant syndrome.
Urinary: urine retention, menstrual irregularities, inhibited lactation.
Skin: photosensitivity reactions, sterile abscesses, rash.
Other: allergic reaction, pain at intramuscular injection site, abnormal growth of breast tissue, ocular changes, blurred vision, transient leukopenia, agranulocytosis, cholestatic jaundice, weight gain.

Onset, Peak, and Duration

Route	Onset	Peak	Duration
Oral, I.M.	Up to several wk	Unknown	Unknown

Massage Considerations

- Because of the sedating effect of this drug on the CNS, deep tissue massage is contraindicated.
- Further cautions and contraindications to massage may be related to the client condition.
- The physician should be consulted before any massage is given.
- The site of intramuscular injection of the drug should not be massaged for up to 4 hours after the drug is administered to avoid increasing the rate of absorption of the drug.
- Side effects of hypotension, dizziness, and drowsiness require care in getting the client on and off the table. Stimulation with effleurage and friction to the legs at the end of the session may help. If the symptoms are severe, using a more stimulating application of massage throughout the session may be needed.
- Constipation may be helped by abdominal massage.

- Rash is a local contraindication to massage and should be reported to the physician immediately. If severe or widespread, massage should be withheld.

---

trihexyphenindyl hydrochloride (trigh-heks-eh-FEEN-ih-dil high-droh-KLOR-ighd)

Apo-Trihex, Trihexy-2, Trihexy-5

Drug Class: Anticholinergic antiparkinsonian drug

Drug Actions

Blocks central cholinergic receptors, improves physical mobility in patients with parkinsonism.

Use

- All forms of parkinsonism and adjunct treatment to levodopa in management of parkinsonism
- Drug-induced extrapyramidal reactions

Side Effects

Cardiovascular: tachycardia.
Gastrointestinal: dry mouth, constipation, nausea, vomiting.
Nervous System: nervousness, dizziness, headache, hallucinations, drowsiness, weakness.
Urinary: urinary hesitancy, urine retention.
Other: blurred vision, mydriasis, increased intraocular pressure.

Onset, Peak, and Duration

Route	Onset	Peak	Duration
Oral	1 hr	2–3 hr	6–12 hr

Massage Considerations

- No cautions or contraindications to massage are related to the actions of this drug. Cautions and contraindications to massage may be related to the client condition.
- The action of this drug blocks peripheral nervous system receptors. This may decrease the relaxation effects of massage in general and decrease the effects of the systemic reflex strokes of rocking, effleurage, and friction. Using these strokes for a longer time than usual may help to achieve the desired effects. Also, using slow, rhythmic effleurage throughout the session may help.
- Side effects of dizziness and drowsiness require care in getting the client on and off the table. Stimulation with friction to the legs at the end of the session may help.
- Constipation may be helped by abdominal massage.

---

trimethobenzamide hydrochloride (trigh-meth-oh-BEN-zuh-mighd high-droh-KLOR-ighd)

Tebamide, T-Gen, Tigan, Triban, Trimazide

Drug Class: Antiemetic

Drug Actions

May act on chemoreceptor trigger zone to inhibit nausea and vomiting

Use

- Nausea, vomiting
- Prevention of postoperative nausea and vomiting

Side Effects

Cardiovascular: hypotension.
Gastrointestinal: diarrhea.
Nervous System: drowsiness, dizziness, headache, disorientation, depression, parkinsonian-like symptoms, coma, seizures.
Skin: hypersensitivity reaction (pain, stinging, burning, redness, swelling at intramuscular injection site), blurred vision, jaundice, muscle cramps.

Onset, Peak, and Duration

Route	Onset	Peak	Duration
Oral	10–20 min	Unknown	3–4 hr
I.M.	15–30 min	Unknown	2–3 hr
Rectal	Unknown	Unknown	Unknown

 Massage Considerations

- Because of the sedating effects of this drug, deep tissue massage should be used with caution.
- Further cautions and contraindications to massage may be related to the client condition.
- The site of intramuscular injection of the drug should not be massaged for at least 2 hours to avoid increasing the rate of absorption of the drug into the body.
- Side effects of hypotension, dizziness, and drowsiness requires care in getting the client on and off the table. Using stimulation with effleurage and tapotement at the end of the session may help. If the symptom is severe, using a more stimulating application of massage throughout the session may be needed.

trimethoprim (trigh-METH-uh-prim)

Alprim, Primsol, Proloprim, Trimpex, Triprim

Drug Class: Antibiotic

Drug Actions

Inhibits growth of certain bacteria

Use

- Acute otitis media
- Uncomplicated urinary tract infections
- Prophylaxis of chronic and recurrent urinary tract infections
- Traveler's diarrhea
- *Pneumocystis carinii* pneumonia

Side Effects

Gastrointestinal: epigastric distress, nausea, vomiting, diarrhea, glossitis.
Nervous System: fever.
Skin: rash, itching, exfoliative dermatitis.
Other: abnormal blood profiles.

Onset, Peak, and Duration

Route	Onset	Peak	Duration
Oral	Unknown	1–4 hr	Unknown

Massage Considerations

- No cautions or contraindications to massage are related to the actions of this drug. Cautions and contraindications to massage may be related to the client condition and severity of infection.
- Side effects of rash, itching, and other skin eruptions are local contraindications to massage and should be reported to the physician immediately. If severe or widespread, massage should be withheld.

triptorelin pamoate (trip-TOE-reh-lin PAM-o-eight)

Trelstar Depot, Trelstar LA

Drug Class: Antineoplastic

Drug Actions

Is a potent inhibitor of gonadotropin secretion, causing testosterone to decline, which decreases effects of sex hormones on tumor growth in the prostate gland.

Use

- Palliative treatment of advanced prostate cancer

Side Effects

Cardiovascular: hypertension.
Gastrointestinal: diarrhea, vomiting.
Nervous System: pain, headache, dizziness, fatigue, insomnia, emotional lability.
Urinary: urine retention, urinary tract infection, impotence.
Skin: itching.
Other: hot flushes, pain at injection site, anemia, skeletal pain, leg pain.

Onset, Peak, and Duration

Route	Onset	Peak	Duration
I.M.	Unknown	Unknown	1 mo

Massage Considerations

- Because of the toxic effects of this drug, deep tissue massage should be used with caution.
- Further cautions and contraindications to massage may be related to the client condition.
- The physician should be consulted before any massage is given, and close collaboration is essential.
- The site of intramuscular injection of the drug should not be massaged for 24 hours.
- Side effects of dizziness require care in getting the client on and off the table. Using stimulation with effleurage at the end of the session may help.
- Itching is a local contraindication to massage and should be reported to the physician immediately. If severe or widespread, massage should be withheld.

U

unoprostone isopropyl (yoo-noh-PROST-ohn igh-soh-PROH-pul)

Rescula

Drug Class: Antiglaucoma agent

Drug Actions

Thought to increase the outflow of aqueous humor and reduce intraocular pressure

Use

- Reduction of intraocular pressure (IOP) in patients with open-angle glaucoma or ocular hypertension

Side Effects

Cardiovascular: hypertension.
Nervous System: dizziness, headache, insomnia, pain.
Other: accidental injury, allergic reaction, flulike syndrome, abnormal vision, blepharitis, cataracts, conjunctivitis, corneal lesion, dry eyes, eye discharge, eye burning or stinging, eye discomfort, eye irritation, eye hemorrhage, decreased length of eyelashes, increased length of eyelashes, eyelid disorder, foreign body sensation, keratitis, lacrimal disorder, pharyngitis, photophobia, rhinitis, sinusitis, vitreous disorder, eye itching, injection of eye, diabetes mellitus, back pain, bronchitis, increased cough, pharyngitis, increased cough.

Onset, Peak, and Duration

Route	Onset	Peak	Duration
Ophthalmic	Unknown	Unknown	Unknown

Massage Considerations

- There are no cautions or contraindications to massage related to this drug.
- Side effects of dizziness requires care in getting the client on and off the table.
- Stimulation with effleurage or tapotement at the end of the session may help.

ursodiol (ur-sih-DIGH-al)

Actigall

Drug Class: Bile acid

Drug Actions

A bile acid that dissolves cholesterol gallstones

Use

- Dissolution of gallstones smaller than 20 mm in diameter in patients who are poor candidates for surgery or who refuse surgery.
- Prevention of gallstone formation in obese patients experiencing rapid weight loss

Side Effects

Gastrointestinal: nausea, vomiting, painful digestion, metallic taste, abdominal pain, biliary pain, cholecystitis, diarrhea, constipation, stomatitis, gas.
Nervous System: headache, fatigue, anxiety, depression, dizziness, sleep disorders.
Urinary: urinary tract infections.
Skin: itching, rash, dry skin, hives, hair thinning, sweating.
Other: rhinitis, joint pain, muscle pain, back pain, cough.

Onset, Peak, and Duration

Route	Onset	Peak	Duration
Oral	Unknown	1–3 hr	Unknown

 Massage Considerations

- The physician should be consulted before any massage is given.
- There are no cautions or contraindications to massage related to the actions of this drug.
- There may be cautions or contraindications to massage related to the client condition.
- Side effects of dizziness require care in getting the client on and off the table. Stimulation with effleurage or tapotement at the end of the session may help. Constipation and gas may be helped by abdominal massage. Rash, itching, or hives are local contraindications to massage, and should be reported to the physician immediately. If severe or widespread, massage should be withheld.

V

valacyclovir hydrochloride (val-ay-SIGH-kloh-veer high-droh-KLOR-ighd)

Valtrex

Drug Class: Antiviral

Drug Actions

Antiviral that innhibits viral replication and growth of herpes zoster

Use

- Herpes zoster (shingles)
- Recurrent genital herpes
- Chronic suppression of recurrent genital herpes
- Chronic suppression of recurrent genital herpes in HIV-infected individuals
- Cold sores (herpes labialis)

Side Effects

Gastrointestinal: nausea, vomiting, diarrhea, abdominal pain.
Nervous System: headache, dizziness, depression.
Other: dysmenorrhea, joint pain.

Onset, Peak, and Duration

Route	Onset	Peak	Duration
Oral	30 min	Unknown	Unknown

Massage Considerations

- There are no cautions or contraindications to massage related to the actions of this drug.
- There may be cautions or contraindications to massage related to the client condition.
- Side effects of dizziness requires care in getting the client on and off the table.
- Stimulation with effleurage or taptotement at the end of the session may help.

---

valganciclovir (val-gan-SYE-kloh-veer)

Valcyte

Drug Class: Antiviral

Drug Actions

Antiviral action inhibits Cytomegalovirus

Use

- Active Cytomegalovirus retinitis in patients with AIDS
- Inactive Cytomegalovirus retinitis
- Prevention of Cytomegalovirus in kidney, heart, and pancreas-kidney transplants

Side Effects

Gastrointestinal: diarrhea, nausea, vomiting, abdominal pain.
Nervous System: pyrexia, headache, insomnia, peripheral neuropathy, paresthesia, seizures, psychosis, hallucinations, confusion, agitation.
Other: catheter-related infection, sepsis, local or systemic infections, hypersensitivity reactions, abnormal blood profiles, bone marrow depression, aplastic anemia, retinal detachment.

Onset, Peak, and Duration

Route	Onset	Peak	Duration
Oral	Unknown	1–3 hr	Unknown

Massage Considerations

- There are no cautions or contraindications to massage related to the actions of this drug.
- There may be cautions or contraindications to massage related to the client condition.
- Side effects of peripheral neuropathy or paresthesia are local contraindications to deep tissue massage.

---

valproate sodium (val-PROH-ayt SOH-dee-um)

Depacon, Depakene, Epilim, Valpro

valproic acid

Depakene

divalproex sodium

Depakote, Depakote ER, Depakote Sprinkle, Epival

Drug Class: Anticonvulsant

Drug Actions

Inhibits nerve impulses in CNS to prevent and treat certain types of seizure activity

Use

- Simple and complex absence seizures
- Mixed seizure types (including absence seizures)
- Mania
- Prevention of migraine headache
- Complex partial seizures

Side Effects

Gastrointestinal: nausea, vomiting, indigestion, diarrhea, abdominal cramps, constipation, increased appetite and weight gain, anorexia, pancreatitis.
Nervous System: sedation, emotional upset, depression, psychosis, aggressiveness, hyperactivity, behavioral deterioration, muscle weakness, tremor, ataxia, headache, dizziness, incoordination.
Skin: rash, hair loss, itching, photosensitivity reactions, erythema multiforme, Stevens-Johnson syndrome.
Other: flulike syndrome, infection, nystagmus, double vision, petechiae, bruising, eosinophilia, hemorrhage, bone marrow suppression, toxic hepatitis, hepatotoxicity, abnormal blood profiles.

Onset, Peak, and Duration

Route	Onset	Peak	Duration
Oral	Unknown	1–4 hr	Unknown
I.V.	Unknown	Unknown	Unknown

Massage Considerations

- Because of the sedating effects of this drug, deep tissue massage should be used with great caution, if at all.
- There may be further cautions or contraindications to massage related to the client condition.
- Side effects of sedation and dizziness require care in getting the client on and off the table. Stimulation with effleurage and tapotement at the end of the session may help. If the symptom is severe, using a more stimulating and rapid manner of application of massage throughout the session may be needed. Constipation may be helped by abdominal massage. Bruising is a contraindication to deep tissue massage. Rash and itching are local contraindications to massage, and should be reported to the physician immediately. If severe or widespread, massage should be withheld. Hair loss is a contraindication to scalp massage if the client is disturbed by hair loss during the session or if the scalp is tender.

valsartan (val-SAR-tin)

Diovan

Drug Class: Antihypertensive

Drug Actions

Antihypertensive that blocks angiotensin, dilates blood vessels, and lowers blood pressure

Use

- Hypertension
- Heart failure

Side Effects

Cardiovascular: edema, hypotension, postural hypotension, syncope.
Gastrointestinal: abdominal pain, diarrhea, nausea, painful digestion.
Nervous System: fatigue, dizziness, headache, insomnia.
Urinary: renal impairment.
Other: viral infection, angioedema, pharyngitis, rhinitis, sinusitis, blurred vision, neutropenia, hyperkalemia, joint pain, back pain, cough, upper respiratory tract infection.

Onset, Peak, and Duration

Route	Onset	Peak	Duration
Oral	Within 2 hr	2–4 hr	24 hr

 Massage Considerations

- There are no contraindications to massage related to the actions of this drug; however, because this drug dilates blood vessels, the vasodilating effects of massage may be increased. Side effects of dizziness and hypotension may result.
- There may be cautions or contraindications to massage related to the client condition.
- Side effects of hypotension and dizziness require care in getting the client on and off the table. Stimulation with effleurage and tapotement at the end of the session may help.

---

vancomycin hydrochloride (van-koh-MIGH-sin high-droh-KLOR-ighd)

Vancocin, Vancoled

Drug Class: Antibiotic

Drug Actions

Antibiotic action kills susceptible bacteria

Use

- Severe *staphylococcal* infections
- Endocarditis prophylaxis for dental procedures
- Antibiotic-related pseudomembranous and *staphylococcal enterocolitis*

Side Effects

Cardiovascular: hypotension.
Gastrointestinal: nausea.
Nervous System: fever, pain.
Urinary: nephrotoxicity, pseudomembranous colitis.
Skin: "red-neck" or "red-man" syndrome (maculopapular rash on face, neck, trunk, and limbs with rapid I.V. infusion; itching and hypotension with histamine release).
Other: chills, anaphylaxis, superinfection, thrombophlebitis at injection site, ringing in the ears, ototoxicity, eosinophilia, leukopenia, wheezing, shortness of breath.

Onset, Peak, and Duration

Route	Onset	Peak	Duration
Oral	Unknown	Unknown	Unknown
I.V.	Immediate	Immediate	Unknown

Massage Considerations

- There are no cautions or contraindications to massage related to the actions of this drug.
- There may be cautions or contraindications to massage related to the client condition and severity of infection.
- Side effects of hypotension require care in getting the client on and off the table.
- Stimulation with effleurage and tapotement at the end of the session may help.
- Thrombophlebitis is a complete contraindication to massage.

vardenafil hydrochloride (var-DEN-ah-phill high-droh-KLOR-ighd)

Levitra

Drug Class: Erectile dysfunction drug

Drug Actions

Erectile dysfunction drug that prolongs smooth muscle relaxation promoting the flow of blood and penile erection

Use

- Erectile dysfunction

Side Effects

Cardiovascular: flushing.
Gastrointestinal: painful digestion, nausea.
Nervous System: headache, dizziness.
Other: flulike syndrome, rhinitis, sinusitis, back pain.

Onset, Peak, and Duration

Route	Onset	Peak	Duration
Oral	Immediate	30–120 min	Unknown

Massage Considerations

- Although the duration of action of this drug is unknown, the peak effect is 2 hours and the half-life is 5 hours. Because of the cardiovascular effects of this drug, no massage should be given for at least 5 hours after this drug is taken.
- Side effects of dizziness require care in getting the client on and off the table. Stimulation with effleurage or tapotement at the end of the session may help.

vasopressin (ADH) (VAY-soh-preh-sin)

Pitressin

Drug Class: Posterior pituitary hormone ADH (antidiuretic hormone)

Drug Actions

Posterior pituitary hormone that promotes reabsorption of water and produces concentrated urine (antidiuretic hormone effect) and stimulates GI motility.

Use

- Neurogenic diabetes insipidus
- Postoperative abdominal distention
- To expel gas before abdominal X-ray
- Provocative testing for growth hormone and corticotropin release
- G.I. hemorrhage

Side Effects

Cardiovascular: angina in patients with vascular disease, vasoconstriction, arrhythmias, cardiac arrest, myocardial ischemia, circumoral pallor, decreased cardiac output.
Gastrointestinal: abdominal cramps, nausea, vomiting, gas.
Nervous System: tremor, dizziness, headache.
Skin: cutaneous gangrene, sweating.
Other: water intoxication (drowsiness, listlessness, headache, confusion, weight gain, seizures, coma), hypersensitivity reactions

Onset, Peak, and Duration

Route	Onset	Peak	Duration
Subcutaneous Injection, I.M., Intranasal	Unknown	Unknown	2–8 hr

Massage Considerations

- The physician should be consulted before any massage is given.
- There are no cautions or contraindications to massage related to the actions of this drug.
- There may be cautions or contraindications to massage related to the client condition.
- The site of subcutaneous or I.M. injection of the drug should not be massaged for at least 2 hours.
- Side effects of dizziness require care in getting the client on and off the table.
- Stimulation with tapotement at the end of the session may help. Gas may be helped by abdominal massage.

venlafaxine hydrochloride (ven-leh-FAKS-een high-droh-KLOR-ighd)

Effexor, Effexor XR

Drug Class: Antidepressant

Drug Actions

Antidepressant that blocks reuptake of norepinephrine and serotonin into neurons in CNS and relieves depression.

Use

- Depression
- Generalized or social anxiety disorder
- Prevention of major depressive disorder relapse

Side Effects

Cardiovascular: hypertension.
Gastrointestinal: nausea, constipation, vomiting, dry mouth, anorexia, diarrhea, painful digestion, gas.
Nervous System: weakness, headache, sleepiness, dizziness, nervousness, insomnia, anxiety, tremor, abnormal dreams, paresthesia, agitation.
Urinary: abnormal ejaculation, impotence, urinary frequency, impaired urination.
Skin: sweating, rash.
Other: yawning, chills, infection, blurred vision, weight loss.

Onset, Peak, and Duration

Route	Onset	Peak	Duration
Oral	Unknown	Unknown	Unknown

Massage Considerations

- There are no cautions or contraindications to massage related to the actions of this drug.
- There may be cautions or contraindications to massage related to the client condition.
- Side effects of sleepiness and dizziness require care in getting the client on and off the table. Stimulation with effleurage and tapotement at the end of the session may help.
- Paresthesia is a local contraindication to deep tissue massage. Constipation and gas may be helped by abdominal massage. Urinary frequency may require the client to get up in the middle of the session. Privacy and quick access to the bathroom is needed. Water fountains or music that may stimulate the urge to urinate should be avoided. Rash is a local contraindication to massage and should be reported to the physician.

---

verapamil hydrochloride (veh-RAP-uh-mil high-droh-KLOR-ighd)

Anpec, Anpec SR, Apo-Verap, Calan, Calan SR, Cordilox, Cordilox SR, Covera-HS, Isoptin, Isoptin SR, Novo-Veramil, Nu-Verap, Veracaps SR, Verahexal, Verelan, Verelan PM

Drug Class: Calcium channel blocker

Drug Actions

Calcium channel blocker that decreases myocardial contractility and oxygen demand and dilates coronary arteries and arterioles thus relieving angina, lowering blood pressure

Use

- Vasospastic angina
- Classic chronic, stable angina pectoris
- Unstable angina
- Chronic atrial fibrillation
- Supraventricular arrhythmias
- Prevention of recurrent PSVT
- Chronic atrial flutter or atrial fibrillation
- Hypertension

Side Effects

Cardiovascular: transient hypotension, heart failure, bradycardia, AV block, ventricular asystole, ventricular fibrillation, peripheral edema.
Gastrointestinal: constipation, nausea.

Nervous System: dizziness, headache, weakness.
Skin: rash.
Other: pulmonary edema.

Onset, Peak, and Duration

Route	Onset	Peak	Duration
Oral	1–2 hr	1–9 hr	8–24 hr
I.V.	Rapid	Immediate	1–6 hr

Massage Considerations

- There are no cautions or contraindications to massage related to the actions of this drug.
- There may be cautions or contraindications to massage related to the client condition.
- Side effects of hypotension and dizziness require care in getting the client on and off the table. Stimulation with effleurage and tapotement at the end of the session may help
- Constipation may be helped by abdominal massage. Rash is a local contraindication to massage and should be reported to the physician.

---

vinblastin sulfate (VLB) (vin-BLAH-steen SUL-fayt)

Velban, Velbe

Drug Class: Antineoplastic

Drug Actions

Antineoplastic drug that inhibits replication of certain cancer cells

Use

- Breast or testicular cancer
- Hodgkin's and non-Hodgkin's lymphoma
- Choriocarcinoma
- Lymphosarcoma
- Mycosis fungoides
- Kaposi's sarcoma
- Histiocytosis
- Letterer-Siwe disease (histiocytosis X)
- Hodgkin's disease
- Testicular germ cell carcinoma

Side Effects

Cardiovascular: hypertension, heart attack, phlebitis.
Gastrointestinal: nausea, vomiting, ulcer, bleeding, constipation, ileus, anorexia, diarrhea, abdominal pain, stomatitis.
Nervous System: depression, paresthesia, peripheral neuropathy and neuritis, numbness, loss of deep tendon reflexes, seizures, CVA, headache.
Urinary: oligospermia, aspermia, urine retention.
Skin: reversible hair loss, vesiculation, cellulitis, necrosis with extravasation.
Other: pharyngitis, abnormal blood profiles, hyperuricemia, weight loss, uric acid nephropathy, muscle pain and weakness, acute bronchospasm, shortness of breath.

Onset, Peak, and Duration

Route	Onset	Peak	Duration
I.V.	Unknown	Unknown	Unknown

Massage Considerations

- Antibiotic action kills susceptible bacteria
- The physician should be consulted before any massage is given and close collaboration is essential.
- Because of the toxic effects of this drug, deep tissue massage is contraindicated and circulatory massage with effleurage should be used with caution and limited.
- There may be further cautions and contraindications to massage related to the client condition.
- The drug is usually given every 1–2 weeks. Massage is best given in the weeks that the drug is not being administered or at least 24 hours after the drug has been given.
- Side effects of paresthesia, neuropathy, and neuritis require care in depth and pressure of massage and contraindicate deep tissue massage. If severe, they may contraindicate massage completely. Constipation may be helped by abdominal massage. Hair loss contraindicates scalp massage if the client is disturbed by hair loss during the massage or if the scalp is tender.
- The best approach to this client is to use the systemic and local reflex strokes of rocking, gentle friction, stretching, tractions, and vibration. Pétrissage and myofascial massage techniques also may be used.

---

vincristine sulfate (vin-KRIH-steen SUL-fayt)

Oncovin, Vincasar PFS

Drug Class: Antineoplastic

Drug Actions

Antineoplastic that inhibits replication of certain cancer cells

Use

- Breast cancer
- Acute lymphoblastic and other leukemias
- Hodgkin's disease
- Non-Hodgkin's lymphoma
- Neuroblastoma
- Rhabdomyosarcoma
- Wilms' tumor

Side Effects

Cardiovascular: hypotension, hypertension, phlebitis.
Gastrointestinal: diarrhea, constipation, cramps, ileus that mimics surgical abdomen, nausea, vomiting, anorexia, painful digestion, intestinal necrosis, stomatitis.
Nervous System: fever, peripheral neuropathy, sensory loss, loss of deep tendon reflexes, paresthesia, wristdrop and footdrop, headache, ataxia, cranial nerve palsies, jaw pain, hoarseness, vocal cord paralysis, seizures, coma, permanent neurotoxicity.
Urinary: urine retention, painful urination, acute uric acid neuropathy, frequent urination.
Skin: rash, reversible hair loss, cellulitis at injection site, severe local reaction with extravasation.
Other: SIADH, visual disturbances, double vision, optic and extraocular neuropathy, ptosis, abnormal blood profiles, hyponatremia, hyperuricemia, weight loss, muscle weakness and cramps, acute bronchospasm.

Onset, Peak, and Duration

Route	Onset	Peak	Duration
I.V.	Unknown	Unknown	Unknown

Massage Considerations

- The physician should be consulted before any massage is given and close collaboration is essential.
- Because of the toxic effects of this drug, deep tissue massage is contraindicated and circulatory massage with effleurage should be used with caution and limited.
- There may be further cautions and contraindications to massage related to the client condition.
- The drug is usually given weekly and has a long half-life of up to 85 hours. Massage is best given the day before the drug is given.
- Side effects of paresthesia, neuropathy, and sensory loss require care in depth and pressure of massage and contraindicate deep tissue massage. If severe, they may contraindicate massage completely. Hypotension may be helped by using friction to the legs at the end of the session. Urinary frequency requires privacy and quick access to the bathroom if the client needs to go during the session. Water fountains and music that may stimulate the urge to urinate should be avoided. Constipation may be helped by abdominal massage. Rash is a local contraindication to massage, and should be reported to the physician immediately. If severe or widespread, massage should be withheld. Hair loss contraindicates scalp massage, if the client is disturbed by hair loss during the massage or if the scalp is tender.
- The best approach to this client is to use the systemic and local reflex strokes of rocking, gentle friction, stretching, tractions, and vibration. Pétrissage and myofascial massage techniques also may be used.

---

vinorelbine tartrate (vin-oh-REL-been TAR-trayt)

Navelbine

Drug Class: Antineoplastic

Drug Actions

Antineoplastic that inhibits replication of selected cancer cells

Use

- Non-small-cell lung cancer
- Breast cancer

Side Effects

Gastrointestinal: nausea, vomiting, anorexia, diarrhea, constipation, stomatitis.
Nervous System: peripheral neuropathy, weakness, fatigue.
Skin: hair loss, rash.
Other: SIADH, injection site pain or reaction, bone marrow suppression, bilirubinemia, jaw pain, chest pain, muscle pain, joint pain, loss of deep tendon reflexes, shortness of breath.

Onset, Peak, and Duration

Route	Onset	Peak	Duration
I.V.	Unknown	Unknown	Unknown

Massage Considerations

- The physician should be consulted before any massage is given and close collaboration is essential.
- Because of the toxic effects of this drug, deep tissue massage is contraindicated and circulatory massage with effleurage should be used with caution and limited.

- There may be further cautions and contraindications to massage related to the client condition.
- The drug is usually given weekly and has a long half-life of up to 43 hours. Massage is best given before the drug is administered, or at least 48 hours after it has been given.
- Side effects of neuropathy require care in depth and pressure of massage and contraindicate deep tissue massage. If severe, it may contraindicate massage completely.
- Constipation may be helped by abdominal massage. Rash is a local contraindication to massage, and should be reported to the physician immediately. If severe or widespread, massage should be withheld. Hair loss contraindicates scalp massage, if the client is disturbed by hair loss during the massage or if the scalp is tender.
- The best approach to this client is to use the systemic and local reflex strokes of rocking, gentle friction, stretching, tractions, and vibration. Pétrissage and myofascial massage techniques also may be used.

voriconazole (vhor-i-KHAN-a-zawl)

Vfend

Drug Class: Antifungal

Drug Actions

Antifungal that kills susceptible fungi

Use

- Invasive aspergillosis
- Serious infections caused by *Fusarium* species and *Scedosporium apiospermum*

Side Effects

Cardiovascular: tachycardia, hypertension, hypotension, peripheral edema, vasodilation.
Gastrointestinal: abdominal pain, nausea, vomiting, diarrhea.
Nervous System: fever, headache, hallucinations, dizziness.
Urinary: acute renal failure.
Skin: rash, itching.
Other: chills, abnormal vision, photophobia, chromatopsia, dry mouth, cholestatic jaundice, hypokalemia, hypomagnesemia.

Onset, Peak, and Duration

Route	Onset	Peak	Duration
Oral, I.V.	Immediate	1–2 hr	12 hr

Massage Considerations

- There are no cautions or contraindications to massage related to the actions of this drug.
- There may be cautions or contraindications to massage related to the client condition.
- Side effects of hypotension or dizziness require care in getting the client on and off the table. Stimulation with effleurage or tapotement at the end of the session may help. Rash and itching are local contraindications to massage and should be reported to the physician immediately. If severe or widespread, massage should be withheld.

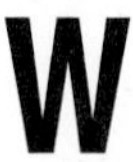

warfarin sodium (WAR-feh-rin SOH-dee-um)

Coumadin, Warfilone

Drug Class: Anticoagulant

Drug Actions

Inhibits clotting factors formed in liver and reduces ability of blood to clot

Use

- Pulmonary embolism related to deep vein thrombosis
- Heart attack
- Rheumatic heart disease with heart valve damage
- Prosthetic heart valves
- Chronic atrial fibrillation

Side Effects

Gastrointestinal: anorexia, nausea, vomiting, cramps, diarrhea, mouth ulcerations, sore mouth, melena.
Nervous System: headache, fever.
Urinary: hematuria, excessive menstrual bleeding.
Skin: hives, necrosis, gangrene, hair loss, rash.
Other: hemorrhage with excessive dosage, easy bruising, hepatitis, jaundice.

Onset, Peak, and Duration

Route	Onset	Peak	Duration
Oral	$^1/_2$–3 days	Unknown	2–5 days
I.V.	Unknown	Unknown	2–5 days

Massage Considerations

- The physician should always be consulted before any massage is given.
- This drug decreases the clotting ability of the blood. If the drug is given because of the presence of an actual blood clot (thrombus or embolus), massage is completely contraindicated until the physician certifies that the blood clot is resolved. If the drug is given to prevent blood clots, massage may be given, but deep tissue massage is contraindicated completely and circulatory massage with effleurage should be used with caution and limited. Myofascial massage techniques should be used with caution, and are contraindicated if they cause bruising or petechea.
- Side effects of hives or rash are local contraindications to massage, and should be reported to the physician immediately. If severe or widespread, massage should be withheld. Hair loss is a contraindication to scalp massage, if the client is disturbed by hair loss during the massage or if the scalp is tender. Bruising requires care in depth and pressure of massage in general and, if severe, should be reported to the physician immediately and massage withheld.
- The best approach to this client is to utilize the local reflex strokes and mechanical strokes of stretching, tractions, vibration, gentle compression, gentle friction, and pétrissage. Rocking may be used.

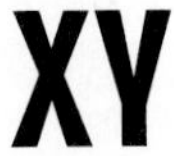

xylometazoline hydrochloride (zigh-loh-met-uh-ZOH-leen high-droh-KLOR-ighd)

Otrivin

Drug Class: Sympathomimetic, decongestant

Drug Actions

Mimics the SNS in the nasal arterioles, reducing blood flow and nasal congestion.

Use

- Nasal congestion

Side Effects

Other: transient burning, stinging; dryness or ulceration of nasal mucosa; sneezing; rebound nasal congestion or irritation (with excessive or long-term use).

Onset, Peak, and Duration

Route	Onset	Peak	Duration
Intranasal	5–10 min	Unknown	5–6 hr

Massage Considerations

- There are no cautions or contraindications to massage related to this drug.

Z

zafirlukast (zay-FEER-loo-kast)

Accolate

Drug Class:Bronchodilator

Drug Actions

Blocks inflammatory action in the lungs, inhibits bronchoconstriction, and improves breathing.

Use

- Chronic asthma
- Seasonal allergic rhinitis

Side Effects

Gastrointestinal: nausea, diarrhea, abdominal pain, vomiting, painful digestion.
Nervous System: headache, weakness, dizziness, pain, fever.
Other: infection, accidental injury, muscle pain, back pain.

Onset, Peak, and Duration

Route	Onset	Peak	Duration
Oral	Unknown	3 hr	Unknown

 Massage Considerations

- There are no cautions or contraindications to massage related to the actions of this drug.
- There may be cautions or contraindications to massage related to the client condition.
- Side effects of dizziness require care in getting the client on and off the table. Stimulation with effeurage and tapotement at the end of the session may help.

zalcitabine (ddC, dideoxycytidine) (zal-SIGH-tuh-been)

Hivid

Drug Class: Antiviral

Drug Actions

Antiviral action reduces symptoms linked to advanced HIV infection

Use

- Advanced HIV infection

Side Effects

Cardiovascular: cardiomyopathy, heart failure, chest pain.
Gastrointestinal: nausea, vomiting, diarrhea, abdominal pain, anorexia, constipation, stomatitis, esophageal ulcer, glossitis, pancreatitis.
Nervous System: peripheral neuropathy, headache, fatigue, dizziness, confusion, seizures, impaired concentration, amnesia, insomnia, depression, tremor, hypertonia, weakness, agitation, abnormal thinking, anxiety, fever.
Skin: itching; night sweats; rash, hives.
Other: pharyngitis, ocular pain, abnormal vision, ototoxicity, nasal discharge, abnormal blood profiles, cough, muscle pain, joint pain.

Onset, Peak, and Duration

Route	Onset	Peak	Duration
Oral	Unknown	1–2 hr	Unknown

 Massage Considerations

- The physician should be consulted before any massage is given.
- Although there are no cautions or contraindications to massage related to the actions of this drug, there will be cautions and contraindications to massage related to the client condition.
- Side effects of neuropathy are a contraindication to deep tissue massage. Dizziness requires care in getting the client on and off the table. Stimulation with effleurage or tapotement at the end of the session may help. Constipation may be helped by abdominal massage. Itching, rash, or hives are local contraindications to massage and should be reported to the physician immediately. If severe or widespread, massage should be withheld.

zaleplon (ZAL-eh-plon)

Sonata

Drug Class: Sedative/hypnotic

Drug Actions

Produces sedative effects in the CNS and promotes sleep

Use

- Short-term treatment of insomnia

Side Effects

Cardiovascular: chest pain, peripheral edema.
Gastrointestinal: constipation, dry mouth, anorexia, painful digestion, nausea, abdominal pain, colitis.
Nervous System: headache, amnesia, dizziness, sleepiness, depression, hypertonia, nervousness, depersonalization, hallucinations, difficulty concentrating, anxiety, paresthesia, hypesthesia, tremor, weakness, migraine, malaise, fever.
Skin: itching, rash, photosensitivity reactions.
Other: abnormal vision, conjunctivitis, eye pain, ear pain, abnormal sensitivity to sound, nose bleed, abnormal sense of smell, dysmenorrhea, arthritis, muscle pain, back pain, bronchitis.

Onset, Peak, and Duration

Route	Onset	Peak	Duration
Oral	1 hr	1 hr	3–4 hr

Massage Considerations

- Because of the sedating effect of this drug on the CNS, deep tissue massage should be used with caution.
- Side effects of dizziness or sleepiness require care in getting the client on and off the table. Stimulation with effleurage and tapotement at the end of the session may help. If the symptoms are severe, use of more stimulating massage techniques throughout the session may be needed. Paresthesia and hypesthesia are contraindications to deep tissue massage. Constipation may be helped by abdominal massage. Itching and rash are local contraindications to massage and should be reported to the physician.

zanamivir (zah-NAM-ah-veer)

Relenza

Drug Class: Antiviral

Drug Actions

Antiviral effects shorten the symptoms of influenza

Use

- Influenza

Side Effects

Gastrointestinal: diarrhea, nausea, vomiting.
Nervous System: headache, dizziness.
Other: bronchitis, cough, nasal signs and symptoms; sinusitis; ear, nose, and throat infections.

Onset, Peak, and Duration

Route	Onset	Peak	Duration
Inhalation	Unknown	1–2 hr	Unknown

 Massage Considerations

- This drug is given during the active phase of the flu. Massage should not be given until symptoms are resolved and the drug is no longer being taken.

zidovudine (azidothymidine, AZT) (zigh-DOH-vyoo-deen)

Apo-Zidovudine, Novo-AZT, Retrovir

Drug Class: Antiviral

Drug Actions

Antiviral effects reduce symptoms of HIV infection

Use

- HIV infection
- Prevention of maternal-fetal HIV transmission
- Postexposure prophylaxis after occupational exposure to HIV

Side Effects

Gastrointestinal: nausea, anorexia, abdominal pain, vomiting, constipation, diarrhea, painful digestion, taste perversion.
Nervous System: weakness, headache, seizures, paresthesia, malaise, insomnia, dizziness, sleepiness, fever.
Skin: rash, sweating.
Other: severe bone marrow suppression (resulting in anemia), abnormal blood profiles, lactic cidosis, muscle pain.

Onset, Peak, and Duration

Route	Onset	Peak	Duration
Oral	Unknown	30–90 min	Unknown
I.V.	Immediate	30–90 min	Unknown

Massage Considerations

- There are no cautions or contraindications to massage related to the actions of this drug.
- There may be cautions and contraindications to massage related to the client condition.
- Side effects of dizziness and sleepiness require care in getting the client on and off the table. Stimulation with effleurage or tapotement at the end of the session may help. Paresthesia is a local contraindication to deep tissue massage. Constipation may be helped by abdominal massage. Rash is a local contraindication to massage and should be reported to the physician immediately. If severe or widespread, massage should be withheld.

ziprasidone (zi-PRAY-si-done)

Geodon

Drug Class: Antipsychotic

Drug Actions

May block serotonin and dopamine neurotransmittors in the CNS, thus relieving psychotic signs and symptoms of schizophrenia

Use

- Schizophrenia

Side Effects

Cardiovascular: tachycardia, vasodilation, orthostatic hypotension; hypertension, bradycardia.
Gastrointestinal: nausea, constipation, painful digestion, diarrhea, dry mouth, anorexia; abdominal pain, rectal hemorrhage, vomiting.
Nervous System: speech disorders, dystonia, akathisia, sleepiness, dizziness, extrapyramidal symptoms, hypertonia, weakness; headache, anxiety, insomnia, agitation, cogwheel rigidity, paresthesia, personality disorder, psychosis, suicide attempt.
Urinary: priapism.
Skin: injection site pain, furunculosis, sweating, rash.
Other: back pain, muscle pain, flulike syndrome, tooth disorder, abnormal vision, dysmenorrhea, cough, rhinitis.

Onset, Peak, and Duration

Route	Onset	Peak	Duration
Oral	1–3 days	6–8 hr	12 hr
I.M.	Unknown	1 hour	Unknown

Massage Considerations

- The physician should be consulted before any massage is given.
- Because of the sedating effect of this drug on the CNS, deep tissue massage should be used with caution.
- In most cases, there will be further cautions and contraindications to massage related to the client condition.
- The site of I.M. injection of the drug should not be massaged for at least 1 hour to avoid increasing the rate of absorption of the drug into the body.
- Side effects of hypotension, dizziness, and sleepiness require care in getting the client on and off the table. Stimulation with effleurage or friction to the legs at the end of the session may help. Paresthesia is a contraindication to deep tissue massage. Constipation may be helped by abdominal massage. Rash is a local contraindication to massage and should be reported to the physician immediately. If severe or widespread, massage should be withheld.

zoledronic acid (zoe-LEH-druh-nick ASS-id)

Zometa

Drug Class: Antihypercalcemic

Drug Actions

Inhibits calcium release into the blood and lowers blood calcium levels in malignant disease

Use

- Hypercalcemia related to malignancy
- Multiple myeloma
- Bone metastases of solid tumors
- Prostate cancer

Side Effects

Cardiovascular: hypotension, leg edema.
Gastrointestinal: nausea, constipation, diarrhea, abdominal pain, vomiting, anorexia, increased appetite, difficulty swallowing.
Nervous System: headache, sleepiness, anxiety, confusion, agitation, insomnia, fever, depression, paresthesia, hypesthesia, fatigue, weakness, dizziness.
Urinary: urinary tract infections, candidiasis.
Skin: hair loss, rash.
Other: progression of cancer, infection, abnormal blood profiles, dehydration, skeletal pain, joint pain, shortness of breath, cough, pleural effusion, weight loss, muscle pain, back pain, rigors.

Onset, Peak, and Duration

Route	Onset	Peak	Duration
I.V.	Unknown	Unknown	7–28 days

Massage Considerations

- The physician should be consulted before any massage is given and close collaboration is essential.
- Although there are no cautions or contraindications to massage related to the actions of this drug, there will be cautions and contraindications to massage related to the client condition.
- Side effects of hypotension, sleepiness, and dizziness require care in positioning the client and getting them on and off the table. Stimulation with gentle friction to the legs at the end of the session may help. Paresthesia and hypesthesia are contraindications to deep tissue massage and, if severe, may contraindicate massage completely. Constipation may be helped by abdominal massage. Rash is a local contraindication to massage and should be reported to the physician immediately and if severe or widespread, massage should be withheld. Hair loss is a contraindication to scalp massage if the client is disturbed by hair loss during the massage or if the scalp is tender.
- The best approach to this client is to use the systemic reflex strokes of rocking, effleurage, and gentle friction. Pétrissage also may be used.

zolmitriptan (zohl-muh-TRIP-tan)

Zomig, Zomig-ZMT

Drug Class: Antimigraine drug

Drug Actions

Constricts cranial blood vessels, inhibits inflammation, and relieves migraine headache pain

Use

- Acute migraine headache

Side Effects

Cardiovascular: palpitations, coronary artery vasospasm, transient myocardial ischemia, heart attack, ventricular tachycardia, ventricular fibrillation; pain, tightness, pressure, or heaviness in chest.
Gastrointestinal: dry mouth, painful digestion, difficulty swallowing, nausea.
Nervous System: sleepiness, dizziness, hypesthesia, paresthesia, weakness, pain.
Skin: sweating.
Other: warm or cold sensations, pain, tightness, or pressure in the neck, throat, or jaw, muscle pain, myasthenia.

Onset, Peak, and Duration

Route	Onset	Peak	Duration
Oral	Unknown	2 hr	3 hr
Orally Disintegrating	Unknown	2 hr	Unknown

Massage Considerations

- The sedating effect of this drug on the CNS requires that deep tissue massage be used with caution. Because this drug is given at the time of a migraine headache, the client may not be able to receive massage at all.
- Side effects of dizziness and sleepiness require care in getting the client on and off the table. Stimulation with effleurage or tapotement at the end of the session may help. If symptoms are severe, more stimulating massage techniques throughout the session may be needed.

zolpidem tartrate (ZOHL-peh-dim TAR-trayt)

Ambien

Drug Class: Sedative/hypnotic

Drug Actions

Exhibits sedating effects in the CNS and promotes sleep

Use

- Short-term management of insomnia

Side Effects

Cardiovascular: palpitations.
Gastrointestinal: nausea, vomiting, diarrhea, painful digestion, constipation, abdominal pain, dry mouth.
Nervous System: daytime drowsiness, light-headedness, abnormal dreams, amnesia, dizziness, headache, hangover effect, sleep disorder, lethargy, depression.
Skin: rash.
Other: flulike syndrome, hypersensitivity reactions, sinusitis, pharyngitis, back or chest pain, muscle pain, joint pain.

Onset, Peak, and Duration

Route	Onset	Peak	Duration
Oral	Rapid	30 min–2 hr	Unknown

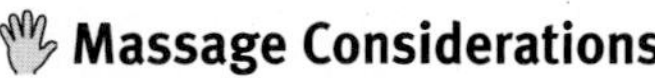

Massage Considerations

- Because of the sedating effect of this drug on the CNS, deep tissue massage should be used with caution.
- Side effects of drowsiness, light-headedness, or dizziness require care in getting the client on and off the table. Stimulation with rapid effleurage or tapotement at the end of the session may help. If the symptom is severe, using more stimulating massage techniques throughout the session may be needed. Constipation may be helped by abdominal massage. Rash is a local contraindication to massage and should be reported to the physician.

---

zonisamide (zon-ISS-a-mide)

Zonegran

Drug Class: Anticonvulsant

Drug Actions

Stabilizes CNS cell membranes to prevents and stop seizure activity

Use

- Partial seizures in adults with epilepsy

Side Effects

Gastrointestinal: anorexia, nausea, diarrhea, painful digestion, constipation, dry mouth, taste perversion, abdominal pain.
Nervous System: headache, dizziness, ataxia, nystagmus, paresthesia, confusion, difficulties in concentration and memory, mental slowing, agitation, irritability, depression, insomnia, anxiety, nervousness, schizophrenic or schizophreniform behavior, sleepiness, fatigue, speech abnormalities, difficulties in verbal expression.
Skin: bruising, rash.
Other: flulike symptoms, double vision, rhinitis, weight loss.

Onset, Peak, and Duration

Route	Onset	Peak	Duration
Oral	Unknown	Unknown	Unknown

Massage Considerations

- The depressant effect of this drug on the CNS requires that deep tissue massage be used with caution.
- There may be further cautions or contraindications to massage related to the client condition.
- The actions of this drug may decrease the effectiveness of the local reflex strokes of stretching, traction, compression, and vibration as well as the effectiveness of deep tissue massage. Using these strokes for longer than usual periods of time may achieve the desired effects. Using the mechanical strokes of pétrissage, effleurage, and friction may be more effective. The effects of the systemic reflex strokes of rocking, rhythmic effleurage, or friction may be increased. Using these strokes in a more rapid and stimulating manner may help balance out the effects either at the end of the session or throughout the session.
- Side effects of dizziness and sleepiness may be addressed as noted earlier. Paresthesia is a contraindication to deep tissue massage. Constipation may be helped by abdominal massage. Bruising is a contraindication to deep tissue massage. Rash is a local contraindication to massage and should be reported to the physician.

Appendix: Guide to Abbreviations

Abbreviation	Definition
ACE	angiotensin-converting enzyme
ACT	activated clotting time
ADH	antidiuretic hormone
AIDS	acquired immunodeficiency syndrome
ALT	alanine transaminase
APTT	activated partial thromboplastin time
AST	aspartate transaminase
AV	atrioventricular
b.i.d.	twice daily
BPH	benign prostatic hyperplasia
BUN	blood urea nitrogen
cAMP	cyclic adenosine monophosphate
CBC	complete blood count
CK	creatine kinase
CMV	cytomegalovirus
CNS	central nervous system
COMT	catechol-O-methyltransferase
COPD	chronic obstructive pulmonary disease
CPK	creatine phosphokinase
CSF	cerebrospinal fluid
CV	cardiovascular
CVA	cerebrovascular accident
CYP	cytochrome P450
DIC	disseminated intravascular coagulation
D_5W	dextrose 5% in water
dl	deciliter
DNA	deoxyribonucleic acid

Abbreviation	Definition
ECG	electrocardiogram
EEG	electroencephalogram
EENT	eyes, ears, nose, throat
FDA	Food and Drug Administration
g	gram
G	gauge
GABA	gamma-aminobutyric acid
GFR	glomerular filtration rate
GGT	gamma-glutamyltransferase
GI	gastrointestinal
gtt	gtt drops
GU	genitourinary
G6PD	glucose-6-phosphate dehydrogenase
H	histamine
HDL	high-density lipoprotein
HIV	human immunodeficiency virus
HMG-CoA	beta-hydroxy-beta-methylglutaryl coenzyme A
hr	hour
h.s.	at bedtime
ICU	intensive care unit
I.D.	intradermal
I.M.	intramuscular
INR	international normalized ratio
IPPB	intermittent positive-pressure breathing
IU	international unit
I.V.	intravenous
kg	kilogram
L	liter
lb	pound
LDH	lactate dehydrogenase
LDL	low-density lipoprotein
M	molar
m^2	square meter
MAO	monoamine oxidase
mcg	microgram
mEq	milliequivalent
mg	milligram
MI	myocardial infarction
min	minute
ml	milliliter
mm^3	cubic millimeter
Na	sodium

Abbreviation	Definition
NG	nasogastric
NSAID	nonsteroidal anti-inflammatory drug
OTC	over-the-counter
oz	ounce
PABA	para-aminobenzoic acid
$PaCO_2$	carbon dioxide partial pressure
PaO_2	oxygen partial pressure
PCA	patient-controlled analgesia
P.O.	by mouth
P.R.	by rectum
p.r.n.	as needed
PT	prothrombin time
PTT	partial thromboplastin time
PVC	premature ventricular contraction
q	every
q.i.d.	four times daily
RBC	red blood cell
RDA	recommended daily allowance
REM	rapid eye movement
RNA	ribonucleic acid
RSV	respiratory syncytial virus
SA	sinoatrial
S.C.	Subcutaneous
SIADH	syndrome of inappropriate antidiuretic hormone
S.L.	Sublingual
SSRI	selective serotonin reuptake inhibitor
T3	Triiodothyronine
T4	Thyroxine
tbs	Tablespoon
t.i.d.	three times daily
tsp	teaspoon
USP	United States Pharmacopeia
UTI	urinary tract infection
WBC	white blood cell

Glossary

A

Adrenergic receptors: Relating to the nerve fibers that release epinephrine or norepinephrine; sympathomimetic or mimicing the sympathetic nervous system.

Agranulocytosis: An abnormal blood condition, characterized by a severe reduction in the number of granulocytes, basophils, eosinophils, and neutrophils, resulting in high fever, exhaustion, and bleeding ulcers of the throat, mucous membranes, and G.I. tract. It is an acute disease and may be an adverse reaction to drug or radiation therapy.

Allergic reaction: A local or general reaction after exposure to an allergen to which the patient has already been exposed and sensitized. Reaction may range from localized dermatitis to anaphylaxis.

Alopecia: Absence or loss of hair.

Angioedema: A potentially life-threatening condition characterized by sudden swelling of tissue involving the face, neck, lips, tongue, throat, hands, feet, genitals, or intestine.

Anaphylaxis: A form of allergic or hypersensitivity reaction to an allergenic antigen mediated by the interactions between factors released from mast cells and immunoglobulin E.

Aplastic anemia: A deficiency of all of the formed elements of the blood related to bone marrow failure. It may be caused by neoplastic bone marrow disease or by destruction of the bone marrow by exposure to toxic chemicals, radiation, or certain medications. Also known as pancytopenia.

Arthralgia: Any pain that affects a joint.

Azotemia: A toxic condition caused by renal insufficiency and subsequent retention of urea in the blood. Also called uremia.

B

Bradycardia: An abnormally slow heart rate.

Bradykinesia: Extreme slowness of movement.

Bronchodilation: Dilation of the bronchi.

Bronchospasm: An abnormal narrowing with partial obstruction of the lumen of the bronchi as a result of spasm of the peribronchial smooth muscle. Clinically, this is accompanied by coughing and wheezing.

C

Cholinergic receptors: Relating to nerve endings that release acetylcholine; parasympathomimetic or mimicing the parasympathetic nervous system.

Chorea: A nervous condition marked by involuntary muscular twitching of limbs or facial muscles.

Cushing syndrome: A metabolic disorder caused by an increased production of adrenocorticotropic hormone from a tumor of the adrenal cortex or of the anterior lobe of the pituitary gland, or by excessive intake of glucocorticoids. It is characterized by central obesity, "moon face," glucose intolerance, growth suppression in children, and weakening of the muscles.

D

Disseminated intravascular coagulation (DIC): A life-threatening coagulopathy resulting from overstimulation of the body's clotting and anticlotting processes in response to disease, septicemia, neoplasms, obstetric emergencies, severe trauma, prolonged surgery, and hemorrhage.

Dyskinesia: A defect in the ability to perform voluntary movement sometimes accompanied by discomfort or pain.

E

Embolism: Obstruction of a blood vessel by a blood clot.

Eosinophilia: An increase in the number of eosinophils in the blood accompanying many inflammatory conditions. Substantial increases are considered a reflection of an allergic response.

Erythema: Redness of the skin caused by dilation and congestion of the superficial capillaries, often a sign of inflammation or infection.

F

Fibrillation: Abnormal quivering or spontaneous contraction of heart muscle fibers that are ineffective in pumping blood from the heart.

G

Gray baby syndrome: A possibly fatal condition that can occur in newborns (especially premature babies) who are given chloramphenicol for a bacterial infection, such as meningitis. Symptoms usually appear 2 to 9 days after therapy has been initiated. They include vomiting, loose green stools, refusal to suck, hypotension, cyanosis, low body temperature, and CV collapse. The baby becomes limp and has a gray coloring.

H

Hemolytic anemia: A disorder characterized by the premature destruction of RBCs. Anemia may be minimal or absent, reflecting the ability of the bone marrow to increase production of RBCs.

Hepatitis: Inflammation of the liver, usually from a viral infection but sometimes from toxic agents.

Hirsutism: Excessive growth of dark, coarse body hair, distributed in a male characteristic pattern.

Hypercalcemia: Greater-than-normal amounts of calcium in the blood. Signs and symptoms include confusion, anorexia, abdominal pain, muscle pain, and weakness.

Hyperglycemia: Greater-than-normal amounts of glucose in the blood. Classic signs and symptoms include excessive hunger, thirst, and frequent urination. Others include fatigue, weight loss, blurred vision, and poor wound healing.

Hyperkalemia: Greater-than-normal amounts of potassium in the blood. Signs and symptoms include nausea, fatigue, weakness, and palpitations or irregular pulse.

Hypermagnesemia: Greater-than-normal amounts of magnesium in the blood. Toxic levels in the blood may cause cardiac arrhythmias and may depress deep tendon reflexes and respiration.

Hypernatremia: Greater-than-normal amounts of sodium in the blood. Signs and symptoms include confusion, seizures, coma, dysrhythmic muscle twitching, lethargy, tachycardia, and irritability.

Hyperplasia: An increase in the number of cells.

Hypersensitivity reaction: An abnormal and undesireable reaction in response to a foreign agent. Classified by the mechanism involved and the time that it takes to occur, these reactions are assigned a rating of 1 through 4 (Types I, II, III, IV).

Hyperesthesia: An increased sensitivity of sensory stimuli, such as pain or touch.

Hypertonia: An excess of muscular tonus.
Hypesthesia: A decrease in sensitivity to touch.
Hypocalcemia: Less-than-normal amounts of calcium in the blood. Signs and symptoms of severe hypocalcemia include cardiac arrhythmias and muscle cramping and twitching as well as numbness and tingling of the hands, feet, lips, and tongue.
Hypoesthesia: A dulled sensitivity to touch.
Hypoglycemia: Less-than-normal amounts of glucose in the blood. Signs and symptoms include weakness, drowsiness, confusion, hunger, and dizziness. Patients may be pale, irritable, shaky, sweaty, and have a cold, clammy feeling and complain of headache and a rapid heart beat. Left untreated, delirium, coma, and death may occur.
Hypokalemia: Less-than-normal amounts of potassium in the blood. Signs and symptoms include palpitations, muscle weakness or cramping, paresthesias, G.I. complaints such as constipation, nausea or vomiting, and abdominal cramping. Patient also may experience frequent urination, delirium, and depression.
Hypomagnesemia: Less-than-normal amounts of magnesium in the blood. Signs and symptoms include nausea, vomiting, muscle weakness, tremors, tetany, and lethargy.
Hyponatremia: Less-than-normal amounts of sodium in the blood. Signs and symptoms may range from mild anorexia, headache, or muscle cramps to obtundation, coma, or seizures.

L

Leukocytosis: An abnormal increase in the number of circulating WBCs. Kinds of leukocytosis include basophilia, eosinophilia, and neutrophilia.
Leukopenia: An abnormal decrease in the number of WBCs to fewer than 5,000 cells/mm^3.

M

Myalgia: Diffuse muscle pain, usually associated with malaise.

N

Nephrotic syndrome: An abnormal kidney condition characterized by marked proteinuria, hypoalbuminemia, and edema.
Neuroleptic malignant syndrome: The rarest and most serious of the neuroleptic-induced movement disorders. It is a neurologic emergency in most cases. Signs and symptoms include fever, rigidity, and tremor. Mental status changes such as drowsiness and confusion can progress to stupor and coma. Other symptoms may include seizures and cardiac arrhythmias.
Neutropenia: An abnormal decrease in the number of circulating neutrophils in the blood.
Nocturia: Increased urination during the night.

P

Palpitations: An abnormally rapid throbbing or fluttering of the heart. The palpitation is perceptible to the client.
Pancytopenia: A deficiency of all of the formed elements of the blood related to bone marrow failure. It may be caused by neoplastic bone marrow disease or by destruction of the bone marrow after exposure to toxic chemicals, radiation, or certain medications. Also known as aplastic anemia.
Paresthesia: Abnormal sensation, sometimes experienced as numbness, tingling, or prickling, or a heightened sensitivity to touch.
Pharmacodynamics: The study of drug action in the body at the tissue site including uptake, movement, binding, and interactions.
Pharmacokinetics: The study of the action of drugs within the body, including the routes and mechanisms of absorption and excretion, the rate at which a drug's action begins and the duration of the effect, the biotransformation of the substance in the body, and the effects and routes of excretions of the metabolites of the drug.

Pseudomembranous colitis: A complication of antibiotic therapy that causes severe local tissue inflammation of the colon. Signs and symptoms include watery diarrhea, abdominal pain or cramping, and low-grade fever.
Pseudotumor cerebri: Benign intracranial hypertension, most common in women between the ages of 20 and 50, caused by increased pressure within the brain. Symptoms include headache, dizziness, nausea, vomiting, and ringing or rushing sound in the ears.
Pruritus: Itching.
Psoriasis: A common skin disorder characterized by the eruption of red, silvery-scaled maculopapules, predominantly on the elbows, knees, scalp, and trunk.
Reye's syndrome: An encephalopathy that affects children of all ages. Although the cause and cure are unknown, research has established a link between the use of aspirin and other salicylate-containing medications, as well as other causes. The syndrome may follow an upper respiratory infection or chicken pox. Its onset is rapid, usually starting with irritable, combative behavior and vomiting, and progressing to semiconsciousness, seizures, coma, and possibly death.

S

Serotonin syndrome: A typically mild, yet potentially serious, drug-related condition most often reported in patients taking two or more medications that increase CNS serotonin levels. The most common drug combinations associated with serotonin syndrome involve the MAO inhibitors, SSRIs, and the tricyclic antidepressants. Signs and symptoms include confusion, agitation, restlessness, rapid heart rate, muscle rigidity or twitching, tremors, and nausea.
Serum sickness: An immune complex disease appearing 1 or 2 weeks after infection of a foreign serum or serum protein, with local and systemic reactions, such as urticaria, fever, general lymphadenopathy, edema, arthritis, and occasionally albuminuria or severe nephritis.
Syncope: A brief loss of consciousness caused by oxygen deficiency to the brain, often preceded by a feeling of dizziness. Having the patient lie down or place his head between his knees may prevent it.

T

Tachycardia: An abnormal rapidity of heart action, usually defined as a resting heart rate of >100 beats per minute in adults.
Thrombocytopenia: An abnormal decrease in the number of platelets in the blood, predisposing the patient to bleeding disorders.
Thrombocytopenic purpura: A bleeding disorder characterized by a marked decrease in the number of platelets, causing multiple bruises, petechiae, and hemorrhage into the tissues.
Thrombosis: The formation, development, or existence of a blood clot or thrombus within the vascular system.
Thrombophlebitis: Inflammation of a vein in conjunction with the formation of a blood clot.
Thrombus: A blood clot.
Tinnitus: Sound in one or both ears, such as buzzing, ringing, or whistling, occurring without external stimuli. It may be caused by an ear infection, the use of certain drugs, a blocked auditory tube or canal, or head trauma.

U

Urticaria: An itchy skin condition characterized by pale wheals with well-defined red edges. This may be the result of an allergic response to insect bites, food, or drugs.

Index

D

E

G

H

I

J

K

L

M

N

O

P

Q

R

S

T

U

V

W

X

Y

Z